# Prevention of Venous Thromboembolism

# Prevention of Venous Thromboembolism

EDITED BY

David Bergqvist MD PhD
Professor of Vascular Surgery
Department of Surgery
Uppsala University
Uppsala, Sweden

Antony J. Comerota MD
Professor of Vascular Surgery
Temple University
Philadelphia, Pennsylvania, USA

Andrew N. Nicolaides MS FRCS FRCSE
Professor of Vascular Surgery
Honorary Consultant Vascular Surgeon
Director, Irvine Laboratory for Cardiovascular Investigation and Research
St. Mary's Hospital Medical School
Imperial College of Science, Technology and Medicine
London, UK

John H. Scurr FRCS
Consultant Surgeon
University and Middlesex School of Medicine
Middlesex Hospital
London, UK

MED-ORION PUBLISHING COMPANY
LONDON    LOS ANGELES    NICOSIA

MED-ORION PUBLISHING COMPANY
LONDON    LOS ANGELES    NICOSIA

Distributed in Europe by
Med-Orion Publishing Company
Kypros House, 262 Seven Sisters Road,
DX Box No. 57450, Finsbury Park,
London, N4 2HY, UK  (Fax: 071-281 4371)
and associated companies, branches and
representatives throughout the world.

Distributed in the United States by
Med-Orion Publishing Company
P.O.Box 1134, Sunland, Ca 91041, USA
Fax: (818) 767-7318

©1994 Med-Orion Publishing Company

All rights reserved; no part of this publication may be reproduced, stored in a retrieval system, or transmitted in any form or by any means electronic, mechanical, photocopying, recording or otherwise, without the prior written permission of the Publishers (Med-Orion Publishing Company, Julia House, 3 Th Dervis Street, P.O. Box 3589, Nicosia, Cyprus).

First published 1994

ISBN 9963-592-52-X

**British Library Cataloguing in Publication Data**
Prevention of Venous Thromboembolism
   I. Bergqvist, David
   616.1

Typeset by Caradoc Books (Cyprus) Ltd
Nicosia, Cyprus

Printed by Zavallis Litho Limited
Nicosia, Cyprus

# FOREWORD

The past decade has witnessed a remarkable progress in the diagnosis and clinical management of venous thrombosis. Besides a clearer understanding of the pathophysiology, the prophylaxis and therapy of venous thormbosis has been a subject of major focus throughout the world. These advances have already made an impact on day-to-day patient care. However, as in the case of many developments in medicine, current progress has also prompted a debate on the relative merits of the newer approaches. Periodic reviews and consensus meetings have provided a forum for establishing accepted guidelines via an open, objective and collective appraoch from physicians, surgeons, research scientists and public advocates.

A Consensus conference was held in Bethesda, Maryland in 1986 under the auspices of the National Heart, Lung and Blood Institute. In this meeting, the magnitude of the problem of venous thromboembolism was discussed in terms of its impact to society. At that time, it was stated that nearly one million individuals in the US alone experience some sort of venous thromboembolic event. Of these, 5-10% may have serious outcomes, being at a high risk to develop pulmonary embolism, potentially leading to a fatal outcome if not treated properly. The identification of venous thrombosis as one of the major health problems after surgery and in several medical conditions was a major accomplishment by this group of experts. This consensus meeting provided, for the first time, certain guidelines on the recommended forms of prophylaxis in these patient groups.

While the 1986 consensus proposed the use of unfractionated heparin via the subcutaneous route for prophylaxis of post-surgical thromboembolic complications, the subsequent introduction of low molecular weight heparins has provided another antithrombotic approach. In the third Consensus conference of the American College of Chest Physicians, both the use of heparin and a low molecular weight heparin was strongly endorsed for prophylaxis of thromboembolism.

The European Consensus conference held in 1991 at Windsor, U.K., and published as the European Consensus Statement in 1992 was organised to develop an updated and more defined consensus statement on the prevention of thromboembolism. The members of the consensus panel represented noted experts in the field from Europe, North America and Australia being comprised of physicians, surgeons and epidemiologists from academic, experimental, industrial and private institutions. These experts from various disciplines contributed their experiences and independent views. In an objective manner, this panel has provided clearly defined and concise statements on the major health problems, clinical screening protocols, risk categories and the prophylactic modalities for each risk group.

This book consists of an integrated and updated account of the evidence presented and discussed at Windsor and on which the European Consensus Statement was based. Many surgeons and physicians continue to raise doubts on the value of prophylaxis having put forward valid arguments regarding safety/efficacy issues, patient compliance, long-term benefits and cost. However, it is clear from the manuscripts in this book that optimised prophylaxis using pharmacologic agents and other means is certainly a major factor in reducing mortality/morbidity due to venous thrombosis. Furthermore, this text contains practical information for both clinicians and surgeons which would otherwise be unavailable or difficult to obtain. Thus, this book will become a handy reference for those involved in the management of thromboembolic disorders. The availability of the individual manuscripts, along with the consensus statement will provide the readers with a true sense of the need for proper diagnosis and prophylaxis.

Professor Andrew Nicolaides and his colleagues are to be congratulated for both organising an objective consensus conference on the subject of thromboembolism and for sensing the need of wide dissemination of the outcome of this meeting. Needless to say, this book represents the first comprehensive and practical account of the diagnostic methods and clinical management of patients with thromboembolism. Rightfully, this text will readily fill a gap in providing much-needed information to clinicians and surgeons with the ultimate benefit going to the patient. This book is undoubtedly a major step forward towards the better understanding of thromboembolism and its prevention.

Jawed Fareed Ph.D
Professor of Pathology and Pharmacology
Hemostasis and Thrombosis Research Laboratories
Loyola University Medical Center
Maywood, IL 60153 USA.

# PREFACE

Although our knowledge of the pathogenesis and prevention of deep vein thrombosis and pulmonary embolism has increased considerably during the last few years, venous thromboembolism remains an important cause of morbidity and mortality in various groups of patients, not least after surgical procedures. In 1986 the NIH Consensus conference and publication dealt with venous thromboembolic problems with special emphasis on prophylaxis. The conclusions concerning the necessity for prevention were firm and several methods were recommended. Despite this, there are indications that the use of prophylaxis is still suboptimal, emphasising the need to continue the educational process.

An important addition to the prophylactic arsenal has occurred after the NIH Consensus conference. This is the low molecular weight glycosaminoglycans (various low molecular weight heparins and Org 10172). Thus, besides the educational motivation, these new prophylactic modalities are an important reason to review the present-day knowledge as well as to define remaining questions which must be urgently elucidated. The European Consensus Statement published in 1992 and circulated to over 100,000 doctors in nine different languages has gone a long way in achieving this. Unlike most consensus statements, it was considered important to scrutinise the data supporting the statements or emphasise the lack of data. The evidence considered has now been updated and summarised in this book. It is presented in four parts. Part I deals with new aspects of aetiology, pathophysiology and methods of detection, Part II with methods of primary prevention, Part III with primary prevention in individual patient groups (general surgical, urological, obstetric and gynaecological, orthopaedic, medical, stroke and neurosurgical), and Part IV with secondary prevention. The European Consensus Statement is reproduced in Part V.

The editors believe that this volume is an update of what we know today about prevention of deep vein thrombosis and pulmonary embolism. It is aimed both at research workers and clinicians who are anxious to incorporate the conclusions of recent clinical studies into their practice, thus bridging the gap between established textbooks and original papers.

D.B
A.J.C.
A.N.N.
J.H.S.

# Contributors

**Juan I. Arcelus** MD PhD
Research Fellow
The Glenbrook Hospital
Glenview Illinois, USA.

**Gianni Belcaro** MD
Director Microcirculation Laboratory,
Cardiovascular Institute,
Chieti University Italy and
Irvine Laboratory for Cardiovascular
Investigation and Research,
St Mary's Hospital Medical School,
London, UK.

**D. Bergqvist** MD PhD
Professor of Vascular Surgery
Department of Surgery
Uppsala University
Uppsala, Sweden.

**Lars C. Borris** MD
Senior Registrar
Department of Orthopaedics
Aalborg Hospital
Aalborg, Denmark.

**D.P.M. Brandjes** MD
Fellow of the Royal Dutch Academy of Arts
and Sciences,
Centre for Haemostasis Thrombosis
Atherosclerosis and Inflammation Research
Academic Medical Centre
Amsterdam, The Netherlands.

**M. De Buysere** BSc
Research Fellow
Department of Cardiovascular Diseases
University Hospital
Gent, Belgium.

**Harry R. Büller** MD PhD
Fellow of the Royal Dutch Academy of Arts
and Sciences
Centre for Haemostasis Thrombosis
Atherosclerosis and Inflammation Research
Academic Medical Centre
Amsterdam, The Netherlands.

**Joseph A. Caprini** MD FACS
Professor of Clinical Surgery
Chief of Surgery
Northwestern University Medical School
Louis W. Biegler Chair of Surgery
The Glenbrook Hospital
Glenview, Illinois, USA.

**Dimitris Christopoulos** MD PhD
Vascular Surgeon
Senior Lecturer
University of Thessaloniki
B2 Surgical Unit
Hippokrateion Hospital
Thessaloniki, Greece.

**D.L. Clarke-Pearson** MD
Professor of Obstetrics and Gynecology
Director Gynecologic Oncology
Duke University Medical Center
Durham, North Carolina, USA.

**D.L. Clement** MD PhD
Professor of Cardiology and Angiology
Department of Cardiovascular Diseases
University Hospital
Gent, Belgium.

**A.T. Cohen** MD
Senior Research Fellow
Thrombosis Research Unit
Kings College Hospital
London, U.K.

**Graham A. Colditz** MD PhD
Associate Professor of Medicine
Harvard Medical School,
Boston, Massachusetts, USA.

**P.D. Coleridge Smith** FRCS
Senior Lecturer and Consultant Surgeon
Department of Surgery
University College of London Medical School
The Middlesex Hospital
London, UK.

**A.J. Comerota** MD
Professor of Vascular Surgery
Temple University
Philadelphia
Pennysylvania, USA.

**J. Conard** MD
Maître des Conferences Université
Praticien Hospitalier
Hôtel Dieu Broussais/Paris
University of Paris VI
Director of Central Laboratory of Haematology
Hôtel-Dieu Hospital,
Paris, France.

**E.D. Cooke** MB BCh BAO MD
Director Thermographic Laboratory
St Bartholomews Hospital
London, UK.

**E. Dekker** MD
Fellow of the Royal Dutch Academy of Arts and Sciences,
Centre for Haemostasis Thrombosis
Atherosclerosis and Inflammation Research
Academic Medical Centre
Amsterdam, The Netherlands.

**D. Duprez** MD
Professor of Cardiology
Deparment of Cardiology and Angiology
University Hospital
Gent, Belgium.

**R. Eichlisberger** MD
Senior Registrar
Division of Angiology
University of Basel
Medical School
Kantonsspital Basel
Basel, Switzerland.

**Bo Eklöf** MD PhD
Visiting Professor of Surgery
University of Hawaii
Vascular Surgeon
Straub Clinic and Hospital
Medical Director
Straub Pacific Health Foundation
Honolulu, Hawaii, USA.

**Charles M. Fisher** MBBS BSc (Med) FRACS
Consultant Vascular Surgeon
Royal North Shore Hospital
St Leonards, Sydney, Australia

**P. Gheeraert** MD
Consultant Cardiologist
Deparment of Cardiology and Angiology
University Hospital
Gent, Belgium.

**Lazar J. Greenfield** MD
Frederick A. Coller Professor and Chairman
Department of Surgery
University of Michigan Hospitals
Ann Arbor, Michigan, USA.

**Peter Haas** MD PhD
Normannenstr 34A
Munich, Germany.

**Sylvia Haas** MD
Professor of Medicine
Institut für Experimentelle Chirurgie der
Technischen Universität München
Munich, Germany.

**J. Hirsh**
Professor and Chairman
Department of Medicine
McMaster University
Hamilton, Ontario, Canada.

**D.W. Hommes** MD
Fellow of the Royal Dutch Academy of Arts and Sciences,
Centre for Haemostasis Thrombosis
Atherosclerosis and Inflammation Research
Academic Medical Centre
Amsterdam, The Netherlands

**M.H. Horellou**
Maîre des Conferences Université
Praticien Hospitalier
Hôtel Dieu Broussais/Paris
University of Paris VI
Director of Central Laboratory of Haematology
Hôtel-Dieu Hospital,
Paris, France.

**Russell D. Hull** MBBS MSc
Professor of Medicine
Head Division of General Internal Medicine
Faculty of Medicine
University of Calgary
Calgary, Alberta, Canada.

**V.V. Kakkar** FRCS FRCSE
Professor of Surgical Sciences and Director
Thrombosis Research Institute
Chelsea, London, UK.

**Evi Kalodiki** MD BA
Senior Vascular Research Fellow,
Irvine Laboratory for Cardiovascular
Investigation and Research,
Department of Vascular Surgery
St. Mary's Hospital Medical School
Imperial College of Science Technology and Medicine
London, UK

**Michael R. Lassen** MD
Senior Registrar
Department of Orthopaedics
Aalborg Hospital
Aalborg, Denmark

**Jacques R. Leclerc** MD FRCP
Director of Hematology
Montreal General Hospital
Associate Professor of Medicine
McGill University
Montreal, Quebec, Canada

**Anthonie W.A. Lensing** MD PhD
Assistant Professor of Internal Medicine
Centre for Haemostasis Thrombosis
Atherosclerosis and Inflammation Research
Academic Medical Centre
Amsterdam, The Netherlands

**Bengt Lindblad** MD PhD
Associate Professor of Surgery
Department of Surgery
University of Lund General Hospital
Malmö, Sweden

**Andrew N. Nicolaides** MS FRCS FRCSE
Professor of Vascular Surgery,
Honorary Consultant Vascular Surgeon,
Director Irvine Laboratory for Cardiovascular
Investigation and Research,
St. Mary's Hospital Medical School
Imperial College of Science Technology and Medicine
London, UK.

**M.T. Nurmohamed** MD
Fellow of the Royal Dutch Academy of Arts and Sciences,
Centre for Haemostasis Thrombosis
Atherosclerosis and Inflammation Research
Academic Medical Centre
Amsterdam, The Netherlands

**Andre Planes** MD
Orthopaedic Surgeon
Dept of Orthopaedic Surgery
Clinique Radio-Chirurgicale du Mail
La Rochelle France

**G. Ramaswami** FRCS
Senior Research Registrar
Irvine Laboratory for Cardiovascular
Investigation and Research,
St. Mary's Hospital Medical School Academic Surgical Unit
Imperial College of Science Technology and Medicine
London, UK.

**Meyer Michel Samama** MD
Professor of Haematology
Hôtel Dieu Broussais/Paris
University of Paris VI
Director of Central Laboratory of Haematology
Hôtel-Dieu Hospital,
Paris, France.

**Arthur A. Sasahara** MD
Venture Head Thrombolytics Research
Abbott Laboratories Abbott Park Illinois,
Professor of Medicine (on leave)
Harvard Medical School
Senior Physician (on leave)
Brigham and Women's Hospital,
Boston, Massachusetts, USA.

**H.E. Schmitt** MD
Professor of Radiology
University of Basel Medical School
Kantonsspital Basel
Basel, Switzerland

**J.H. Scurr** FRCS
Consultant Surgeon
University and Middlesex School of Medicine
Middlesex Hospital
London, UK.

**Marc Silsiguen**
Biostatistician
Rhone Poulenc Rorer
Antony, France

**Jan W. ten Cate** MD PhD
Professor Chair of the Netherlands Thrombosis
Foundation
Centre for Haemostasis Thrombosis
Atherosclerosis and Inflammation Research
Academic Medical Centre
Amsterdam, The Netherlands

**F. Toulemonde** MD
Hotel Dieu Broussaia/Paris
University of Paris VI
Hotel-Dieu Hospital
Paris, France

**Clara J. Traverso** MD PhD
Research Fellow
The Glenbrook Hospital
Glenview, Illinois, USA

**A.G.G. Turpie** MB FRCP (Lond Glasg) FACP
FACC FRCPC
Professor of Medicine
McMaster University
Hamilton, Ontario, Canada.

**Nicole Vochelle** MD
Anaesthetist
Dept of Orthopaedic Surgery
Clinique Radio-Chirurgicale du Mail
La Rochelle, France

**L.K. Widmer** MD PhD
Professor of Medicine
Division of Angiology
University of Basel Medical School
Kantonsspital Basel
Basel, Switzerland

**M. Th. Widmer** MD
Division of Angiology
University of Basel Medical School
Kantonsspital Basel
Basel, Switzerland

**E. Zemp** MD MPH
Senior Research Fellow
Institute of Social and Preventive Medicine
University of Basel
Basel, Switzerland

# Contents

Foreword     v
Preface     vii
Contributors     ix

## Part I: New aspects of aetiology pathophysiology and methods of detection

1. Incidence of venous thromboembolism in medical and surgical patients     3
   D. Bergqvist, B. Lindblad

2. Incidence of late sequelae of deep vein thrombosis     17
   L. Widmer, M. Th. Widmer, H.E. Schmitt, R. Eichlisberger, E. Zemp, K. Jäger

3. Operative venous dilatation and its relationship to postoperative deep vein thrombosis     31
   A.J. Comerota

4. Coagulation abnormalities predisposing to the development of deep vein thrombosis     43
   M. Samama, J. Conard, M.H. Horellou, F. Toulemonde

5. Venous stasis and trauma in hip surgery     57
   A. Planes, N. Vochelle

6. DVT diagnostic tests in the screening of asymptomatic patients     63
   A.J. Comerota

7. Diagnosis of deep vein thrombosis in asymptomatic patients     73
   A.W.A. Lensing, H.R. Büller, J. Hirsh, J.W. ten Cate

8. The contribution of colour flow imaging to postoperative surveillance for DVT     93
   A. N. Nicolaides, E. Kalodiki

9. Venography in asymptomatic patients having total hip replacement: interobserver variation     103
   L.C. Borris, M.R. Lassen

10. The natural history of deep vein thrombosis     109
    G. Ramaswami, A. N. Nicolaides

## Part II: Methods of primary prevention

11. The current practice of prevention     123
    E.D. Cooke

12. Low dose heparin with and without dihydroergotamine — 131
V.V. Kakkar, A.T. Cohen

13. Low molecular weight heparins: mode of action and dosage — 143
M.M. Samama

14. The efficacy of low molecular weight heparin — 149
S. Haas, P. Haas

15. Low molecular weight heparin versus standard heparin in general and orthopaedic surgery: a meta-analysis — 163
M.T. Nurmohamed, H.R. Büller, E. Dekker, D.W. Hommes, J.W. ten Cate

16. Orgaran (Org 10172) a low molecular weight heparinoid — 175
A.G.G. Turpie

17. Dextran — 181
D. Bergqvist

18. Oral anticoagulants and antiplatelet drugs — 199
A.G.G. Turpie

19. Graduated compression stockings for the prevention of venous thromboembolism — 203
J. Scurr

20. Intermittent pneumatic compression — 209
J.A. Caprini, C.J. Traverso, J.I. Arcelus

21. Combined methods — 225
A.N. Nicolaides

# Part III: Prevention in individual patient groups

22. Pre-operative risk factors in the prediction of postoperative venous thromboembolism — 235
D.W. Hommes, H.R. Büller, D.P.M. Brandjes, J.W. ten Cate

23. General surgery — 243
D. Bergqvist

24. Obstetrics and gynaecology — 249
D.L. Clarke-Pearson

25. Elective hip surgery — 271
A. Planes, M. Silsiguen, N. Vochelle

26. Thromboprophylaxis in hip fracture patients — 281
M.R. Lassen, L.C. Borris

27. Combined modalities for hip surgery — 297
J.I. Arcelus, J.A. Caprini, C.I. Traverso

28. Knee surgery — 309
C.I. Traverso, J.I. Arcelus, J.A. Caprini

29. Medical patients — 319
D.I. Clement P. Gheeraert, M. De Buysere, D. Duprez

30. Stroke and neurosurgical patients — 327
A.G.G. Turpie

31. Urologic surgery — 333
G. Belcaro, A.N. Nicolaides

32. A protocol plan for preventing deep vein thrombosis — 339
P. Coleridge-Smith

## Part IV: Secondary prevention

33. The combination of liquid crystal thermography and duplex scanning: accuracy and cost-effectiveness — 349
E. Kalodiki, C.M. Fisher, A.N. Nicolaides

34. The value of thrombectomy — 357
B. Eklof

35. The value of fibrinolysis in secondary prevention — 373
A. Sasahara

36. Air plethysmography — 381
D. Christopoulos, A.N. Nicolaides

37. Indications and efficacy of vena caval filters — 393
L.J. Greenfield

38. Cost effectiveness of prevention — 405
G.A. Colditz

39. Prevention of venous thromboembolism: key questions that need to be answered — 421
R.D. Hull

40. Anticoagulant therapy — 429
R.D. Hull

## Part V European Consensus Statement

41. Prevention of thromboembolism: European Consensus Statement — 443
The European Consensus Statement Faculty

Index — 457

PART I

# New Aspects of Aetiology, Pathophysiology and Methods of Detection

CHAPTER 1

# Incidence of Venous Thromboembolism in Medical and Surgical Patients

David Bergqvist
Bengt Lindblad

## Introduction

There has been an increased interest in venous thromboembolism complicating various disorders and surgical interventions during this century, but not until objective diagnostic methods became available did it become possible to establish the magnitude of the problem. The aim of this chapter is to present and discuss the frequency of thromboembolic phenomena in various groups of patients where specific prophylactic methods have not been used.

## Diagnostic Methodology and Different Endpoints

Although it falls outside the scope of this article to discuss various diagnostic methods in detail, the latter must be mentioned because data on frequencies are based on diagnostic methodology. The problem is fairly simple when we deal with nonorthopaedic surgery or nonoperated groups of patients. The majority of studies have been performed using the fibrinogen uptake test (FUT) and the data are reliable, the test having a good diagnostic accuracy when compared with venography. The situation is more complicated, however, when the interest is focused on orthopaedic patients and especially those undergoing extremity surgery. Although the overall frequency does not differ between studies having used the FUT and studies having used venography (Bergqvist, 1983) there are two conditions which make the FUT less reliable. First, haematoma in the field of surgery gives a false positive test because of the accumulation of radiolabelled fibrin in the haemorrhagic clot. Second, in hip surgery there are two pathogenetic mechanisms for the development of thrombosis: stasis and activation of coagulation factors causing calf vein thrombosis just

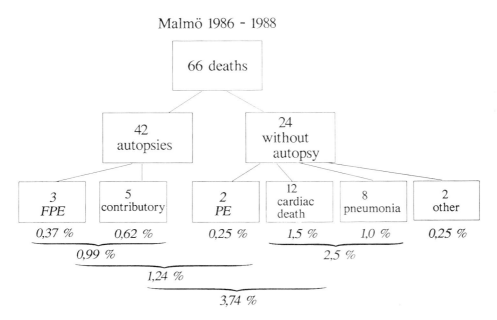

Fig. 1.1 Causes of death after hip fracture in Malmö

as in any kind of surgery and femoral vein damage by the surgical procedure causing isolated proximal thrombosis (Stamatakis et al, 1977; Planes et al, 1990; Binns and Pho, 1990; Hogevold et al, 1990). The FUT is not accurate in detecting the latter (Fauno et al, 1990), nor is $^{99m}$mTc-plasmin test (Christensen et al, 1987). The combination of plethysmographic methods and the FUT also tend to underestimate the frequency (Paiement et al, 1988; Comerota et al, 1988; Cruickshank et al, 1989). The use of B-mode ultrasound may be useful (Froehlich et al, 1989; Woolson et al, 1990; Comerota et al, 1990) but more data are needed, and at least some studies show a poor agreement with venography for surveillance (Borris et al, 1989). Moreover, to exclude DVT in a surveillance situation, the method takes time. Thus, the only reliable method so far in patients with hip surgery is venography. However, one problem with bilateral venography is that some 15% of legs cannot be investigated for various reasons (Bergqvist et al, 1991). Another problem is that venography is hardly suitable for repeated examinations. A third problem is the unreliability within certain anatomic areas such as the internal iliac veins and the deep femoral vein.

With regard to pulmonary embolism, a few studies have been performed using scintigraphic techniques, either the combination of perfusion scintigraphy and pulmonary X-ray, or, in rare cases, the combination of perfusion and ventilation scintigraphy (see Table 1.10). Probably this technology gives the frequency of fairly large pulmonary emboli, but the accuracy compared with pulmonary angiography has been questioned (PIOPED, 1990). Systematic studies where routine pulmonary angiography has been used have not been published.

An important end-point when discussing prophylactic methods is fatal pulmonary embolism. One problem in this context is the diagnostic criteria. We have used a classification of three categories: fatal, contributory and incidental (Bergqvist and Lindblad, 1985). The autopsy rate is of vital importance when discussing causes of death and this is especially

**Table 1.1**
Venous thromboembolism during 1987 in the city of Malmö
Figures within brackets show the total number of investigations made

|  | Number of patients | Per 100,000 population |
|---|---|---|
| Deep vein thrombosis |  |  |
|    Venography (n=1007) | 366 | 159 |
|    Autopsy (n=1323) | 284 | 123 |
| Pulmonary Embolism |  |  |
|    Scintigraphy (n=233) | 45 | 19 |
|    Autopsy (n=1323) | 321 | 139 |
| Fatal or contributory |  |  |
|    pulmonary embolism | 218 | 94 |
|    pulmonary embolism postop. | 19 | 8 |

true for pulmonary embolism as it is known to be one of the most difficult premortal diagnoses (Sheppeard et al, 1981). An illustration of the problem is given in figure 1.1 with data from a study on mortality after hip fracture surgery (Bergqvist and Fredin, 1991).

# Frequency of Venous Thromboembolism on a Population Basis

The problem of venous thromboembolism within a well defined population with only one hospital for emergencies was investigated in 1987 in the city of Malmö, Sweden (236,000 inhabitants). Table 1.1 shows the incidence of venous thromboembolism diagnosed with various methodologies, also recalculated per 100,000 inhabitants. It is remarkable that

**Table 1.2**
Background factors in 366 patients with phlebographically verified deep vein thrombosis during 1987 in the city of Malmö

|  | n | Per cent |
|---|---|---|
| Heredity | 21 | 6 |
| Hormone therapy | 11 | 3 |
| Smoking | 92 | 25 |
| Heavy alcohol consumption | 18 | 5 |
| Known malignancy | 71 | 19 |
| Malignancy developed within one year after diagnosis of DVT | 19 | 5 |
| Previous thromboembolism | 97 | 27 |
| Surgery within 30 days | 101 | 28 |
| Fracture within 30 days | 38 | 10 |
| Infection within 30 days | 33 | 9 |
| Other chronic disease | 231 | 63 |
| No clinical risk factor | 7 | 2 |

**Table 1.3**
Frequency (%) of deep vein thrombosis in various non-operated patient groups

| | |
|---|---|
| Infectious diseases | 5 |
| General internal medicine | 10–15 |
| Myocardial infarction | 5–20 |
| Stroke, paralyzed leg | 60-70 |
| Non-paralyzed leg | 10 |
| Preoperative hospitalisation | 5–20 |
| Radiation therapy | 40 |

The above frequencies are averages based on several studies, using FUT or venography for diagnosis

pulmonary embolism was clinically suspected in 233 patients but scintigraphically verified in only 45 cases. In table 1.2 the incidence of the various background factors in patients with venographically verified DVT (336 positive venograms out of 1007 performed with suspected DVT) is presented.

# Frequency of DVT in Non-surgical Patients

Table 1.3 shows the frequency of DVT in non-surgical patients as well as before operation in surgical patients. The highest incidence is found in stroke patients, where the paralysed leg has a very high frequency of DVT, which also illustrates one important pathogenic factor — the absence of a functioning calf muscle pump. Most of the studies on myocardial infarction are fairly old and in newer ones the frequency seems to have decreased, the changing attitude towards early mobilisation probably being one important factor explaining the decrease.

Pregnancy related DVT constitutes a special problem. The frequency is very low but nontheless several times higher than in nonpregnant women of the same age. In table 1.4 the frequency of pregnancy related DVT is shown. The frequency of fatal pulmonary embolism is fortunately extremely low — 1 in 250,000 pregnancies (Dixon, 1987).

Another potential risk situation, although also with a very low frequency, is contraceptive medication. With decreasing amount of oestrogen the incidence seems to be diminished (Table 1.5).

**Table 1.4**
Frequency (%) of pregnancy related deep vein thromboses

| | |
|---|---|
| During pregnancy | 1% |
| During puerperium | << 1% |
| After Caesarean section | 1–2%[*] |

There seems to be no great difference between the trimesters. There is a clear left sided dominance
[*]Bergqvist et al, 1979

**Table 1.5**
Data of venous thromboembolism in oral contraceptive users in relation to oestrogen content. From Gerstman et al (1991) analysing 2,739,400 oral contraceptive prescriptions received by 234,218 women

| Oestrogen defined cohorts (µg) | Rate/10,000 person-years |
|---|---|
| <50 | 4.2 |
| 50 | 7.0 |
| >50 | 10.0 |
| All | 5.8 |

Relative risk estimates adjusted for age and calendar period were 1.5 (p<0.04) for intermediate-dose formulations and 1.7 (p<0.06) for high-dose formulations

## Frequency of Postoperative DVT

Table 1.6 gives data in non-orthopaedic surgery based on FUT and table 1.7 in orthopaedic surgery based on venography. As there is a decreasing number of studies with untreated control groups most of the data in the tables are fairly old. However, there are some recent prophylactic studies with untreated control groups, indicating that there is no reason to believe in a spontaneous decrease of the problem (Table 1.8). Table 1.9 shows frequencies after some specialised types of surgery.

**Table 1.6**
Frequency (%) of deep vein thrombosis after non-orthopaedic surgical procedures based on the FUT

| | |
|---|---|
| Transvesical prostatectomy | 40 % |
| General abdominal surgery | 30 % |
| Non-cardiac thoracic surgery | 30 % |
| Gynaecologic surgery | 25 % |
| Neurosurgery | 25 % |
| Transvesical prostatic resection | 10 % |
| Herniorrhaphy | 5 % |

The above frequencies are averages based on a number of studies. The interstudy variations are great, in general surgery from 13% to 59% (Bergqvist 1983)

**Table 1.7**
Frequency (%) of deep vein thrombosis after hip and knee surgery, based on venography

| | |
|---|---|
| Knee surgery | 75 % |
| Hip fracture surgery | 60 % |
| Elective hip arthroplasty | 55 % |

The above frequencies are averages based on a number of studies. The interstudy variations in frequency do not seem to be as great as in general surgery

**Table 1.8**
Frequency (%) of deep vein thrombosis (DVT) in studies from the 1980s where untreated control groups have been included

| Author | Type of surgery | Number of patients | DVT | Frequency % | Diagnostic method |
|---|---|---|---|---|---|
| Lindstrom et al, 1982 | General | 40 | 12 | 30 | FUT |
| Turpie et al, 1986 | THR | 50 | 21 | 42 | FUT + pleth + venography |
|  |  | 39 | 20 | 51 | Venography |
| Lassen et al, 1988 | THR | 116 | 53 | 46 | Plasmin + venography |
| Ockelford et al, 1989 | General | 88 | 14 | 16 | FUT |
| Torholm et al, 1989 | THR | 54 | 19 | 35 | FUT |
| Jorgensen et al, 1989 | Hip fract | 38 | 22 | 58 | FUT |
| Lassen et al, 1989 | Hip fract | 54 | 23 | 43 | Plasmin + venography |
| Hull et al, 1990 | THR | 158 | 77 | 49 | Venography |
| Hoeck et al, 1990 | THR | 99 | 56 | 57 | Venography |

## Frequency of Non-fatal Postoperative Pulmonary Embolism

Table 1.10 gives the frequency of scintigraphically detected pulmonary embolism. The clinical relevance of these emboli is poorly understood and should be studied further. There is also a great need for systematic studies where pulmonary angiography is used to establish the true frequency of postoperative pulmonary embolism.

## The Frequency of Postoperative Fatal Pulmonary Embolism

Data on fatal pulmonary embolism is summarised in Table 1.11. The frequency is admittedly low in most studies but still this is one of the single most important causes of death after operation. As already stated, the autopsy rate is extremely important, and in studies on prophylaxis it should be kept as high as possible. Otherwise conclusions on an effect on fatal pulmonary embolism is hardly reliable.

**Table 1.9**
Frequency (%) of deep vein thrombosis after some specialised types of surgery

| | |
|---|---|
| Renal transplantation | 20–30 |
| Aortoiliac reconstruction | 20–30 |
| Femoropopliteal reconstruction | 8–20 |
| Leg fracture | 40–50 |
| Amputation | 60–70 |
| Meniscectomy | 10–25 |
| Spinal cord injury | 50–100 |

**Table 1.10**
Frequency (%) of non-fatal pulmonary embolism based on scintigraphic diagnosis

| Author | Type of surgery | Number of patients | Patients with perfusion defect | Defect frequency (%) |
| --- | --- | --- | --- | --- |
| Allgood et al, 1970 | General | 64 | 9 | 14 |
| Bergqvist et al, 1979 | Elective Hip | 71 | 14 | 20 |
| Bergqvist et al, 1980 | Elective Hip | 150 | 19 | 13 |
| Browse et al, 1974 | General | 40 | 7 | 18 |
| Buttermann et al, 1977 | General | 175 | 41 | 23 |
|  | Urology | 100 | 10 | 10 |
| Hartsuck and Greenfield, 1973 | Abdominal, Pelvic | 196 | 114 | 58 |
| Johansson et al, 1975 | Abdominal | 49 | 13 | 27 |
| Lahnborg et al, 1974 | Abdominal | 54 | 24 | 44 |
| Murphy et al, 1972 | Urology | 59 | 8 | 14 |
| Salzman and Axilrod, 1971 | Urology | 51 | 4 | 8 |

**Table 1.11**
Frequency (%) of postoperative fatal pulmonary embolism when no prophylaxis is used

| General surgery | 0.5–1 % |
| --- | --- |
| Hip arthroplasty | 2% |
| Hip fracture | 5–7 % |

# Reasons for Variations in the Frequency of Venous Thromboembolism between Different Studies

Taking the studies on general surgery with the average frequency of 30% in table 1.6 there was a variation in frequency from 13% to 59% in the individual studies (Bergqvist, 1983). One important question is how this wide range may be explained. Some potential reasons are given in Table 1.12.

**Table 1.12**
Potential reasons for interstudy variations in the frequency of postoperative DVT

1. Distribution of risk factors
2. Type of anaesthesia
3. Geographic differences
4. Fluctuations over time
5. Diagnostic differences
6. Differences in general care of patients
7. Representativeness
8. Statistical reasons

## Distribution of risk factors
Discussion of risk factors falls outside the scope of this presentation. However, it is obvious that differences in the distribution of risk factors will have a great impact. Age is such a factor as is the type of surgery. Above 40-45 years of age, the risk increases rapidly and therefore the number of patients in various age strata is important. General abdominal surgery includes everything from herniorrhaphy and cholecystectomy to abdomino--perineal resection for rectal carcinoma, with frequencies varying from less than 10% to above 40%.

## Type of anaesthesia
The few randomised studies available indicate that epidural/spinal anaesthesia in itself lowers the frequency of DVT compared with general anaesthesia (Modig et al, 1981, 1983, 1985; McKenzie et al, 1985; Hendolin et al, 1981; Davis et al, 1981, 1989). The relative frequency of epidural/spinal versus general anaesthesia therefore seems to be of importance for the overall frequency of deep vein thrombosis within a group of patients.

## Geographic differences
There are several theoretical reasons why there should be geographical differences such as differences in age, general health and nutritional state, genetic factors, and environmental factors, climatological factors and dietary habits. In fact, most studies from non-western countries show a low frequency of postoperative deep vein thrombosis although variations are great also here (Bergqvist, 1990). There may also be seasonal variations in at least fatal pulmonary embolism (Wroblewski et al, 1990; Colantonio et al, 1990), which also may show a circadian distribution (Colantonio et al, 1989).

## Fluctuations over time
Fluctuations over time do not seem to be important (Table 1.8), although the number of studies with untreated patients are diminishing because of ethical considerations.

## Diagnostic differences
Although the FUT has been used in most studies in general surgery it must be stressed that the diagnostic methodology is important for the frequency of detected DVT. Also, even

### Table 1.13
Frequency (%) of deep vein thrombosis after hip fracture surgery detected by venography. No prophylaxis

| Author | Time venography was performed | Frequency (%) |
| --- | --- | --- |
| Ahlberg et al, 1968 | 2-10 m | 36 |
| Borgstrom et al, 1965 | 3-4 m | 56 |
| Culver et al, 1970 | <4 m | 40 |
| Freeark et al, 1967 | 12.3 d | 41 |
| Hamilton et al, 1970 | 5-12 d | 47 |
| Johnson et al, 1968 | <3 m | 52 |
| Myhre, Holen, 1969 | 21 d | 36 |
| Smyrnis et al, 1973 | 6-10 d | 60 |
| Stevens et al, 1968 | 9-21 d | 30 |

when using the same diagnostic method different criteria and interpretations are a reality. In this context the importance of defining the time for follow-up must also be stressed and differences here might easily explain differences in incidence of DVT between studies. Table 1.13 illustrates the time for postoperative venography in studies on hip fracture surgery. When using the FUT it is important to state in detail for how long the patients are followed up and if reinjection of fibrinogen is used.

**Differences in general care of patients**
This is difficult to quantify but seems to have to do with the degree and length of preoperative immobilisation, fluid balance, atraumatic surgical technique, differences in surgical technique, the time for and aggressiveness of early mobilisation — factors that are only rarely stated in the various studies.

**Representativeness**
Only rarely is it possible to know how representative the patients are for the whole surgical population from which they have been recruited and ideally the background population should be defined. Otherwise differences in exclusion and inclusion criteria may have an impact on the frequency of DVT and therefore on differences between studies which at first glance seem similar.

**Statistical reasons**
Finally, most of the studies are fairly small, meaning that the confidence limits are wide, and the difference between studies may not be that great. The studies in general surgery with variations in frequency from 13 to 59% are illustrated in figure 1.2 with 95% confidence limits included.

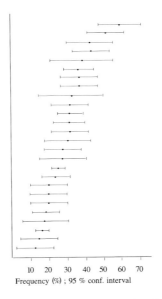

Figure 1.2  The incidence and 95% confidence intervals of DVT in studies of 26 patients having general surgery without thrombophylaxis

## Conclusion

The overwhelming amount of studies on venous thromboembolism are made in postoperative patients. Without prophylaxis deep vein thrombosis is a frequent complication and pulmonary embolism an important cause of death. The frequencies given undoubtedly motivate one to practice prophylaxis and to search for information on how and when to use it.

## References

Ahlberg Å, Nylander G, Robertson B, Cronberg S, Nilsson IM. Dextran in prophylaxis of thrombosis in fractures of the hip. Acta Chir Scand Suppl 387:83, 1968

Allgood R., Cook J, Weedn R, Speed HK, Whitcomb W, Greenfield L. Prospective analysis of pulmonary embolism in the post-operative patient. Surgery 68:116, 1970

Bergqvist D. Prophylaxis of postoperative thromboembolic complications with low-dose heparin. An analysis of different administration levels. Acta Chir Scand 145:7, 1979

Bergqvist D. Postoperative thromboembolism. Frequency, etiology, prophylaxis. Springer-Verlag, Berlin, Heidelberg, New York, 1983

Bergqvist D. Prophylaxis against postoperative venous thromboembolism — a survey of surveys. Thromb Haemorrh Disorders 2:69, 1990

Bergvist D, Efsing HO, Hallöök T, Lindhagen A. Analysis of preoperative and postoperative lung scintigraphy in patients undergoing elective hip surgery. VASA 9:311, 1980

Bergvist D, Efsing HO, Hallöök T, Hedlund T. Thromboembolism after elective and post-traumatic hip surgery — a controlled prophylactic trial with dextran-70 and low-dose heparin. Acta Chir Scand 145:213, 1979

Bergqvist D, Fredin H. Fatal pulmonary embolism and mortality in patients with fractured hip — a prospective consecutive series during routine thromboprophylaxis. Eur J Surg 157:571, 1991

Bergqvist D, Kettunen K, Fredin H, Fauno P, Suomalainen O, Soimakallio S, Karjalainen P, Cederholm C, Jensen LJ, Justesen T, Stiekema JCJ. Thromboprophylaxis in hip fracture patients — a prospective randomised comparative study between Org 10172 and Dextran 70. Surgery 109:617, 1991

Bergqvist D, Lindblad B. A 30-year survey of pulmonary embolism verified at autopsy: an analysis of 1,274 surgical patients. Br J Surg 72:105, 1985

Bergström S, Greitz T, van der Linden W, Molin J, Rudics I. Anticoagulant prophylaxis of venous thrombosis in patients with fractured neck of the femur. A controlled clinical trial using venous phlebography. Acta Chir Scand 129:500, 1965.

Binns M, Pho R. Femoral vein occlusion during hip arthroplasty. Clin Orthop 255:168, 1990

Borris LC, Christensen HM, Lassen MR, Olsen AD, Schott P. Comparison of real-time B-mode ultrasonography and bilateral ascending venography for detection of postoperative deep vein thrombosis following elective hip surgery. Thromb Haemost 61:363, 1989

Browse NL, Clemenson G, Croft DN. Fibrinogen-detectable thrombosis in the legs and pulmonary embolism. Br Med J 1:603, 1974

Butterman G, Theisinger W, Weidenbach A, Hartung H, Welzel D, Pabst HW. Quantitative Bewertung der postoperativen Thromboembolieprophylaxe. Vergleichende Untersuchungen uber Thrombose- und Emboliehaufigkeiten unter Acetylsalicylsaure, Dextran, Dihydroergotamin, Heparin sowie der fixen Kombination von Heparin und Dihydroergotamin. Med Clin 72:1624, 1977

Christensen SW, Wille-Jorgensen P, Kjaer L, Stadeager C, Widding A, Vestergaard Aa, Bjerg-Nielsen A. Contact thermography, $^{99m}$Tc-plasmin scintimetry and $^{99m}$Tc-plasmin scintigraphy as screening methods for deep venous thrombosis following major hip surgery. Thromb Haemost 58:831, 1987

Colantonio D, Casale R, Abruzzo BP, Lorenzetti G, Pasqualetti P. Circadian distribution in fatal pulmonary embolism. Am J Cardiol 64:403, 1989

Colantonio D, Casale R, Natali G, Pisqualetti P. Seasonal periodicity in fatal pulmonary thromboembolism. Lancet 335:56, 1990

Comerota AJ, Katz ML, Grossi RJ, Czeredarczuk M, Bowman G, DeSai S, Vujic I. The comparative value of noninvasive testing for diagnosis and surveillance of deep vein thrombosis. J Vasc Surg 7:40, 1988

Comerota AJ, Katz ML, Greewald LL, Leefmans E, Czeredarczuk M, White JV. Venous Duplex imaging: should it replace hemodynamic tests for deep venous thrombosis? J Vasc Surg 11:53, 1990

Cruickshank MK, Levine MN, Hirsh J, Turpie AGG, Powers P, Jay R, Gent M. An evaluation of impedance plethysmography and $^{125}$I-fibrinogen leg scanning in patients following hip surgery. Thromb Haemost 62:830, 1989

Culver D, Crawford JS, Gardiner JH, Wiley AM. Venous thrombosis after fractures of the upper end of the femur. A study if incidence and site. J Bone Joint Surg 52.B:61, 1970

Davis FM, Laurenson VG. Spinal anaesthesia or general anaesthesia for emergency hip surgery in elderly patients. Anaesth Intens Care 9:352, 1981

Davis FM, Laurenson VG, Gillespie WJ, Seagar D. Leg blood flow during total hip replacement under spinal or general anaesthesia. Anaesth Intens Care 17:136, 1989

Dixon JE. Pregnancies complicated by previous thromboembolic disease. Br J Hosp Med 449, 1987

Fauno P, Suomalainen O, Bergqvist D, Fredin H, Kettunen K, Soimakallio S, Cederholm C, Karjalainen P, Vissinger H, Justesen T. The use of fibrinogen uptake test in screening for deep vein thrombosis in patients with hip fracture. Thromb Res 60:185, 1990

Freeark R, Boswik J, Fardin R. Posttraumatic venous thrombosis. Arch Surg 95:567, 1967

Froehlich JA, Dorfman GS, Cronan JJ, Urbanek PJ, Herndon JH, Aaron RK. Compression ultrasonography for the detection of deep venous thrombosis in patients who have a fracture of the hip. J Bone Joint Surg 71-A:249, 1989

Gerstmann BP, Piper JM, Tomita DK, Ferguson WJ, Stadel BV, Lundin FE. Oral contraceptive estrogen dose and the risk of deep venous thromboembolic disease. Am J Epidemiol 133:32, 1991

Hamilton HW, Crawford JS, Gardiner JH, Wiley AM. Venous thrombosis in patients with fracture of the upper end of the femur. A phlebographic study of the effect of prophylactic anticoagulation. J Bone Joint Surg 52.B:268, 1970

Hartsuck J, Greenfield L. Postoperative thromboembolism. A clinical study with $^{125}$I-fibrinogen and pulmonary scanning. Arch Surg 107:733, 1973

Hendolin H, Mattila MAK, Poikolainen E. The effect of lumbar epidural analgesia on the development of deep vein thrombosis of the legs after open prostatectomy. Acta Chir Scand 147:425, 1981

Hoek JA, Nurmohamed MT, ten Cate JW. Prevention of deep vein thrombosis following total hip replacement by a low molecular weight heparinoid (Org 10172). Thromb Haemost 62:1637, 1989

Hogevold HE, Hoseth A, Reikeras O. Deep vein thrombosis after total hip replacement. A venographic study. Acta Radiol 31:571, 1990

Hull RD, Raskob GE, Gent M. Effectiveness of intermittent leg compression for preventing deep vein thrombosis after total hip replacement. JAMA 263:2313, 1990

Johansson E, Ericson K, Asard P. Postoperative leg vein thrombosis and pulmonary embolism after upper abdominal operations. A prospective study with $^{125}$I-fibrinogen test and pulmonary scintigraphy. Acta Chir Scand 141:522, 1975

Jørgensen PS, Knudsen JB, Broeng L et al. The thromboprophylactic effect of a low molecular weight heparin (Fragmin) in hip fracture surgery: a placebo controlled study. Clin Orthop 278:95, 1992

Lahnborg G, Bergstrom K, Friman L, Lagergren H. Effect of low-dose heparin on incidence of postoperative pulmonary embolism detected by photoscanning. Lancet I:329, 1974

Lassen MR, Borris LC, Christiansen HM et al. Prevention of thromboembolism in hip-fracture patients. Comparison of low-dose heparin and low-molecular weight heparin combined with dihydroergotamine. Arch Orthop Trauma Surg 108:10, 1989

Lassen MR, Borris LC, Christiansen HM et al. Prevention of thromboembolism in 190 hip arthroplasties. Comparison of LMW heparin and placebo. Acta Orthop Scand 62:33, 1991

Lindström B, Holmdal D, Jonsson O, Korsan-Benstsen K, Lindberg S, Petrusson B, Petterson S, Wikstrand J, Wojciehowski J. Prediction and prophylaxis of postoperative thromboembolism — a comparative study of calf muscle stimulation with group of impulses and dextran 40. Br J Surg 69:633, 1982

McKenzie PJ, Wishart HY, Gray I, Smith G. Effects of anaesthetic technique on deep vein thrombosis. A comparison of subarachnoid and general anaesthesia. Br J Anaesth 57:853, 1985

Modig J. The role of lumbar epidural anaesthesia as antithrombotic prophylaxis in total hip replacement. Acta Chir Scand 151:589, 1985

Modig J, Hjelmstedt A, Sahlstedt B, Maripuu E. Comparative influences of epidural and general anaesthesia on deep venous thrombosis and pulmonary embolism after total hip replacement. Acta Chir Scand 147:125, 1981

Modig J, Borg T, Bagge L, Saldeen T. Role of extradural and of general anaesthesia in fibrinolysis and coagulation after total hip replacement. Br J Anaesth 55:625, 1983

Murphy M, Dalrymple G, Rivarola C. Silent pulmonary embolism in the elderly surgical patient. Geriatrics 27:87, 1972

Myhre H, Holen A. Thrombosis prophylaxis. Dextran or sodium warfarin? A controlled clinical study. Nord Med 82:1534, 1969

Ockelford PA, Patterson J, Johns AS. A double-blind randomized placebo-controlled trial of thromboprophylaxis in major elective general surgery using once daily injections of a low molecular weight heparin fragment (Fragmin). Thromb Haemost 62:1046, 1989

Paiement G, Wessinger SJ, Waltman AC, Harris WH. Surveillance of deep vein thrombosis in asymptomatic total hip replacement patients. Am J Surg 155:400, 1988

The PIOPED Investigators. Value of the ventilation/perfusion scan in acute pulmonary embolism. Results of the Prospective Investigation of Pulmonary Embolism Diagnosis (PIOPED). JAMA 263, 2753,1990

Planes A, Vochelle N, Fagola M. Total hip replacement and deep vein thrombosis. A venographic and necropsy study. J Bone Joint Surg 72-B:9, 1990

Salzman A, Axilrod H. The value of preoperative lung scanning in the assessment of postoperative perfusion abnormalities. J Urol 106:581, 1971

Sheppeard H, Henson J, Ward DJ, Connor BTO. A clinico-pathological study of fatal pulmonary embolism in a specialist orthopaedic hospital. Arch Orthop Traumat Surg 99:65, 1981

Smyrnis SA, Kolios AS, Agnantis JK. Deep-vein thrombosis in patients with fracture of the upper part of the femur. A phlebographic study. Br J Surg 60:447, 1973

Stamatakis JD, Kakkar VV, Sagar S, Lawrence D, Nairn D, Bentley PG. Femoral vein thrombosis and total hip replacement. Br Med J 2:223, 1977

Stevens J, Fardin R, Freeark R. Lower extremity thrombophlebitis in patients with femoral neck fractures. A venographic investigation and a review of the early and late significance of the findings. J Trauma 8:527, 1968

Tørholm C, Broeng L, Jørgensen PS et al. Thromboprophylaxis by low-molecular-weight heaprin in elective hip surgery. A placebo controlled study. J Bone Joint Surg (BR)73.B:434, 1991

Turpie, AGG, Levine MN, Hirsch J et al. A randomized controlled trial of a low molecular weight heparin (Enoxaparin) to prevent deep-vein thrombosis in patients undergoing elective hip surgery. N Engl J Med 315:925, 1986

Woolson ST, McCrory DW, Walter JF, Maloney WJ, Watt JM, Cahill PD. B-mode ultrasound scanning in the detection of proximal venous thrombosis after total hip replacement. J Bone Joint Surg 72-A:983, 1990

Wroblewski BM, Siney P, White R. Seasonal variation in fatal pulmonary embolism after hip arthroplasty. Lancet 335:56, 1990

CHAPTER 2

# Incidence of Late Sequelae of Deep Vein Thrombosis
# Comparison of thrombolysis with anticoagulation

Leo K Widmer
M-Th Widmer
Hans-E Schmitt

Remy Eichlisberger
Elisabeth Zemp
Kurt Jäger

## Introduction

The notion that leg ulcers might be of post-thrombotic origin was first voiced by Gay, an English surgeon (1812-1885), who observed that ulcers may be due to "conditions which involve obstruction of the trunk veins, deep and superficial, from impediments on the venous side" and not to varices. In the period which preceded the discovery of anticoagulation, the late sequelae, especially the post-thrombotic syndrome (PTS) were very severe (Bauer, 1942; Widmer, 1977; Widmer, 1984). Anticoagulants helped to reduced the incidence of post-thrombotic syndrome but did not eliminate it. This is why Tillet's discovery, that streptokinase produced by beta-streptococci could be used to lyse thrombi, evoked much enthusiasm, particularly after Fletcher had developed a method of purifying the enzyme (van de Loo et al, 1983).

## Acute Phase

Thrombolysis of deep vein thrombosis (DVT) in the lower extremities was introduced at the Basle Medical Clinic in 1962. DVT was diagnosed clinically, by noninvasive procedures

Our thanks to PD Dr G. Marbet, Coagulation Laboratory, Prof. Dr. R. Ritz, Division of Intensive Care, Medical Department, University, CH-4031 Basle.

**Table 2.1**
Contraindications to SK therapy (modified from NIH) (Minar et al, 1984)

*Absolute contraindications*
Active internal bleeding or haemorrhagic diathesis
Previous cerebrovascular accident or other active intracranial process

*Relative contraindications*

| Major | Minor |
|---|---|
| Surgery, obstetrical delivery, organ biopsy, puncture of non-compressible vessels, serious trauma, cardiopulmonary resuscitation: < 10 days. | Menstruation (First 20 hours) |
| Vascular, neurosurgical, eye operations in the previous weeks | Abnormal haemostatic screening |
| Recent serious GI bleeding | Bacterial endocarditis |
| Arterial hypertension (diastolic ≥ 110) or grade 4 retinopathy | Puncture of non-compressible vessels < 10 days |
| Diabetic haemorrhagic retinopathy | Age > 70 years |
| 1st trimester of pregnancy | Previous SK therapy within 3-6 months |

and confirmed by ascending venography as described by Schmitt (1972). Most of the thrombi involved several levels (see below). The leading causes of DVT in men were surgery, trauma, and exertion. In women aged less than 50, hormonal contraception was the main cause (Brandenberg, 1982; Widmer, 1984; Widmer et al, 1985).

At that time, thrombolysis was the treatment of choice (Schmutzler and Koller, 1965; Schmulzler, 1966; Koller and Duckert, 1983; Koller and Marbet, 1983). Patients in good health with extensive thrombi received thrombolysis with titrated doses of streptokinase for 4 to 6 days in the intensive care unit, followed by anticoagulation. Our experience with urokinase or TPA lysis is limited (Duckert et al, 1975; 1978). Elderly patients with limited DVT and those with contraindications (Table 2.1) were anticoagulated with heparin (Initial dose 5,000 IU, maintenance dose approx 25,000 IU per day) and Marcoumar. The effect of treatment was assessed by venography on the 5th (max. 14th) day. In the course of hospitalisation, patients were given a general examination and fitted with a compression stocking. Follow-up treatment, including anticoagulation (recommended for 6 months) was performed by the patient's general practitioner.

**Success rate**
Partial clearance was observed in 69%, complete clearance in 17%, no clearance in 14%. The figures are at the lower range of those reported by others (Table 2.2). The success rate was dependent upon the age of the thrombus and its adherence to the wall of the vein (Schmitt, 1972).

**Side effects**
In thrombolysis, haemorrhagic events from puncture sites were frequent. In 12% treatment was stopped because of macrohaematuria. The initially frequent allergic reaction disappeared after the thrombolytic agent had been purified. There were four severe complications out of 549 patients treated: one fatal lung embolism, one fatal paradoxic embolus. Two nonfatal intracerebral haemorrhages occurred in a 40 year old woman with hemianopsia and a 64 year old man with epileptic attacks under control with phenytoin. Non fatal

**Table 2.2**
Success of Thrombolysis: Acute Stage

|  |  |  | Success of thrombylosis (%) | | |
| --- | --- | --- | --- | --- | --- |
| Author | Year | n | Complete | Partial | Without Success |
| Jarvinen | 1978 | 36 | 17 | 69 | 14 |
| Ehringer | 1984 | 55 | 42 | 20 | 38 |
| Marbet | 1986 | 154 | 44 | 31 | 25 |
| Trübestein | 1986 | 336 | 43 | 37 | 20 |
| Theiss | 1989 | 94 | 28 | 38 | 34 |
| Jacobson | 1990 | 839 | 70 | | 30 |
| Review Studies | | | | | |
| Hess | 1967 | 161 | 62 | | 38 |
| Breddin | 1982 | 855 | 35 | 42 | 23 |
| Schulman | 1985 | 143 | 29 | 39 | 32 |
| Stehle | 1986 | 228 | 40 | 32 | 28 |

pulmonary embolism was observed in 4% and fatal in 0.2% (Table 2.3). The fatal complications were similar to those observed by Jakobson and Trübestein (1989). Schulman (1985) reported fatal complications in 1.8% of 1127 thrombolyses vs 0.6% in 2305 anticoagulated patients.

# Follow-up Examination

Follow-up examinations should include reexamination of a sufficient number of consecutive (not selected) patients examined after a sufficient time interval (Amacher and Widmer, 1981).

Mortality, interim recurrence of thromboembolism, incidence of post-thrombotic syndrome, personal and sociomedical consequences were analysed in three studies of patients with unilateral DVT, reexamined after 5, 6 (341 survivors) and 13 years (223 survivors).

**Table 2.3**
Experiences of severe complications (549 patients treated since 1962 in Basle[*])

|  | n | % |
| --- | --- | --- |
| Non-fatal intracerebral haemorrhage | 2 | 0.36 |
| Fatal pulmonary embolism | 1 | 0.18 |
| Fatal paradoxic embolism | 1 | 0.18 |
| Total | 4 | 0.72 |

[*] Personal communication by PD Dr G Marbet

## Mortality and cause of death
The data are based on the patient's death certificate completed by the treating physician and filed at the Swiss Central Office of Statistics. The certificate provides information about age, sex, direct cause of death, concomitant diseases and post-mortem examination (if performed) (Brandenberg, 1982).

## Surviving patients
Surviving patients were interviewed with regard to history of previous venous disease, interval treatment, thromboembolic recurrence, personal and sociomedical considerations. Information on thromboembolic recurrence and leg ulcers was substantiated and validated by consultation with the family doctor or the relevant hospital. The venological examination included a clinical check-up and Polaroid documentation of the lower leg/foot region. A blind technique was used, i.e., the interviewing physician ignored the actual venological status and the examining physician ignored the type of treatment performed during the acute phase. In order to exclude cases of chronic venous insufficiency due to other causes, a scoring system taking into account pronounced oedema and trophic changes was used in the five year follow-up (Brandenberg, 1982; Widmer, 1984).

## Analysis
Mortality, DVT recurrence, post-thrombotic syndrome incidence, symptoms and sociomedical consequences depended upon the initial extent of DVT. Surviving patients were therefore subdivided into a negative and a positive group. The negative group comprised patients whose initial and control venograms were identical, i.e., who had been treated with heparin or, unsuccessfully, with thrombolysis. This group more or less reflected the natural course of DVT. The positive group comprised of patients with partial or complete thrombolysis.

## Five year follow-up: Mortality in 278 patients
In 1977, 278 consecutive patients who had been treated by anticoagulation or thrombolysis at least three years before, were sent invitations to attend a follow-up examination (Brandenberg, 1982; Widmer, 1984). All patients could be reached. At entry patients were 55.5 years old. Forty-five patients had died within 5.4 years, 31 men and 14 women at a mean age of 68.8 years. This was significantly sooner than the general life expectancy at the time, men 76, women 81 years. The immediate cause of death was cardiovascular disease (36%: 10 coronary heart disease, 6 pulmonary embolism), tumours (56%) and other diseases (8%). Tumours, detected in 12 patients during the acute phase and in 13 during the interval were localised for women mainly in the urogenital tract and the lymphatic system (4 cases), in men in the stomach and the bronchi (9 cases) as described by Minar and Wegmann (Wegmann 1981; Minar et al, 1984). No pulmonary hypertension was mentioned in either the death certificates or the postmortem examinations (19 patients). A leg ulcer was observed during lifetime in 6.3% of the men and 5.6% of the women.

## Six Year follow-up of 341 surviving patients
226 men and 115 women (aged 52.0±16 years at entry), were reexamined 6.2 years after the acute event. Thrombosis had been localised in 193 on the left and 148 on the right side. Two hundred and eight patients were treated with thrombolysis and 133 with anticoagulants (Widmer et al, 1985).

**Table 2.4**
Extent of DVT at entry in the negative and positive groups
*6 years*

| DVT extent at entry | Negative Group (Anticoagulation and unsuccessful lysis) (n = 194) | | Positive Group (Successful lysis) (n = 147) | |
|---|---|---|---|---|
| | n | % | n | % |
| Special | 10 | 5 | 12 | 8 |
| Lower Leg | 35 | 18 | 2 | 1 |
| L Popliteal | 32 | 17 | 28 | 19 |
| L P Femoral | 60 | 31 | 50 | 34 |
| L P F Pelvic | 57 | 29 | 55 | 38 |

A significant correlation was observed between the DVT at entry, the thromboembolic recurrence and the incidence of post-thrombotic syndrome. Consequently the patients were subdivided into a negative group with anticoagulation and unsuccessful thrombolysis, reflecting the natural course, and a positive group with successful lysis (Table 2.4).

*The Negative Group*
In spite of the prevalence of patients whose prognosis was favourable (i.e., DVT at 1 to 2 levels), 7.7% had leg ulcers and 16% had post-thrombotic syndrome without ulceration.

*The Positive Group*
Prognosis was less favourable due to the prevalence of DVT at 3 or 4 levels (Table 2.4). Since comparison is only meaningful if the extent of DVT is similar at entry, the groups were compared "étage by étage". The result of this comparison between the positive and the negative group is shown in figure 2.1.

### 13-year follow-up of 223 surviving patients

The 341 patients participating in the 6-year follow-up were invited for a second re-examination in 1980.

*Mortality*
In the period between the 5 and 13 year follow-up examinations, 58 men and 20 women had died. Fifty-one belonged to the negative and 27 to the positive group. One patient had been bilaterally amputated because of occlusive peripheral arterial disease. Of 262 patients 39 could not be traced, so that the drop-out rate is 14.8%. The death rate was correlated to

**Table 2.5**
Extent of DVT at entry and mortality in the period between the 6 and 13 year follow-up

| Extent of DVT | n | Mortality |
|---|---|---|
| Special | 22 | 1 (4%) |
| Lower Leg | 37 | 7 (19%) |
| L Popliteal | 60 | 8 (13%) |
| L P Femoral | 110 | 25 (23%) |
| L P F Pelvic | 112 | 37 (33%) |

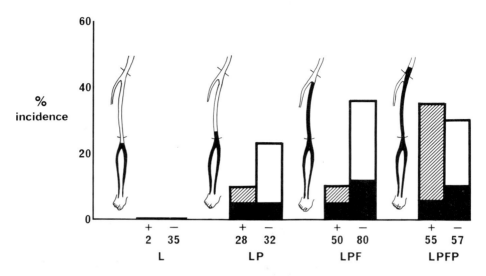

Figure 2.1  Incidence of post-thrombotic syndrome in the positive and negative groups at 6 years

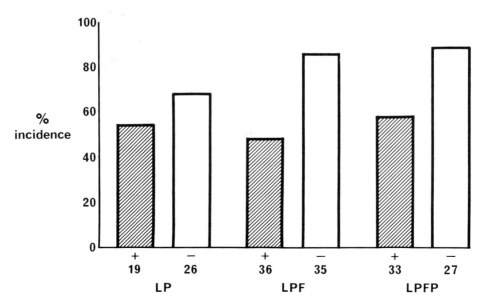

Figure 2.2  Incidence of severe symptoms (leg pain, oedema and incapacity) in the positive and negative groups at 13 years

**Table 2.6**
Extent of DVT at entry in the negative and positive groups
*13 years*

| DVT extent at entry | 123 Negative | 100 Positive |
| --- | --- | --- |
| Special     | 4  (3%)  | 11 (11%) |
| Lower Leg   | 28 (23%) | 1  (1%)  |
| L Popliteal | 26 (21%) | 19 (19%) |
| L P Femoral | 36 (29%) | 36 (36%) |
| L P F Pelvic| 29 (24%) | 33 (33%) |

the extent of DVT at entry. Of 22 patients who had leg ulcers after 5 years, 7 had died (Table 2.5).

*The Surviving Patients*
One hundred and fifty-one men and 72 women (aged 61.7 ± 14.7 years) survived. One hundred and forty-four had been thrombolysed and 79 anticoagulated. Re-examination was performed after 13 ± 1.4 years. Once again, the extent of DVT at entry in the negative group was different from that in the positive group (Table 2.6).

*Negative Group*
The negative group was 63.9 ± 14.9 years old. It consisted of 79 anticoagulated and 44 unsuccessfully thrombolysed. 9.8% had leg ulcers, 29.3% had post-thrombotic syndrome without ulcers, 25.0% had mild, not considered changes, and 35.9% showed no change.

*Positive Group*
The positive group was 59.4 ± 13.9 years old (75 partially and 25 complete successful thrombolyses). At interview, leg pain, swelling and impairment were significantly less frequent than in the negative group (Fig. 2.2).

*Incidence of Post-thrombotic Syndrome*
The comparison "étage by étage" yields no difference for specially located, lower leg and 2-level thrombosis. On the other hand, the incidence of post-thrombotic syndrome is significantly lower for thromboses on 3 and 4 levels (Fig. 2.3).

*Group with Leg Ulcers*
The group consisted of 14 men and 2 women aged 59.7 years. Many patients had previous venous disease (31%), i.e., venous disease which occurred before the actual thrombosis which determined their inclusion into this study. The group was also characterised by a high recurrence rate (25%). Leg ulcers occurred mainly in extended DVT. Interestingly, involvement of the popliteal vein seemed to be a determinant of leg ulcers (Table 2.7).

*Complete clearance by thrombolysis*
Complete clearance by thrombolysis was obtained in 14 men and 11 women at an age of 52.6 years. Clearance was complete in patients with DVT in a special location and in 1/5 of those with 4-level DVT. Only 4% had previous venous disease, 20% had recurrence of DVT in the interval; 28% used regular compression (Table 2.8)

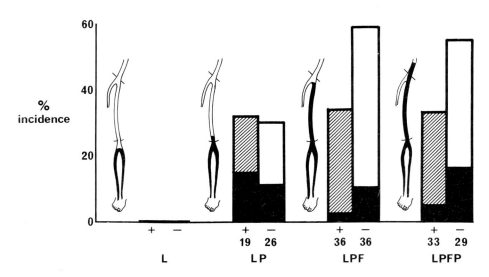

Figure 2.3  Incidence of post-thrombotic syndrome in the positive and negative groups at 13 years

**Table 2.7**
Extent of DVT at entry and incidence of leg ulcers
*13 years*

| Extent of DVT at entry | 223 patients n | 17 leg ulcers n |
|---|---|---|
| Special | 15 | 0 |
| Lower Leg | 29 | 0 |
| L Popliteal | 45 | 6 |
| L P Femoral | 72 | 5 |

**Table 2.8**
Extent of partial and complete clearance by thrombolysis
*13 years*

Men : women  14 : 11
Age  52.6

| Extent of DVT | Successfully Thrombolysed n | Complete Clearance n |
|---|---|---|
| Special | 11 | 10 (91%) |
| Lower Leg | 1 | 1 |
| L Popliteal | 19 | 5 (26%) |
| L P Femoral | 36 | 2 ( 6%) |
| L P F Pelvic | 33 | 7 (21%) |

## Discussion

**Methodological difficulties**
There is no consensus of opinion about late sequelae of DVT. Longterm studies are difficult to perform (Widmer et al, 1983; Theiss, 1990).
 Even in the acute phase, DVT is of a protean nature. It is difficult to ascertain when thrombus formation starts and thus to determine the age of the latter. Furthermore, DVT has many aetiologies. Because heparin is used for mild DVT and for cases where streptokinase is contraindicated, the number of thrombolysis candidates available for re-examination is considerably reduced.
 *Follow-up* examination several years after the acute event presents a number of different obstacles. The first is *the recruiting of a sufficient number of patients after a sufficient interval*. The second is the *problem of drop-outs* well known in cardiovascular epidemiology (Amacher and Widmer, 1981). For example, our group observed leg ulcers in only 3.7% of patients who accepted the first invitation. This rate rose to 12.4% when, after repeated invitations, the remaining patients came for follow-up examination. A high drop-out rate gives an incomplete picture which is often false. One author, who re-examined only 97 out of 143 patients two years after the acute event, observed that the incidence of post-thrombotic syndrome after limited and extended thromboses was the same. With a 32.1% drop-out rate, how much significance, if any at all, could be attached if no difference has been found in a comparison between 88 anticoagulated and 29 thrombolysed patients? Another influential factor is *patients with chronic venous insufficiency of different origin*, e.g., varicose veins, especially if post-thrombotic syndrome and varicose veins occur at the same time (Browse et al, 1968; Browse et al, 1980). Nowadays it would be much simpler to define post-thrombotic syndrome by noninvasive procedures such as continuous wave Doppler or Doppler ultrasound (Norgren and Gjöres, 1977; Partsch et al, 1980; Franzeck et al, 1991; Obernosterer et al, 1991). However such techniques were not available when our study was started.

## Our Study

Our study was not randomised, but the criteria for inclusion and exclusion were strictly adhered to and the dropout rate was very low. Post-thrombotic syndrome was defined according to strict criteria on the basis of the interview and photographic documentation. This allowed the reappraisal of post-thrombotic syndrome ensuring that only pronounced changes were considered.

**Acute phase of treatment**
Our results are in the lower ranges of clearance rates found in table 2.1, probably because many patients with previous venous disease and patients with thrombi older than five days were included in the study. Whether better results would have been obtained with streptokinase — or urokinase —regimens is debatable. Many techniques have been applied in different centres, including continuous or intermittent, fixed or individually titrated streptokinase or urokinase treatment, ultra-high streptokinase etc (Duckert et al, 1975; Gallus et al, 1975; Duckert et al, 1978; Marbet et al, 1982; Minar et al, 1984; Martin and Fiebach, 1985; Marbet and Duckert, 1986; Trübestein et al, 1986). Despite the longstanding experi-

**Table 2.9**
Long-term results in randomised clinical trials between heparin and streptokinase

|  | Patients |  | Duration of follow-up (months) | Asymptomatic Patients | Normal Venogram |
|---|---|---|---|---|---|
|  | No. | Therapy |  |  |  |
| Johansson et al, 1979 | 8 | SK | 134 | 4 |  |
|  | 6 | H | 106 | 2 |  |
| Common et al, 1976 | 15 | SK | 7 | 10 | 6 |
|  | 12 | H | 7 | 6 | 1 |
| Arnesen et al, 1982 | 17 | SK | 76 | 13 | 7 |
|  | 18 | H | 77 | 6 | 0 |
| Elliot et al, 1979 | 23 | SK | 19 | 15 | 10 |
|  | 21 | H | 19 | 2 | 0 |
|  | 63 | SK | 46 | 42 (67%) |  |
|  | 57 | H | 44 | 16 (28%) |  |

ence only a few multicentre studies with different streptokinase regimens have been published (van de Loo et al, 1983a; Schulman et al, 1984; Heinrich, 1991).

*Side effects*
In many quarters, thrombolysis is considered to be risky. This is because it was promulgated in the 1970s at numerous meetings as a technique for every hospital, and even for general practices. Consequently there were many avoidable instances of severe side effects. Thrombolysis fell out of favour and was even added to the list of prohibited treatments. Side effects cannot be ruled out even if thrombolysis is "controlled". But severe complications are very rare, the prevalence is less than 0.5% (Schulman, 1985). This figure has to be offset against protracted suffering, thromboembolic recurrence and sociomedical consequences.

## Long term studies
Little information on mortality, thromboembolic recurrence, leg pain and sociomedical consequences is available because most long-term studies have concentrated upon the incidence of post-thrombotic syndrome.

*Mortality*
The high 5-year mortality rate was mainly due to tumours and pulmonary embolism. The mean age at death was 8 years below the life expectancy for 1978. It is of interest that pulmonary hypertension was not reported as a cause of death either in death certificates or in post-mortem findings. This indicates that DVT rarely causes "cor pulmonale".

*Incidence of post-thrombotic syndrome*
Randomised studies are few and have involved only very small groups of patients (Table 2.9).

The correlation between the extent of DVT at entry and the incidence of post-thrombotic syndrome initially surprised us. However our findings were by no means revolutionary: they merely confirmed what Bauer, Zilliakus and Halse had published decades ago (Bauer, 1942; Zilliakus, 1946; Halse, 1954). Further confirmation has been given recently by several teams (Browse et al, 1968; Thiele et al, 1989; Theiss, 1990). It is absolutely essential for any study to include adequate information on the extent of DVT at entry.

The incidence of post-thrombotic syndrome in the negative group (33%) corresponds to recent observations also (Theiss, 1990; Obernosterer et al, 1991). It is much higher than the figures of Franzeck who examined mainly short thromboses (Franzeck et al, 1991). Not only was reduction of post-thrombotic syndrome incidence by successful thrombolysis observed but also a reduction in leg pain and need for interval treatment, sociomedical consequences and parameters which have not received much attention.

As could be expected, the best results were achieved with complete thrombolysis; the incidence of post thrombotic syndrome being 8% (4% with and 4% without ulcers). This contrasts strongly to the natural history group with a corresponding incidence of 39.1%. In addition to a decrease in the incidence of post-thrombotic syndrome, there were also considerable reductions in thromboembolic recurrence, leg pain and impairment.

### Interval treatment
It could be argued that treatment of DVT during the acute phase is unnecessary, since post-thrombotic syndrome can be prevented by a consequent compression treatment. This may be true, although our study revealed that many patients find compression treatment very cumbersome. Many disregarded the consequences and discontinued when they felt no relief and saw no improvement. This was the case frequently in the negative group. Furthermore, 24% of the patients with leg ulcers admitted that they had abandoned compression.

### Socio-economic consequences
Incapacity was generally limited to the period of hospitalisation and the short recovery phase, 1½ months in all. Five patients were incapacitated in the first 5 years and an additional four in the 13-year follow-up stage. All had been treated by anticoagulation.

### Risk factors for Post-thrombotic Syndrome
The study seems to show that one of the major determinants for the evolution of post-thrombotic syndrome is *previous venous disease*, i.e., of disease which occurred before the thrombus that led to inclusion into the study. Incidence of previous venous disease was lowest in patients who were completely thrombolysed and highest in the negative group. *Thromboembolic recurrences*, which were observed in a third of our patients, constitute another risk factor. These factors should be taken into account when a decision has to be made as to whether a patient should be treated with anticoagulants or thrombolysis.

# Recommendations

Long-term sequelae continue to occur with an excess mortality and frequent thromboembolic recurrence. The post-thrombotic syndrome is, in 10% of cases, accompanied by ulceration, and in 22% by pronounced changes in the skin and veins. In some instances it causes years of suffering thromboembolic recurrence and sociomedical consequences. Thrombolysis should be "controlled", i.e., DVT should be venographically confirmed, streptokinase or urokinase should be administered for 3 to 5 days. This treatment should, however, be given when there are no contraindications and only in hospitals where coagulation parameters can be determined and where 24-hour care is available.

We still await a predictive test for efficacy of thrombolysis and of haemorrhage, which will ensure good results in the following patient groups:

Patients below 50 years of age in whom there are no contraindications

Patients with no previous venous disease including thromboembolic episodes, and without underlying malignant disease

Patients presenting with fresh thrombi up to a maximum of 5 days, with pronounced stasis.

# References

Amacher A, Widmer LK. Allgemeine Daten. In: Venen-Arterien-Krankheiten, koronare Herzkrankeit bei Berufstatigen — Basler Studie. Eds Widmer LK, Stahelin HB, Nissen C, da Silva A: 30, Huber, Berne, 1981

Anning ST. Historical Survey. In: The Pathology and Surgery of the Veins of the Lower Extremity. Eds Dodd H, Cockett FB: 6, Livingstone, Edinburgh and London, 1956

Arnesen H, Heilo A et al. A prospective study of streptokinase and heparin in the treatment of deep vein thrombosis. Acta Med Scand 203:57, 1978

Arnesen H, Hoiseth A, Bernt L. Streptokinase or heparin in the treatment of deep vein thrombosis. Acta Med Scand 211:65, 1982

Bauer G. A roentgenologic and clinical study of the sequelae of thrombosis. Acta Chir Scand 86:Suppl. 76, 1942

Brandenberg E. Venenthrombose und post-thrombotisches syndrom. 5-jahres follow-up bei 278 patienten. Diss., Basel, 1982

Browse NL, Thomas ML, Rim HP. Streptokinase and deep vein thrombosis. Br Med J 3:717, 1968

Browse NL, Clemenson G, Thomas ML. Is the post-phlebitic leg always post-phlebitic? Relation between phlebographic appearances of deep vein thrombosis and late sequelae. Brit Med J 281:1167, 1980

Common HH, Seaman AJ et al. Deep vein thrombosis treated with streptokinase or heparin. Follow-up of a randomised study. Angiology 27:645, 1976

Duckert F, Müller G et al. Treatment of deep vein thrombosis with streptokinase. Brit Med J 1:479, 1975

Duckert F, Marbet GA, Malter M et al. Thrombolytic treatment with a streptokinase low dose regimen. In: New Concepts in streptokinase therapy. Eds Martin H, Schoop W, Hirsch J: 83-86. Huber, Berne, 1978

Eichlisberger R, Widmer M-Th, Widmer LK, Zemp E. Spätfolgen nach becken-beinvenenthrombose — Basler Erfahrungen in fortschritte angiologie 1987. Eds Eringer, Holzner, Heidrich, Mahler, Minar. VASA Suppl. 20, Huber, Berne, 1987

Eichlisberger R, Zemp E, Widmer M-Th et al. Late sequelae of deep leg vein thrombosis. 13-year follow-up. In: Abst. 12B2. Ed. Partsch. 5th Europ-Am Symp Ven Dis 1990

Franzeck UK, Schalch I et al. Prospektive 5-jahres verlaufsuntersuchung haemodynamischer und klinischen parameter nach tiefer bein-beckenvenenthrombose. In: Angiology 91. Eds Rudofsky G, Pilger E, Jäger K: 228, VASA Suppl 33, Huber, Bern, 1991

Gallus AS, Hirsh J, Cade JF et al. Thrombolysis with a combination of small doses of streptokinase and full doses of heparin. Thromb Haemostas 2:14, 1975

Halse Th. Das postthrombotische Syndrom — pathogenese, diagnostik, behandlung und verhütung von akuter beinvenen-thrombose. Steinkopf, Darmstadt, 1954

Heinrich U. Ergebnisse der nord-badischen venen-lyse-studie. Randomisierte prüfung der wirkung von UHSK versus konventionell dosierter streptokinase. In: Angiologie 1991. Eds Rudofsky G, Pilger J, Jäger K: VASA Suppl 33, Huber, Bern, 1991

Jacobsen B. Thrombolytic treatment in venous thromboembolism. In: Controversies in the Management of Venous Disorders. Butterworth, London, 1989

Johansson L, Nylander G et al. Comparison of streptokinase with heparin: late results in the treatment of deep venous thrombosis. Acta Med Scand 206:93, 1979

Kakkar VV, Lawrence D. Haemodynamic and clinical assessment after therapy of acute deep vein thrombosis. Am J Surg Suppl 150:54, 1985

Koller F, Duckert F. Thrombose und embolie. Schattauer, Stuttgart 1983

Koller F, Marbet GA. Kontraindikationen. In: Thrombose und Embolie. Eds. Koller F, Duckert F: 439, Schattauer, Stuttgart, 1983

Marbet GA, Eichlisberger R, Duckert F et al. Side effects of thrombolytic treatment with porcine plasmin and low dose of streptokinase. Thromb Haemostas 48:196, 1982

Marbet GA, Duckert F. The development of thrombolytic treatment in venous thrombosis. Experiences with SK-based regimens. VASA 15:359, 1986

Martin M, Fiebach BJO (Hrsg). Die streptokinase-behandlung peripherer arterien — und venenverschlüsse unter besonderer Berücksichtigung der ultrahohen Dosierung. Huber, Bern, 1985

Minar E, Ehringer H, Marosi L, Sommer G, Deutsch E. Thrombolyse mit Urokinase bei akuter phlebothrombose. VASA 13:41, 1984

Norgren L, Gjöres JE. Venous function in previously thrombosed legs. A follow-up of streptokinase-treated patients. Acta Chir Scand 143:421, 1977

Obernosterer A, Decrinis N, Pilger E et al. Inzidenz eines postthrombotischen syndroms nach systematischer fibrinolyse von tiefenvenenthrombosen. In: Angiologie 91. Eds Rudofsky G, Pilger E, Jäger K: VASA Suppl. 33:120, 1991

Partsch H, Weidinger et al. Funktionelle Spätergebnisse nach thrombektomie, fibrinolyse und konservativer therapie von bein-beckenvenenthrombosen. VASA 9:53, 1980

Rudofsky G, Pilger E, Jäger K. Eds Angiologie 91, VIII. Gemeinsame Jahrestagung der Oesterreichischen, Schweizerischen und Deutschen Gesellschaft für Angiologie. VASA Suppl. 33:59, 1991

Schmitt HE. Aszendierende Phlebographie bei tiefer Venenthrombose. Huber, Bern, 1972

Schmutzler R. Klinik der thrombolytischen behandlung. Internist 10:21, 1969

Schulman S. Studies on the medical treatment of deep vein thrombosis. Acta Med Scand, Suppl. 704, 1985

Schulman S, Lockner D, Granqvist S et al. A comparative randomised trial of low-dose versus high-dose streptokinase in deep vein thrombosis of the thigh. Thromb and Haemostas 51:261, 1984

Theiss W. Scientific acceptability of longterm follow-up in deep leg thrombosis. In: Abst. 12B2. Ed. Partsch. 5th Europ-Am Symp Ven Dis, 1990

Thiele C, Theiss W, Kurfürst-Seebauer R. Langzeitergebnisse nach fibrinolytischer behandlung tiefer venenthrombosen im becken-bein-bereich. VASA 18:48, 1989

Trübestein G and R, Wilgalis M et al. Die fibrinolytische therapie mit streptokinase und urokinase bei tiefer venenthrombose. Med Klinik 3:79, 1986

Trübestein G. Fibrinolytische therapie. Indikationen und Durchführung. Dtsch Med Wchr 110:1417, 1985

van de Loo JCW, Prentice CRM, Beller LK. The thromboembolic disorders. Schattauer, Stuttgart, 1983

van de Loo JCW, Kreissmann A, Trübestein G et al. Controlled multicenter pilot study of urokinase-heparin and streptokinase in deep vein thrombosis. Thromb Haemostas 50:660, 1983a

Wegmann J. Paraneoblastische thrombose — eine mortalitätsstatische untersuchung. VASA 10:111, 1981

Widmer LK. Treatment of venous thrombosis: angiological aspects. Sandoz Triangle 16:47, Basle, 1977

Widmer LK, Brandenberg E, Widmer M-Th. Venenthrombose und postthrombotisches syndrom — methodische probleme bei der nachkontrolle von thrombose-patienten. In: Fibrinolytic Therapy. Eds Trübestein, Etzel. Schattauer, Stuggart, 1983

Widmer LK, Zemp E et al. Late results in deep vein thrombosis of the lower extremity. VASA 14:264, 1985

Widmer M-Th. Venenthrombose — postthrombotisches syndrom nach thrombolyse und antikoagulation. Diss. Basel 1984

Zilliacus H. On specific treatment of thrombosis and pulmonary embolism with anticoagulants, with particular reference to post-thrombotic sequelae: results of 5 years treatment of thrombosis and pulmonary embolism at a series of Swedish hospitals during the years 1940-1945. Acta Med Scand, Suppl. 171:13, 1946

CHAPTER 3

# Operative Venous Dilatation and its Relationship to Postoperative Deep Vein Thrombosis

Anthony J Comerota

## Introduction

Postoperative deep vein thrombosis (DVT) is a well recognised major problem encountered by patients undergoing thoracic, abdominal and orthopaedic procedures (NIH Consensus Conference 1986). Undoubtedly, prevention is the most effective means of dealing with the problem. It is implicitly evident that to provide effective prophylaxis one must have a clear understanding of the causes of postoperative DVT, so that the responsible factors can be controlled.

## Virchow's triad

The factors which cause venous thrombosis in the absence of direct venous injury have been of interest for more than a century. In 1856 Virchow presented his classic triad, where he stated that changes in blood elements (hypercoagulable states), a reduced blood flow velocity (stasis) and venous wall injury (endothelial damage) combined to create an environment which promoted thrombus formation.

### Hypercoagulability
The effect of hypercoagulable states and the existence of stasis have been summarised by Stead (1985). It has been shown that an increased risk of thrombosis is associated with an increase in procoagulant activities in the plasma including increases in platelet count and adhesiveness, changes in the coagulation cascade and endogenous fibrinolytic activity (Hirsh et al, 1980). Additionally, deficiencies of antithrombin III, protein C and protein S

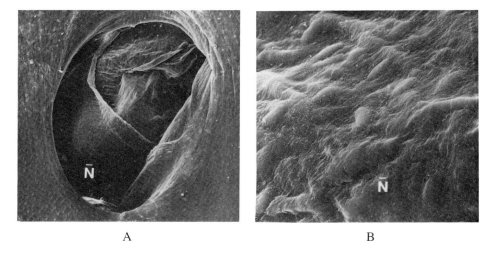

Fig. 3.1 Scanning electron micrographs of the luminal surface of the jugular vein of a dog which was anaesthetised but not operated on. Both low power (A) and high power (B) magnification demonstrate an intact endothelial monolayer without evidence of damage

as well as the presence of a lupus anticoagulant indicate either primary or secondary hypercoagulable states.

### Stasis

It is widely accepted by clinicians that stasis is a major factor in the cause of DVT. The occurrence of stasis has been demonstrated radiographically (Almen and Nylander, 1968) with femoral vein flow measurements (Clark and Cotton, 1968) and with radioisotopic techniques (Nicolaides and Kakkar, 1971). In an autopsy study Gibbs (1957) has shown the soleal sinuses to be the principle site of venous thrombosis.

Although the evidence indicates that stasis occurs in patients, and it is logical that reduced flow might prolong the contact time of activated platelets and clotting factors with the vein wall thereby permitting thrombus formation, in no study has stasis alone been causally related to DVT.

The hypercoagulable state and stasis seem to have been well accepted in the aetiological theories of postoperative DVT. However, the role of venous injury in initiating thrombosis has received little attention. Few would argue that direct venous wall injury either at the operative site or by penetrating and/or blunt trauma would lead to thrombus formation. As one examines the overall problem, it is clear that the more distant veins are not directly damaged during major operations, yet these are the most common sites of postoperative DVT.

### Endothelial Damage

To study the possibility that acute damage to venous endothelium may be caused by a distant operation, animal models have been developed. The development of endothelial damage in veins distant from the operative wound has been investigated by Schaub et al (1978) in canine models of abdominal operations and by Stewart et al (1983) in canine models of total hip replacement. In canine models of three different types of abdominal surgery, which included hysterectomy, splenectomy and anastomosis of the small intestine, Schaub et al (1978) found that leucocytes adhered to and invaded the wall of jugular and femoral veins

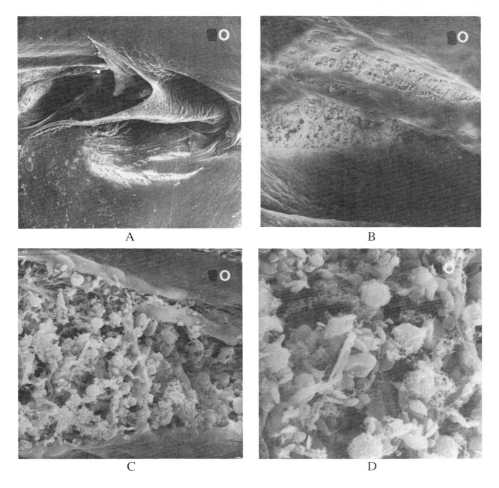

Fig. 3.2 Scanning electron photomicrographs of a dog's jugualr vein which underwent total hip replacement with significant operative venodilatation. Note that under low power magnification (A) an endothelial tear is located in the area of a valve cusp. With progressively higher power magnification, it appears that the endothelial damage ocurred as a stretching (tearing) mechanism (B). The damage extends through the endothelium and basement membrane exposing highly thrombogenic subendothelial collagen. One can appreciate the adherence of red blood cells, white blood cells, platelets and fibrin strands to the area of damage (C and D)

along their entire length. They theorised that these lesions were induced by blood-borne substances which were released at the operative site, gaining entry into the blood stream through capillaries and lymphatics, and then circulating throughout the body. Based upon these possibilities, they studied the effects of a continuous intravenous infusion of a low level of histamine and bradykinin (both of which are released from injured tissues) on canine jugular and femoral veins. Subsequent experiments by Stewart and her associates (1983) demonstrated that mild endothelial damage occurred after abdominal operations and that much more serious endothelial damage was found after total hip replacement. These endothelial lesions occurred as multiple microtears around the junction of small side branches with the major receiving veins, that is, jugular and femoral veins (Figs 3.1 and 3.2). These tears extended through the endothelium and through the basement membrane

**Table 3.1**
Incidence of venous endothelial lesions occurring according to percentage of dilatation of the jugular vein during total hip replacement in dogs

| Veins Examined* | Percent dilatation from Baseline | | |
|---|---|---|---|
| | 0%<br>(3 dogs) | 4-11%<br>(4 dogs) | 17-43%<br>(3 dogs) |
| Jugular | 17± 8 | 16± 6 | 60± 7 |
| R. Femoral | 11±10 | 25±26 | 24±21 |
| L. Femoral (operated side) | 16±17 | 26±18 | 43±12 |

* Veins examined with scanning electron microscopy

exposing the subendothelial collagen. The lesions were infiltrated with leucocytes and platelets. The appearance of the lesions suggested several likely hypotheses. First, the lesions could serve as sites for the initiation of venous thrombi. Second, the constant location of the endothelial damage to the venous confluence, (side branch) which is usually adjacent to a valve cusp, suggested that a structural weakness existed in this area, a theory subsequently proven by Stone and Stewart (1988) and described later in this chapter. Third, the endothelial damage could have been caused by dilatation of the vein wall beyond the ability of the endothelium and basement membrane to accommodate. On the basis of the possibility that intraoperative venous dilatation might occur, and that this might be a means of causing intimal damage, Stewart and colleagues (1987) developed a system for monitoring venous diameter noninvasively. With this system, the jugular veins of dogs were monitored during total hip replacement. It was found that dilatation beyond a certain critical point correlated with an increased incidence of venous lesions in this canine model, when the jugular and femoral veins were examined (Table 3.1). It was interesting to note that the incidence of endothelial lesions in dogs which showed no dilatation of the jugular vein was the same as controls for the jugular and femoral veins. Dilatation of 4-11% from baseline diameter caused no increase in the incidence of lesions in the jugular veins but approximately a two-fold increase in the incidence of lesions in the femoral veins. However, dilatation of 17-43% caused an increase of more than three-fold in the incidence of lesions in the jugular veins and a further increase in incidence in the femoral veins on the operated side. These observations indicate that the jugular and femoral veins are damaged as a result of operative venodilatation, though they may differ somewhat in their ability to withstand dilatation, with the femoral veins being more sensitive than the jugular veins. It also appears that the femoral vein on the operated side sustained a higher incidence of lesions than the femoral vein on the nonoperated side, which is likely to be the result of the local concentration of vasoactive amines generated in the wound. This observation is consistent with the findings of Hume (1978), that isolated thigh vein thrombi occur on the operated side in about 90% of all patients with isolated thigh vein thrombosis. One can speculate that the amount of venodilatation of the femoral vein might substantially exceed that observed and recorded from the jugular vein, due to the local concentration of vasoactive amines, and thus the endothelial damage in femoral veins would be expected to be greater.

Interestingly, these observations in animals appeared to correlate with our own clinical observations (Comerota et al, 1989) when we monitored the cephalic vein of patients who underwent total hip replacement and the observations of Stewart et al (1990), who monitored patients undergoing both total hip and total knee replacement. The findings indicated that dilatation of the cephalic vein, on the nonoperated side, beyond a critical point correlated with subsequent development of venographically proven DVT. Stewart (1987) has postulated that vasoactive substances generated at the operative site entered the circulation and survived long enough to cause distant veins to dilate. There is substantial clinical evidence supporting the importance of operative venodilation as a cause of postoperative DVT, especially as one integrates studies evaluating prophylaxis. Observations by Kakkar et al (1979), the Multicenter Trial Committee (1984), and Biesaw et al (1988) have shown that the addition of a venotonic agent, dihydroergotamine (DHE) to low dose heparin significantly improves efficacy of DVT prophylaxis (see chapter 11).

With the information at hand, several important questions arise which could potentially be answered in a prospective evaluation: 1) Does operative venodilatation correlate with the development of postoperative DVT in patients undergoing total hip replacement? 2) Can operative venodilatation be prevented by the use of the venotonic agent DHE; and, 3) Does modification of operative venodilatation prevent postoperative DVT?

## Design of a Study Evaluating Operative Venodilatation

An ultrasound device was specifically designed to continuously monitor venous diameter throughout the operation (following induction of anaesthesia). Since monitoring of leg veins directly would be cumbersome and fraught with position artifact, the cephalic vein was chosen. The ultrasonographic device was modified from a commercially available real time instrument with A, B, and C-mode capabilities. The B-mode image was used to identify the vein and establish optimal probe position. The A-mode had two electronic gates which were used for the tracking of venous diameter. One gate was electronically fixed to the superficial wall of the vein and the second to the deep wall. An analog signal proportional to the distance between the gates was obtained and continuously recorded on a strip chart recorder (Fig. 3.3). The instrument was previously tested and the accuracy and resolution established (Stewart et al, 1987). The axial resolution of the probe was 0.3 mm with excellent long-term stability, and readings of a phantom varying 0.05 mm only over one hour. Discrepancy of measurements of known diameter plastic tubing varied from 1.1% to 4.6%, an acceptable variability. On the basis of these validation studies it appeared that this technique could reliably detect venous diameter changes of the magnitude found in patients having surgery.

Patients undergoing elective total hip replacement were randomised in a prospective double blind study of DVT prophylaxis using DHE (0.5 mg) plus heparin (5000 units) given subcutaneously two hours before operation and every eight hours after operation or a placebo group which received a similar volume of NaCl. All nonsteroidal anti-inflammatory agents were avoided for three days prior to operation and during the postoperative period all anticoagulants, elastic stockings and external pneumatic compression devices were avoided.

The afternoon prior to total hip replacement, each patient's arm contralateral to the operative side was fitted with a long-arm plaster case which was bivalved and fixed to a specially designed table. The support table was designed with a low friction top upon which the ultrasonic probe was mounted. On the day of operation, after induction of general anaesthesia the patient's arm was stabilised by placing it within the plaster cast. This enabled the patient's arm and ultrasonic probe to move as a single unit during cephalic vein monitoring, thereby maintaining the relative position of vein to probe during the operation (Fig. 3.4).

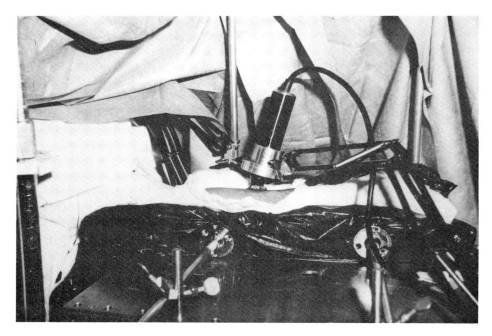

Fig. 3.3 An operative photograph of a patient's right cephalic vein being continuously monitored during a left total hip replacement

The baseline venous diameter was considered to be the diameter of the vein after induction of general anaesthesia but before skin incision. Maximal venodilation and maximal venoconstriction were calculated from the strip chart recording as the percentage change from baseline (Fig. 3.5). After operation, all patients had ascending venography performed on the operated leg. This was on the seventh postoperative day, or sooner, if routine fibrinogen uptake monitoring indicated acute thrombus formation.

**Correlations with Venoreactivity**
Significant variation occurred in the degree of venodilatation and venoconstriction. Interestingly, the degree of venoreactivity was independent of blood pressure, duration of operation, blood loss and intravenous fluid replacement (Table 3.2). Anaesthetic agents, sedatives and muscle relaxants were also examined, and no correlation could be established with either venoreactivity, outcome, or any other observed variable.

The correlation of operative venodilatation with outcome (DVT or no DVT) and treatment group (DHE/Hep or placebo) is illustrated in figure 3.5 as has previously been reported (Comerota et al, 1989). It was clearly evident that differences in venodilatation were present in patients suffering postoperative DVT compared to those who did not. Interestingly, those patients with excess dilatation were also significantly older than those patients with minimal or no dilatation. A mean dilatation of 28.9% ± 3.9% and a mean age of 67.7 ± 2.3 years were found in patients in whom DVT developed compared with 11.6% ± 1.6% and 58.4 ± 3.6 years in those in whom DVT did not develop, both of these differences being statistically significant. It is interesting that an inverse relationship was observed with operative duration; however, we believe this to be an incidental finding and not representative of a trend indicating a cause and effect relationship.

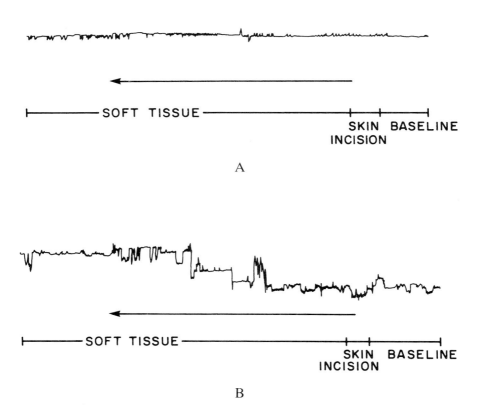

Fig. 3.4 A strip chart recording of cephalic vein diameter in a patient undergoing total hip replacement who did not experience operative venodilatation (A). Postoperative ascending phlebography failed to demonstrate DVT. The strip chart recording of the cephalic vein diameter in a patient undergoing total hip replacement who had a 33% operative venodilatation (B). This patient developed venographically proven deep venous thrombosis within one week after operation.

In an attempt to group patients according to operative venodilatation, patients having dilatation greater than 20% of baseline diameter were termed excess dilators and those dilating less than 20% were termed minimal dilators. Of nine patients with excess dilatation, 100% (9/9) developed postoperative DVT, which was a statistically significant difference. The mean age of patients with excess dilatation was 68 ± 2.8 years and those with minimal dilatation was 59.8 ± 3.1 years, a value which did not quite reach statistical significance (p=0.07), probably because of the small number of the patients studied. It was most interesting that the two patients who were classified as minimal dilators but who developed postoperative DVT were 65 and 68 years old respectively (mean 66.5 years) whereas the

**Table 3.2**
Mean values (±sd) for patients categorised according to outcome (+ or - DVT) treatment group (Placebo or DHE/hep) and venous response (Dilatation or Nondilatation)

| Group | Age | Blood Loss | IV Fluids | Op Duration | Constriction | Dilatation | DVT |
|---|---|---|---|---|---|---|---|
| +DVT | 67.7±2.3 | 947.7±160.9 | 3359±383 | 186±9 | 19.5%±4.4 | 28.9%±3.9 | NA |
| -DVT | 58.4±3.6 | 1007±126.9 | 3845±391 | 217±9 | 22.3%±4.8 | 11.6%±1.6 | NA |
| p-Value | 0.037 | 0.78 | 0.39 | 0.022 | 0.68 | 0.001 | NA |
| *Excess | 68±2.8 | 936.1±180.3 | 3528±429 | 187±11 | 14.7%±3.6 | 32.9±3.6 | 100% (9/9) |
| *Minimum | 59.8±3.1 | 1005.8±121.6 | 3637±367 | 210±9 | 25.5%±4.6 | 11.5±1.3 | 16.7% (2/12) |
| p-Value | 0.07 | 0.74 | 0.85 | 0.11 | 0.09 | 0.001 | 0.001 |
| Placebo | 64.9±3.1 | 956.8±147.9 | 3682±369 | 192±10 | 15.7%±3.3 | 28.6%±4.1 | 81.8% (9/11) |
| DHE/Hep | 61.5±3.5 | 997±145.3 | 3490±421 | 210±10 | 26.5%±5.3 | 11.9%±1.5 | 20% (8/10) |
| p-Value | 0.46 | 0.85 | 0.73 | 0.23 | 0.09 | 0.002 | 0.001 |

* Dilatation

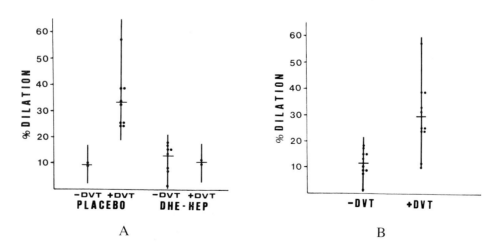

Fig. 3.5 (A) Relationship of operative venodilatation to outcome (proven by venography). The correlation of excessive operative venodilation with postoperative DVT is statistically significant (p=0.001). (B) It is evident that DHE/heparin had a significant influence on preventing operative venodilatation (p=0.002) and postoperative DVT (p=0.001) compared with placebo (from Comerota A.J. et al 1989, reproduced with permission).

**Table 3.3**
Maximal venoreactivity (dilatation and constriction) from time of skin incision and the tissue handled at the time of maximal response

| Response | Time(min) | TISSUE HANDLED Soft Tissue | Bone | p-Value |
|---|---|---|---|---|
| Max. Dilatation | 21.7±6.48 | 95% (20/21) | 5% (1/21) | <0.0001 |
| Max. Constriction | 58.8±8.08 | 21% (4/19) | 79% (15/19) | <0.005 |
| p-Value | <0.001 | <0.001 | <0.0001 | |

mean age of the remaining minimal-dilatation group, all of whom did not develop postoperative DVT, was 58.4 years.

It was evident that DHE had a significant effect on venous tone. Mean operative venodilatation in patients receiving DHE was 11.9% ± 1.5% compared with 28.6% ± 4.1% in those receiving placebo. When controlled for age, the treatment patients received was significantly related to venodilatation. Mean venoconstriction in patients receiving DHE was 26.5% ± 5.3% compared with 15.7% ±3.3% in those receiving placebo. This was indeed a definite trend, however the p-value is not quite statistically significant.

The time from skin incision to maximal venous response and the tissue which was being handled at the time of maximal venous response is shown in table 3.3. The mean time to maximal venodilatation was 21.7 ± 6.48 minutes and to maximal venoconstriction, 58.8 ± 8.08 minutes. These differences were statistically significant. In 95% of the patients, maximal venodilatation occurred while work was being performed on soft tissue, especially the muscle, whereas in 79%, maximal venoconstriction occurred while work was being performed on bone.

# Clinical Implications and Correlations

The observations have demonstrated that operative venodilatation can occur during operations, specifically during total hip replacement and that excessive venodilatation is directly correlated with postoperative deep vein thrombosis. It is postulated that the mechanism involves endothelial damage resulting in the exposure of highly thrombogenic subendothelial collagen. Interestingly, patients who had developed DVT were significantly older than those who had not, and two patients in the DHE/Heparin group who did not have excessive venodilatation in whom DVT developed were also appreciably older than the remaining patients in that same group. Likewise, the only two patients in the placebo group in whom DVT did not develop had only minimal venodilatation, and both of these patients were substantially younger than the remaining patients in that group. These findings correlate with the many clinical observations that increased age is a significant risk factor for postoperative DVT. These observations also suggest that a major component of the older patient's risk is excessive venodilatation, and this complements the report by Clarke (1933) that increased venous compliance occurs with increasing age. Likewise, current observations indicate that postoperative DVT in paediatric patients is unusual, despite the presence of commonly accepted risk factors observed in older adults. Whether the changes occurring with age are due to modification of venous smooth muscle response to tissue injury or to changes in the mediators themselves is not known.

It is postulated that the observed venodilatation is a humoral response to mediators released at the wound site during operation. The mediators are unknown, but perhaps some clue can be gleaned by the observation that the majority of patients had maximal venodilatation while work was being done on the soft tissue, predominantly muscle, whereas maximal venoconstriction occurred at the time of bone resection or reaming of the marrow. Many vasoactive mediators have been studied and may play a role in significantly influencing venomotor activity, venous endothelial damage and ultimately, venous thrombosis. Many other vasoactive amines may play a role and interact in additive, synergistic, or an inhibitory fashion.

Although humoral mediation is the proposed mechanism, it is evident that the smooth muscle response is segmental and does not occur in a simultaneous fashion affecting all veins. No changes in blood pressure were observed during the time of maximal venodilatation or maximal venoconstriction. Although the cephalic vein may be a marker of what is occurring in the deep venous system, it would be premature to assume that the quantitative response in any other portion of the venous system is equivalent.

In summary, excessive operative venodilatation is a new and important aetiologic factor leading to postoperative DVT. It appears that veins distant from the site of injury dilate in response to trauma, and animal data suggest that this dilatation is accompanied by substantial endothelial damage. This damage occurs within the valve cusp in the area of venous side branches. The vein wall is attenuated in these areas, most likely predisposing to stretch injury. In humans, excess operative dilation is followed by postoperative deep vein thrombosis. It appears that maximal venodilation occurs relatively early in the course of an operation while soft tissue (muscle) is being handled. Interestingly, the degree of operative venodilatation can be pharmacologically controlled with the use of low doses of dihydroergotamine, known to selectively increase venous smooth muscle tone. It is accepted that postoperative DVT originates within valve cusps, and the recent data blend the venodilatation data with clinical observations and recent anatomical studies suggesting that vein wall attenuation in the area of the venous confluence leads to inherent susceptibility to vein wall injury with operative venodilatation. Our increasing awareness and understanding of these pathophysiologic mechanisms will undoubtedly improve our ability to offer more effective prophylaxis and avoid the morbid and potentially lethal complications of postoperative DVT.

# References

Almen T, Nylander G. Serial phlebography of the normal lower leg during muscular contraction and relaxation. Acta Radiol 57:264, 1961

Biesaw NE, Comerota AJ, Groth HE, et al. Dihydroergotamine/heparin in the prevention of deep vein thrombosis after total hip replacement. J Bone Joint Surg (Am) 70-A(1):2, 1988

Clark C, Cotton LT. Blood flow in deep veins of the legs. Recording technique and evaluation of methods to increase flow during operation. Br J Surg 55:211, 1968

Clarke JH. The elasticity of veins. Am J Physiol 105:418, 1933

Comerota AJ, Stewart GJ, Alburger PD, Smalley K, White JV. Operative venodilation. A previously unsuspected factor in the cause of postoperative deep vein thrombosis. Surgery 106:301, 1989

Gibbs NM. Venous thrombosis of the lower limb with particular reference to bed-rest. Br J Surg 45:209, 1957

Hirsh J, Barlow GH, Swaan HC, Salzman EW. Diagnosis of prethrombotic state in surgical patients. Contemp Surg 16:65, 1980

Hume M. Sex, aspirin, and venous thrombosis. Orthop Clin N Am 9:761, 1978

Kakkar VV, Stamatakis JD, Bentley PG, Lawrence D, DeHass HA, Ward VP. Prophylaxis for postoperative deep vein thrombosis. Synergistic effect of heparin and dihydroergotamine. JAMA 241:39, 1979

The Multicenter Trial Committee. Dihydroergotamine/heparin prophylaxis of postoperative deep vein thrombosis. JAMA 251:2960, 1984

Nicolaides AN, Kakkar VV, Renney JTG. The soleal sinuses and stasis. Br J Surg 58:307, 1971

Prevention of venous thrombosis and pulmonary embolism. NIH Consensus Development Conferences. Bethesda, Maryland: National Institutes of Health. JAMA 256:744, 1986

Schaub RG, Lynch PR, Stewart GJ. The response of canine veins to three types of abdominal surgery: a scanning and transmission electron microscopic study. Surgery 83:411, 1978

Stead RB. The Hypercoagulable State. In: Pulmonary Embolism and Deep Venous Thrombosis. Ed: SZ Goldhaber, p. 161. W.B. Saunders, Philadelphia, 1985

Stewart GJ, Alburger PD, Stone EA, Soszka TW. Total hip replacement induces injury to remote veins in a canine model. J Bone Joint Surg 65(A):97, 1983

Stewart GJ. Venous Pathophysiology. In: Vascular Diseases: Current Research and Clinical Applications. Eds: DE Strandness, P Didisheim, A Clowes, J Watson, p. 429. Grune and Stratton, New York, 1987

Stewart GJ, Ziskin MC, Schaub RG et al. Use of ultrasound for noninvasive study of blood vessel responsiveness. Am J Physiol 253:H671, 1987

Stewart GJ, Lachman JW, Alburger PD, Ziskin MC, Philips CM, Jensen K. Intraoperative venous dilation and subsequent development of deep vein thrombosis in patients undergoing total hip or total knee replacement. Ultrasound in Med and Biol 16:133, 1990

Stone EA, Stewart GJ. Architecture and structure of canine veins with special reference to confluences. Anat Rec 222:154, 1988

Virchow R. Neuer fall von todlicher emboli der lungenarterie. Arch Pathol Anat 10:225, 1856

CHAPTER 4

# Coagulation Abnormalities Predisposing to the Development of Deep Vein Thrombosis

Michel M Samama  Jacqueline Conard
Marie Helene Horellou  Francis Toulemonde

## Introduction

Clinicians have long recognised that certain patients are prone to thromboembolic episodes. Multiple factors are usually present to account for such thrombophilic states. In certain pathological conditions, *in vivo* activation of coagulation occurs, while in others, well defined congenital deficiency in coagulation inhibitors or alterations in fibrinogen or plasminogen structures are considered as predisposing. These inherited disorders represent the cause of thrombophilia in only a minority of patients with thromboembolic antecedents.

Among the acquired causes, many are known to be associated with diseases such as cancer, lupus erythematosus, ulcerative colitis, and paroxysmal nocturnal haemoglobinuria. In others, no underlying conditions can be found (idiopathic thrombosis). In all these conditions, the search for a laboratory diagnostic test for a "hypercoagulable" state has been

**Table 4.1**
Inherited risk factors predisposing to thromboembolism

*Deficiency in natural "inhibitors" of coagulation:*
    Antithrombin III deficiency
    Protein C deficiency
    Protein S deficiency
    Heparin cofactor II deficiency?
*Disorders of the fibrinolytic system:*
    Abnormal fibrinogen — dysfibrinogenaemias
    Alteration of the fibrinolytic activators or inhibitors
*Vascular damage:*
    Homocystinuria

the object of extensive research. Most of the published tests lack predictive value. However, some recently developed tests are promising and will be discussed.

A thrombosis may result either from an increased tendency to clot formation or from a reduced clot dissolution. Conversely, a physiological balance, involving factors and inhibitors of coagulation and fibrinolysis is the prerequisite to prevent both thrombosis and bleeding.

# Hypercoagulable States

### Inherited risk factors predisposing to thromboembolism
Among the inherited conditions are those associated with the congenital deficiency of the physiological inhibitors of coagulation such as antithrombin III, proteins C and S, dysfibrinogenaemia and abnormalities of the fibrinolytic system (Egeberg, 1965; Samama et al, 1988). Other inherited abnormalities include endothelial damage from homocystinuria (Harker et al, 1974), and platelet damage in paroxysmal nocturnal haemoglobinuria (Dixon and Ross, 1977) (Table 4.1).

The subject is often controversial, since multiple factors are involved in thrombogenesis and alterations in many of the commonly measured coagulation parameters do not always specifically imply a high risk for thrombosis. Many coagulation changes are secondary to the concurrent diseases occurring in the patient, while others are products of ongoing coagulation processes taking place. Some of the latter changes reflect an intravascular coagulation.

The causal relationship between antithrombin III (At-III), Protein C and Protein S deficiency and thrombosis is well documented. These genetic alterations are transmitted as an autosomal dominant trait. They have some clinical features in common: first episode of thrombosis between 20 and 40 years of age in most cases, unusual site of thrombosis (such as mesenteric vein thrombosis) and increased tendency to recurrence.

The causal relationship is not well established for the other conditions listed above, except for homocystinuria.

On clinical grounds alone, there are many conditions that carry a high risk for thrombosis. Knowledge of these conditions is helpful in the assessment of a patient suspected to have thromboembolic conditions. Some of these risk factors are associated with inherited deficiencies of proteins with antithrombotic functions (listed above), while others are found with various acquired diseases.

### Acquired risk factors predisposing to venous thromboembolism
The acquired conditions (Table 4.2) are grouped into those associated with changes in the coagulation and fibrinolytic functions, those with abnormal platelet functions, and those with stasis or abnormal blood flow. This classification is, however, not all-inclusive, because frequently, in a single individual patient, more than one factor is at work.

In patients with the nephrotic syndrome, there is an increased incidence of venous thromboembolic complications. A common form of thrombosis involves the renal vein, which in turn will add to the severity of the syndrome (Kendall et al, 1971). The loss of antithrombin III in the urine has been considered an important causative factor for thrombogenesis.

**Table 4.2**
Acquired risk factors predisposing to thromboembolism

*Changes in coagulation factors and fibrinolytic functions*
    Pregnancy and puerperium
    Cancer
    Inflammatory bowel disease
    Nephrotic syndrome
    Infusion of activated prothrombin complex concentrates
    Lupus anticoagulant
*Platelet abnormalities*
    Myeloproliferative disorders, essential thrombocytosis
    Diabetes mellitus
    Hyperlipidaemia
    Heparin-associated thrombocytopenia
*Stasis or aberrant blood flow*
    Advanced age
    Perioperative state
    Immobilisation
    Pregnancy
    Congestive heart failure
    Stroke
    Obesity
*Increased blood viscosity*
    Polycythemia vera, sickle cell disease
    Dehydration
    Paraproteinuria
*Endothelial damage*
    Radiation
    Drugs, chemotherapy, contrast media
    Behchet's disease
    Artificial surfaces
*Miscellaneous*
    Oral contraceptives
    Thrombotic thrombocytopenic purpura

The platelet abnormalities seen in myeloproliferative disorders are usually those of a platelet dysfunction resulting in an increased bleeding tendency (Murphy, 1983; Schafer, 1984). Paradoxically, thrombotic complications are also common. The thromboses are both venous and arterial, and may be seen in unusual anatomical sites such as splenic, hepatic, portal and mesenteric vessels, as well as in the microvasculature involving the cerebral and digital circulation (Singh and Wetherley-Mein, 1977; Jabaily et al, 1983). The concurrent high haematocrit and high platelet count are probably both important in the thrombogenesis. However, a high platelet count alone may not necessarily be associated with an increased risk of thrombosis. For many years it was believed that postsplenectomy thrombocytosis is thrombogenic (Hirsh et al, 1966), but this was not substantiated by later studies (Coon et al, 1978; Boxer et al, 1987).

## Alterations of Fibrinogen and Fibrinolysis

A normal fibrin clot may be dissolved by plasmin originating from activation of the fibrinolytic system. Thus, a decreased fibrinolysis or a structural alteration of the clot inducing its resistance to lysis may be responsible for an increased risk of thrombosis due to a defect in fibrin elimination. Another mechanism is also postulated and concerns decreased thrombin binding to abnormal fibrin possibly leading to an increase in circulating thrombin.

### Alterations of fibrinogen

Functional alterations of fibrinogen (dysfibrinogenaemias) are usually asymptomatic. However, in about 10% of the reported cases, thromboembolic manifestations have been observed, mostly without a familial history (Samama et al, 1987). Although such an association may seem paradoxical, different mechanisms have been proposed that may explain this apparent coincidence: 1) increased activity of fibrinogen as cofactor for platelet aggregation, as in Fibrinogen Oslo (Thorsen et al, 1986); 2) increased thrombin binding to fibrin as in Fibrinogen Malmoe (Soria et al, 1985), Milano (Haverkate et al, 1983), or Pamplona (Fernandez et al, 1986); 3) hypofibrinolysis due to decreased plasminogen induced activation by abnormal fibrin as Fibrinogen Dusard (Lijnen et al, 1984) or due to resistance to plasmin degradation of the abnormal fibrinogen as in Fibrinogen Chapell Hill (Carrell et al, 1983). In addition, in Fibrinogen New York I, a combined defective thrombin and tPA binding to fibrin has been postulated to explain the predisposition to venous thromboembolism. A recent review has been devoted to this topic (Samama et al, 1988).

### Alterations of the fibrinolytic system

In addition to dysfibrinogenaemias with clot resistance to lysis, different abnormalities may lead to hypofibrinolysis: they are related either to plasminogen, or to an alteration in tPA or factor XII dependent fibrinolysis pathways, or to an alteration of the protein C system.

*Deficiency in plasminogen*

Few constitutional hypo- or dysplasminogenaemias associated with thrombosis have been reported (Aoki et al, 1978; Wohl et al, 1979; Kazama et al, 1981; Soria et al, 1983; Lottenberg et al, 1985; Mannucci et al, 1986; Scharrer et al, 1986). However, familial studies are seldom convincing since the association of the anomaly with thrombosis is often found in the propositus only, and even a homozygous patient may be asymptomatic (Aoki, 1984).

*Alterations of the tPA fibrinolytic pathway*

The tPA fibrinolytic pathway is considered to be the main pathway of fibrinolysis in vivo. Normally, tissue plasminogen activator or tPA, present in endothelial cells, is released in blood after anoxia or after administration of a vasopressin derivative (DDAVP), and an inhibitor balances this activator: the Plasminogen Activator Inhibitor or PAI-1.

An impaired fibrinolysis after stimulation is a frequent finding in patients with a history of deep vein thrombosis (Nilsson et al, 1985) but very few families with such an alteration associated with thrombosis have been reported (Johansson et al, 1978; Jorgensen et al, 1982; Stead et al, 1983), suggesting that the abnormality is more frequently acquired than congenital. In addition, a decreased fibrinolytic response to a stimulation may result from a decreased synthesis or release of tPA and/or from an elevated PAI-1 level (Nilsson et al, 1985). Until recently, increased PAI-1 level was the most frequent finding (Juhan-Vague et al, 1987; Nguyen et al, 1988) and in many cases was associated with an inflammatory process, obesity or hypertriglyceridaemia.

*Deficiency in contact factors*

A deficiency in a contact factor could, at least theoretically, predispose to thrombosis since the intrinsic activation of fibrinolysis requires factor XII, prekallicrein and high molecular weight kininogen. Although Mr Hageman died from pulmonary embolism, the incidence of thromboembolic episodes in factor XII deficiency does not seem to be significantly increased, although few venous thrombotic accidents have been reported (Goodenough et al, 1983). Thrombosis is even less frequent in the deficiencies of other contact factors. Thus, although it is not clear whether these alterations predispose to venous thromboembolism, it is important to stress that deficient patients are not protected from thrombotic accidents.

As there is some evidence that hypofibrinolysis may be a risk factor for postoperative thromboembolism, it was tempting to establish a relationship between fibrinolytic impairment and postoperative deep vein thrombosis. Unfortunately, specific enhancement of fibrinolysis, which is depressed in the post-operative period, using Stanazolol does not reduce the frequency of thrombosis, indicating that this defect *per se* is not of major importance (Blamey et al., 1983).

Anyhow, defects in fibrinolysis have been taken into account for establishing at least 3 predictive indices: Clayton et al (1976), using euglobulin lysis time, Sue-Ling et al (1986) using the same index and Rocha et al (1988) using PAI, tPA and FDP levels.

Particularly, PAI-1 increase has been considered more recently as a predictive factor of postoperative thromboembolism in orthopaedic surgery (Rocha et al, 1988; Grimaudo et al, 1989) but this finding has to be confirmed in a prospective study.

# Thrombosis in Relation to Coagulation Abnormalities in Different Clinical Conditions

Several fields in vascular diseases may be associated with one or several abnormalities in coagulation or fibrinolysis.

## Role of Previous DVT

A defect in coagulation inhibitors is much more often present when a patient has recurrences of DVT, compared with normal individuals. The percentage of deficiencies of AT-III, Protein C and Protein S in patients with a history of thrombosis is altogether about 10% (Juillet et al, 1978; Thaler and Lechner, 1981; Spahn-Attenhofer and von Felten, 1985; Samama et al, 1986; Andersson et al, 1987; Bertina et al, 1987; Engesser et al, 1987; Broekmans and Conard, 1988; Heijboer et al, 1990) (Table 4.3).

As the risk of DVT in patients with a history of previous DVT is said to be multiplied by 2.5 (Janssen index) (Janssen et al, 1987), it may be that these recurrences were in relation to undetected deficiency of these inhibitors.

## Precipitating factors of the first thrombotic episode

In patients with AT-III or Protein C deficiencies, several situations may be triggering factors for DVT appearance. They have been checked in several studies, mainly by Thaler (Thaler and Lechner, 1981) for AT-III and Broekmans for Protein C (Broekmans and Conard, 1988) (Table 4.4).

**Table 4.3**
Incidence of Deficiencies in AT-III, Protein C, Protein S and HC II in normal individuals and patients with a history of DVT

| Deficiency | In normal Individuals | In patients with history of DVT | References |
|---|---|---|---|
| AT III | 0.02% | 3-4% | Juillet et al, 1978; Thaler and Lechner, 1981 |
| Protein C | 0.3% | 4-8% | Broekmans and Conard, 1988; Samama et al, 1986; Spahn-Attenhofer and Von Felten, 1985 |
| Protein S |  | 2-8% | Engesser et al, 1987 |
| HC II* | 0.9% | 0.7% | Andersson et al, 1987; Bertina et al, 1987 |

* Thus HC II deficiency may not be an important risk factor

### Presence of cancer
In the previously mentioned Janssen Index (Janssen et al, 1987), the risk of DVT in patients suffering from cancer is multiplied by 2.5.

It is classical to describe two different mechanisms for hypercoagulation in cancer. First, direct activation of FXa by cancer cell activity; second, through a tissue endogenous factor with the same activation process.

In the clinical field, it is well known that one of the major causes of death in cancer patients are thromboembolic phenomena. The corollary of this finding is that patients with thromboembolic phenomena of unknown origin should have adequate medical follow-up in order to detect the presence of a yet undeclared carcinoma.

### Lupus with circulating anticoagulant presents a broad heterogeneity
Antiphospholipid syndrome is defined as the ensemble of clinical features (venous and/or arterial thromboses, thrombocytopenias, repeated abortions) associated to a lupus anticoagulant and/or an anticardiolipin antibody.

The most common changes in biological values are:
- Prolonged APTT, prolonged dilute Russel viper venom time (DRVVT) and to a lesser extent prolongation of KCCT. If a highly sensitive cephalin reagent is used, the APTT seems to be a very good screening test for the presence of lupus anticoagulant.

**Table 4.4**
The incidence of factors triggering the first thrombotic episode in patients with Antithrombin III (AT-III) and Protein C deficiency

| Triggering Factors | AT-III Deficiency | Protein C Deficiency |
|---|---|---|
| Pregnancy | 28 % | 20 % |
| Surgery | 13 % | 15 % |
| Oral Contraceptives | 4 % | 7 % |
| Immobilisation | — | 9 % |
| Others | — | 3 % |
| Unknown | 42 % | 46 % |

**Table 4.5** Main clinical studies comparing operated patients with and without oral contraceptives

|  | Number of patients | Type of surgery | Method of diagnosis | Treatment | DVT (%) | Comparison with control |
|---|---|---|---|---|---|---|
| Sigel et al, 1974 | 1655 | Various | FUT | Nil | 4.7 | NS |
| Clarke-Pearson et al, 1987 | 411 | Gynaec | FUT | Nil | 17.5 | NS |
| Clarke-Pearson et al, 1983 | 281 | Gynaec/KC | Clinical | ± Heparin | 7.8 | NS |
| Veth et al, 1985 | 358 | General | FUT | ± Hep/DHE ± Sulfinpy. | 12.87 17.5 | NS |
| Stringer et al, 1989 | 312 | Knee | Venog. | Nil | 28.2 | NS |

- No change in protein C plasma level; however, lupus anticoagulant fraction may inhibit thrombomodulin (via Protein C inactivation) leading to the thrombophilic tendency in these patients).

Thrombotic complications are common. Bowie et al (1963) were the first to report an increased risk of thrombosis in patients with lupus anticoagulant. The cumulative literature suggests approximately 30% of patients with lupus anticoagulant have at least one thrombotic event (Lechner, 1987).

## Hormonal Treatments

*Oral contraceptives*

The increased risk of venous thromboembolism associated with oral contraceptives has been demonstrated in different studies and the relative risk is approximately 4 (Stadel, 1981). It is probably dependent on the dose of ethinyl oestradiol and lower with the newly developed preparations containing less than 50 µg (40, 30 and even 20 µg). The risk is not related to the duration of use, and is restricted to current users (Vessey et al, 1986).

The increase in the risk of postoperative venous thrombosis attributed to oral contraceptives, is still controversial but coagulation modifications have been found to persist at least 4 weeks after surgery (Robinson et al, 1991). For these reasons, it is recommended to stop oral contraceptives 4 weeks before surgery or to protect the patient after surgery with prophylactic methods, even if, to date, the risk of post surgical DVT in these patients appears to be rather low (Table 4.5).

*Use of oestrogens in post-menopausal women*

Oestrogens used in replacement therapy are either conjugated either equine oestrogen given by oral route or natural oestrogen (17 β oestradiol) by oral or percutaneous route. Some modifications of coagulation have been observed when these compounds are administered orally but not with the percutaneous route. At present, no data are available on the risk of postoperative thrombosis in women taking hormone replacement therapy, but it appears to be lower than with oral contraceptives.

## New markers of blood coagulation activation

More recent tests for markers of the activation of coagulation have been designed based on our knowledge of the mechanisms of blood coagulation. In brief, early activation of blood coagulation is associated with the *in vivo* formation of activated coagulation factors with normally rapid clearance rates.

*A. Thrombin formation*

An abnormal persistence of activated coagulation factors will induce prothrombin activation resulting in a thrombin formation leading to the release of a small prothrombin fragment called F1+2. Its presence, at an abnormally high concentration, is an indirect marker of hypercoagulation (Lau et al, 1979; Lau and Rosenberg 1980; Teitel et al, 1982). This test is very sensitive, but its availability is restricted to a few laboratories.

*B. Thrombin/Fibrinogen Interaction*

Thrombin formation will have multiple consequences. Thrombin-antithrombin III complexes may form *in vivo*, and can be detected in plasma with an Elisa method. The increase in thrombin-AT III complexes is not limited to prethrombotic or thrombotic states such as acute promyelocytic leukaemia, but may also be found in septicaemia (Bauer et al, 1983; Bauer and Rosenberg, 1984).

Thrombin, once formed, will react on plasma fibrinogen resulting in the formation of fibrin monomers and of fibrinopeptides A and B, released from the parent molecule. Fibrinopeptide A can be measured in plasma by an Elisa method or a radio-immunoassay and it is a very specific marker of hypercoagulation. However, its main limitation is the in-vitro activation of blood coagulation during blood sample collection, giving rise to a false-positive result.

Fibrin monomers, once formed, can bind to fibrinogen itself or fibrin degradation products (FDP) to form soluble complexes. The presence of soluble complexes in the blood is an early sign of disseminated intravascular coagulation (DIC). The ethanol gelation test, protamine precipitation, and Largo's method are almost routinely used, but their limited sensitivity restricts their usefulness in DIC (Godal and Abildgaard, 1966; Largo et al, 1976).

*C. Activation of fibrinolysis*

The presence of soluble fibrin in plasma triggers the fibrinolytic system resulting in the generation of variable amounts of plasmin. This enzyme can be indirectly detected in plasma, by the presence of $\alpha_2$-antiplasmin-plasmin complexes and by fibrinogen-FDP resulting from the enzyme proteolytic activity.

Fibrinogen/fibrin fragment E was recently studied with a radio-immunoassay in patients with thromboembolism, DIC, and various nonthromboembolic diseases (Mombelli et al, 1987). It has been shown that its use in parallel with fibrinopeptide A measurement could be useful in the investigation of intravascular thrombin and fibrin formation (Zielinsky et al, 1982) but the fragment E antigen assay is too time consuming and cannot be used in clinical practice.

Another significant new test called D-dimer test uses a special antibody which is able to detect cross-linked D-fragments or D-dimer in plasma. Since it does not react with fibrinogen, its specificity is limited to D-dimer and some larger fibrin degradation fragments containing this D-dimer (Elms et al, 1983; Whitaker et al, 1984). An increase in the plasma D-dimer level is a good, but indirect, evidence of fibrin formation. It is often positive in thrombotic states, although these cross-linked degradation products have been found after multiple trauma and are, thus, limited in their specificity. A normal D-dimer test especially with the Elisa method has a negative predictive value higher than 90% as demonstrated in many studies (Goldhaber et al, 1988; Bounameaux et al, 1989; Boneu et al, 1991).

**Table 4.6**
Mean values (± sd) of T-AT complexes (ng/ml) in patients receiving two different prophylactic regimens (Bogaty-Yver and Samama, 1989)

| Time | Heparin Group | LMW Heparin Group |
|---|---|---|
| 12 h before surgery | 1.99 ± 0.44 | 2.00 ± 0.66 |
| 12 h after surgery | 9.47 ± 11.96 | 9.25 ± 13.80 |
| Day 2 | 5.80 ± 8.65 | 2.96 ± 0.83 |
| Day 4 | 2.50 ± 0.75 | 2.65 ± 0.75 |
| Day 7 | 3.05 ± 0.89 | 4.20 ± 4.66 |

When fibrinogen reacts with plasmin, certain degradation fragments are identified and used as sensitive markers for low-grade *in vivo* fibrinolysis. The fragments are derived from the ß chain of fibrinogen and are known as the Bß 1-42- and Bß 15-42- related peptides. Immunologic methods for their quantitation are available in commercial kits (Nossel, 1981; Walenga et al, 1984).

*D. Interest of these new markers in post surgery*
It has been known, for a long time, that shortening of APTT was common after operation but without relationship to DVT occurence on an individual basis. The same is valid for fibrinogen level (Gallus et al, 1973).

More recent assays showed evidence of hypercoagulation in such patients. It is the case for thrombin-antithrombin (T-AT) complexes (Bogaty-Yver and Samama, 1989).

The mean postoperative values of T-AT complexes in patients receiving two different prophylactic regimens (unfractionated and LMW heparin) are shown in table 4.6. However, T-AT complexes rose in the same way in DVT positive and DVT negative patients, as shown by the Hoek study (Hoek et al, 1989) in patients treated with ORG 10172, a heparinoid, after hip surgery (Table 4.7). The results indicate a clear tendency to hypercoagulation mainly on day 1, but there is not a clearcut difference between positive DVT and negative DVT patients. In another study (Kroneman et al, 1991), in which 239 patients were tested for possible DVT, plethysmograms confirmed the presence of DVT in 60. The sensitivity and specificity of FDP, DD and T-AT assays are summarised in table 4.8. Thus correlations have been established for these new tests and the presence of DVT.

**Table 4.7**
Mean (± sd) of T-AT Complexes (ng/ml) in DVT positive and DVT negative patients treated by Org 10172 (Hoek et al, 1989)

| TAT | DVT +ve<br>n = 13 | DVT -ve<br>n = 80 |
|---|---|---|
| Pre-operative | 2.8 ± 0.6 | 2.6 ± 0.2 |
| Day 1 | 9.9 ± 1.0 | 7.6 ± 0.6 |
| Day 4 | 6.2 ± 0.7 | 4.5 ± 0.5 |

**Table 4.8**
The sensitivity and specificity of FDP, DD and T-AT assays in 239 patients studied with plethysmography. Plethysmography was positive (i.e., thrombosis proximal to the calf) in 60.

|        | Sensitivity | Specificity |
|--------|-------------|-------------|
| F.D.P. | 95          | 16          |
| D.D.   | 92          | 80          |
| T-A T. | 37          | 88          |

# Conclusion

Some inherited coagulation abnormalities predisposing to thrombosis are well documented. In contrast, although many batteries of laboratory tests have been devised in order to define the acquired coagulation abnormalities leading to or associated with thrombosis, none has been experimentally verified or has stood the test of time. Since the hypercoagulable state is not a single disease entity, but rather a clinical spectrum which may result from a wide variety of underlying conditions, it is probably naive to expect that a single workable laboratory test protocol could detect all of the diverse processes which might result in an increased thrombotic tendency. Despite this practical problem, there are a variety of conditions which have a well-established relationship to thrombosis. When these entities are suspected, selective laboratory evaluation can be of great value.


# References

Andersson TR, Larsen ML, Abildgaard U. Low heparin cofactor II associated with abnormal crossed immuno-electrophoresis pattern in two Norwegian families. Thromb Res 47:243, 1987

Aoki N. Genetic abnormalities of the fibrinolytic system. Semin Thromb Hemost 10:42, 1984

Aoki N, Moroi M, Sakata Y, Yoshida N, Matsuda M. Abnormal plasminogen. A hereditary molecular abnormality found in a patient with recurrent thrombosis. J Clin Invest 61:1186, 1978

Bauer KA, Rosenberg RD. Thrombin generation in acute promyelocytic leukemia. Blood 65:791, 1984

Bauer KA, Kass BL, Beller DL et al. The detection of protein C activation in humans. Blood 62 (Suppl. I, Abstr):297, 1983

Bertina RM, Van Der Linder IK, Engesser L, Muller HP, Brommer EJP. Hereditary heparin cofactor II deficiency and the risk of development of thrombosis. Thromb Haemost 57:196, 1987

Blamey SL, McArdle BM, Burns P, Lowe GDO, Forbes CD, Carter DC, Prentice CRM. Prevention of fibrinolytic shutdown after major surgery by intramuscular stanozolol. Thromb Res 31:451, 1983

Bogaty-Yver J, Samama M. Thrombin-antithrombin III complexes for the detection of postoperative hypercoagulable state in surgical patients receiving heparin prophylaxis. Thromb Haemost 61:538, 1989

Boneu B, Bes G, Pelzer H, Sie P, Boccalon H. D-dimers, thrombin antithrombin III complexes and prothrombin fragments 1+2: diagnostic value in clinically suspected deep vein thrombosis. Thromb Haemost 65:28, 1991

Bounameaux H, Schneider PA, Reber G, De Moerloose P, Krahenbuhl B. Measurement of plasma D-dimer for diagnosis of deep venous thrombosis. Am J Clin Pathol 91:82, 1989

Bowie EJW, Thompson JH, Pascuzzi CA et al. Thrombosis in systemic lupus erythematosus despite circulating anticoagulants. J Lab Clin Med 62:416, 1963

Boxer MA, Braun J, Ellman L. Thromboembolic risk of postsplenectomy thrombocytosis. Arch Surg 113:808, 1987

Broekmans AW, Conard J. Hereditary protein C deficiency. In: Bertina (Ed). Protein C and related proteins, 160; Churchill Livingstone, Edinburgh, London, 1988

Carrell N, Gabriel DA, Blatt P, Carr ME, McDonagh J. Hereditary dysfibrinogenemia in a patient with thrombotic disease. Blood 62:439, 1983

Clarke-Pearson DL, Jelovsek FR, Creasman WT. Thromboembolism complicating surgery for cervical and uterine malignancy: incidence, risk factors and prophylaxis. Obst Gynecol 61:87, 1983

Clarke-Pearson DL, Delong ER, Synan IS, Coleman RE, Creasman WT. Variables associated with postoperative deep venous thrombosis: a prospective study of 411 gynecology patients and creation of a prognostic model. Obstet Gynecol 69:146, 1987

Clayton K, Anderson JA, McNicol GP. Pre-operative prediction of postoperative deep vein thrombosis. Br Med J 2:910, 1976

Conard J, Veuillet-Duval A, Horellou MH, Samama M. Etude de la coagulation et de la fibrinolyse dans 131 cas de thromboses veineuses récidivantes. Nouv Rev Franç Hématol 24:205, 1982

Coon WW, Penner J, Clagett GP et al. Deep venous thrombosis and postsplenectomy thrombocytosis. Arch Surg 113:429, 1978

Dixon RH, Ross WF. Mechanism of complement-mediated activation of human blood platelets in vitro: comparison of normal and paroxysmal nocturnal hemoglobinuria platelets. J Clin Invest 59:360, 1977

Egeberg O. Inherited antithrombin deficiency causing thrombophilia. Thromb Diath Haemorrh 13:516, 1965

Elms MJ, Bunce IH, Bundesen PG et al. Measurement of crosslinked fibrin degradation products, an immunoassay using monoclonal antibodies. Thromb Haemost 50:591, 1983

Engesser L, Broekmans AW, Briet E, Brommer EJP, Bertina RM. Hereditary protein S deficiency — clinical manifestations. Ann Intern Med 106:677, 1987

Fernandez J, Paramo JA, Cuesta B, Aranda A, Rocha E. Fibrinogen Pamplona II. A new congenital dysfibrinogenaemia with abnormal fibrin-enhanced plasminogen activation and defective binding of thrombin to fibrin. In: Muller-Berghaus G, Scheefers-Borchel U, Selmayr E, Menschen A. (eds) Exerpta Medica, 25, 1986

Gallus AS, Hirsh J, Gent M. Relevance of preoperative and post-operative blood tests to detect postoperative leg-vein thrombosis. Lancet 13:805, 1973

Godal HC, Abildgaard U. Gelation of soluble fibrin in plasma by ethanol. Scan J Haematol 3:342, 1966

Goldhaber SZ, Vaughan DE, Tumch SS, Loscalzo J. Utility of cross-linked fibrin degradation products in the diagnosis of pulmonary embolism. Am Heart J 116:505, 1988

Goodenough LT, Saito H, Ratnoff OD. Thrombosis or myocardial infarction in congenital clotting factor abnormalities and chronic thrombocytopenias: a report of 21 patients and a review of 50 previously reported cases. Medicine 62:248, 1983

Grimaudo V, Kruithof EKO, Stiekema JCJ, Bachmann F. High pre-operative plasminogen activator inhibitor levels are correlated with post-operative deep vein thrombosis in total hip replacement. Thromb Hemost 62 (Abstract), 96, 1989

Harker LA, Slichter SJ, Scott CR et al. Homocystinemia: vascular injury and arterial thrombosis. N Engl J Med 291:537, 1974

Haverkate F, Mannucci CM, d'Angelo A. An abnormal fibrinogen (Milan II) with defective thrombin binding and thrombin clotting time, but normal reptilase and arvin times. Thromb Haemost 50 (Abst.):337, 1983

Heijboer H, Brandjes DPM, Buller HR, Sturk APh, Ten Cate JW. Deficiencies of coagulation-inhibiting and fibrinolytic proteins in outpatients with deep-vein thrombosis. N Engl J Med 29:1512, 1990

Hirsh J, McBridge JA, Dacie JV. Thromboembolism and increased platelet adhesiveness in post-splenectomy thrombocytosis. Australas Ann Med 15:122, 1966

Hoek JA, Nurmohamed MT, Ten Cate JW, Buller HR, Knipscheer HC, Hamelynch KJ, Marti RK, Sturk A. Thrombin-antithrombin III complexes in the prediction of deep vein thrombosis following total hip replacement. Thromb Haemost 62:1050, 1989

Jabaily J, Iland HJ, Laszlo J et al. Neurologic manifestations of essential thrombocythemia. Ann Intern Med 99:513, 1983

Janssen HF, Schachner J, Hubbard J, Hartman JT. The risk of deep venous thrombosis: a computerised epidemiologic approach. Surgery 101:205, 1987

Johansson L, Hedner U, Nilsson IM. A family with thromboembolism disease associated with deficient fibrinolytic activity in vessel wall. Acta Med Scand 203:477, 1978

Jorgensen M, Mortensen JZ, Madsen AG, Thorsen S, Jacobsen B. A family with reduced plasminogen activator activity in blood associated with recurrent venous thrombosis. Scand J Haematol 29:217, 1982

Juhan-Vague I, Valadier J, Alessi MC, Aillaud MF, Ansaldi J, Philip-Joet C, Holvoet P, Serradimigni A, Collen D. Deficient tPA release and elevated PA inhibitor levels in patients with spontaneous or recurrent deep venous thrombosis. Thromb Haemost 57:67, 1987

Juillet Y, Aiach M, Fiessinger JN, LeClerc M, Housset E. Antithrombine III et thromboses veineuses. Nouv. Presse Méd 7:367, 1978

Kazama M, Tahara C, Suzuki K, Gohchi K, Abet T. Abnormal plasminogens, a cause of recurrent thrombosis. Thromb Res 21:517, 1981

Kendall AG, Lohmann RC, Dossetor JB. Nephrotic syndrome a hypercoagulable state. Arch Intern Med 127:1021, 1971

Kroneman H, Van Bergen PFMM, Knot EAR, de Maat MPM. Is D-dimer useful to predict deep venous thrombosis? Thromb Haemost 65 (Abstr.):979, 1991

Largo R, Heller V, Straub PW. Detection of soluble intermediates of the fibrinogen-fibrin conversion using erythrocytes coated with fibrin monomers. Blood 47:991, 1976

Lau HK, Rosenberg RD. The isolation and characterisation of a specific antibody population directed against the thrombin-antithrombin complex. J Biol Chem 255:5885, 1980

Lau HK, Rosenberg JS, Beeler DL et al. The isolation and characterisation of a specific antibody population directed against the prothrombin activation fragments F2 and F1+2. Biol Chem 254:8751, 1979

Lechner K. Lupus anticoagulants and thrombosis. In: Verstraete M, Vemylen J, Lijnen R, Arnout J. (eds). Thrombosis and Haemostasis, 525. Leuven University Press, Leuven, Belgium, 1987

Lijnen HR, Soria J, Soria C, Collen D, Caen JP. Dysfibrinogenemia (fibrinogen Dusard) associated with impaired fibrin-enhanced plasminogen activation. Thromb Haemost 51:108, 1984

Lottenberg R, Dolly FR, Kitchens CS. Recurrent thromboembolic disease and pulmonary hypertension associated with severe hypoplasminogenemia. Am J Hematol 19:181, 1985

Mannucci PM, Kluft C, Traas DW, Seveso P, d'Angelo A. Congenital plasminogen deficiency associated with venous thromboembolism. Therapeutic trial with stanozolol. Br J Haematol 63:753, 1986

Mombelli G, Monotti R, Haeberti AN et al. Relationship between fibrinopeptide and fibrinogen/fibrin fragment E in thromboembolism, DIC and various non-thromboembolic diseases. Thromb Haemostas 58:758, 1987

Murphy S. Thrombocytosis and thrombocythaemia. Clin Haematol 12:89, 1983

Nguyen G, Horellou MH, Kruithof EKO, Conard J, Samama M. Residual plasminogen activator inhibitor activity after venous stasis as a criterion for hypofibrinolysis: a study in 83 patients with confirmed deep vein thrombosis. Blood 72:601, 1988

Nilsson IM, Ljungner H, Tengborn L. Two different mechanisms in patients with venous thrombosis and defective fibrinolysis: low concentration of plasminogen activator or increased concentration of plasminogen activator inhibitor. Br Med J 290:1453, 1985

Nossel HL. Relative proteolysis of the fibrinogen Bß chain by thrombin and plasmin as a determinant of thrombosis. Nature 291:165, 1981

Robinson GE, Burren T, Mackie IJ, Bounds W, Walshe K, Faint R, Guillebaud J, Machin SJ. Changes in haemostasis after stopping the combined contraceptive pill: implications for major surgery. Br Med J 302:269, 1991

Rocha E, Alfaro MJ, Paramo JA, Canadell JM. Pre-operative identification of patients at high risk of deep venous thrombosis despite prophylaxis in total hip replacement. Thrombosis Haemost 59:93, 1988

Samama M, Horellou MH, Van Dreden P, Bara L, Conard J. Clinical and laboratory findings in 335 patients with history of idiopathic venous thrombosis. 9th World Congr Phlebol (Abstr.):14, 1989

Samama M, Conard J, Horellou MH, Nguyen G, Van Dreden P, Soria J. Abnormalities of fibrinogen and fibrinolysis in familial thrombosis. Thromb Haemost 58:249, 1987

Samama M, Conard J, Soria J. Congenital dysfibrinogenemia and thrombosis. Fibrinolysis 2 (Sup. 2):18, 1988

Schafer AL. Bleeding and thrombosis in the myeloproliferative disorders. Blood 64:1, 1984

Scharrer IM, Wohl RC, Hach V, Sinio L, Boreisha I, Robbins KC. Investigation of a congenital abnormal plasminogen. Frankfurt I and its relationship to thrombosis. Thromb Haemost 55:396, 1986

Sigel B, Ipsen J, Felix WR. The epidemiology of lower extremity deep venous thrombosis in surgical patients. Ann Surg 179:278, 1974

Singh AK, Wetherley-Mein G. Microvascular occlusive lesions in primary thrombocythaemia. Br J Haematol 36:553, 1977

Soria J, Soria C, Bertrand O, Dun F, Drouet L, Caen JP. Plasminogen Paris I: congenital abnormal plasminogen and its incidence in thrombosis. Thromb Res 32:229, 1983

Soria J, Soria C, Hedner U, Nilsson IM, Bergqvist D, Samama M. Episodes of increased fibronectin level observed in a patient suffering from recurrent thrombosis related to congenital hypodysfibrinogenemia (Fibrinogen Malmoe). Br J Haematol 61:727, 1985

Spahn-Attenhofer CH, Von Felten A. Coagulation studies in 100 consecutive patients with severe thromboembolic disease to identify an increased risk of rethrombosis. Thromb Haemost 54 (Abstr.):234, 1985

Stadel BV. Oral contraceptives and cardiovascular disease. N Engl J Med 305:612, 1981

Stead NW, Bauer KA, Kinner TR, Lewis JG, Campbell EE, Shikfman MA, Rosenberg RD, Pizzo SV. Venous thrombosis in a family with defective release of vascular plasminogen activator and elevated plasma factor VIII/von Willebrand factor. Am J Med 74:33, 1983

Stringer MC, Steadman CA, Hedges AR, Thomas EM, Morley TR, Kakkar VV. Deep vein thrombosis after elective knee surgery. J Bone and Joint Surg 71b:492, 1989

Sue-Ling HM, Johnston D, McMahon MJ, Philips PR, Andrew-Davis J. Pre-operative identification of patients at high risk of deep venous thrombosis after elective major abdominal surgery. Lancet ii:1173, 1986

Teitel JM, Bauer KA, Lau HK et al. Studies of the prothrombin activation pathway utilising radioimmunoassays for the F2/F1+2 fragment and thrombin-antithrombin complex. Blood 59:1086, 1982

Thaler E, Lechner K. Antithrombin III deficiency and thromboembolism. In: Prentice CRM (ed.) Clinics in haematology, 369. WB Saunders, London, 1981

Thorson TI, Brosstad F, Solum O, Stormorken H. Increased binding to ADP-stimulated platelets and aggregation effect of the dysfibrinogen Oslo I as compared with normal fibrinogen. Scand J Haematol 36:203, 1986

Vessey M, Mant D, Smith A, Yeates D. Oral contraceptives and venous thromboembolism: findings in a large prospective study. Br Med J 292:526, 1986

Veth G, Meuwissen O, Van Houwelingen H, Sixma JJ. Prevention of postoperative deep vein thrombosis by a combination of subcutaneous heparin with subcutaneous dihydroergotamine or oral sulphinpyrazone. Thromb Haemost 54:570, 1985

Walenga JM, Fareed J, Mariani G et al. Diagnostic efficacy of a simple radioimmunoassay test for fibrinogen/fibrin fragments containing the Bß 15-42 sequence. Semin Thromb Haematol 10:252, 1984

Whitaker AN, Elms MJ, Masci PP et al. Measurement of crosslinked fibrin derivatives in plasma: an immunoassay using monoclonal antibodies. J Clin Pathol 37:882, 1984

Wohl RC, Sumaria L, Robbins KC. Physiological activation of the human fibrinolytic system. Isolation and characterisation of human plasminogen variants Chicago I and Chicago II. J Biol Chem 254:9063, 1979

Zielinsky A, Hirsh J, Straumanis G et al. The diagnostic value of the fibrinogen/fibrin fragment E antigen assay in clinically suspected deep vein thrombosis. Blood 59:346, 1982

CHAPTER 5

# Venous Stasis and Trauma in Hip Surgery

**Andre Planes**
**Nicole Vochelle**

## Introduction

That venous stasis is induced by anaesthesia was demonstrated by Clark and Cotton(1968) when they inserted a thermal dilution flow probe into the femoral and external iliac veins of patients undergoing surgery, both before and during operation. Their most striking conclusion was that the induction of general anaesthesia was followed by a profound fall in venous flow, reducing by half the flow in the external iliac vein and probably causing similar effects more distally. When measured with ultrasound (Makin, 1970) both the pulsatility and velocity of the venous flow in the leg veins were demonstrated to decrease during operation, with the most profound slowing occurring during the induction. By comparison, spinal anaesthesia was followed by a less intense depression (Modig et al, 1980; Poikolainen and Hendolin, 1983).

The association of stasis with the systemic "hypercoagulability" (activation of coagulation and inhibition of fibrinolysis) forms the basis for the mechanism believed to produce the general thrombo-embolic disease associated with all operations. The disease has an equal repartition in both legs and in general surgical patients varies in meta-analyses between 27% (Colditz, 1986); 22.4% (Collins et al, 1988) and 25% (Clagett and Reisch, 1988). When the fibrinogen uptake test is confirmed by venography, the incidence is 19.1% (Clagett and Reisch, 1988). In the meta-analysis by Clagett (1988), the rate of proximal DVT was 6.9%.

When a venographic assessment was used after hip replacement, the incidence of DVT appeared higher with a 50% overall incidence of DVT, 22.7% to 28% of these being proximal.

The fact that two diseases can occur after hip surgery, along with local trauma to the femoral vein, was demonstrated by Stamatakis and his colleagues (Stamatakis et al, 1977).

Using a perioperative venographic examination of the femoral vein, they demonstrated that the femoral vein appeared angulated and narrowed. The maximum distortion was found at the level of the lesser trochanter in patients having an anterior approach. With a posterior approach the femoral vein was narrowed with an appearance of torsion at the level of the lesser trochanter. There was also a slowing of blood flow often with a filling of the long saphenous vein. Johnson et al (1978) used an anterior approach and the same venographic assessment, noting at the time of dislocation "... a considerable kinking of the femoral veins and a slowing of blood flow on both sides though much more marked on the operated side ...". Nillius and Nylander (1979) in their venographic study were the first to explicitly state that after total hip replacement there are two types of thrombosis. First, a post-operative thrombosis (as previously defined, seen after all types of surgery) and second, a proximal type resulting from damage to the wall of the femoral vein during hip surgery.

## Three Recent Studies

The question remained as such for many years and was renewed recently by three studies addressing the mechanism of femoral vein aggression during elective hip surgery.

### The Study of Wuh
Wuh et al (1989) worked perioperatively on five consecutive patients undergoing total hip replacement. The patients were in lateral decubitus position, and wore thigh high intermittent sequential pneumatic compression devices intraoperatively (6-chambers device: Kendall Corporation). A postero-lateral surgical approach to the hip joint was used and both the anterior and posterior capsules were excised. Venous blood velocity was studied with a portable, continuous wave, bi-directional Doppler ultrasonic instrument and spectrum analyser with a sterile pencil probe operating at a transmission frequency of 5 mHz. A spectral display of the Doppler shift wave forms was generated and recorded with an attached video-recorder and printer. The Doppler probe was placed over the common femoral vein in the groin region using sterile acoustic gel as interface. The angle producing the maximum magnitude of spectral display was maintained during measurements. Measurements were taken before skin incision, following surgical exposure and femoral neck osteotomy with the hip in anterior and posterior dislocation. Measurements were made with the compression device on and off.

During posterior dislocation there was no blood flow detectable, indicating total or near total obstruction. Bursts of rapid flow were detected when the hip was released from the posteriorly dislocated position.

During anterior dislocation there was a 23% average decrease in flow velocity and the velocity wave form changed into a continuous pattern indicating partial obstruction.

During intermittent sequential compression, blood velocity increased on average by 71% with the hip reduced. With anterior dislocation it increased by 30%. With posterior dislocation a detectable flow was established in one patient.

### The study of Planes
We have recently performed a necropsy study on five fresh cadavers (10 hips) (Planes et al, 1990). With the body lying supine, an incision was made along the line of the femoral vessels in the proximal thigh. The femoral vessels were visualised without disturbing their

close anatomical connections. Then for alternate hips either a posterior (Moore) or an anterior (Hardinge) approach to the hip was made.

For the posterior approach, the body was turned onto its side. After posterior dislocation of the hip and section of the neck of the femur, the body was replaced into the supine position with a block of wood under the buttock. The femoral vessels were then examined with the leg in the position used during an operation for total hip replacement, first in medial rotation of 90° to 110° and then with various degrees of adduction and/or flexion of the hip adding medial rotation to simulate the positions needed for the preparation of the acetabulum and the femoral shaft.

The anterior approach was made with the patient supine. After anterior dislocation of the hip and section of the neck of the femur, the femoral vessels were examined with the leg in the appropriate operating positions, first retracted backwards to expose the acetabulum, then crossed over the body with flexion, adduction and lateral rotation, again in the position used for the preparation of the femoral canal.

*Results*

In every case the femoral vein had the appearance of a soft rubber tube, and after resection of the neck of the femur, it appeared too long for the shortened thigh and tended to fold, starting on the vein itself or over a transverse branch of the femoral artery. The exact level varied but was always in the proximal third of the thigh. Folding was induced by certain defined positions of the hip. After a posterior approach and dissection, internal rotation of 90° or even 100° to 110° did not induce a fold when the hip remained in extension. But when the thigh was flexed and even more so when it was adducted, a fold appeared and increased dramatically to become a kink at extreme position. The fold disappeared when the hip was extended and the thigh elongated. After an anterior approach, a fold appeared when the hip was adducted and flexed, after the thigh had been brought across the body and the femoral neck had been sectioned. The fold became smaller when these forced positions were relaxed and disappeared when the hip was replaced in its anatomical position. This study did not assess the transtrochanteric lateral or Charnley approach.

## The Study of Binns and Pho

Binns and Pho (1990) also reported a necropsy study on 20 adult anatomic specimens. In ten hips they assessed the posterior approach and in the other ten they used an anterolateral approach. On each specimen they inserted a plastic tube into the femoral vein on one side behind the knee and a second into the external iliac vein in the pelvis through an extraperitoneal approach. Saline was injected into the popliteal vein by a standard intravenous infusion set at normal physiologic values for a supine subject under general anaesthesia of 0.5 litres per minute at a pressure of 10 cm of water. Saline drained freely from the tube in the external iliac vein. After having dislocated the hip anteriorly or posteriorly they manipulated the femur to investigate the point where the cessation of flow occurred. After flow studies, micro-opaque x-ray contrast medium was injected by the same route and the joint held in extreme degrees of positioning during a posterior or anterior approach. An anteroposterior roentgenogram of the pelvis was then taken to observe the position and pattern of any venous occlusion. Thereafter the popliteal vein was injected with either Batson's acrylic or neoprene latex. The femur was held in the same extreme position for 48 hours to allow the injected medium to solidify. After amputation of each limb through the sacro-iliac joint and symphysis pubis, the soft tissues were dissected and corroded away from the femoral vein in 10% hypochlorite solution and any occlusive pattern observed.

*Results*

After posterior dislocation in 10 specimens, flow ceased at mean values of 82° flexion, 64° adduction, 83° internal rotation. Roentgenograms after the injection of contrast medium consistently showed an absence or attenuation of medium at the level of the femoral neck. The corrosion and dissection studies of acrylic-injected specimens showed a 3 cm segment of filling discontinuity just distal to the femoral sheath, with oblique cut off of acrylic both distally and proximally. Dissection of the latex-injected specimen showed that dislocation produced about 4 cm of shortening of the femoral vein in the relatively unsupported segment distal to the femoral sheath, which then buckles and kinks. Also adduction and internal rotation caused the distal part of this unsupported segment to lie perpendicularly across the proximal segment with a kink at the apex, convex laterally. Also, a tethering action of the circumflex and profunda branches of the common femoral vein was found in the femoral triangle. When the femur was internally rotated byond 80°, the scissoring action increased considerably.

After anterior dislocation, external rotation had no effect on flow, but extreme position of flexion (>71%) and adduction (>38%) stopped the flow. Roentgenographic studies showed the same attenuation or occlusion that was previously described with the posterior approach. Dissection showed the same shortening of about 4 cm of the femoral vein and in extreme positioning the same pattern of kinking and buckling with the convexity based laterally.

## Interpretation and Synthesis of the Three Studies

At the time of the operation the common femoral vein is under considerable strain. There is a characteristic folding of the femoral vein (convex laterally) which appears in certain forced positions of the hip. These forced positions are imposed at the time of the preparation of the femoral canal. After a posterior approach, extreme rotation, flexion or adduction should be avoided. After anterior approach, external rotation is better tolerated, but a fold appears when the hip is brought across the body and forced into flexion and adduction.

The extent of harm to the vessel wall remains speculative. Direct endothelial damage at the level of the kink is possible in some patients. Also obstruction of the femoral vein may induce a distension of the vein resulting in vascular damage, or after repeated manipulations the fibrinolytic activity of the vein wall in that region may be reduced. Defective fibrinolytic activity could predispose the patient to DVT. This hypothesis is based upon research using specific trials of fibrinolytic variables and has recently attracted much interest. Some authors found a relationship between high pre-operative levels of PAI-1 activity and post-operative DVT (Paramo et al, 1985; Rocha et al, 1988; Ericksson et al, 1989; Grimaudo et al, 1989). Others found no correlation in both general surgery and in hip replacement surgery, when a mandatory bilateral venographic examination was performed and the results of a single mode of prophylaxis assessed (Mellbring et al, 1985; Sue-Ling et al, 1987; Kluft et al, 1986; Sorensen et al, 1990).

In favour of a defective endothelial protection against DVT is the observation of Johnson and his team (Johnson et al, 1978). They performed a post-operative bilateral venographic assessment between day 7 and the 4th week on 34 patients operated on for total hip replacement. They observed no thrombi at 7 days, but the longer after operation the venograms were performed, the higher the incidence of thrombus formation. Moreover, in a further series of 14 patients they performed two successive bilateral venographic assessments. 14 were examined on the 7th postoperative day and 11 were normal. At 14 days these 11 patients were reassessed and 9 had a thrombus in the "sensitive" segment. The common femoral segment is the most "sensitive". Kakkar et al (1985) made the same observation of delayed appearance of DVT between the 15th and the 24th postoperative day.

## Conclusions

It is now well demonstrated and acknowledged that after total hip replacement, two types of thromboembolic venous disease are observed. These are general and local, proximal, in the operated leg.

Damage to the common femoral vein can occur at the time of the operation and particularly when forced positions applied to the hip at the time of preparation of the femoral canal. These extreme positons should be avoided or, if not, minimised.

The extent of vessel damage is still unknown but defective thrombo-resistance of the endothelium is probable and is possibly prolonged for several weeks after surgery.

## References

Binns M, Pho R. Femoral vein occlusion during hip arthroplasty. Clin Orthop 255:168, 1990

Clagett GP, Reisch JS. Prevention of venous thromboembolism in general surgical patients. Ann Surg 208:227, 1988

Clark C, Cotton LT. Blood flow in deep veins of the legs. Recording technique and evaluation of methods to increase flow during operation. Br J Surg 55:211, 1968

Colditz GA, Tuden RL, Oster G. Rates of venous thrombosis after general surgery: combined results of randomized clinical trials. Lancet ii:143, 1986

Collins R, Scrimgeour A, Yusuf S, Peto R. Reduction in fatal pulmonary embolism and venous thrombosis by perioperative administration of subcutaneous heparin. New Engl J Med 318:1162, 1988

Ericksson BI, Ericksson E, Gyzander E, Teger-Nilsson AC, Risberg B. Thrombosis after hip replacement. Relationship to the fibrinolytic system. Acta Orthop Scand 60:159, 1989

Grimaudo V, Kruithof EKO, Stiekema JCJ, Bachmann F. High pre-operative plasminogen activator inhibitor levels are correlated with postoperative deep vein thrombosis in total hip replacement. Thromb Haemost 62:96, 1989

Johnson R, Carmichael JHE, Almond HGA, Loynes RP. Deep venous thrombosis following Charnley arthroplasty. Clin Orthop 132:24, 1978

Kakkar VV, Fok PJ, Murray WJG, Paes T, Merrenstein D, Dodds R, Farrell R, Crellin RQ, Thomas EM, Morley TR, Price AJ. Heparin and dihydroergotamine prophylaxis against thromboembolism after hip arthroplasty. J Bone and J Surg 67B:538, 1985

Kluft C, Jie AFH, Lowe GDO, Blamey SL, Forbes CD. Association between postoperative hyper-response in t-PA inhibition and deep vein thrombosis. Thromb Haemostas 56:107, 1986

Makin GS. The effect of surgical operation on the velocity of venous return from the legs. Br J Surg 10:513, 1970

Mellbring G, Dahlgren S, Wieman B, Sunnegardh O. Relationship between preoperative status of the fibrinolytic system and occurrence of deep vein thrombosis after major abdominal surgery. Thrombosis Res 39:157, 1985

Modig J, Malmberg P, Karlstrom G. Effect of epidural versus general anaesthesia on calf blood flow. Acta Anaesth Scand 24:305, 1980

Nillius AS, Nylander G. Deep vein thrombosis after total hip replacement. A clinical and venographic study. Br J Surg 66:324, 1979

Paramo JA, Alfaro MJ, Rocha E. Postoperative changes in the plasmatic levels of tissue-type plasminogen activator and its fat-acting inhibitor. Relationship to deep vein thrombosis and influence of prophylaxis. Thromb Haemostas 54:713, 1985

Planes A, Vochelle N, Fagola M. Total hip replacement and deep vein thrombosis. A venographic and necropsy study. J Bone Joint Surg 72-B:9, 1990

Poikolainen E, Hendolin H. Effects of lumbar epidural analgesia and general anaesthesia on flow velocity in the femoral vein and postoperative deep vein thrombosis. Acta Chir Scand 149:361, 1983

Rocha E, Alfaro MJ, Paramo JA, Canadell JM. Preoperative identification of patients at high risk of deep vein thrombosis despite prophylaxis in total hip replacement. Thromb Haemostas 59:93, 1988

Sorensen JV, Lassen MR, Borris LC, Jorgensen PS, Sholt P, Weber S, Murphy R, Walenga J. Postoperative deep vein thrombosis and plasma levels of tissue plasminogen activator inhibitor. Thromb Research 60 247:1990

Stamatakis JD, Kakkar VV, Sagar S, Lawrence D, Nairn D, Bentley PG. Femoral vein thrombosis and total hip replacement. Br Med J 2:223, 1977

Sue-Ling HM, Johnston D, Verheijen JH, Kluft C, Philips PR, Davies JA. Indicators of depressed fibrinolytic activity in pre-operative prediction of deep venous thrombosis. Br J Surg 74:275, 1987

Wuh HCK, Woolson ST, McCrory DW. Intra-operative ultrasonic measurement of common femoral venous blood flow during total hip replacement. Trans Orthop Res Soc 14:423, 1989

CHAPTER 6

# DVT: Diagnostic Tests in the Screening of Asymptomatic Patients

Anthony J Comerota

## Introduction

Most physicians today acknowledge that the signs and symptoms of acute deep vein thrombosis (DVT) are nonspecific and that the clinical diagnosis is unreliable. Therefore an accurate diagnosis of DVT is essential, before treating this potentially lethal and frequently morbid disease if patients are to be cared for properly.

Ascending venography has been shown to be highly sensitive and specific and has been accepted as the "gold standard" for the diangosis of DVT. However, venography is invasive, causes patient discomfort and is associated with allergic reactions and renal toxicity. It cannot be performed in pregnant women and cannot be frequently repeated. Because of its intrinsic morbidity, which includes severe local tissue destruction if contrast extravasation occurs and the possibility of post-phlebographic thrombosis (although rare when modern non-ionic contrast media are used), alternative forms of accurate diagnosis are highly desirable.

A variety of diagnostic methods have been introduced during the past three decades in an attempt to overcome the disadvantages of venography (Comerota et al, 1988b). This review will address the most commonly used noninvasive techniques which have generally been recognised as the most reliable.

Impedance plethysmography (IPG) and phleborheography (PRG) are noninvasive tests that have been refined to such a degree that the reported diagnostic sensitivities are in excess of 90%. (Cranley et al, 1976; Comerota et al, 1982; Hull et al, 1985; Wheeler and Anderson, 1985) and it has been suggested that such tests could be used to replace ascending venography. However, these studies conflict with the data reported by others that document high false negative and high false positive rates (Vaccaro et al, 1987; Young et al, 1978). The latter reports seriously questioned the diagnostic reliability of the noninvasive tests and generated concerns on the part of referring physicians as to how to integrate the results of the noninvasive tests with patient care. At Temple University Hospital, we noticed an unacceptably low sensitivity for detecting proximal venous thrombosis with IPG and PRG compared to our experience in Cincinatti which was previously reported (Comerota et al, 1982). We also observed that the noninvasive tests and venography were being performed more commonly on asymptomatic patients at high risk for DVT, namely those undergoing total joint replacement, compared to our previous experience. Attempting to resolve the dichotomy in our results compared to others, it became evident that most centres reporting excellent diagnostic sensitivities and predictive values were evaluating symptomatic patients. We therefore thought that there could be a difference in the results of the noninvasive tests when evaluating symptomatic patients compared to those who were asymptomatic, but at high risk for DVT. If this were true, it should reflect a difference in the distribution of these two patient groups, differences in the size and extent of thrombi, as well as differences in the incidence of occlusive versus nonocclusive thrombi.

Noninvasive studies continued to develop and evolve into direct imaging techniques. Duplex scanning has been studied and now appears to be superior to that of haemodynamic tests for deep vein thrombosis (Elias et al, 1987; Comerota et al, 1988a). However, the question has remained whether venous duplex imaging has the same limitations as the haemodynamic noninvasive studies when applied to those asymptomatic patients at high risk for DVT. Duplex scanning with colour flow imaging has recently emerged as the newest technological advancement in the noninvasive evaluation of vascular disease (Persson et al, 1989) and has recently been applied to the study of venous disease. It is expected that further improvements in diagnostic sensitivity and predictive values would be provided by the addition of colour. In order to place the noninvasive methods of the diagnosis of acute DVT into proper perspective, a number of important questions need to be answered:

1. Does patient selection influence diagnostic reliability of noninvasive haemodynamic testing for DVT?
2. Is there a difference in the incidence of DVT in symptomatic patients compared to asymptomatic patients at high risk for DVT?
3. Does the addition of the fibrinogen uptake test (FUT) improve the diagnostic sensitivity enough to make the noninvasive results of symptomatic and asymptomatic patients comparable?
4. Is there a difference in the location of thrombi in these two patient groups?
5. Is there a difference in the extent of thrombi in these two patient groups?
6. Is the diagnostic reliability of duplex scanning better than haemodynamic testing for acute DVT?
7. Does the addition of colour flow imaging improve the sensitivity and predictive values compared to conventional duplex scanning?

## Methods Used to Evaluate the Problems and the Results

Two consecutive, prospective analyses have been performed to determined whether patient selection influences diagnostic reliability and whether the incidence of DVT is different in symptomatic compared to asymptomatic patients. In the first study (Comerota et al, 1988a) a prospective analysis of 351 patients having IPG, PRG, fibrinogen uptake testing (FUT), and ascending venography has been performed. All patients had at least one noninvasive diagnostic test and ascending venography during the same 24 hour period. All patients were categorised into one of three groups on the basis of their ascending venogram. Those without

**Table 6.1**
Impedance plethysmography compared with venography (n=308)

|      | Overall      | Diagnostic    |    | Surveillance   | p Value |
|------|--------------|---------------|----|----------------|---------|
| SPEC | 85% (119/140)| 81% (66/81)   | vs | 90% (53/ 59)   | NS      |
| SENS | 49% (83/168) | 71% (69/97)   | vs | 20% (14/ 71)   | <0.001  |
| A/K  | 68% (79/116) | 83% (68/82)   | vs | 32% (11/ 34)   | <0.001  |
| B/K  | 8%  (4/ 52)  | 7%  (1/15)    | vs | 8%  (3/ 37)    | NS      |
| -PV  | 58% (119/204)| 70% (66/94)   | vs | 48% (53/110)   | <0.005  |
| +PV  | 80% (83/104) | 82% (69/84)   | vs | 70% (14/ 20)   | NS      |

SPEC = specificity    SENS = sensitivity
-PV = negative predictive value    +PV = positive predictive value

evidence of DVT were categorised as normal, those with isolated calf vein thrombosis as B/K and patients with proximal vein thrombosis (whether or not calf vein thrombus was present) as A/K. By convention, all patients with thrombus in the popliteal vein were considered to have proximal (A/K) DVT, even if the thrombus was limited to the distal popliteal vein, below the knee joint. Patients who had symptoms of acute deep vein thrombosis had the noninvasive studies to confirm the clinical suspicion of acute DVT, and these patients were classified as the "diagnostic group". Those patients who were asymptomatic but at high risk for postoperative DVT because they were orthopaedic patients undergoing total hip replacement had noninvasive studies as part of a surveillance programme. These patients were classified as the "surveillance group".

In the surveillance group, 120 patients had the FUT performed. No patients in the diagnostic group had the FUT as part of the diagnostic evaluation. Of the 120 patients having the FUT, 111 had an IPG and 103 had a PRG performed.

The results of IPG compared with venography are listed in table 6.1 and the results of PRG compared with venography are listed in table 6.2. While the PRG appears to be a more sensitive test than IPG, both analyses demonstrate that these haemodynamic tests are more sensitive in detecting blood clots in symptomatic patients compared to asymptomatic patients. The sensitivity for the diagnosis of acute DVT is unacceptably low for both tests when they are used to evaluate asymptomatic patients as part of a surveillance programme.

**Table 6.2**
Phleborheography compared with venography (n=302)

|      | Overall       | Diagnostic    |    | Surveillance | p Value  |
|------|---------------|---------------|----|--------------|----------|
| SPEC | 78% (116/134) | 81% (65/ 80)  | vs | 94% (51/54)  | <0.05    |
| SENS | 59%  (99/168) | 78% (82/105)  | vs | 20% (14/71)  | <0.0001  |
| A/K  | 78%  (88/113) | 92% (79/ 86)  | vs | 33%  (9/27)  | <0.0001  |
| -PV  | 63% (116/185) | 74% (65/ 88)  | vs | 53% (51/97)  | <0.001   |
| +PV  | 85%  (99/117) | 85% (82/ 97)  | vs | 85% (17/20)  | NS       |

SPEC = specificity    SENS = sensitivity
-PV = negative predictive value    +PV = positive predictive value

**Table 6.3**
Comparison of the venographic results between patient groups

| Location | Diagnostic n = 212 | Surveillance n = 139 | p Value |
|---|---|---|---|
| No thrombi | (94/212) 44% | (63/139) 45% | NS |
| A/K | (99/212) 47% | (36/139) 26% | <0.0001 |
| B/K | (19/212) 9% | (40/139) 29% | <0.0001 |

**Table 6.4**
Occluding versus nonoccluding thrombi in patients with proximal DVT (n = 100)

| | Diagnostic n = 69 | Surveillance n = 31 | p Value |
|---|---|---|---|
| Occluding | 84% (58/69) | 23% (7/31) | <0.0001 |
| Nonoccluding | 16% (11/69) | 77% (24/31) | <0.0001 |

Insight as to why the results are so different between these two patient groups might be obtained by analysis of the venographic characteristics of the thrombi; that is, the distribution of a thrombus and the severity of occlusion. This information is shown in tables 6.3 and 6.4 respectively. Although there is no difference in the incidence of DVT between patient groups, there is a significant difference in the percentage of patients with proximal (A/K) thrombi in the diagnostic group (84% — 99/118) compared with those in the surveillance group (47% — 36/76) (p<0.001). We would intuitively expect that occluding thrombi in the deep venous system would create haemodynamic abnormalities and therefore would more likely cause symptoms; whereas, nonoccluding thrombi would not alter venous return and would likely remain asymptomatic (Table 6.5). Available venograms in patients with A/K thrombi were reviewed to determine whether the thrombus was occluding or nonoccluding (Table 6.4). Eighty-four percent of A/K thrombi in the diagnostic group (58/69) were occluding compared with 23% in the surveillance group (7/31) (p<0.0001).

The timing of postoperative venography in the surveillance group is important when assessing the extent of thrombi. The shorter the interval between operation and postoperative venography in any surveillance programme, the more likely one is to diagnose calf vein thrombosis and nonoccluding thrombi. In the patients reported here, 94% had the venogram performed within the first 7 postoperative days. The effect of FUT on improving the sensitivity of diagnosing postoperative DVT is appreciated by examining the data in tables

**Table 6.5**
Haemodynamic abnormalities of proximal thrombi by patient group (n = 94)

| IPG/PRG | Diagnostic n = 69 | Surveillance n = 25 | p Value |
|---|---|---|---|
| Neither positive | 3% (2/69) | 58% (13/25) | <0.01 |
| One positive | 97% (67/69) | 48% (12/25) | <0.001 |
| Both positive | 74% (51/69) | 20% (5/25) | <0.01 |

*Note: All patients had IPG and PRG and venography in the same 24-hour period

**Table 6.6a**
Combined impedance plethysmography and fibrinogen uptake test versus venography (n = 111)

|      | FUT alone   | IPG alone   | IPG+FUT     | p Value* |
|------|-------------|-------------|-------------|----------|
| SPEC | 71% (39/55) | 91% (50/55) | 67% (37/55) | <0.005   |
| SENS | 73% (41/56) | 16% (9/56)  | 77% (43/56) | <0.0001  |
| A/K  | 63% (15/24) | 25% (6/24)  | 71% (17/24) | <0.001   |
| B/K  | 81% (26/32) | 9% (3/32)   | 81% (26/32) | <0.0001  |
| -PV  | 72% (39/54) | 52% (50/97) | 74% (37/50) | <0.005   |
| +PV  | 72% (41/57) | 64% (9/14)  | 71% (43/61) | NS       |

* Significance of difference between IPG alone and IPG/FUT

6.6a and 6.6b. The FUT significantly improves overall sensitivity as well as the sensitivity of diagnosing A/K and B/K thrombi for both IPG and PRG. Because of the false positive results associated with the FUT, the specificity is reduced compared to that obtained by the noninvasive test alone. Likewise the negative predictive value of the combination of tests is significantly better compared with either IPG or PRG alone. Although adding the IPG or PRG to the FUT appears to improve the sensitivity for detecting A/K thrombi compared with the FUT alone, this difference is not significant.

To determine whether patient selection influences the results of the combination of tests (IPG plus FUT) the surveillance data in the current series were compared with both diagnostic and surveillance data published previously by Hull (Table 6.7). Similar observations were made with the results of the combination of tests as with the noninvasive tests alone. The FUT plus IPG has significantly better sensitivity when used in symptomatic patients compared to asymptomatic patients in an intensive surveillance programme (Table 6.7). The same trend is observed with the combination of studies compared to the IPG alone. There is significantly better sensitivity in the diagnostic group of patients compared to those in the surveillance group.

A second prospective study was performed to determine whether the same limitations occurred with venous duplex imaging as with the haemodynamic tests for DVT (Comerota et al, 1990). This study evaluated duplex scanning, PRG (the most sensitive haemodynamic test, and ascending venography within the same 24 hour period. The results are listed in

**Table 6.6b**
Combined phleborheography and fibrinogen uptake test versus venography (n = 103)

|      | FUT alone   | PRG alone   | PRG+FUT     | p Value* |
|------|-------------|-------------|-------------|----------|
| SPEC | 74% (37/50) | 94% (47/50) | 68% (34/50) | <0.001   |
| SENS | 70% (37/53) | 26% (14/53) | 77% (41/53) | <0.0001  |
| A/K  | 52% (11/21) | 33% (7/21)  | 67% (14/21) | <0.05    |
| B/K  | 81% (26/32) | 22% (7/32)  | 84% (27/32) | <0.0001  |
| -PV  | 70% (37/53) | 55% (47/86) | 74% (34/46) | <0.01    |
| +PV  | 74% (37/50) | 82% (14/17) | 72% (41/57) | NS       |

* Significance of difference between PRG alone and PRG/FUT

**Table 6.7**
Comparison of IPG + fibrinogen uptake tests done for surveillance vs diagnosis of DVT

|  | Diagnostic<br>Hull et al, 1980 | Surveillance<br>Hull et al, 1990 | Comerota et al, 1990 |
|---|---|---|---|
| SPEC | 95% (154/160) | 93% (140/150) | 67% (37/55)[*] |
| SENS | 90% (103/114) | 46% (50/109)[*] | 77% (43/56)[*] |
| A/K | 100% (78/ 78) | 48% (30/ 63)[*] | 71% (17/24)[*] |
| B/K | 69% (25/ 36) | 43% (20/ 46)[*] | 81% (26/32) |
| -PV | 93% (103/111) | 93% (140/150) | 74% (37/50)[*] |
| +PV | 93% (103/111) | 70% (140/199)[*] | 71% (43/61)[*] |

[*] Indicates that difference compared to diagnostic testing is significant (p<0.01)


**Table 6.8**
Duplex scanning and phleborheography compared to ascending venography

|  | Duplex scanning | Phleborheography | p-Value |
|---|---|---|---|
| A. All patients (n = 110) |  |  |  |
| SENS |  |  |  |
| All | 96% (51/53) | 55% (29/53) | <0.001 |
| A/K | 100% (44/44) | 66% (29/44) | <0.001 |
| B/K | 78% ( 7/ 9) | 0% ( 0/ 9) | <0.001 |
| +VE PV | 93% (51/55) | 83% (29/35) | NS |
| SPEC | 93% (53/57) | 89% (51/57) | NS |
| -VE PV | 96% (53/55) | 68% (51/75) | <0.001 |
| B. Diagnostic patients (n = 72) |  |  |  |
| SENS |  |  |  |
| All | 98% (43/44) | 61% (27/44) | <0.001 |
| A/K | 100% (37/37) | 66% (27/37) | <0.01 |
| B/K | 86% (6/ 7) | 0% (0/ 7) | <0.01 |
| +VE PV | 91% (43/47) | 82% (27/33) | NS |
| SPEC | 86% (24/28) | 79% (22/28) | NS |
| -VE PV | 96% (24/25) | 56% (22/39) | <0.001 |
| C. Surveillance patients (n = 38) |  |  |  |
| SENS |  |  |  |
| All | 89% (8/ 9) | 22% (2/ 9) | <0.05 |
| A/K | 100% (7/ 7) | 29% (2/ 7) | <0.05 |
| B/K | 50% (1/ 2) | 0% (0/ 2) | NS |
| +VE PV | 100% (8/ 8) | 100% (2/ 2) | NS |
| SPEC | 100% (29/29) | 100% (29/29) | NS |
| -VE PV | 97% (29/30) | 81% (29/36) | NS |

table 6.8. The overall sensitivity of duplex scanning is 96% (51/53) compared to 55% (29/53) for the PRG (p<0.001). Duplex scanning detected 100% (44/44) of A/K thrombi compared to 66% (29/44) detected by PRG (P<0.001). It is interesting to note that duplex scanning detected 78% (7/9) of B/K thrombi compared to 0% (0/9) detected by PRG (p<0.001). Although the positive predictive value and specificity between the two noninvasive tests were not different, the negative predictive value was significantly better for the duplex examination.

## Discussion

The data reported here indicate that there are significant differences in the ability of noninvasive tests to accurately diagnose DVT in patients who have symptoms compared to asymptomatic patients in surveillance programmes. These data reported by Comerota et al in 1988 and 1990 have been supported by Hull et al in 1981 and 1990, and by Paiement et al in 1990. Patient selection has a profound influence on the diagnostic sensitivity of haemodynamic testing, and these tests are unreliable when used in surveillance programmes. That being the case, noninvasive studies relying on haemodynamic principles cannot determine the true incidence of postoperative DVT, even when combined with the FUT. Therefore, anatomic studies continue to be a necessary requirement for a complete surveillance programme after total joint replacement. These data indicate that noninvasive haemodynamic testing is inadequate as an endpoint for generating reliable epidemiologic data. Additionally, studies evaluating the efficacy of DVT prophylaxis cannot use haemodynamic tests to determine whether DVT exists, and therefore will continue to require anatomic studies as an endpoint.

The reasons for these observations is that there is a significant difference in the location of thrombi as well as the extent of thrombi in these two patient groups. Patients in the surveillance programme had more B/K thrombi and nonoccluding thrombi than symptomatic patients as mentioned previously. This makes intuitive sense, since thrombi which do not affect venous haemodynamics in the lower limb are unlikely to create symptoms.

The location and extent of postoperative thrombi will be affected by the regimen of DVT prophylaxis given to patients. Therefore, subsequent studies evaluating patients in surveillance programmes may show differences in incidence, distribution or extent of thrombi, depending upon the type of prophylaxis they receive.

Duplex scanning did not have the same limitations as the haemodynamic tests for DVT. There was no difference between those patients evaluated in the surveillance group and those in the diagnostic group. Duplex scanning detected 100% of proximal (A/K) thrombi in both diagnostic and surveillance groups and 78% (7/9) of all isolated below knee thrombi. Duplex scanning was more sensitive than PRG for detecting both above and below knee thrombi, (p<0.001) and, most important, the negative predictive value of duplex was higher than that for PRG (p<0.001). Based upon these observations it appears that duplex scanning offers superior noninvasive diagnostic acumen without the limitations of traditional haemodynamic techniques. Duplex scanning reliably diagnosed nonocclusive and infrapopliteal thrombi, thereby offering superior epidemiologic and natural history capability in patients with acute DVT. In experienced vascular laboratories, duplex scanning may be more sensitive than ascending venography. This is most certainly true when all patients requiring diagnostic evaluation are considered, since some patients are excluded from venography due to access problems, contrast toxicity or allergic reactions. Duplex scanning may become the new diagnostic standard for deep vein thrombosis.

Whether the addition of colour flow imaging to duplex scanning improves the diagnostic sensitivity is discussed in the next chapter (Chapter 7). It appears that both experience and colour flow imaging improve sensitivity in patients in a surveillance programme (Mattos et al, 1992). One cannot assume that excellent results can be obtained with all instruments, nor can one assume that instruments are interchangeable. Additionally, the dedication of the physician interpreting the examination and the ability and persistence of the technologist performing the examination are the keys to reproducibly good results.

# References

Comerota AJ, Cranley JJ, Cook SE et al. Phleborheography — a 10-year experience. Surgery 91:573, 1982

Comerota AJ, Katz ML. The diagnosis of acute deep venous thrombosis by duplex venous imaging. Semin Vasc Surg 1:32, 1988

Comerota AJ, Katz ML, Grossi RJ et al. The comparative value of noninvasive testing for diagnosis and surveillance of deep vein thrombosis. J Vasc Surg 7:40, 1988a

Comerota AJ, Knight LC, Maurer AH. The diagnosis of acute deep venous thrombosis: noninvasive and radioisotopic techniques. Ann Vasc Surg 4:406, 1988b

Comerota AJ, Katz ML, Greenwald LL, Leefmans E, Czeredarczuk M, White JV. Venous duplex imaging: should it replace hemodynamic tests for deep venous thrombosis? J Vasc Surg 11:53, 1990

Cranley JJ. Phleborheography. In: Kempczinski RF, Yao JST (eds) Practical Noninvasive Vascular Diagnosis, 2nd ed: 438, Year Book Med Publishers, Chicago, 1987

Elias A, Le Corff G, Bouvier JL, Benichou M, Serradimigni A. Value of real-time B-mode ultrasound imaging in the diagnosis of deep vein thrombosis of the lower limbs. Int Angiol 6:175, 1987

Huisman MV, Buller HR, Cate JV, Vreeken J. Serial impedance plethysmography for suspected deep venous thrombosis in outpatients. N Engl J Med 314:823, 1986

Hull R, Hirsh J, Sackett DL, Taylor DW, Carter C, Turpie AGG, Zielinsky A, Powers P, Gent M. Replacement of venography in suspected venous thrombosis by impedance plethysmography and $^{125}$I-fibrinogen leg scanning. Ann Intern Med 94:12, 1981

Hull RD, Hirsh J, Carter CJ, Jay RM, Ockelford PA, Buller HR, Turpie AG, Powers P, Kinch D, Dodd PE, Gill GJ, Leclerc JR, Gent M. Diagnostic efficacy of impedance plethysmography for clinically suspected deep vein thrombosis. Ann Intern Med 102:21, 1985

Hull RD, Raskob GE, Gent M, McLoughlin D, Julian D, Smith FC, Dale NI, Reed-Davis R, Lofthouse RN, Anderson C. Effectiveness of intermittent pneumatic leg compression for preventing deep vein thrombosis after total hip replacement. JAMA 263:2213, 1990

Mattos MA, Londrey GL, Lentz DW, Hodgson KJ, Ramsey DE, Barkmeier LD, Stuaffer ES, Spadone DP, Sumner DS. Colour flow duplex scanning for the surveillance and diagnosis of acute deep venous thrombosis. J Vasc Surg 2:366, 1992

Paiement G, Wessinger SJ, Waltman AC, Harris WH. Surveillance of deep vein thrombosis in asymptomatic total hip replacement patients. Amer J Surg 400, 1990

Persson AV, Jones C, Zide R, Jewell ER. Use of the triplex scanner in diagnosis of deep venous thrombosis. Arch Surg 124:593, 1989

Stallworth JM, Plonk GW, Horne JB. Negative phleborheography: Clinical follow-up in 593 patients. Arch Surg 116:795, 1981

Vaccaro P, Van Aman M, Miller S, Fochman J, Smead WL. Shortcomings of physical examination and impedance plethysmography in the diagnosis of lower extremity deep venous thrombosis. Angiology 232:5, 1987

Wheeler HB, Anderson FA. The diagnosis of venous thrombosis by impedance plethysmography. In: Bernstein EF (ed), Noninvasive Diagnostic Techniques in Vascular Disease, 3rd End: 755, CV Mosby Co, St Louis, 1985

Young AE, Henderson BS, Phillips DA, Couch NP. Impedance plethysmography: its limitations as a substitute for phlebography. Cardiovasc Radiol 1:233, 1978

CHAPTER 7

# Diagnosis of Deep Vein Thrombosis in Asymptomatic Patients

Anthonie WA Lensing    Harry R Buller
Jack Hirsh    Jan Wouter ten Cate

## Introduction

The estimated frequency of venous thrombosis and pulmonary embolism after major knee or hip surgery without thromboprophylaxis has been reported to be between 40-50% and 2-5% respectively (Gallus et al, 1973). Although prophylactic agents are effective in reducing the frequency of venous thrombosis, approximately 12-25% of these patients still develop venous thrombosis despite prophylaxis (Francis et al, 1983; Leyvraz et al, 1983; Turpie et al, 1986; Hirsh et al, 1988). Therefore, even with prophylaxis patients are being discharged from hospital with undetected clinically important thrombi unless accurate objective tests are performed.

Contrast venography is widely accepted as the reference standard for the diagnosis of deep vein thrombosis. However, because of its invasiveness, side-effects associated with the use of contrast material, and costs, venography is not widely accepted as a screening test for venous thrombosis (Lensing et al, 1990; Buller et al, 1991). In contrast to the established role of noninvasive tests for the detection of venous thrombosis in symptomatic patients, the role of noninvasive tests for the screening of high risk patients is controversial (Büller et al, 1991). The difference between the accuracy of noninvasive tests in symptomatic patients and their questionable accuracy in asymptomatic patients is related to the specific features of thrombi in these patients. As indicated in the previous chapter (Chapter 6), venous thrombi are usually asymptomatic, frequently nonocclusive, relatively small, and predominantly involve the calf veins. These characteristics potentially influence the accuracy indices (sensitivity, specificity, and predictive values) of the various diagnostic tests. Moreover, the frequency of obtaining an interpretable test result may be hampered by the comorbid conditions of the patients. Therefore, screening tests for patients at high risk for asymptomatic deep vein thrombosis should meet the following two requirements: 1) They should be capable of detecting non-obstructive small thrombi, mainly localised in the calf veins, and 2) they should be easy to perform in large numbers of postoperative and medical patients with a minimum of discomfort.

In this article we critically review the evidence for the use of the fibrinogen uptake test (FUT), impedance plethysmography (IPG), and real-time B-mode ultrasonography in the diagnosis of venous thrombosis in asympatomatic postoperative patients. We also review studies that report on the combined use of these diagnostic tests. To minimise the effects of bias on the study outcomes, we have established criteria a priori to distinguish studies with potential for bias from those without.

## Methods

### Selection and classification of clinical studies

We critically reviewed articles published in the English literature that evaluated the accuracy of noninvasive screening tests (i.e., FUT, IPG, and real-time B-mode ultrasonography) for the diagnosis of venous thrombosis. A best effort was made to identify all articles. This included carrying out a Medline search of the literature, reviewing bibliographies of appropriate publications, and searching recent journals using Current Contents to find reports that may not have been included in the Medline search. In addition, we searched for unpublished articles by contacting experts in the field. Because the FUT, IPG and real-time B-mode ultrasonography were introduced as diagnostic tools for venous thrombosis in 1965, 1976, and 1984, respectively (Atkins and Hawkins, 1965; Hull et al, 1976; Raghavendra et al, 1984), the search was conducted from these time points through June 1991. Reports selected for review were those that (1) compared fibrinogen uptake testing, impedance plethysmography or real-time B-mode ultrasonography results (or the combined use of these tests) with the results of contrast venography in all patients (true accuracy studies); or that performed venography only in patients with abnormal noninvasive test results (positive predictive value studies); and (2) included at least 50 legs. Studies on the accuracy of real-time B-mode ultrasonography were categorised into those which used real-time imaging only, duplex scanning, and colour coded Doppler imaging.

### Evaluation of study methodology

All potentially eligible reports were reviewed to determine whether they included the essential design features required to evaluate whether the accuracy or the positive predictive value of a diagnostic test (Sackett et al, 1985); these criteria are listed in table 7.1. Three of these methodologic criteria were considered to be mandatory since their absence from the study design introduces biases which invalidate the results of the studies. The mandatory design features are (1) explicitly defined criteria for a normal and an abnormal test result for leg scanning, IPG, or real-time ultrasonography. In addition the criteria for the interpretation of the gold standard (venography) needed to be specified; (2) an independent and blind comparison of the results of the noninvasive test(s) and venography by observers who had no knowledge of the other test result; (3) the inclusion of consecutive patients. The interpretation of noninvasive tests and venography have subjective elements so that failure to define the criteria used for a normal and an abnormal test result and failure to ensure that the results of each test are interpreted independently and without knowledge of the other test result introduces a number of biases which could invalidate the findings. Failure to include consecutive patients can result in the exclusion of patients in certain risk categories

**Table 7.1**
Essential design features for the evaluation of a diagnostic test for venous thrombosis

*Mandatory Criteria*
1. Establishment of a priori objective criteria for a normal and an abnormal test result
2. Independent comparison with the gold standard for venous thrombosis
3. Inclusion of consecutive patients

*Other Criteria*
4. Description of the tactics for carrying out the tests in sufficient detail to permit their exact replication
5. Identification of patients selected for study
6. Determination of the reproducibility of the test result and its interpretation

and so produce false estimates of efficacy. The other criteria for the evaluation of a diagnostic test listed in table 7.1 are desirable but their absence from the study report does not necessarily invalidate the observed findings. A study was considered to have included consecutive patients if this methodologic requirement was explicitly mentioned in the article or if the exclusion criteria were described in sufficient detail to allow this judgement to be made.

Reports which included all three mandatory criteria were classified as level 1 studies, while reports which did not include all three criteria were classified as level 2 studies. Reports from which the positive predictive value of the noninvasive tests could be assessed, were graded as level 1 studies if in at least 70% of the patients with an abnormal noninvasive test result an interpretable venogram was obtained. Moreover, the diagnostic criterion for leg scanning had to be an increase of more than 20% from that sustained for at least 48 hours at any point on the leg, compared with readings at adjacent points in the same leg or at a corresponding point in the opposite leg. The indices of diagnostic efficacy are calculated as follows: sensitivity is assessed by dividing the proportion of patients with an abnormal result by the total number of patients with venographically proven venous thrombosis; specificity is assessed by dividing the proportion of patients with a normal test result by the total number of patients with normal venograms; the positive predictive value is determined by dividing the proportion of patients with a true normal result by the total number of patients with a normal result. For leg scanning, sensitivity was calculated for both isolated calf and total venous thrombosis, whereas for IPG and real-time ultrasonography sensitivity was calculated for proximal vein thrombosis. The 95% confidence intervals (CI) are calculated according to standard methods. The chi square test was used to calculate statistical significance.

# Results

### Fibrinogen uptake test
Fibrinogen uptake testing as a screening method for the detection of postoperative venous thrombosis is well established (Nanson et al, 1965; Flanc et al, 1968; Kakkar, 1972). Initially the test was considered to be highly accurate for demonstrating the presence or absence of asymptomatic venous thrombosis, especially those thrombi confined to the calf or distal

**Table 7.2**
Correlation of FUT with contrast venography in orthopaedic surgical patients

| Investigators | No. of Patients | Prev-alence | Sensitivity C.V.T. | Sensitivity Total D.V.T. | Specificity | Positive Predictive Value | Negative Satisfied Value | Criteria |
|---|---|---|---|---|---|---|---|---|
| Level 1 | | | | | | | | |
| Harris et al, 1976 | 78* | 23% | 75% (6/8) | 37% (7/19) | 90% (53/59) | 54% (7/13) | 82% (53/65) | 1,2,3,4,5 |
| Sautter et al, 1979 | 146* | 34% | 59% (23/39) | 58% (29/50) | 70% (67/96) | 50% (29/58) | 76% (67/88) | 1,2,3,4 |
| Sautter et al, 1983 | 117 | 50% | 59% (14/24) | 34% (20/50) | 79% (47/59) | 63% (20/32) | 55% (47/85) | 1,2,3,4,5 |
| Paiement et al, 1988 | 937* | 14% | 59% (78/133) | 44% (84/190) | 96% (769/804) | 69% (78/113) | 93% (769/824) | 1,2,3,4,5 |
| Cruickshank et al, 1989 | 951* | 18% | 51% (59/116) | 45% (78/115) | 95% (737/776) | 67% (78/117) | 88% (737/834) | 1,2,3,4,5 |
| Fauno et al, 1990 | 255* | 13% | 50% (30/60) | 44% (12/27)** | 87% (368/423) | 35% (30/85) | 93% (368/398) | 1,2,3,4,5 |
| Total | 2484 | | 55% (210/380) | 45% (230/511) | 92% (2041/2217) | 58% (242/418) | 89% (2041/2294) | |
| Level 2 | | | | | | | | |
| Field et al, 1972 | 63* | 43% | ? | 93% (25/27) | 81% (29/36) | 78% (25/32) | 94% (29/31) | 1,4,5 |
| Myrvold et al, 1973 | 82* | 34% | ? | 89% (25/28) | 93% (50/54) | 86% (25/29) | 94% (50/53) | 1,3,4,5 |
| Flicoteaux et al, 1977 | 77* | 18% | ? | 86% (12/14) | 95% (60/63) | 80% (12/15) | 97% (60/62) | 1,3,4,5 |
| Loudon et al, 1978 | 170* | 43% | 94% (34/36) | 93% (68/73) | 67% (65/97) | 68% (68/100) | 93% (65/70) | 1,2,4 |
| Moskovitz et al, 1978 | 118* | 11% | ? | 53% (10/19) | 86% (85/99) | 42% (10/24) | 90% (85/94) | 1,3,4,5 |
| Suomalainen et al, 1985 | 97* | 27% | ? | 73% (19/26) | 63% (19/30) | 35% (12/34) | 92% (183/195) | 1,4,5 |
| Comerota et al, 1988 | 111 | 51% | 81% (26/32) | 73% (41/56) | 71% (39/55) | 72% (41/57) | 72% (39/54) | 1,4,5 |
| Total | 718 | | 88% (60/68) | 82% (200/243) | 79% (322/400) | 66% (193/291) | 91% (511/559) | |

* Data presented in limbs instead of patients
** Results reported only for the non-operated leg

thigh veins (Kakkar, 1975; Kakkar, 1977). However, several years' experience has led to dissatisfaction with its precision in arriving at a positive diagnosis of venous thrombosis in many centres (Harris et al, 1975; Roberts, 1975; Harris et al, 1976; Harris et al, 1977, Sautter et al, 1979; Harris, 1980; Sautter et al, 1983; Paiement et al, 1988; Cruickshank et al, 1989; Hull et al, 1990). A potential limitation of the test is that it is impossible to interpret the fibrinogen leg scan result over the operated thigh or knee in patients who have hip or knee surgery because the extravasated blood from the operative wound can produce a falsely positive result; this limitation is of importance because approximately 30% of thrombi in hip surgery patients are localised in the femoral vein on the operated side and proximal thrombi in knee surgery patients are usually extensions of calf vein thrombi.

## Fibrinogen uptake test (FUT) — accuracy studies

FUT was compared with venography in 13 studies (all in orthopaedic surgical patients), of which six were classified as level 1 (Harris et al, 1976; Sautter et al, 1979; Suatter et al, 1983; Paiement et al, 1988; Cruickshank et al, 1989; Faunø et al, 1990) and 7 as level 2 (8 in orthopaedic surgical patients) (Field et al, 1972; Myrvold et al, 1973; Flicoteaux et al, 1977; Loudon et al, 1978; Moskovitz et al, 1979; Suomalainen et al, 1985; Comerota et al, 1988)(Table 7.2). A total of 2,484 legs were assessed by both leg scanning and venography in the six level 1 studies. Calf vein thrombosis was detected in 380 legs by venography and it was identified by FUT in 210, for a sensitivity of 55% (95% CI, 50 to 60%). Calf or proximal vein thrombosis was detected in 511 legs and was identified by leg scanning in 230, for a sensitivity of 45% (95% CI, 41 to 49%). The venogram was normal in 2041 legs; the FUT was falsely positive in 176, for a specificity of 92% (95% CI, 91 to 93%). The positive and negative predictive values of FUT were 58% and 89% respectively (95% CIs, 53 to 63% and 55 to 93%, respectively).

A total of 718 legs were assessed by both FUT and venography in the seven level 2 studies (all in orthopaedic surgical patients). Isolated calf vein thrombosis was detected in 68 legs by venography and it was identified by FUT in 60 (sensitivity, 88%). Calf or proximal vein thrombosis was found in 243 legs and was demonstrated by FUT in 200 (sensitivity, 82%). The venogram was normal in 408 legs of which leg scanning was falsely positive in 86 (specificity, 79%). The positive and negative predictive values of FUT in the level 2 studies were 66% and 91% respectively. The observed differences between the level 1 and 2 studies were statistically significant for all indices of accuracy: sensitivity to calf vein thrombosis (p<0.00001), sensitivity to calf or proximal vein thrombosis (p<0.00001), specificity (p<0.00001), positive and negative predictive values (p<0.00001 and <0.02, respectively) (Table 7.3).

### Table 7.3
Accuracy indices, ranges, and 95% confidence intervals of FUT, IPG and ultrasonography for the diagnosis of venous thrombosis in postoperative patients

| Accuracy Indices | %age | Range % | 95% Confidence Interval | p Value Level 1 vs 2 |
| --- | --- | --- | --- | --- |
| *FUT versus Venography* | | | | |
| Level 1 studies | | | | |
| Sensitivity CVT | 55 | 50- 75 | 50- 60 | <0.00001 |
| Sensitivity Total DVT | 45 | 34- 58 | 41- 49 | <0.00001 |

| Accuracy Indices | %age | Range % | 95% Confidence Interval | p Value Level 1 vs 2 |
| --- | --- | --- | --- | --- |
| Specificity | 92 | 70- 96 | 91- 93 | <0.00001 |
| Positive Predictive Value | 58 | 35- 69 | 53- 63 | <0.0001 |
| Negative Predictive Value | 89 | 55- 93 | 87- 90 | <0.02 |
| Level 2 studies | | | | |
| Sensitivity CVT | 88 | 81 -94 | 78- 93 | |
| Sensitivity Total DVT | 82 | 53- 93 | 79- 91 | |
| Specificity | 79 | 63- 95 | 76- 83 | |
| Positive Predictive Value | 66 | 35- 86 | 51- 81 | |
| Negative Predictive Value | 91 | 72- 97 | 89- 94 | |
| *FUT and IPG versus Venography* | | | | |
| Level 1 studies | | | | |
| Sensitivity CVT | 48 | 43- 75 | 39- 56 | <0.01 |
| Sensitivity Total DVT | 48 | 46- 74 | 43- 53 | <0.001 |
| Specificity | 94 | 93- 97 | 93- 95 | <0.00001 |
| Positive Predictive Value | 69 | 62- 88 | 64- 75 | p= 0.97 |
| Negative Predictive Value | 87 | 70- 92 | 85- 89 | <0.02 |
| Level 2 studies | | | | |
| Sensitivity CVT | 81 | — | 63- 92 | |
| Sensitivity Total DVT | 77 | — | 63- 87 | |
| Specificity | 67 | — | 54- 81 | |
| Positive Predictive Value | 71 | — | 57- 81 | |
| Negative Predictive Value | 74 | — | 59- 85 | |
| *IPG versus Venography* | | | | |
| Level 1 studies | | | | |
| Sensitivity Proximal DVT | 23 | 25- 83 | 16- 31 | <0.02 |
| Specificity | 98 | 95- 99 | 97- 99 | <0.0001 |
| Positive Predictive Value | 48 | 47- 53 | 35- 61 | p = 0.3 |
| Negative Predictive Value | 93 | 76- 98 | 92- 94 | <0.00001 |
| Level 2 studies | | | | |
| Sensitivity Proximal DVT | 32 | — | 21- 43 | |
| Specificity | 90 | — | 79- 96 | |
| Positive Predictive Value | 70 | — | 47- 93 | |
| Negative Predictive Value | 48 | — | 80- 84 | |
| *Ultrasonography versus Venography* | | | | |
| Level 1 studies | | | | |
| Sensitivity Proximal DVT | 54 | 38-100 | 44- 64 | <0.00001 |
| Specificity | 92 | 91- 99 | 90- 94 | <0.0001 |
| Positive Predictive Value | 71 | 53- 92 | 61- 79 | <0.02 |
| Negative Predictive Value | 81 | 69- 97 | 78- 83 | <0.00001 |
| Level 2 studies | | | | |
| Sensitivity Proximal DVT | 92 | 83-100 | 81- 98 | |
| Specificity | 98 | 96-100 | 96- 99 | |
| Positive Predictive Value | 88 | 63-100 | 77- 95 | |
| Negative Predictive Value | 99 | 99-100 | 96-100 | |

CVT = (isolated) calf vein thrombosis
Total DVT = (isolated) calf and proximal vein thrombosis
95% CI = 95% Confidence Interval

Paiement and his colleagues demonstrated that the sensitivity of FUT for calf vein thrombosis was critically dependent on the size of the thrombus; the test had a sensitivity of 83% for large thrombi in the calf and a sensitivity of 73% and 40% for medium sized and small sized clots, respectively (Paiement et al, 1988).

### Fibrinogen uptake testing (FUT) — positive predictive value studies

A total of 53 studies were retrieved that evaluated the predictive value of an abnormal FUT result by direct comparison with venography. Of these, 39 studies were classified as level 1 and 14 as level 2 studies (Table 7.4). More than 7,500 legs were screened by FUT in level

**Table 7.4**
Positive predictive value of FUT for the screening of venous thrombosis in postoperative patients

| Investigators | Type of Surgery | % patients with Positive Scan (limbs) | Positive Predictive Value | Diagnostic Criterion |
|---|---|---|---|---|
| **Level 1** | | | | |
| Kakkar et al, 1969 | General | 30% (40/132) | 98% (39/40) | 20% |
| Kakkar et al, 1972 | General | 36% (32/88) | 89% (32/36) | 20% |
| Bonnar et al, 1972 | Abdominal | 6% (16/260) | 100% (16/16) | 20% |
| Myrvold et al, 1973 | Hip | 34% (29/82)* | 86% (25/29) | 20% |
| Gallus et al, 1973 | Major | 56% (34/61) | 91% (31/34) | 20% |
| Becker et al, 1973 | General | 21% (24/116) | 29% (7/24) | 20% |
| Abernethy et al, 1974 | Major | 6% (7/125) | 67% (4/6) | 20% |
| Covey et al, 1975 | General | 13% (14/105) | 60% (6/10) | 20% |
| Harris et al, 1976 | Hip | 17% (13/78)* | 54% (7/13) | 20% |
| Gallus et al, 1976 | Major | 9% (72/820) | 89% (64/72) | 20% |
| Flicoteaux et al, 1977 | Hip | 18% (14/77) | 86% (12/14) | 20% |
| Moskovitz et al, 1978 | Hip | 20% (24/118) | 42% (10/24) | 20% |
| Coe et al, 1978 | Urologic | 23% (19/81) | 71% (12/17) | 20% |
| Skillman et al, 1978 | Neurosurgery | 22% (21/95) | 74% (14/19) | 20% |
| Kakkar et al, 1978 | Major | 9% (18/190) | 66% (12/18) | 20% |
| Xabregas et al, 1978 | Hip | 28% (14/50) | 100% (14/14) | 20% |
| Loudon et al, 1978 | Hip | 41% (70/170)* | 68% (65/70) | 20% |
| Sautter et al, 1979 | Hip | 40% (58/146)* | 50% (29/58) | 20% |
| Hull et al, 1979 | General | 5% (34/630) | 79% (27/34) | 20% |
|  | Hip | 50% (79/158) | 86% (68/79) | 20% |
| Salzman et al, 1980 | Urologic | 11% (11/100) | 63% (5/8) | 20% |
| Nandi et al, 1980 | Major | 3% (4/150) | 100% (4/4) | 20% |
| Hendolin et al, 1982 | Abdominal | 9% (9/98) | 33% (3/9) | 20% |
| Kakkar et al, 1982 | Major | 4% (6/150) | 33% (2/6) | 20% |
| Fredin et al, 1982 | Hip | 29% (20/69) | 70% (14/20) | 20% |
| Sautter et al, 1983 | Hip | 29% (20/69) | 70% (14/20) | 20% |
| Suomalainen et al, 1985 | Hip | 30% (29/97)* | 86% (25/29) | 20% |
| Alfaro et al, 1986 | Hip | 17% (20/120) | 80% (16/20) | 20% |
| Sasahara et al, 1986 | Abdominal | 10% (27/269) | 100% (21/21) | 20% |
| Ockelford et al, 1987 | General | 10% (18/183) | 83% (15/18) | 20% |
| Paiement et al, 1988 | Hip | 12% (113/937)* | 69% (78/113) | 20% |

| Investigators | Type of Surgery | % patients with Positive Scan (limbs) | Positive Predictive Value | Diagnostic Criterion |
|---|---|---|---|---|
| Fricker et al, 1988 | Abdominal | 3% (2/80) | 0% (0/2) | 20% |
| Eriksson et al, 1988 | Hip | 36% (36/98) | 89% (32/36) | 20% |
| Comerota et al, 1988 | Hip | 51% (57/111) | 72% (41/57) | 20% |
| Kakkar et al, 1989 | Abdominal | 11% (20/179) | 95% (18/19) | 20% |
| Pini et al, 1989 | Hip | 24% (12/49) | 100% (12/12) | 20% |
| Baumgartner et al, 1989 | General | 16% (28/176) | 46% (13/28) | 20% |
| Cruickshank et al, 1990 | Hip | 14% (117/834)* | 67% (78/117) | 20% |
| Mätzsch et al, 1990 | Hip | 32% (31/96) | 58% (11/19) | 20% |
| Faunø et al, 1990 | Hip | 33% (85/255)* | 35% (30/85) | 20% |
| Total | | 17% (1309/7750) | 73% (932/1284) | |
| Level 2 | | | | |
| Flanc et al, 1968 | General | 14% (18/130)* | 94% (17/18) | |
| Negus et al, 1968 | Major | 34% (32/93) | 95% (18/19) | 15% |
| Lambdie et al, 1970 | General | 95% (40/42)* | 91% (36/40) | 15% |
| Pinto, 1970 | Hip | 34% (17/50) | 88% (15/17) | 15% |
| Milne et al, 1971 | General | 25% (37/150)* | 78% (18/23) | 15% |
| Tsapogas et al, 1971 | Major | 12% (11/95) | 73% (8/11) | 15% |
| Field et al, 1972 | Hip | 74% (75/102)* | 78% (25/32) | 20% |
| Hume et al, 1972 | Hip | 24% (12/50) | 83% (10/12) | 15% |
| Wu et al, 1977 | Abdominal | 5% (7/134) | 100% (5/5) | 20% |
| Butson, 1981 | General | 8% (10/119) | 100 (7/7) | ? |
| Borow et al, 1981 | General | 19% (96/500) | 89% (42/47) | ? |
| Onarheim et al, 1986 | Abdominal | 8% (4/52) | 25% (1/4) | 15% |
| Encke et al, 1988 | Abdominal | 4% (70/1909) | 88% (23/26) | 20% |
| Hartl et al, 1990 | Abdominal | 7% (18/250) | 56% (10/18) | ? |
| Total | | 12% (447/3675) | 84% (235/279) | |

* Data presented in limbs instead of patients

1 studies; an abnormal FUT result was obtained in 1,309 of which 1,284 (98%) had a venogram which was adequate for interpretation. The venogram was abnormal in 932 legs for a positive predictive value of 73% (95% CI, 70 to 75%).

More than 3,500 legs were screened by FUT in the level 2 studies. Abnormal results were observed in 447. Venograms that were interpretable were obtained in only 279 (62%) and demonstrated venous thrombosis in 235 instances (positive predictive value, 84%; Table 7.4). The pooled results for positive predictive value of level 1 studies were statistically significantly lower when compared with those studies which did not fulfil the essential methodologic criteria (p<0.0001).

**Fibrinogen Uptake Testing (FUT) and Impedance Plethysmography (IPG)**
The use of the combination of FUT and IPG for the screening of high risk patients is less well-established than that of FUT alone. The rationale for the combined use of these methods in this patient category is based on the assumption that FUT is sensitive for isolated calf vein thrombosis and IPG is sensitive for thrombosis of the popliteal, femoral or iliac veins (proximal veins) but is relatively insensitive to calf vein thrombosis. Therefore, the

**Table 7.5**
Correlation of the combined use of FUT and IPG with contrast venography in postoperative patients

| Investigators | Type of Surgery | Number of Patients | Prevalence | Sensitivity CVT | Sensitivity Total DVT | Specificity | Positive Predictive Value | Negative Predictive Value | Criteria |
|---|---|---|---|---|---|---|---|---|---|
| **Level 1** | | | | | | | | | |
| Harris et al, 1976 | Hip | 78* | 24% | 75% (6/8) | 74% (14/19) | 97% (57/59) | 88% (14/16) | 92% (57/62) | 1,2,3,4,5 |
| Paiement et al, 1988 | Hip | 937* | 20% | ? | 46% (86/188) | 94% (708/751) | 67% (86/129) | 87% (708/810) | 1,2,3,4,5 |
| Cruickshank et al, 1989 | Hip | 824* | 17% | 48% (43/90) | 50% (69/139) | 94% (643/685) | 62% (69/111) | 90% (643/713) | 1,2,3,4,5 |
| Hull et al, 1990 | Hip | 259 | 42% | 43% (20/46) | 46% (50/109) | 93% (140/150) | 83% (50/60) | 70% (140/199) | 1,2,3,4,5 |
| Total | | 2098 | | 48% (69/144) | 48% (219/455) | 94% (1548/1645) | 69% (219/316) | 87% (1548/1784) | |
| **Level 2** | | | | | | | | | |
| Comerota et al, 1988 | Hip | 111 | 50% | 81% (26/32) | 77% (43/56) | 67% (37/55) | 71% (43/61) | 74% (37/50) | 1,4,5 |

* Data presented in limbs instead of patients     CVT = calf venous thrombi

combination of both tests could have an optimal sensitivity for venous thrombosis. In symptomatic patients, it has been shown that IPG is relatively insensitive for small and nonocclusive thrombi, whereas the combination of IPG and FUT was shown to be an accurate strategy in patients with symptomatic venous thrombosis (Buller et al, 1991).

### Fibrinogen Uptake Testing and Impedance Plethysmography — Accuracy studies

The combined use of FUT and IPG was compared with contrast venography in five studies in orthopaedic surgical patients (Table 7.5), of which four were graded as level 1 (Harris et al, 1976; Paiement et al, 1988; Cruickshank et al, 1989; Hull et al, 1990) and one as level 2 (Comerota et al, 1988). The pooled sensitivity of the level 1 studies for isolated calf vein thrombosis was 48% (95% CI, 39 to 56%), the sensitivity for isolated calf and proximal vein thrombosis was also 48% (95% CI, 43 to 53%), and the specificity was 94% (95% CI, 93 to 95%). The sensitivity for isolated calf vein thrombosis in the single level 2 study was 81%, the sensitivity for isolated calf and proximal vein thrombosis was 77%, and the specificity was 67%. The sensitivity for both isolated calf and isolated calf plus proximal vein thrombosis and the specificity were significantly different for the level 1 studies as compared with the level 2 study (p<0.01).

Cruickshank et al (1989) could not detect a statistically significant difference for either the sensitivity or the specificity of the combined results of leg scanning and impedance plethysmography between the operated and non-operated leg.

### IPG compared with venography in asymptomatic post-operative patients — Accuracy studies

Impedance plethysmography was compared with venography in four studies (in all orthopaedic surgical patients) of which three were graded as level 1 (Paiement et al, 1988;

**Table 7.6**
Correlation of IPG with contrast venography in postoperative patients

| Investigators | Type of Surgery | Number of Patients | Prevalence | Sensitivity Proximal DVT | Specificity | Positive Predictive Value | Negative Predictive Value | Criteria |
|---|---|---|---|---|---|---|---|---|
| **Level 1** | | | | | | | | |
| Paiement et al, 1988 | Hip | 937* | 20% | 12% (9/73) | 99% (856/864) | 53% (9/17) | 93% (856/920) | 1,2,3,4,5 |
| Cruickshank et al, 1989 | Hip | 681* | 20% | 45% (14/31) | 98% (767/784) | 45% (14/31) | 98% (767/784) | 1,2,3,4,5 |
| Ginsberg et al, 1990 | Hip | 247 | 26% | 26% (7/26) | 95% (146/154) | 47% (7/15) | 76% (146/192) | 1,2,3,4,5 |
| Total | | 1865* | | 23% (30/131) | 98% (1769/1802) | 48% (30/63) | 93% (1769/1896) | |
| **Level 2** | | | | | | | | |
| Comerota et al, 1988 | Hip | 130 | 32% | 32% (11/34) | 90% (53/59) | 70% (14/20) | 48% (53/110) | 1,4,5 |

*Data presented in limbs instead of patients

Cruickshank et al, 1989; Ginsberg et al, 1991) and one study as level 2 (Comerota et al, 1988). In the level 1 studies, IPG detected 30 of the 131 patients with proximal vein thrombosis (sensitivity, 23%; 95% CI 16 to 31%). Normal IPG results were obtained in 1,769 of the 1,802 patients with normal venograms (specificity, 98%; 95% CI 97 to 99%). Venous thrombosis could be confirmed in 30 of the 63 patients with an abnormal IPG test (positive predictive value, 48%; 95% CI 35 to 61%, Table 7.6). In the single level 2 study, the sensitivity for proximal vein thrombosis was 32%. The specificity, and positive predictive value were 90% and 70%, respectively. Although the level 1 studies and the level 2 study demonstrated that IPG has a very poor sensitivity for proximal vein thrombosis, the accuracy indices of IPG for the detection of asymptomatic venous thrombosis were significantly different (with the exception of the positive predictive value) for the level 1 studies as compared with the level 2 study (Table 7.3).

No studies could be identified that assessed only the predictive value of an abnormal impedance plethysmography test result.

**Real-Time B-mode Ultrasonography**
Since real-time B-mode ultrasonography has been introduced as a reliable diagnostic tool for venous thrombosis in symptomatic patients, the method has gained widespread popularity. An accurate, objective and simple criterion for the presence of deep vein thrombosis is non-compressibility of the vein under gentle probe pressure (compression ultrasound), whereas the visualisation of the thrombus and the extension of vein diameter during a Valsalva manoeuvre are subjective (Buller et al, 1991). The currently available ultrasound equipment allows adequate evaluation of the proximal veins (with the exception of the iliac vein) but the visualisation of the calf veins is complicated by the small size of these vessels. In contrast to the use of real- time ultrasonography in symptomatic patients, opinions are divided about its value for the diagnosis of asymptomatic thrombosis. The addition of

**Table 7.7**
Correlation of real-time B-mode, duplex, and colour-coded Doppler ultrasonography with contrast venography in postoperative patients

| Investigators | Type of Surgery | Number of Patients | Prevalence | Sensitivity Proximal DVT | Specificity | Positive Predictive Value | Negative Predictive Value | Criteria |
|---|---|---|---|---|---|---|---|---|
| **Level 1** | | | | | | | | |
| Borris et al, 1989 (US) | Hip | 60 | 47% | 63% (15/24) | 91% (29/32) | 83% (15/18) | 69% (29/42) | 1-5 |
| Froelich et al, 1989 (D) | Hip | 40 | 15% | 100% (5/5) | 97% (33/34) | 83% (5/6) | 97% (33/34) | 1-5 |
| Agnelli et al, 1991 (US) | Hip | 187[*] | 26% | 55% (12/22) | 99% (137/138) | 92% (12/13) | 79% (137/174) | 1,2,,,5 |
| Ginsberg et al, 1992 (US) | Hip | 247[*] | 25% | 52% (11/21) | 99% (184/186) | 89% (16/18) | 80% (184/229) | 1-5 |
| Davidson et al, 1992 (D) | Hip/Knee | 169 | 30% | 50% (5/10) | 92% (128/169) | 56% (14/25) | 89% (128/144) | 1-5 |
| Davidson et al, 1992 (CD) | Hip/Knee | 319 | 25% | 38% (8/21) | 94% (225/239) | 53% (16/30) | 78% (225/289) | 1-5 |
| Total | | 1022 | | 54% (56/103) | 92% (736/798) | 71% (78/110) | 81% (736/912) | |
| **Level 2** | | | | | | | | |
| Barnes et al, 89 (D) | Hip/Knee | 153[*] | 19% | 83% (10/12) | 96% (135/141) | 63% (10/16) | 99% (135/137) | 1,4,5 |
| Comerota et al, 90 (D) | Hip/Knee | 36 | 25% | 100% (7/7) | 100% (29/29) | 100% (7/7) | 100% (29/29) | 3,4,5 |
| Woolson et al, 90 (US) | Hip | 152[*] | 19% | 89% (17/19) | 100% (133/133) | 100% (17/17) | 99% (133/135) | 1,4,5 |
| Dorfman et al, 90 (US) | Hip | 93 | 19% | 100% (14/14) | 100% (75/75) | 100% (14/14) | 100% (75/75) | 1,3,4,5 |
| Total | | 434[*] | | 92% (48/52) | 98% (372/378) | 88% (48/54) | 99% (372/376) | |

US = Performed with real-time ultrasonography; D = Performed with duplex ultrasonography; CD = Performed with colour coded Doppler; [*] = Legs instead of patients; [**] = Calculated for all patients

Doppler (duplex) or colour coded Doppler images to compression ultrasound may eventually allow a more accurate evaluation of these smaller veins.

### Real-Time B-mode Ultrasonography — Accuracy studies
A total of 13 studies (all in orthopaedic surgical patients) could be identified that reported on the accuracy of real-time B-mode ultrasonography for the diagnosis of post-operative venous thrombosis. Of these, three were excluded from the analysis since results were reported for both asymptomatic post-operative patients and patients with clinically suspected venous thrombosis (Nix et al, 1989; Mussurakis et al, 1990) or pulmonary embolism (Monreal et al, 1989). An additional study was excluded because venography was performed only in patients with an abnormal ultrasound or IPG test result (White et al, 1990). Of the remaining studies, five were graded as level 1 (Borris et al, 1989; Froelich et al, 1989; Ginsberg et al, 1992; Agnelli et al, 1991; Davidson, 1992) and four as level 2 (Barnes

et al, 1989; Comerota et al, 1990; Dorfman et al, 1990; Woolson et al, 1990) (Table 7.7). A total of 1,022 legs/patients underwent both ultrasonography and venography in the level 1 studies. Ultrasonography detected 56 of the 103 legs with proximal vein thrombosis (sensitivity 54%, 95% CI 44 to 64%). An abnormal ultrasonography test occurred in 62 legs with a a normal venogram (specificity, 92%; 95% CI 90 to 94%). The predictive value of an abnormal and normal ultrasound result was 71% and 81% respectively (95% CIs, 61 to 79% and 78 to 83%, respectively)

The combined results of all level 2 studies suggest that ultrasonography is sensitive for proximal vein thrombosis (92%; 48/52), is specific (98%; 372/378), and has a positive and negative predictive values of 88% and 99% respectively. The observed differences between the level 1 and 2 studies are significantly higher as compared with those obtained in the level 1 studies (Table 7.3; p<0.0002)

Ginsberg and his colleagues assessed the value of adding IPG to the real-time ultrasonography evaluation and demonstrated that the combination had comparable sensitivity for proximal vein thrombosis as real-time ultrasonography alone, whearese the combination of these tests led to decreased specificity (Ginsberg et al, 1991). The addition of Doppler (duplex) or colour-coded Doppler to the real-time B-mode images did not result in an improvement of accuracy for proximal vein thrombosis (Table 7.7)

**Contrast Venography**
Ascending contrast venography for the diagnosis of deep vein thrombosis was introduced in 1940 (Bauer, 1940). With adequate technique, venography outlines the entire deep venous system of the leg, including the common iliac vein and inferior vena cava and is, therefore, widely accepted as the reference method for establishing the presence or absence of deep vein thrombosis (Haeger, 1969). Despite carefully defined diagnostic criteria (Rabinov and Paulin, 1972), there are three important limitations with respect to its applicability. First, venograms cannot be obtained in 5-10% of patients. Second, the interpretation of venograms is subject to considerable observer variation (13-26%) (McLachlan et al, 1979), and finally inadequate studies are observed in 5-12% of patients (Hull et al, 1976; Hull et al, 1981; Hull et al, 1985; Huisman et al, 1986; Huisman et al, 1989). The clinical implications of the limitations of the interpretation of venography are disturbing and potentially dangerous since there is the potential that anticoagulant treatment will be incorrectly withheld from patients with deep vein thrombosis, and therapy will be initiated unnecessarily in patients who have falsely abnormal or inadequate tests results.

The venographic method according to Rabinov and Paulin is widely used. An alternative venographic technique applies long- leg films, instead of spot films, and is performed using a larger amount of radio-opaque contrast material. In a large prospective cohort study, the latter method was not associated with serious contrast related side-effects (Lensing et al, 1990). Both techniques are fully comparable with respect to the radiation exposure. In a recent study, these two techniques were compared with respect to the percentage of inadequate venograms and the magnitude of variation in the interpretation of the test results. Two experienced and independent radiologists assessed both series of venograms. The results clearly indicate that the interpretation of Rabinov and Paulin (1972) venograms by two observers is subject to substantial interobserver variation (21%) and that a significant percentage of the tests results are adjudicated inadequate for interpretation. In contrast, using long-leg films, the same two observers agreed almost entirely on the interpretation (observer variation, 4%) and the frequency of inadequate venograms was negligible. The differences with respect to the interobserver variation and inadequacy rate between the two venographic techniques were both statistically significant.

## Conclusions

The results of our review demonstrate that striking differences exist between the accuracy indices for postoperative venous thrombosis by the FUT, IPG, and real-time ultrasonography observed in the level 1 studies as compared with those in level 2 studies and indicate that all these tests (separate or in combination) are unreliable for the screening of high risk patients.

Although FUT, IPG and real-time ultrasonography are considered to be objective tests, their interpretation is in part subjective and can be problematic. Thus, unless the results of each test are interpreted independently and without knowledge of the outcome of venography, the interpretation of the test results is susceptible to bias. The major difference in the design of the level 1 and level 2 studies did not ensure that the diagnostic tests were interpreted independently of each other. Therefore, we conclude that the (high) estimates of sensitivity of the level 2 studies and the much lower estimates of sensitivity of the level 1 studies are caused by falsely high estimates of the level 2 studies due to bias.

Surprisingly, the poor sensitivity of FUT observed in the level 1 studies was not only due to failure to detect proximal vein thrombi (as would be expected) but also due to failure to detect calf vein thrombosis. Although there were no level 1 studies in general surgical or medical patients, the poor sensitivity of leg scanning for calf vein thrombi observed in hip surgery indicates that this screening test may also have limitations in non-orthopaedic surgical patients.

Although IPG and real-time ultrasonography have been demonstrated to be highly accurate tests for the diagnosis of proximal vein thrombosis in symptomatic patients, it is known that the tests have poor sensitivity for symptomatic isolated calf vein thrombosis (Huisman et al, 1989; Buller et al, 1991). In the screening of asymptomatic postoperative patients, however, both tests have poor sensitivity for proximal vein thrombosis (sensitivity IPG 23%; sensitivity real-time ultrasonography 54%). Even the combination of FUT with IPG or the combination of IPG with real-time ultrasonography are not effective strategies since more than 50% and 40% of the patients with deep vein thrombosis had normal test results, respectively. It is most likely that differences in characteristics of the thrombi account for the different sensitivities of IPG and real-time ultrasonography in postoperative (orthopaedic) patients compared with symptomatic patients. Indeed, in symptomatic patients thrombi are usually large, occlusive and are extended in the proximal veins, whereas in asymptomatic postoperative patients thrombi are often small, nonocclusive, and confined to the calf veins. Moreover, in asymptomatic patients thrombi are usually fresher than in symptomatic patients, a property that can account for less echogenicity of the thrombus and normal compressibility if evaluated with real-time ultrasonography.

What are the major implications of these analyses? First, it is important for physicians to realise that the occurrence of a normal result of FUT, IPG, or real-time ultrasonography does not exclude the presence of all proximal vein thromboses and most isolated calf vein thrombi in postoperative patients at a high risk for venous thrombosis. Second, meta-analyses which evaluated the efficacy of prophylactic methods for venous thrombosis and included reports that used FUT as the outcome measure, are subject to bias unless the test result is interpreted without knowledge of the outcome of the reference method and the treatment group to which the patient has been assigned. Furthermore, there is also evidence from one large study that the sensitivity of FUT is inversely proportional to the size of the thrombus, the sensitivity for small calf thrombi being 40% and for large calf thrombi 80% (Paiement et al, 1988). Moreover, the sensitivity of leg scanning is influenced by the location of the thrombosis, being less sensitive to thigh vein thrombi than calf vein thrombi. Therefore, prophylactic agents which reduce the size of a thrombus or the incidence of calf vein thrombosis preferentially without altering the incidence of proximal vein thrombosis would produce falsely high estimates of efficacy. For these reasons, FUT is likely to produce false estimates of efficacy even when a randomised trial is double-blinded. All of these shortcomings render the interpretation of meta-analyses of prophylactic studies which use FUT as the primary outcome measure highly questionable.

FUT was developed in the 1960's, was evaluated as a diagnostic test for detection of sub-clinical venous thrombosis in the 1970's and was accepted enthusiastically as an accurate screening test. Although the introduction of this noninvasive approach to screen postoperative patients has provided a convenient method for evaluating new approaches to prophylaxis, it is now clear that this method has serious limitations for the detection of venous thrombosis. Although the diagnostic value of IPG in postoperative patients has never been reported to be comparable with that obtained in symptomatic patients, the results of this analysis excludes any additional role of IPG when used in combination with other noninvasive diagnostic tests. Unfortunately, real-time ultrasonography does not demonstrate a comparable accuracy in postoperative as in symptomatic patients.

At present, venography is the only proven accurate method for the detection of asymptomatic deep vein thrombosis in high risk patients as long as care is paid to its performance and interpretation. It should be noted, however, that this method has several potential drawbacks, in particular its invasiveness and high frequency of inadequate or non-available test results. Therefore, further efforts should be undertaken to optimise the diagnosis of deep vein thrombosis in asymptomatic patients.

# References

Abernethy EA, Hartsuck R. Postoperative pulmonary embolism. Am J Surg 128:739, 1974

Agnelli G, Volpato R, Radicchia S et al. Accuracy of real-time B-mode ultrasonography in the diagnosis of asymptomatic deep vein thrombosis in hip surgery patients. Thromb Haemostas 65:1728, 1991

Aitken AGF, Godden DJ. Real-time ultrasound diagnosis of deep vein thrombosis: a comparison with venography. Clin Radiol 38:309, 1987

Alfaro MJ, Paramo JA, Rocha E. Prophylaxis of thromboembolic disease and platelet changes following total hip replacement: a comparative study of aspirin and heparin-dihydroergotamine. Thromb Haemostas 56:53, 1986

Appelman PT, de Jong TE, Lampman LE et al. Deep venous thrombosis of the leg: US findings. Radiology 163:743, 1987

Atkins P, Hawkins LA. Detection of venous thrombosis in the legs. Lancet 1217, 1965

Barnes RW, Nix ML, Barnes CL et al. Perioperative asymptomatic venous thrombosis: role of duplex scanning versus venography. J Vas Surg 9:251, 1989

Bauer G. A venographic study of thromboembolic problems. Acta Chir Scand 4 (Suppl 161):1, 1940

Baumgartner A, Jacot N, Moser G, Krahenbuhl B. Prevention of postoperative deep vein thrombosis by only one daily injection of low molecular weight heparin and dihydroergotamine. VASA 18:152, 1989

Becker J, Schampi B. The incidence of postoperative venous thrombosis of the legs. Acta Chir Scand 139:357, 1973

Bonnar J, Walsh J. Prevention of thrombosis after pelvic surgery by British Dextran 70. Lancet i:614, 1972

Borow M, Goldson H. Postoperative venous thrombosis. Am J Surg 141:245, 1981

Borris LC, Christiansen HM, Lassen MR et al. Comparison of real-time B-mode ultrasonography and bilateral ascending phlebography for detection of postoperative deep vein thrombosis following elective hip surgery. Thromb Haemost 61:363, 1989

Büller HR, Lensing AWA, Hirsh J, ten Cate JW et al. Deep vein thrombosis: new noninvasive diagnostic tests. Thromb Hemostas 66:133, 1991

Büller HR, Lensing AWA, Hirsh J, ten Cate JW et al. Management of clinically suspected acute venous thrombosis in outpatients with serial impedance plethysmography in a community hospital setting. Arch Int Med 149:511, 1989

Butson ARC. Intermittent pneumatic calf compression for prevention of deep venous thrombosis in general abdominal surgery. Am J Surg 142:525, 1981

Coe NP, Collins REC, Klein LA et al. Prevention of deep vein thrombosis in urological patients: a controlled randomised trial of low dose heparin and external pneumatic compression boots. Surg 83:230, 1978

Comerota AJ, Katz ML, Grossi RJ et al. The comparative value of noninvasive testing for diagnosis and surveillance of deep vein thrombosis. J Vasc Surg 7:40, 1988

Comerota AJ, Katz ML, Greenwald LL et al. Venous duplex imaging: should it replace haemodynamic tests for deep venous thrombosis. J Vasc Surg 11:53, 1990

Covey TH, Sherman L, Baue AE. Low dose heparin in postoperative patients. Arch Surg 110:1021, 1975

Cruickshank MK, Levine MN, Hirsh J et al. An evaluation of impedance plethysmography and $^{125}$I-fibrinogen leg scanning in patients following hip surgery. Thromb Haemostas 62:830, 1989

Davidson B., Elliott CG, Lensing AWA. Low accuracy of colour Doppler ultrasound in the detection of proximal leg vein thrombosis in asymptomatic high-risk patients. Ann Intern Med 117:735, 1992

Dorfman GS, Froehlich JA, Cronan JJ, Urbanek PJ, Herndon JH. Lower-extremity venous thrombosis in patients with acute hip fractures. AJR 154:851, 1990

Encke A, Breddin K. Comparison of a low molecular weight heparin and unfractionated heparin for the prevention of deep vein thrombosis in patients undergoing abdominal surgery. Br J Surg 75:1058, 1988

Eriksson BI, Zachrisson BE, Teger-Nilsson AC, Risberg B. Thrombosis prophylaxis with low molecular weight heparin in total hip replacement. Br J Surg 75:1053, 1988

Faunø P, Suomalainen O, Bergqvist D et al. The use of the fibrinogen uptake test in screening for deep vein thrombosis in patients with hip fracture. Thromb Res 60:185, 1990

Field ES, Nicolaides AN, Kakkar VV, Crelin RQ. Deep vein thrombosis in patients with fractures of the femoral neck. Br J Surg 59:377, 1972

Flanc D, Kakkar VV, Clarke MB. Detection of venous thrombosis of the legs using $^{125}$I-labelled fibrinogen. Br J Surg 55:742, 1968

Flicoteaux H, Kher A, Jean N et al. Comparison of low dose heparin and low dose heparin combined with aspirin in prevention of deep vein thrombosis after total hip replacement. Path Biol 25:55, 1977

Francis CW, Marder VJ, Evarts CM, Yaukoolbodi S. Two step warfarin therapy: prevention of postoperative venous thrombosis without excessive bleeding. JAMA 249:374, 1983

Fredin HO, Nillius SA, Bergqvist D. Prophylaxis of deep vein thrombosis in patients with fracture of the femoral neck. Acta Orthop Scand 53:413, 1982

Fricker JP, Vergnes Y, Schach R et al. Low dose heparin versus low molecular weight heparin in the prophylaxis of thromboembolic complications of abdominal oncological surgery. Eur J Clin Inv 18:561, 1988

Froelich JA, Dorfman GS, Cronan JJ et al. Compression ultrasonography for the detection of deep venous thrombosis in patients who have a fracture of the hip. J Bone Joint Surg 71:249, 1989

Gallus AS, Hirsh J, Tuttle RJ et al. Small subcutaneous doses of heparin in prevention of venous thrombosis. N Engl J Med 288:545, 1973

Gallus AS, Hirsh J, O'Brien S et al. Prevention of venous thrombosis with small, subcutaneous doses of heparin. JAMA 235:1980: 1976

Ginsberg JS, Caco CC, Brill-Edwards P et al. Venous thrombosis in patients who have undergone major hip or knee surgery: Detection with compression US and impedance plethysmography. Radiology 181, 1991

Haeger K. Problems of acute deep venous thrombosis I. The interpretation of signs and symptoms. Angiology 20:219, 1969

Harris WH. Thromboembolic disease in total hip replacement. N Engl J Med 297:1246, 1977

Harris WH, Athanasoulis C, Waltman AC, Salzman EW. Cuff-impedance phlebography and $^{125}$I fibrinogen leg scanning versus roentgenographic phlebography for diagnosis of thrombophlebitis following hip surgery. J Bone Joint Surg 58:939, 1976

Harris WH, Salzman EW, Athanasoulis CA et al. Comparison of $^{125}$I-fibrinogen count scanning for detection of venous thrombi after elective hip surgery. N Engl J Med 292:665, 1975

Harris WH, Salzman EW, Athanasoulis CA et al. Aspirin prophylaxis of venous thromboembolism after total hip replacement. N Engl J Med 297:1246, 1977

Hartl P, Brucke P, Dienstl E, Vinazzer H. Prophylaxis of thromboembolism in general surgery: comparison between standard heparin and fragmin. Thromb Res 57:577, 1990

Hendolin H, Tuppurainen T, Lathinen J. Thoracic epidural analgesia and deep vein thrombosis in cholecystectomised patients. Acta Chir Scand 148:405, 1982

Hirsh J, Levine M. Prevention of venous thrombosis in patients undergoing major orthopaedic surgical procedures. Br J Clin Pract 65 (Suppl):43, 2, 1988

Huisman MV, Buller HR, ten Cate JW, Vreeken J. Serial impedance plethysmography for suspected deep venous thrombosis. The Amsterdam general practitioner study. N Engl J Med 314:823, 1986

Huisman MV, Buller HR, ten Cate JW et al. Management of clinically suspected acute venous thrombosis in outpatients with serial impedance plethysmography in a community hospital setting. Arch Int Med 149:511, 1989

Hull RD, Hirsh J, Carter CJ et al. Diagnostic efficacy of impedance plethysmography for clinically suspected deep-vein thrombosis: a randomised trial. Ann Intern Med 102:21, 1985

Hull R, Hirsh J, Sackett D et al. The value of adding impedance plethysmography to $^{125}$I-fibrinogen leg scanning for the detection of deep vein thrombosis in high risk surgical patients: a comparative study between patients undergoing general and hip surgery. Thromb Res 15:227, 1979

Hull R, Hirsh J, Sackett D et al. Replacement of venography in suspected venous thrombosis by impedance plethysmography and $^{125}$I-fibrinogen leg scanning: a less invasive approach. Ann Intern Med 94:12, 1981

Hull RD, Raskob GE, Gent M et al. Effectiveness of intermittent pneumatic leg compression for preventing deep vein thrombosis after total hip replacement. JAMA 263:2313, 1990

Hull RD, van Aken WG, Hirsh J et al. Impedance plethysmography using the occlusive cuff technique in the diagnosis of venous thrombosis. Circulation 53:696, 1976

Hume M, Gurewich V. Peripheral venous scanning with $^{125}$I-fibrinogen. Lancet 1:845, 1972

Kakkar VV. The diagnosis of deep vein thrombosis using the $^{125}$I-fibrinogen test. Arch Surg 104:152, 1972

Kakkar VV. Deep vein thrombosis. Detection and prevention. Circulation 51:8, 1975

Kakkar VV. Fibrinogen uptake test for detection of deep vein thrombosis - a review of current practice. Sem Nucl Med 7:229, 1977

Kakkar VV, Djazaeri B, Fletcher M et al. Low molecular weight heparin and prevention of postoperative deep vein thrombosis. Br Med J 284:375, 1982

Kakkar VV, Howe CT, Flowe C et al. Natural history of postoperative deep vein thrombosis. Lancet 2:230, 1969

Kakkar VV, Lawrence D, Bentley PG et al. A comparative study of low doses of heparin and a heparin analogue in the prevention of postoperative deep vein thrombosis. Thromb Res 13:111,1978

Kakkar VV, Stringer MD, Hedges AR et al. Fixed combinations of low molecular weight or unfractionated heparin plus dihydroergotamine in the prevention of postoperative deep vein thrombosis. Am J Surg 157:413, 1989

Lambdie JM, Mahafy RG, Barber DC et al. Diagnostic accuracy in venous thrombosis. Br Med J 2:142, 1970

Lensing AWA, Buller HR, Prandoni P et al. Contrast venography, the gold standard for the diagnosis of deep vein thrombosis: improvement in observer agreement. Thromb Haemostas 67:8, 1991

Lensing AWA, Levi MM, Buller HR et al. An objective Doppler method for the diagnosis of deep-vein thrombosis. Ann Intern Med 113:9, 1990

Lensing AWA, Prandoni P, Buller HR et al. Contrast venography: results and side-effects. Radiology 177:503, 1990

Leyvraz PF, Richard J, Bachman F et al. Adjusted versus fixed dose subcutaneous heparin in the prevention of deep vein thrombosis after total hip replacement. N Engl J Med 309:954, 1983

Loudon JR, McCarrity G, Vallance R, Baylis AC, Graham J. The fibrinogen uptake test after hip surgery. Br J Surg 65:616, 1978

Mätzsch T, Bergqvist D, Fredin H, Hedner U. Low molecular weight heparin compared with Dextran as prophylaxis against thrombosis after total hip replacement. Acta Chir Scand 156:445, 1990

McLachlan MSF, Thomson JG, Taylor DW, Kelly ME, Sackett DL. Observer variation in the interpretation of lower limbs venograms. Am J Radiol 132:227, 1979

Milne RM, Griffiths JMT, Gunn AA et al. Postoperative deep venous thrombosis. A comparison of diagnostic techniques. Lancet 1:614, 1971

Monreal M, Montserrat E, Salvador R et al. Real-time ultrasound for diagnosis of symptomatic venous thrombosis and for screening of patients at risk. Angiology 40:527, 1989

Moskovitz PA, Ellenberg SS, Feffer HL et al. Low-dose heparin for prevention of venous thromboembolism in total hip arthroplasty and surgical repair of hip fractures. J Bone Joint Surg 60:1065, 1978

Mussurakis S, Papaioannou S, Voros D, Vrakatselis T. Compression ultrasonography as a reliable imaging monitor in deep venous thrombosis. Surg Gyn Obstet 171:233, 1990

Myrvold HE, Persson JE, Svensson et al. Prevention of thromboembolism with Dextran 70 and heparin in patients with femoral neck fractures. Acta Chir Scand 139:609, 1973

Nandi P, Wong KP, Wei WI et al. Incidence of postoperative deep vein thrombosis in Hong Kong Chinese. Br J Surg 67:251, 1980

Nanson EM, Palko PD, Dick AA et al. Early detection of deep vein thrombosis of the leg using 131-tagged human fibrinogen: a clinical study. Ann Surg 162:438, 1965

Negus D, Pinto DJ, LeQuesne LP et al. $^{125}$I-labelled fibrinogen in the diagnosis of deep vein thrombosis and its correlation with phlebography. Br J Surg 55:835, 1968

Nix ML, Nelson CL, Harmon BH, Ferris EF, Barnes RW. Duplex venous scanning: image vs Doppler accuracy. Soc Vasc Technol 121, 1989

Ockelford PA, Patterson J, Johns AS. A double-blind randomised placebo controlled trial of thromboprophylaxis in major elective general surgery using once daily injections of a low molecular weight heparin fragment. Thromb Haemostas 62:1046, 1987

Onarheim H, Lund T, Heimdal A, Arnesjo B. A low molecular weight heparin for prophylaxis of postoperative deep vein thrombosis. Acta Chir Scand 152:593, 1986

Paiement G, Wessinger SJ, Waltmann AC, Harris WH. Surveillance of deep vein thrombosis in asymptomatic total hip replacement patients. Am J Surg 155:400, 1988

Peters SHA, Jonker JJC, de Boer AC et al. Home diagnosis of deep venous thrombosis with impedance plethysmography. Thromb Haemost 48:297, 1982

Pini M, Tagliaferri A, Manotti C et al. Low molecular weight heparin compared with unfractionated heparin in prevention of deep vein thrombosis after hip fractures. Int Angiol 8:134, 1989

Pinto DJ. Controlled trial of an anticoagulant in prevention of venous thrombosis following hip surgery. Br J Surg 57:349, 1970

Rabinov K, Paulin S. Roengten diagnosis of venous thrombosis in the leg. Arch Surg 104:134, 1972

Raghavendra BN, Horii SC, Hilton S et al. Deep venous thrombosis: detection by probe compression of veins. J Ultrasound Med 5:89, 1986

Raghavendra BN, Rosen RJ, Lam S et al. Deep venous thrombosis: detection by high resolution real-time ultrasonography. Radiology 152:789, 1984

Roberts VC. Fibrinogen uptake scanning for diagnosis of deep vein thrombosis: a plea for standardisation. Br Med J 3:455, 1975

Sackett DL, Haynes RB, Tugwell P. The interpretation of diagnostic data. In: Clinical Epidemiology. A basic science for clinical medicine. Little, Brown and Company, Boston, Toronto, 1985

Salzman EW, Ploetz J, Bettmann M et al. Intraoperative external pneumatic calf compression to afford longterm prophylaxis against deep vein thrombosis in urological patients. Surgery 87:239, 1980

Sasahara AA, Koppenhagen K, Harin R et al. Low molecular weight heparin plus dihydroergotamine for prophylaxis of postoperative deep vein thrombosis. Br J Surg 73:697, 1986

Sautter RD, Larson DE, Bhattacharyya SK et al. The limited utility of fibrinogen $^{125}$-I leg scanning. Arch Intern Med 139:148, 1979

Sautter RD, Koch EL, Myers WO et al. Aspirin-sulfinpyrazone in prophylaxis of deep venous thrombosis in total hip replacement. JAMA 250:2649, 1983

Suomalainen O, Kettunen K, Rissanen V et al. The $^{125}$I-labelled fibrinogen uptake test in elective hip surgery. Ann Clin Res 17:24, 1985

Tsapogas MJ, Goussous H, Peabody RA et al. Postoperative venous thrombosis and the effectiveness of prophylactic measures. Arch Surg 103:561, 1971

Turpie AG, Levine MN, Hirsh J et al. A randomised controlled trial of low molecular weight heparin to prevent deep vein thrombosis in patients undergoing elective hip surgery. N Engl J Med 315:925, 1986

White RH, Goulet JA, Bray TJ et al. Deep vein thrombosis after fracture of the pelvis. J Bone Joint Surg 72A:495, 1990

Woolson ST, McCrory DW, Walter JF et al. B-mode ultrasound scanning in the detection of proximal venous thrombosis after total hip replacement. J Bone Joint Surg 72:983, 1990

Wu TK, Tsapogas MJ, Jordon FR. Prophylaxis of deep venous thrombosis by hydroxychloroquine sulfate and heparin. Surg Gyn Obstet 145:714, 1977

Xabregas A, Gray L, Ham JM. Heparin prophylaxis of deep vein thrombosis in patients with a fractured neck of the femur. Med J Augs 1:620, 1978

CHAPTER 8

# The contribution of colour flow imaging in postoperative surveillance for DVT

**Andrew Nicolaides**
**Evi Kalodiki**

## Introduction

Duplex scanning was developed in the late 1970s by combining real time B-mode imaging and gated Doppler. Compared to today's standards, the resolution of B-mode imaging at that time was relatively poor. Arterial plaques of 2-3 mm were difficult to see in contrast to high resolution modern probes which have a resolution of 0.2 mm. Also, the presence of acoustic shadows from arterial wall calcification made the examination impossible. These problems were overcome by the addition of gated Doppler which enabled the operator to interrogate individual anatomically identified arteries and grade a stenosis on the basis of increased velocities and turbulence. Application of duplex scanning to the venous system became possible with the better resolution provided by the second generation of instruments in the mid and late 1980s. The third generation of instruments offering a high resolution (0.15 to 0.2 mm) and the addition of colour flow imaging have made duplex scanning a very accurate method for the detection of deep vein thrombosis (DVT) in symptomatic patients. Thus, duplex scanning has become the method of choice for the diagnosis of DVT and in hospitals where the facility is available venograms are now rarely performed. There remains the problem of detecting DVT in asymptomatic patients. In the past, the radioactive fibrinogen uptake test (FUT) had fulfilled this role admirably and has enabled us to study the incidence of postoperative DVT and the efficacy of preventive measures in many groups of surgical and medical patients. However, with the advent of AIDS and the increasing risk inherent in the use of blood products, the use of the FUT has become virtually impossible. Also, in orthopaedic patients in whom the FUT is inaccurate because of the surgical wound, venography is the only accurate and acceptable method in clinical trials. A new noninvasive method that would replace both the FUT and venography in screening asymptomatic

**Table 8.1**
Criteria for normal veins or DVT using colour flow imaging

---

Negative scan
    No thrombus visualised
    Spontaneous or augmented flow
    Colour fills entire lumen
    Vein collapses completely with pressure (not in adductor canal)

Positive scan
    Flow absent despite augmentation
    Filling defect present as a definite encroachment on the flow image
    Absence of venous compressibility
    Non-confluence flow image or irregularities of image without consistent areas of encroachment on flow image are highly suggestive of nonocclusive small calf thrombus provided the settings of the instrument are correctly adjusted

---

patients is needed for both practical and financial reasons. It has been the hope of many workers in the field that duplex scanning would become such a method.

The aim of this review is to determine the progress made and the value of duplex scanning in patient surveillance studies. Also, whether the lessons learned from the use of duplex for symptomatic patients can lead to an accurate technique and a practical application in asymptomatic patients.

# Methods of Duplex Scanning for DVT

In some of the early studies, only the B-mode imaging of the duplex scanner was used. This method relied essentially on the ability to make the venous walls approximate each other by compression. It was soon realised that some areas such as the femoral vein in the adductor canal were not compressible and the iliac veins were not visible with the conventional black and white duplex instrument. Thus, pulsed Doppler interrogation of the veins was introduced by some researchers in the field. It is now realised that this is the most important part of the examination, especially in asymptomatic patients (see below). However, it meant that the veins had to be interrogated for spontaneous and augmented flow every few centimetres making the examination very tedious. For this reason, many groups decided not to study the veins below the knee (Table 8.2)

The introduction of colour flow imaging has made the examination much easier. Using the slow flow facility available in all new equipment meant that pelvic and calf veins could be easily visualised so that frequent interrogation using the gated Doppler was not so necessary; also detailed examination of all the veins became possible and the technique was accordingly modified (Table 8.1). Thus, although the scanning routine may be the same, the technical details of the examination and criteria for DVT are different depending on whether one is using a conventional duplex or one with colour flow imaging.

### Position of the Patient and Scanning Routine

It is essential that the legs are lower than the trunk so that the veins are full of blood. This is achieved by tilting the bed 30° or if possible examining the patient in the standing (for

## Table 8.2
Prospective studies evaluating B-mode or conventional duplex in symptomatic patients

|  | Limbs studied | DVT on Venography | B-mode or duplex +ve (sensitivity) | B-mode or duplex -ve (specificity) |
|---|---|---|---|---|
| Appelman et al, 1987[*] | 110 | 50 | 48/ 50 (96%) | 58/ 60 (97%) |
| Cronan et al, 1987[*] | 51 | 28 | 25/ 28 (89%) | 23/ 23 (100%) |
| Aitken & Golden, 1987[*] | 42 | 16 | 15/ 16 (94%) | 26/ 26 (100%) |
| Elias et al, 1987 | 847 | 333 | 325/333 (98%) | 483/514 (94%) |
| Vogel et al, 1987[*] | 53 | 20 | 19/ 20 (95%) | 33/ 33 (100%) |
| Lensing et al, 1989 | 220 | 77 | 70/ 77 (91%) | 142/143 (99%) |
| Mussurakis et al, 1990 | 94 | 36 | 30/ 36 (83%) | 58/ 58 (100%) |
| Fletcher et al, 1990[*] | 44 | 14 | 14/ 14 (100%) | 29/ 30 (97%) |
| van Ramshorst et al 91[*] | 120 | 64 | 58/ 64 (91%) | 53/ 56 (95%) |
| TOTAL | 1581 | 638 | 604/638 (95%) | 905/943 (96%) |
| 95% Confidence Interval |  |  | (92.9%-94.7%) | (94.7%-97.2%) |

[*] Calf veins not studied or not included in the analysis

common and superficial femoral vein) and sitting position (for popliteal and calf veins). Whatever position or positions are adopted, it is essential that the patient is comfortable and that the muscles are relaxed with slight flexion of the hip and knee. It should be remembered that full knee extension occludes the popliteal vein in 20% of normal people (Leon et al, 1992).

One starts the examination at the common femoral vein and proceeds distally to the adductor hiatus. Also, the long saphenous vein is examined at this stage. The patient then changes position, from standing to sitting or from supine to prone with the feet on a pillow to ensure slight knee flexion. If this position is not possible, the lateral decubitus position is an alternative with the leg to be examined uppermost. The popliteal vein and its tributaries are examined systematically; also the short saphenous, gastrocnemius, soleal, posterior tibial, anterior tibial and peroneal veins. All veins are compressed at frequent intervals while imaged in transverse section and the Doppler is used to interrogate the vein if the latter is not compressible or too painful.

The following features and criteria for DVT should be looked for:
- The presence of a clot in the lumen. This may be seen if it is several days old. However, a fresh clot which has the same echogenicity as blood is often not visible.
- Absence of venous compressibility with absence of flow on pulsed Doppler interrogation is the most reliable criterion. The infrapopliteal veins are small and unless modern third-generation high resolution instruments are used, interpretation is difficult.
- Pulsed Doppler interrogation determines whether flow is present. Flow which is spontaneous, phasic with respiration, augmented with distal gentle compression indicates normality. Continuous, non-phasic flow with impaired augmentation on distal compression should warn the examiner that there is an abnormality.
- Partial occlusion at the examined site or complete occlusion more proximally or distally.

**Table 8.3**
Prospective studies evaluating B-mode or conventional duplex for diagnosing symptomatic calf DVT

|  | Limbs studied | DVT on Venography | B-mode or duplex +ve (sensitivity) | B-mode or duplex -ve (specificity) |
|---|---|---|---|---|
| Elias et al, 1987 | 593 | 92 | 84/ 92 (91%) | 483/501 (96%) |
| Fletcher et al, 1990 | 43 | 13 | 11/ 13 (85%) | 25/ 30 (83%) |
| Mitchell et al, 1991 | 49 | 21 | 17/ 21 (81%) | 25/ 28 (89%) |
| TOTAL | 685 | 126 | 112/126 (89%) | 533/559 (95%) |
| 95% Confidence Interval |  |  | (83.4%-94.3%) | (93.6%-97.1%) |

**Colour Flow Scanning Routine**
The same scanning sequence is used as with the conventional duplex and the same criteria for DVT are available. However, with the presence of colour there is less need for compression and the emphasis on the criteria is slightly different. By using the slow-flow facility, spontaneous flow phasic with respiration should be visible in practically all the veins. Only velocities less than 1 cm per second are not visible. By convention, colour is assigned as blue for flow centrally and red for flow distally. In the calf, using the colour, finding the artery and the venae comitantes is relatively easy. Augmentation with gentle calf or foot compression producing visualisation of both venae comitantes clearly and uniformly throughout their length makes compression unnecessary. Absence of visible flow despite augmentation is an indication to use compression. The colour is switched off and compression is applied with the probe held transversely to the artery. Non-confluent filling of the vein or irregular flow with augmentation suggests a partially occluding thrombus provided the settings of the duplex scan are correctly adjusted (Table 8.1)

# Results of Prospective Studies in Symptomatic Patients

The results of prospective studies evaluating B-mode or conventional duplex in symptomatic patients are summarised in tables 8.2 — 8.5. The overall sensitivity and specificity for DVT proximal to the calf using B-mode or conventional duplex are 95% and 96% respectively with 95% confidence intervals in excess of 90%. Those who had instruments with high resolution and looked for calf DVT found sensitivities and specificities in excess of 80% (Table 8.3). With the advent of colour flow imaging more researchers confirmed the value of duplex not only for proximal (Table 8.4) but also for calf DVT (Table 8.5).

Using colour flow imaging, the overall sensitivity and specificity for proximal DVT were 97% and 99% and for calf DVT were 87% and 91% respectively. The examination is much shorter: all the veins can be systematically studied in 30 minutes.

**Results from Postoperative Surveillance Studies**
In contrast to studies in symptomatic patients, B-mode compression was poor for proximal DVT (overall sensitivity 59%) (Table 8.6) and very poor for calf DVT (overall sensitivity 16%) (Table 8.7).

### Table 8.4
Colour-coded duplex for symptomatic DVT (femoropopliteal segment)

|  | Limbs studied | DVT | Duplex +ve (sensitivity) | Duplex -ve (specificity) |
|---|---|---|---|---|
| Foley et al, 1989 | 47 | 19 | 17/ 19 (89%) | 28/ 28 (100%) |
| Persson et al, 1989 | 23 | 15 | 15/ 15 (100%) | 8 /8 (100%) |
| Rose et al, 1990 | 75 | 26 | 25/ 26 (96%) | 49/ 49 (100%) |
| Schindler et al, 1990 | 94 | 55 | 54/ 55 (98%) | 39/ 39 (100%) |
| Mattos et al, 1992 | 77 | 32 | 32/ 32 (100%) | 44/ 45 (98%) |
| Kalodiki et al, 1992 | 100 | 34 | 32/ 34 (94%) | 64/ 66 (97%) |
| TOTAL | 416 | 181 | 175/181 (96.6%) | 232/235 (98.7%) |
| 95% Confidence Interval |  |  | (94%-99.3%) | (97.2%-100%) |

### Table 8.5
Colour-coded duplex for symptomatic DVT (calf veins)

|  | Limbs studied | DVT | Duplex +ve (sensitivity) | Duplex -ve (specificity) |
|---|---|---|---|---|
| Foley et al, 1989 | 16 | 4 | 4/ 4 (100%) | 12/ 12 (100%) |
| Rose et al, 1990 | 74 | 30 | 22/30 (73%) | 38/ 44 (86%) |
| Mattos et al, 1992 | 75 | 33 | 31/33 (94%) | 34/ 42 (81%) |
| Kalodiki et al, 1992 | 100 | 12 | 11/12 ( 92%) | 85/ 88 (97%) |
| TOTAL | 265 | 79 | 68/79 (86%) | 169/186 (91%) |
| 95% Confidence Interval |  |  | (78.4%-93.7%) | (86.7%-95%) |

### Table 8.6
B-mode compression in postoperative surveillance studies (femoropopliteal segment)

|  | Limbs studied | DVT | Duplex +ve (sensitivity) | Duplex -ve (specificity) |
|---|---|---|---|---|
| Borris et al, 1989 | 60 | 24 | 15/24 (63%) | 34/ 36 (94%) |
| Borris et al, 1990 | 61 | 11 | 8/11 (73%) | 48/ 50 (96%) |
| Ginsberg et al, 1991 | 247 | 21 | 10/21 (52%) | 219/226 (97%) |
| Kalodiki et al, 1993 | 44 | 9 | 5/ 9 (55%) | 33/ 35 (94%) |
| TOTAL | 412 | 65 | 38/65 (58%) | 334/347 (96%) |
| 95% Confidence Interval |  |  | (46.5%-70.4%) | (94.2%-98.2%) |

**Table 8.7**
B-mode compression in postoperative surveillance studies (calf veins)

|  | Limbs studied | DVT | Duplex +ve (sensitivty) | Duplex -ve (specificity) |
|---|---|---|---|---|
| Borris et al, 1989 | 60 | 14 | 4/14 (29%) | — |
| Borris et al, 1990 | 61 | 3 | 2/ 3 (67%) | — |
| Ginsberg et al, 1991 | 223 | 37 | 2/37 (5%) | 184/186 (99%) |
| TOTAL | 344 | 54 | 8/54 (16%) |  |
| 95% Confidence Interval |  |  | (5.3%-24.3%) |  |


**Table 8.8**
Conventional duplex in postoperative surveillance studies (femoropopliteal segment)

|  | Limbs studied | DVT | Duplex +ve (sensitivity) | Duplex -ve (specificity) |
|---|---|---|---|---|
| Barnes et al, 1989 | 153 | 12 | 10/12 (83%) | 135/141 (96%) |
| Froelich et al, 1989 | 40 | 5 | 5/ 5 (100%) | 34/ 35 (97%) |
| Woolson et al, 1990 | 150 | 19 | 17/19 (89%) | 131/131 (100%) |
| Comerota et al, 1990 | 36 | 7 | 7/ 7 (100%) | 29/ 29 (100%) |
| White et al, 1990 | 32 | 12 | 11/12 (92%) | 20/ 20 (100%) |
| TOTAL | 412 | 55 | 50/55 (91%) | 349/356 (98%) |
| 95% Confidence Interval |  |  | (83.3%-98.5%) | (96.6%-99.5%) |


**Table 8.9**
Colour coded duplex in postoperative surveillance studies (hip arthroplasty — femoral and popliteal)

|  | Limbs studied | DVT | Duplex +ve (sensitivity) | Duplex -ve (specificity) |
|---|---|---|---|---|
| Mattos et al, 1992 | 92 | 2 | 2/ 2 (100%) | 90/ 90 (100%) |
| Kalodiki et al, 1993 | 107 | 14 | 13/14 N(93%) | 92/ 93 (99%) |
| TOTAL | 199 | 16 | 15/16 (94%) | 182/183 (99%) |
| 95% Confidence Interval |  |  | (82%-100%) | (98.4%-100%) |

**Table 8.10**
Colour coded duplex in postoperative surveillance studies (hip arthroplasty — calf veins)

|  | Limbs studied | DVT | Duplex +ve (sensitivity) | Duplex -ve (specificity) |
|---|---|---|---|---|
| Mattos et al, 1992 | 92 | 24 | 19/24 (79%) | 66/ 68 (97%) |
| Kalodiki et al, 1993 | 107 | 19 | 15/19 (79%) | 85/ 88 (96%) |
| TOTAL | 199 | 43 | 34/43 (79%) | 151/156 (97%) |
| 95% Confidence Interval |  |  | (67%-91%) | (94%-99.5%) |

Conventional duplex for femoropopliteal segment DVT was better with an overall sensitivity of 91% and specificity of 98% (Table 8.8).

Only one study by Comerota et al (1990) addressed the problem of calf DVT using conventional duplex scanning. In 50 limbs there were two isolated calf thrombi of which one was detected. Duplex scanning was negative in all 29 limbs with normal venograms (specificity 100%). In this study the numbers were too small to draw any conclusions.

Two studies have investigated the accuracy of colour coded duplex in postoperative patients having elective hip surgery (Tables 8.9 and 8.10). The data shown in the tables have been obtained by both teams after modifying the conventional technique to that of colour as described above and after they had been through their learning curve. They concluded that the high sensitivities obtained for both proximal and calf thrombi demonstrated the potential for the use of colour coded duplex in postoperative surveillance.

# Discussion and Conclusions

The results published by several teams indicate that accurate results are more difficult to obtain in asymptomatic than symptomatic patients. It is obvious that B-mode compression alone is not enough and although good results can be obtained with conventional duplex scanning for thrombosis proximal to the calf (overall sensitivity 91% and specificity 98% — Table 8.8), colour flow imaging is essential for the detection of calf thrombi. The methodology available would allow clinical trials to be performed in asymptomatic patients with popliteal and femoral thrombosis as an endpoint. Considering that only 20% of the thrombi that start in the calf propagate into the popliteal and more proximal segments, the number of patients that should be included in such studies would be five times the number required when calf thrombosis is the endpoint.

The availability of colour coded duplex scanning to detect calf thrombosis may overcome this problem. However, before one undertakes a surveillance study in asymptomatic patients, one should demonstrate the accuracy of duplex scanning in one's own hands against venography. In addition, until the accuracy of colour duplex scanning is confirmed by several other groups, positive duplex scans in surveillance studies should be confirmed by venography. This was the practice of the 1970s when the FUT test was used. This will be an important factor that would give credibility to the method and to such studies.

# References

Aitken AG, Godden DJ. Real-time ultrasound diagnosis of deep vein thrombosis: a comparison with venography. Clin Radiol 38 (3):309, 1987

Appelman PT, De Jong TE, Lampmann LE. Deep venous thrombosis of the leg: US findings. Radiology 163:743, 1987

Barnes RW, Nix ML, Barnes CL, Lavender RC, Godden WE, Harmon BH, Ferris EJ, Nelson CL. Perioperative asymptomatic venous thrombosis: role of duplex scanning versus venography. J Vas Surg 9:251, 1989

Borris LC, Christiansen HM, Lassen MR, Olsen AD, Schøtt P. Comparison of real-time B-mode ultrasonography and bilateral ascending phlebography for detection of postoperative deep vein thrombosis following elective hip surgery. The Venous Thrombosis Group. Thromb Haemost 61 (3):363, 1989

Borris LC, Christiansen HM, Lassen MR, Olsen AD, Schøtt P. Real-time B-mode ultrasonography in the diagnosis of postoperative deep vein thrombosis in non-symptomatic high-risk patients. Eur J Vasc Surg 4 (5):473, 1990

Comerota AJ, Katz ML, Greenwald LL, Leefmans E, Czeredarczuk M, White JV. Venous duplex imaging: should it replace hemodynamic tests for deep venous thrombosis? J Vasc Surg 11 (1):53-9, discussion 59, 1990

Cronan JJ, Dorfman GS, Scola FH, Schepps B, Alexander J. Deep venous thrombosis: US assessment using vein compression. Radiology 162:191, 1987

Elias A, Le Corff G, Bouvier JL, Benichou M, Serradimigni A. Value of real-time B-mode ultrasound imaging in the diagnosis of deep vein thrombosis of the lower limbs. Int Angiol 6:175, 1987

Fletcher JP, Kershaw LZ, Barker DS, Koutts J, Varnava A. Ultrasound diagnosis of lower limb deep venous thrombosis. Med J Aust 153:453, 1990

Foley WD, Middleton WD, Lawson TL, Erickson S, Quiroz FA, Macrander S. Colour Doppler ultrasound imaging of lower-extremity venous disease. AJR 152:371, 1989

Froelich JA, Dorfman GS, Cronan JJ, Urbanek PJ, Herndon JH, Aaron RK. Compression ultrasonography for the detection of deep venous thrombosis in patients who have a fracture of the hip. J Bone Joint Surg 71:249, 1989

Ginsberg JS, Caco CC, Brill-Edwards P, Panju AA, Bona R, Demers CM, Tuters LM, Nugent P, McGinnis J, Grant BM, Vander Lander Vries MA. Venous thrombosis in patients who have undergone major hip or knee surgery: Detection with compression ultrasonography and impedance plethysmography. Radiology 181:651, 1991

Kalodiki E, Marston R, Volteas N, Leon M, Labropoulos N, Fisher CM, Christopoulos D, Touquet R, Nicolaides AN. The combination of liquid crystal thermography and duplex scanning in the diagnosis of deep vein thrombosis. Eur J Vasc Surg 6:311, 1992

Kalodiki E, Geroulakos G, Nicolaides AN. B-mode and colour flow duplex imaging versus venography in postoperative surveillance of toal hip replacement patients. International Union of Angiology and Societé d'Angiologie de langue Française XXème Congress, Beaune 7-8 Oct 1993 (Abstr)

Legemate DA, Verzijlbergen JF, Hoeneveld H, Eikelboom BC, de Valois JC, Meuwissen OJATh. Duplex scanning in the diagnosis of acute deep vein thrombosis of the lower extremity. Eur J Vasc Surg 5:255, 1991

Lensing AWA, Prandoni P, Brandjes D, Huisman PM, Vigo M, Tomasella G, Krekt J, ten Cate JW, Huisman MV, Büller HR. Detection of deep-vein thrombosis by realtime B-mode ultrasonography. N Engl J Med 320:342, 1989

Leon M, Volteas N, Labropoulos N, Hajj H, Kalodiki E, Fisher CM, Chan P, Belcaro GV, Nicolaides AN. Popliteal entrapment in the normal population. Eur J Vasc Surg 6:623, 1992

Mattos MA, Londrey GL, Leutz DW, Hodgson KJ, Ramsey DE, Barkmeier LD, Stauffer ES, Spadone DP, Sumner DS. Colour-flow duplex scanning for the surveillance and diagnosis of acute deep vein thrombosis. J Vasc Surg 15:366, 1992

Mitchell DC, Grasty MS, Stebbings WS, Nockler IB, Lewars MD, Levison RA, Wood RF. Comparison of duplex ultrasonography and venography in the diagnosis of deep venous thrombosis. Br J Surg 78:611, 1991

Mussurakis S, Papaioannou S, Voros D, Vrakatselis T. Compression ultrasonography as a reliable imaging monitor in deep venous thrombosis. Surg Gyn Obstet 171:233, 1990

Persson AV, Jones C, Zide R, Jewell ER. Use of the triplex scanner in diagnosis of deep venous thrombosis. Arch Surg 124:593, 1989

Rose SC, Zwiebel WJ, Nelson BD, Priest DL, Knighton RA, Brown JW, Lawrence PF, Stults BM, Reading JC, Miller FJ. Symptomatic lower extremity deep venous thrombosis: Accuracy, limitations and role of colour duplex flow imaging in diagnosis. Radiology 175:639, 1990

Schindler JM, Kaiser M, Gerber A, Vailliomenet A, Popovich A, Bertel O. Colour coded duplex sonography in suspected deep vein thrombosis of the leg. Br Med J 301:1369, 1990

Vogel P, Laing FC, Jeffrey RB Jr, Wing VW. Deep venous thrombosis of the lower extremity: US evaluation. Radiology 163 (3):747, 1987

White RH, Goulet JA, Bray TJ, Daschbach MM, McGahan JP, Hartling RP. Deep vein thrombosis after fracture of the pelvis: Assessment with serial duplex ultrasound screening. J Bone Joint Surg 72 (4):495, 1990

Woolson ST, McCroy DW, Walter JF, Maloney WJ, Watt JM, Cahill PD. B-mode ultrasound scanning in the detection of proximal venous thrombosis after total hip replacement. J Bone Joint Surg 72 (7):983, 1990

CHAPTER 9

# Venography in asymptomatic patients having total hip replacement: inter-observer variation

Lars C Borris   Michael R Lassen

## Introduction
At present venography is the only accepted diagnostic method in clinical studies of prophylaxis of DVT in patients undergoing hip or knee operations and it is the standard with which other diagnostic methods are compared. However, although the technique of venography can be highly standardised, the interpretation of a venographic examination depends on the observer. Several studies have reported a considerable intra- and inter-observer variation with rather low Kappa values (McLachlan et al, 1979; Picolet et al, 1990; Lensing et al, 1992). The aim of this chapter is to report the inter-observer variation and its influence in the interpretation of lower limb venograms in a prophylaxis study; in addition, we wish to present the current state of knowledge about the methodological pitfalls of venography.

## Material and methods

### Material
The study comprised 210 patients (Lassen et al, 1991) wearing thigh-length compression stockings who underwent total hip replacement. It was a double-blind, randomised, parallel group study, and the patients were randomly allocated to two groups: In the logiparin group, patients had injections with a low molecular weight heparin (Logiparin[R], Novo Nordisk A/S, Bagsvaerd, Denmark), once daily for 7 postoperative days, starting 2 hours before operation, and in the placebo group, patients had a similar series of injections with saline.

Patients were examined with bilateral ascending venography between days 8 and 10 after operation.

### Venographic Technique
The most commonly used technique or modifications of the technique has been described by Rabinov and Paulin (1972). The patient is placed in a semi-upright position on a tilting fluoroscopic examination table and with the examined leg in a non-weight bearing position. The contrast medium is injected into a dorsal foot vein. It is common practice to use a nonionic contrast medium although it is not yet definitively proven that it causes fewer thrombotic complications. It is well documented that there are fewer local complications with these media compared with the high osmolar ionic media (Laerum and Holm, 1981; Lensing et al, 1990). The volume of contrast medium used is important because if it is too small it will not provide a proper contrast intensity and thereby will obscure the diagnosis. Approximately 75–125 ml is recommended for one leg (Rabinov and Paulin, 1972). One tourniquet or more may be used to improve filling of the deep veins but it is often not necessary. During the examination a number of separate exposures of the calf, popliteal and thigh veins are made in the antero-posterior and lateral views when maximal contrast filling of the veins is present as determined by fluoroscopic means.

The final outcome will depend upon the experience of the examiner, the co-operation of the patient, the quality of the veins and — last but not least — the interpretation of the venograms.

### Diagnostic criteria of deep vein thrombosis
It is uncommon to find a definition of the deep veins of the legs in prophylaxis studies. Most often the deep veins are defined as the deep plantar veins of the foot, the three paired crural veins, the popliteal vein, the superficial and deep femoral veins of the thigh, and finally the common femoral vein to the inguinal ligament. It is not uncommon to find that the deep muscular veins of gastrocnemius and soleus in the lower leg and the numerous communicating veins connecting the superficial and deep veins in the foot and lower leg are not considered to belong to the deep veins. This is despite the fact that the majority of thrombi after surgery are formed in the muscular veins.

The most commonly used diagnostic criterion of fresh postoperative thrombosis is the presence of an intraluminal filling defect (Rabinov and Paulin, 1972; Zachrisson and Jansen, 1973). Most authors also agree that filling defects must be "constant", i.e., have the same position and shape in all projections or in at least two different projections. A number of false signs mimicking filling defects due to inadequate mixing of blood and contrast medium have been previously described (Zachrisson and Jansen, 1973). Non-filling of a vein segment, commonly seen with the deep femoral vein and some crural veins, is only an indirect sign of thrombosis and is not considered to be reliable except when other signs are present. Non-filling may be due to reasons other than thrombosis such as external or internal compression of the vein by muscle contraction, tumours, fracture haematomas, bandages and oedema. However, there does not exist a clear consensus about how the phenomenon must be interpreted.

### Evaluation of Venograms
In our study, all venograms were evaluated by two independent observers without any knowledge of the result of the randomisation. The diagnostic criterion for deep vein thrombosis (DVT) at both evaluations was a constant filling defect. The main endpoint of

**Table 9.1**
The number of patients with or without DVT by the first and second observer

|  | First observer |  |  |  |
|---|---|---|---|---|
|  | Logiparin |  | Placebo |  |
|  | + | — | + | — |
| Second observer |  |  |  |  |
| + | 16 | 0 | 28 | 3 |
| — | 14 | 71 | 16 | 51 |

the study was the presence of a thromboembolic complication (DVT or pulmonary embolism — PE) in the postoperative period.

## Results

28 patients were excluded from the analysis due to the preset criteria of eligibility. None of the patients developed any symptoms of DVT during the study. Two patients (one in each group) developed PE. With respect to the evaluation of the venograms, there was extensive disagreement between the two observers, resulting in a 44% reduction in the total number of thrombi diagnosed at the second compared with the first evaluation (112 thrombi vs. 63). The number of patients with or without the diagnosis of a thromboembolic complication at the first versus the second evaluation is shown in table 9.1. In the logiparin group, the number of patients with thromboembolic complications was reduced from 30 (30%) to 16 (16%) from the first to the second evaluation, and in the placebo group from 44 (45%) patients to 28 (29%). However, this reduction was not significantly different between the two groups (p=0.53).

## Discussion

Despite well defined diagnostic criteria it has been documented that the interpretation of venograms is subject to a considerable degree of intra- and inter-observer variations in previous studies. When agreement is assessed, it is necessary to use the kappa statistic in order to take into account agreement by chance. A kappa value of +1 indicates perfect agreement, whereas a value of O indicates that agreement is entirely due to chance. A kappa value of less than 0.50 is generally accepted as expressing poor concordance. In previous studies on interpretation of venograms kappa values for intra-observer variation for the diagnosis of deep vein thrombosis have been between 0.66 to 0.93 (McLachlan et al, 1979; Picolet et al, 1990) and for interobserver variation between 0.67 and 0.89 (McLachlan et al, 1979; Wille-Jørgensen et al, 1992). These values of kappa are usually considered low for a diagnostic test which is considered to be "the gold standard". It would be reasonable to expect the observer variations to be even more pronounced in the interpretation of venograms from asymptomatic patients, i.e., patients screened postoperatively for deep vein thrombosis in prophylaxis studies because thrombi in such patients are mostly small, non-occluding and exclusively confined to the veins of the calf where they may be difficult to localise (Kälebo et al, 1990)

In a double-blind multicentre study in 1,290 patients undergoing general surgery, the impact of variations in the interpretation of the venograms has been studied also. The study was a three-armed comparison between two doses of a low molecular weight heparin and standard heparin in the prevention of postoperative thromboembolism. DVT was detected by the fibrinogen uptake test and confirmed by venography. The venograms were evaluated twice by two observers at an interval of 4 months. At the final evaluation, all discrepancies were settled by the intervention of a third observer. The result of the final evaluation was used in analysis of the study and it showed that only the highest dose of low molecular weight heparin was as effective as the standard heparin regimen in the prevention of DVT (Liezorovicz et al, 1991). When based on the result of the first reading all three regimens were equally effective (Picolet et al, 1990). Technical differences in equipment between centres and differences in training of the examiners, together with problems during the central reading procedure were emphasised to explain the observed discrepancies in this study.

At present venography is the only reliable diagnostic method to use for screening purposes in postoperative patients especially after hip and knee operations. Different actions can be taken to minimise the variations in the interpretation of venograms. First of all, the venographic procedures must be standardised in all detail and the examinations must be performed in well equipped centres by a limited number of well-trained examiners. In a recently published study it was recommended to use long-leg films instead of spot films based on the findings that the inadequacy rate thereby was significantly reduced from 20% to 2% and the interobserver variation from 21% to 4% which caused the kappa value to increase significantly from 0.65 to 0.92 (Lensing et al, 1992). It is also important to have strictly defined diagnostic criteria. In some studies, reading committees consisting of two or more expert radiologists are used. The members must be given the opportunity to discuss the diagnostic criteria before evaluation of the venograms in order to minimise differences. This approach resulted in an improved agreement between two different observers in a previous study (Zachrisson and Jansen, 1973). In every case of disagreement, members of the reading committee will meet to reach a consensus on the presence or absence of thrombosis.

It is less well recognised but beyond doubt that part of the observed variation between different observers is due to difference in the clinical situation in which the evaluation is carried out. In the daily routine situation where a symptomatic patient is referred to the radiology department for venography, it is obvious that equivocal examinations may often result in a positive diagnosis of DVT in order not to withhold necessary treatment from the patient. This is in contrast to the situation in a clinical study in which venography is carried out in asymptomatic patients for screening purposes. The radiologists evaluating the venograms for the purpose of the study are well aware that the outcome of the evaluation will have no therapeutic consequences to the patients and therefore there may be a tendency towards a more rigorous evaluation in this situation resulting in a higher inadequacy rate and fewer positive diagnoses.

## Conclusions

Variations in the interpretation of venograms may be minimised but cannot be totally avoided. It is therefore important to be aware of these variations when results of prophylaxis studies using venography are considered. Thus, it is the relative risk reduction obtained with a certain prophylactic regimen rather than the actual incidence of deep vein thrombosis that should be used in the conclusions. Most important, however, is the realisation that it is not possible to perform direct comparisons of results of different prophylaxis studies even though the same diagnostic criteria are used in the evaluation of the venograms.

## References

Borris LC, Lassen MR, Hull R, Rascob G. Impact of different evaluations of phlebography in a clinical study. Read before the International Symposium: Low molecular weight heparins and related polysaccharides, Munich, Germany, 1991

Kälebo P, Anthmyr BA, Eriksson BE, Zachrisson BE. Phlebographic findings in venous thrombosis following total hip replacement. Acta Radiol 31:259, 1990

Laerum F, Holm HA. Postphlebographic thrombosis. A double blind study with methylglucamine metrizoate and metrizamide. Radiology 140:651, 1981

Lassen MR, Borris LC, Christiansen HM et al. Prevention of thromboembolism in 190 hip arthroplasties. Comparison of LMW heparin and placebo. Acta Orthop Scand 62:33, 1991

Liezorovicz A, Picolet H, Peyrieux JC, Boissel JP. Prevention of perioperative deep vein thrombosis in general surgery: a multicentre double blind study comparing two doses of Logiparin and standard heparin. Br J Surg 78:412, 1991

Lensing AWA, Büller HR, Prandoni P et al. Contrast venography, the gold standard for the diagnosis of deep vein thrombosis: improvement in observer agreement. Thromb Haemost 67:8, 1992

Lensing AWA, Prandoni P, Büller HR, Casara D, Cogo A, ten Cate JW. Lower extremity venography with Iohexol: results and complications. Radiology 177:503, 1990

McLachlan MSF, Thomson JG, Taylor DW, Kelly ME, Sackett DI. Observer variation in the interpretation of lower limb venograms. AJR 132:227, 1979

Picolet H, Liezorovicz A, Revel D, Chirossel P, Amiel M, Boissel JP. Reliability of phlebographies for the assessment of venous thrombosis in a clinical trial. Haemostasis 20:362, 1990

Rabinov K, Paulin S. Roentgen diagnosis of venous thrombosis in the leg. Arch Surg 104:134, 1972

Wille-Jørgensen P, Borris LC, Jørgensen LN et al. Phlebography as the gold standard in thromboprophylactic studies. Acta Radiol 33:24, 1992

Zachrisson BE, Jansen H. Phlebographic signs in fresh postoperative venous thrombosis of the lower extremity. Acta Radiol (Diagn) 14:82, 1973

CHAPTER 10

# Natural history of deep vein thrombosis

Ganesh Ramaswami   Andrew N Nicolaides

## Introduction

The development of the $^{125}$I-fibrinogen uptake test (FUT) in the late sixties, made possible the early detection of deep vein thrombosis, when the patient was still asymptomatic. It soon came to be realised that in surgical patients the majority of thrombi started in the calf and subsequently approximately 20% underwent proximal extension.

The natural history of any disease process may be defined as the evolution of the disease in the absence of therapeutic intervention. The diagnosis of a thrombus in the deep veins of the calf may be possible when the patient is still asymptomatic with the help of the FUT. Once formed, the thrombus may either (a) lyse spontaneously, (b) extend and propagate proximally in the deep venous system, (c) embolise, resulting in pulmonary embolism which may either be asymptomatic or symptomatic, non-fatal or fatal, (d) recanalise over several weeks or months, causing destruction of venous valves with the development of the post-thrombotic syndrome with resultant pain, swelling, liposclerosis eczema and eventually ulceration of the lower limbs and finally (e) the thrombus may recur.

The aim of this chapter is to provide a review of the overall incidence of deep vein thrombosis (calf and proximal), lysis, progression, and the relationship of these to pulmonary embolism, recurrent DVT and late sequelae, i.e. the post-thrombotic syndrome.

## Pathology and Symptoms

Whatever the nature of the initiating factors, the earliest recognisable event in thrombosis is platelet aggregation, which begins as microscopic nidi in valve cusp pockets, vein junctions or in saccules. These primary thrombi grow by laminated accretion of layers of platelets and fibrin in the direction of blood flow and are firm in consistency. When primary thrombi are large enough to occlude flow, secondary propagation occurs, in most instances antegrade but sometimes in a retrograde manner. Secondary thrombi are less dense than primary thrombi and are composed of a loose homogenous mass of fibrin in which are enmeshed leucocytes, platelets and red cells.

Spontaneous lysis of the thrombi may occur as a result of local fibrinolytic activity (plasminogen activator release) and the condition may resolve without the patient experiencing any symptoms. Although small thrombi may lyse completely, it is uncommon for larger thrombi to do so and incomplete lysis may lead to shrinkage and retraction of organised thrombus with reduction in the luminal diameter of the vein. The presence of these webs within the lumen predisposes to recurrent episodes of thrombosis. Furthermore, incomplete lysis of thrombi leads to mechanical impairment of valve cusps with deep vein reflux and its attendant sequelae, namely pain, swelling, pigmentation and ulceration. Thus, the post thrombotic syndrome is effectively the result of incomplete recanalisation of the deep veins (outflow obstruction) and valve incompetence (reflux).

The onset of symptoms such as pain and swelling are dependent upon the degree and duration of venous obstruction and also on the state of the collateral supply. Two of the earliest clinical signs described are increased warmth of the limb and also dilatation of superficial veins. These are due to collateral filling bypassing a thrombosed vein as well as an inflammatory response. Congestion of the vasa vasorum as a result of this inflammatory response leads to oedema in the perivenous tissue with local discomfort, induration and tenderness. The development of swelling is dependent upon the extent of outflow obstruction. The thrombus may be extensive and still not cause complete obstruction to venous outflow, resulting in the late onset of swelling. However, thrombus occluding a collateral tributary from a vein may lead to the rapid onset of symptoms. The site and extent of swelling will also provide a clue as to the site of thrombus. Swelling of the ankle and foot suggests that the deep veins of the calf are involved. Swelling of the thigh, suggests involvement of the ileofemoral segment, whilst swelling of the groin along with the thigh and calf means the presence of iliac thrombosis extending up to the inferior vena cava.

Virchow realised the relationship between deep vein thrombosis occurring in the lower limb and pulmonary embolism when he wrote "Secondary disturbances are very frequently occasioned by the detachment of larger or smaller fragments from the end of softening thrombus which are carried along by the current of blood and driven into remote vessels. This gives rise to the very frequent process upon which I have endowed the name EMBOLIA. Thus we can see that as a rule all the thrombi from the periphery of the body produce secondary obstruction and metastatic deposits in the lung" (Virchow, 1860).

The lodgement of an embolus in the pulmonary arterial tree leads to reduction of pulmonary arterial bed. If the embolus is large enough, the sudden mechanical occlusion by itself may cause death. With emboli of smaller size, the pulmonary arterial pressure rises with concomitant increased work-load on the right ventricle. Compensatory mechanisms come into play and blood flow to the opposite lung increases along with a fall in peripheral resistance. It must be noted that the reserve capacity is such that more than 50% of the pulmonary arterial bed must be lost before significant hypertension develops. If the myocardium is healthy, local autoregulatory mechanisms cause an increase in coronary blood flow. But, in the presence of impaired cardiovascular reserve, severe cardiorespiratory sequelae arise. The cyanosis and hypoxaemia seen in massive embolism are due to a decrease in cardiac output with widening alveolar arterial oxygen tension and also a failure to ventilate the normal lung which is being overperfused. With smaller emboli and repeated episodes of embolisation, varying degrees of infarction and resolution occur along with

**Table 10.1**
Results of meta-analysis in general surgical patients: venous thromboembolism in control general surgical patients (Clagget and Reisch, 1988)

| Endpoint | No. of trials | Total | Incidence (%) | 95% C.I. |
|---|---|---|---|---|
| DVT (+FUT) | 54 | 4310 | 1084 (25.1%) | 23.9-26.5 |
| Confirmed DVT | 20 | 1507 | 288 (19.1%) | 17.1-21.1 |
| DVT (+ FUT) (Malignant disease) | 16 | 546 | 159 (29.1%) | 25.3-32.9 |
| DVT (+FUT) (Europe) | 37 | 2775 | 824 (29.7%) | 28.0-31.4 |
| DVT (+FUT) (N. America) | 14 | 1111 | 178 (16.1%) | 13.9-18.3 |
| Above Knee DVT | 16 | 1206 | 83 (6.9%) | 5.5- 8.3 |
| All PE | 32 | 5091 | 82 (1.6%) | 1.3- 1.9 |
| Fatal PE | 33 | 5547 | 48 (0.87%) | 0.6- 1.1 |

alveolar hypoventilation, ventilation perfusion abnormalities, pulmonary oedema etc., all of which cause hypoxaemia.

In clinical practice, the diagnosis of pulmonary embolism is difficult because few disease processes are as protean in manifestation. In a study done by Modan et al (1972), the evidence of pulmonary embolism at autopsy correlated poorly to the ante-mortem diagnosis of pulmonary embolic disease and in only one third of cases were the emboli properly diagnosed. This average for a potentially fatal disease is unsatisfactory. Tachypnoea and dyspnoea occur in 80-90% of patients with pulmonary embolism but these findings are not specific. Similarly, cough and pleuritic chest pain are reported in roughly 50%, of patients but these are not diagnostic. Thus, it is important for the clinician to bear a high degree of suspicion in patients developing symptoms in the immediate postoperative period, and in those at high risk because of fractures and prolonged immobilisation, hypercoagulable states and cardiac failure.

Pulmonary embolism secondary to proximal DVT may be either silent, symptomatic or fatal. An embolism in the pulmonary arterial tree may undergo fragmentation, dissolution or may recanalise. Fragmentation of the thrombus may explain the spontaneous improvement seen in some patients. Distal migration of the fragments may result in the development of new symptoms, e.g. pleural irritation with new scintigraphic findings which are not necessarily indicative of further episodes of thromboembolism. Dissolution of the embolus may occur by indigenous fibrinolytic mechanisms. The dissolution and recanalisation process is responsible for the recovery of the patient over a period lasting several days to weeks. The presence of underlying cardiopulmonary disease may delay recovery and in some of these patients, the scintigraphic findings may never return to normal.

# Overall Incidence of Deep Vein Thrombosis

The meta-analysis of Clagett and Reisch (1988), summarised the results of many trials using various methods of prophylaxis over a 10 year period in "general surgical patients". In this review, the "general surgical patient" referred to any patient over 40 years of age undergoing major abdominal surgery and also included those with gynaecologic, urologic, thoracic and vascular procedures. The incidence of isotopically detected venous thrombosis in control "general surgical patients" receiving no treatment is listed in table 10.1. (Clagett and Reisch, 1988). The endpoint in all these studies was the development of DVT as diagnosed either by the FUT or venography. Overall, the incidence of calf deep vein thrombosis in patients undergoing general surgical procedures and not receiving any prophylaxis was 25.1%. The incidence of proximal extension with resultant above-knee DVT was 6.9%. The incidence of pulmonary embolism (PE) was 1.6% and that of fatal PE was 0.87%. A more recent review of eleven trials in patients undergoing elective orthopaedic procedures (total hip replacement), by Planes and Silsiguen (Chapter 25), revealed a 50.5% incidence of deep vein thrombosis in patients not receiving prophylaxis. Also, there was a higher incidence of above knee DVT (24.4%) in these patients.

## Natural history studies

One of the first of the earlier studies on the natural history of deep vein thrombosis was the work of Kakkar et al (1969). They studied 132 consecutive patients undergoing general surgical procedures. Any patient with a history or clinical signs suggestive of recent deep vein thrombosis, or any undergoing operation on their legs or thyroid were excluded. All the patients investigated were screened with the FUT and patients with abnormal scans underwent venography. Of the 132 patients studied, 40 (30%) had abnormal scans and this was confirmed in all but one case by venography, but only 20 of these patients had any clinical signs. In 14 patients (35%) the thrombus lysed spontaneously within 72 hours and in 26 (65%) the thrombus persisted. Of these, the thrombus remained localised to the calf in 19 (73%) and underwent proximal extension in 7 (27%). Clinical pulmonary embolism developed in 4 (57%) It was interesting to note that only one of the four patients with pulmonary embolism had signs of deep vein thrombosis in the leg. Also no proximal extension into the popliteal vein occurred without prior calf DVT and no pulmonary emboli occured without thrombosis proximal to the calf.

An extensive review of the literature on the natural history by Philbrick and Becker (1988) analysed the results of 20 studies in which venography was used for the initial diagnosis of DVT. Calf thrombi were found in 1044 (48.8%) of the 2140 patients studied. The authors found that propagation of calf DVT into the thigh occurred in up to 20% of cases and that propagation invariably occurred before embolisation. No fatal emboli were seen in patients presenting with isolated calf DVT. A recurrence rate of 29% was seen in symptomatic calf DVT and anticoagulation appeared to prevent extension, embolisation and early recurrence.

In the International Multicentre Trial (1975), a total of 1,292 patients with isotopically detected DVT were randomised into treatment or control. Of the 667 patients in the control group 164 (24.6%) developed DVT and in 44 (30%) the thrombus extended proximally.In a more recent study of 75 patients with calf vein thrombi diagnosed by duplex scanning, (Lohr et al, 1991), proximal propagation occured in 24 (32%) and in 11(15%), propagation extended into the popliteal or larger veins of the thigh.

### Incidence of Pulmonary Embolism

In the United States, fatal PE accounts for 200,000 deaths per year and is the third leading cause of death (Bell et al, 1982). It is now generally accepted that fatal PE is the most preventable cause of death in the hospital patient. Recent studies show that a large number of pulmonary emboli are found at autopsy, although the number of fatal PE have declined during the last few years. In a retrospective review of all autopsies done over a 30 year period, (autopsy rate 73-100%) PE was found in 1274 (23.6%) of the 5477 patients who died (Bergqvist et al, 1985). Of the pulmonary emboli found, 349 (27.3%) were considered fatal, 353 (27.7%) contributory to death and 572 (44.8%) incidental. It was interesting to note that 51% of these patients were not operated upon and that in 24 cases (6.9%) of fatal PE, the source was thrombi that had formed around central venous catheters. A recent study by Sandler et al (1989) showed the rate of PE to be around 10% (239 of 2,388 autopsies performed). It was noted that only 83% of these patients had DVT, of whom only 19% had symptoms and only 3% had undergone investigations for the same before death. It must be remembered that autopsy studies show only one aspect of PE and they reflect findings in a selected high-risk group; it is hardly surprising that there is so much discrepancy between this and clinical studies.

The International Multicentre Trial for the prevention of postoperative pulmonary embolism (1975) found the incidence of fatal PE in the control group to be 0.7% with an incidence in the heparin treated group of 0.09%. In a review of trials in general, orthopaedic, and urologic surgery (Collins et al, 1988), the authors reviewed the results of over 70 trials that included 16,000 patients, randomised into treatment or control groups. The reduction in deaths due to PE in the treated group was particularly striking (19 in patients receiving heparin compared to 55 in the control group, $p < 0.001$). The rates of fatal PE in elective hip surgery varied from 1.4% (Johnson et al, 1977) to 3.4% (Coventry et al, 1973).

### Incidence of PE in relation to extent of DVT
Kakkar et al (1969) found no incidence of clinical pulmonary embolism in the 19 patients with thrombi localised to the calf in their study. None of these patients had lung scans and the decision was based on clinical examinaton, chest X-ray and ECG. In contrast, in the 9 patients who had proximal extension, pulmonary embolism was found in 4 (44%). The incidence of PE (high probability lung scan) in relation to the site of DVT is summarised in Fig 10.2. The methods used for the diagnosis of PE and DVT, the patient presentation and the incidence of high probability lung scans is shown. Based on studies using lung scanning, silent pulmonary embolism in patients with calf DVT is probably more common than previously recognised. Symptomatic pulmonary embolism with calf thrombi is an uncommon event and the incidence of fatal pulmonary embolism with related calf thrombi is probably exceedingly low. On the other hand proximal thrombi have a higher association with silent pulmonary emboli. Clinical PE are usually associated with proximal (iliofemoral) DVT. Iliofemoral thrombi are the main cause of fatal pulmonary emboli, as shown by autopsy studies (Diener, 1971).

### Results of treatment on natural history of pulmonary embolism
Barritt and Jordan (1960) conducted the only randomised controlled study in patients with clinically and radiologically diagnosed pulmonary embolism. Patients were randomised into treatment with intravenous heparin and nicoumalon or no treatment. Randomisation ceased after 35 patients because of five deaths in the untreated group (5/19; 26%). All subsequent 38 patients studied received anticoagulant therapy, with only one further death (due to anuria) The results suggested that anticoagulant therapy not only reduced immediate mortality but also reduced the risk of death from further emboli.

The efficacy of thrombolytic agents have been compared with heparin in the Urokinase Pulmonary Embolism Trial (UPET Phase 1 Study, 1970). This multicentre study ran-

**Table 10.2**
Incidence of high probability lung scans in relation to site of DVT

| Reference | Diagnostic test | Patient presentation | Patients n= | Incidence of PE (high probability) on lung scanning Calf DVT | Proximal DVT | No DVT |
|---|---|---|---|---|---|---|
| Kistner et al, 1972 | Venography, Ventilation-perfusion scan, Chest x-ray | Acute Clinical DVT | 52 | 2/7 (28%) | 28/45 (62%) | — |
| Marena-Cabral et al, 1976 | Venography, V/Q scan, pulmonary angiogram | Symptomatic DVT or clinical PE | 54 | 9/27 (33%) | 18/27 (66%) | — |
| Moser and LeMoine, 1981 | Venography, Radiofibrinogen test, IPG, V/Q scan | Symptomatic DVT | 68 | 0/21 (0%) | 8/15 (53%) | 0/32 (0%) |
| Plate et al, 1985 | Venography, perfusion lung scan, chest x-ray | Acute ileofemoral thrombosis | 49 | — | 22/49 (45%) | — |
| Dorfman et al, 1987 | Venography, V/Q scan | Post-operative DVT | 58 | 0/9 (0%) | 17/49 (35%) | — |
| Doyle and Turpie, 1987 | Venography, V/Q scan | Acute thrombophlebitis | 102 | 11/33 (33%) | 35/69 (51%) | — |
| Huisman et al, 1989 | Venography, IPG, V/Q scan, Chest x-ray | Clinical DVT | 128 | 2/11 (18%) | 43/78 (55%) | 2/39 (5%) |
| TOTAL: | | | 511 | 24/108 (22%) | 171/332 (51.5%) | 2/71 (3%) |

domised patients with pulmonary embolism into treatment with urokinase initially and subsequent heparin sodium or heparin alone. It was seen that thrombolytic therapy significantly accelerated the resolution of pulmonary thromboemboli, especially massive emboli at 24 hours as shown by pulmonary angiograms, lung scans and right-sided pressure measurements. Also, younger patients (less than 50 years) and patients with emboli (less than 48 hours old) fared better. The bleeding complication rate was 45% in the urokinase group compared to 27% in the heparin group but this was attributed to the invasive procedures required by the trial protocol. No significant difference in mortality was found between the two groups and this was probably due to the fact that patients who survived long enough to enter a clinical trial, probably made up a group with an improved prognosis since the more severely affected patients would have died before receiving therapy. Secondly, a mortality study would require a larger trial limited to the highest risk patients who are relatively rare, or a trial with a larger number of patients.

The results of treatment of pulmonary embolism also depend upon the presence or absence of previous cardiopulmonary disease. Patients with a permanently compromised cardiovascular reserve may exhibit the signs of massive PE even with small emboli. Also, patients presenting with shock and prolonged hypotension have a poorer prognosis. Miller and Hall (1977) reviewed the outcome of 68 patients with angiographically diagnosed massive PE and found the mortality in patients presenting with shock to be 22% compared with 7% in the non-shock group. Similar results have also been shown by Alpert et al (1975). Thus in the group of patients presenting with shock, a more aggressive approach, either by thrombolysis or thrombectomy is warranted. Recovery from pulmonary embolism may take days to weeks and is dependent on the dissolution and recanalisation of the thrombus. The presence of underlying cardiopulmonary disease may delay the process and in some patients, the scintigraphic findings never return to normal. It has been shown by Tow and Wagner (1979) that approximatgely 50% of patients with sub-massive embolism have a normal perfusion scan by three months.

## Post thrombotic syndrome

The post thrombotic syndrome (PTS) is characterised by the development of pain, swelling, pigmentation and ulceration in patients with DVT. The problem arising in assessing these patients is the variability of the subjective symptoms, such as pain, heaviness in the legs and aching. In their two year follow-up of 53 patients with calf DVT treated either with heparin or streptokinase (Kakkar and Lawrence, 1985), 78% of limbs were asymptomatic or had minimal post-thrombotic changes, 16% had moderate and 8% severe changes. In contrast, Widmer et al (1985) found no post-thrombotic changes with isolated calf thrombi in 37 patients at 5 year follow-up. In 112 patients with proximal thrombi, the ulcer rate was 8% and that of PTS was 26%. Thus, post-thrombotic symptoms are not frequently encountered following isolated calf DVT. With proximal thrombosis, there is a higher incidence of post-thrombotic changes. O'Donnell et al (1977) reviewed 21 patients with venographically documented thrombi in the iliac and femoral veins at 10 years. They found that 75% of the patients at 5 years and 86% of the patients at 10 years had a leg ulcer. Ulcers recurred despite medical and surgical treatment in 16 of the 21 patients. Three patients required below-knee amputations as the recurrent painful ulcers and venous claudication had totally incapacited them. Browse et al (1980) reported a 20% rate of moderate to severe PTS after calf DVT in comparison to a 45% incidence after proximal thrombi. Schulman et al (1986) reviewed the results of treatment with streptokinase (low dose vs high dose) in 36 patients with symptomatic calf DVT at 38 months follow-up. Signs of deep venous insufficiency were noted in 17 (49%) of 35 patients in the high dose streptokinase group in comparison to 26 (74%) of 35 patients receiving low dose streptokinase. Elliot et al (1979) reviewed the results of 19 months follow-up in 51 patients with acute proximal venous thrombosis of less than one week's duration, randomised into treatment with streptokinase or heparin. In the heparin treated group, only 2 of 21 patients had asymptomatic legs. All patients complained of symptoms of aching, 4 had venous claudication and 1 had a venous ulcer. In the streptokinase group 16 of 17 patients who had 80-100% lysis had asymptomatic legs, 12 patients remained asymptomatic and 3 had died of unrelated causes, 1 patient being lost to follow-up. In patients receiving streptokinase and achieving incomplete lysis, 5 out of 9 (55.6 %) complained of aching and oedema, 2(22.2%) had venous claudication, 1 died of carcinoma and 1 was lost to follow-up.

Strandness et al (1983) studied the long term sequelae of deep venous thrombosis in 61 patients (65 limbs). There were 7 limbs with calf thrombi and 58 limbs with proximal thrombi (15 superficial femoropopliteal, 41 iliofemoral). The incidence of oedema/pain in the calf thrombi group was 3/7 limbs (42.9 %), pigmentation 2/7 limbs (28.6 %) and ulcer (0%) at 39 months follow-up. In the proximal DVT group, the incidence of oedema/pain was 36/58 limbs (62.1 %). It was found that the most important factor with regard to prognosis was the status of the distal deep veins. Only 8% of the normal distal veins were found to have pigmentation during follow-up compared to 40% in those with either occlusion or incompetence of valves.

A recent study on the incidence and time of occurrence of venous reflux after DVT by Markel et al (1992), followed up 107 patients (123 legs) over a mean period of 341 days. Patients were subjected to duplex scanning and were studied at intervals of 1 and 7 days, 1

**Table 10.3**
Incidence of reflux in deep veins of the leg following thrombosis (Markel et al 1992)

| Follow-up interval | Number of legs | Reflux (%) | 95% CI |
|---|---|---|---|
| 1 day | 40 | 2 | (5) |
| 1 week | 54 | 9 | (17) |
| 1 month | 54 | 20 | (37) |
| 3 months | 61 | 32 | (52) |
| 6 months | 49 | 26 | (53) |
| 9 months | 36 | 20 | (56) |
| 1 year | 32 | 22 | (69) |
| 2 years | 24 | 15 | (63) |
| 3 years | 10 | 5 | (50) |

month, every three months for the first year and then yearly thereafter (Table 10.3). In addition, duplex examination was carried out in 502 patients with negative duplex study results and no previous history of thrombosis or chronic venous insufficiency. In the group of patients with acute deep venous thrombosis, valvular incompetence was noted in 17 limbs (14%) at the time of the initial study. Reflux was absent in 106 limbs (86%), but 17% of limbs in the group had developed reflux by day 7. By the end of the first month, 37% demonstrated reflux and at the end of 1 year nearly two-thirds of the limbs had developed valvular reflux. The distribution of reflux among different groups was, popliteal vein (58%), superficial femoral vein (37%), great saphenous vein (25%) and posterior tibial vein (18%). Reflux seemed to be more frequent in segments previously affected by deep vein thrombosis. Interestingly, in limbs without deep vein thromboses, 8% of posterior tibial veins showed reflux after 1 year. In the group of patients without deep vein thrombosis, reflux in either the deep or the superficial systems was seen in 60 of 1003 legs (6%).

Thus, one may conclude that the incidence of post thrombotic syndrome is higher in patients with proximal thrombi than in those with isolated calf DVT. It is important to reiterate the point that a combination of incompetent valves and incomplete recanalisation contribute to the syndrome.

**Recurrence of DVT**

Moser and LeMoine (1981) followed up 21 patients with asymptomatic isolated calf thrombus (not treated by heparin) and verified by venography for 3 months and found a very low risk of embolisation in contrast to patients with proximal thrombi. Lagerstedt et al (1985) studied the need for oral anticoagulation in patients with symptomatic calf thrombi in 51 patients (23 received warfarin for 3 months and 28 did not). Both groups received an initial course of heparin and all wore compression stockings. During the first 3 months, 8 patients (29%) in the non-warfarin group developed recurrences in comparison to none in the warfarin group (p <0.001). Of these 8 patients with recurrences, 5 had recurrence with proximal extension and 1 had a pulmonary embolus. At the end of 1 year, 22 of 23 (96%) patients in the warfarin group had not had a recurrence compared to 19 out of 28 (68%) in the non-treatment group. A certain amount of proximal extension may have occurred during the initial therapy with heparin, since extension during heparin use does occur and some of the recurrences may be attributed to inadequately treated proximal thrombi rather than calf DVT. In one prospective study (Hull et al, 1979) patients were randomised to treatment either with low dose subcutaneous heparin or warfarin after initial treatment with heparin.

None of the 32 patients with calf thrombi developed recurrences, whereas patients with proximal thrombi did. Thus, low-dose heparin was sufficient treatment for calf thrombus but not for proximal thrombus. In another study by Hull et al (1986), continuous intravenous heparin was compared with subcutaneous heparin in the initial treatment of proximal thrombi. 115 patients with venographically confirmed proximal DVT were randomised into treatment either with continuous intravenous heparin therapy for 10 days or daily therapeutic subcutaneous doses of heparin for the same period. During a 3 month follow-up, 11 of the 52 patients (19%) in the subcutaneous heparin group developed recurrent thrombi in comparison to 3 of 58 patients (5%), receiving continuous intravenous heparin. Thus, inadequately treated proximal thrombi lead to recurrence.

Modern noninvasive investigations may be used to follow up asymptomatic calf thrombi so that treatment can be commenced if proximal extension occurs. Symptomatic calf DVT needs to be treated adequately to prevent proximal extension.

# References

Alpert JS, Smith RE, Ockene IS, Askenazi J, Dexter L, Dalen JE. Treatment of massive pulmonary embolism: The role of pulmonary embolectomy. Am Heart J 89:413, 1975

Barrit DW, Jordan SC. Annticoagulant drugs in the treatment of pulmonary embolism. A controlled trial. Lancet 1:1309, 1960

Bell, WR, Simon TL. Current status of pulmonary thromboembolic disease: Pathophysiology, diagnosis, prevention and treatment. Am Heart J 103:239, 1982

Bergqvist D, Lindblad B. A 30-year survey of pulmonary embolism verified at autopsy: an analysis of 1,274 surgical patients. Brit J Surg 72:105, 1985

Bone RC. Ventilation/Perfusion Scan in Pulmonary Embolism: 'The Emperor is Incompletely Attired'. JAMA 263 (20):2794, 1990

Browse NL, Clemenson G, Croft DN. Fibrinogen-detectable thrombosis in the legs and pulmonary embolism. Br Med J 1: 604, 1974

Browse NL Clemenson G, Thomas ML. Is the post-phlebitic leg always postphlebitic? Relation between phlebographic appearances of deep vein thrombosis and late sequelae. Br Med J 2: 1167, 1980

Clagett GP, Reisch JS. Prevention of venous thromboembolism in general surgical patients. Ann Surg 208: 227, 1988

Clarke-Pearson DL et al. The natural history of postoperative venous thromboemboli in gynecologic oncology: A prospective study of 382 patients. Am J Obstet Gynecol 148: 1051, 1984

Collins R, Scrimgeour A, Yusuf S et al. Reduction in fatal pulmonary embolism and venous thrombosis by perioperative administration of subcutaneous heparin. New Engl J Med 318:1162, 1988

Coventry MB, Nolan DR, Beckenbauigh RD. Delayed prophylactic anticoagulation. A study of results and complications in 2012 total hip arthroplasties. J Bone J Surg 55A: 1487, 1973

Diener, L. Intraosseous phlebography of the lower limb. Acta Radiol suppl 304:1, 1971

Dorfman GS, Cronan JJ, Tupper TB, Messersmith RN, Denny DF, Lee CH. Occult pulmonary embolism: a common occurrence in deep venous thrombosis. AJR 148: 263, 1987

Doyle DJ, Turpie AGG, Hirsh J et al. Adjusted subcutaneous heparin or continuous intravenous heparin in patients with acute deep vein thrombosis. Ann Int Med 107:441, 1987

Elliot MS, Immelman J, Jeffery P et al. A comparative randomized trial of heparin versus streptokinase in the treatment of acute proximal venous thrombosis: an interim report of a prospective trial. Br J Surg 66:838, 1979

Huisman MV, Büller MR, ten Cate JW. Unexpected high prevalence of silent pulmonary embolism in patients with deep venous thrombosis. Chest 95: 498, 1989

Hull RD et al. Warfarin sodium versus low dose heparin in the longterm treatment of venous thrombosis. N Engl J Med 301: 855, 1979

Hull RD, Hirsh J, Carter CJ et al. Pulmonary angiography, ventilation lung scanning, and venography for clinically suspected pulmonary embolism with abnormal perfusion lung scan. Ann Int Med 98:891, 1983

Hull RD et al. Continuous intravenous heparin compared with intermittent subcutaneous heparin in the initial treatment of proximal vein thrombosis. N Engl J Med 315: 1109, 1986

International Multicentre Trial. Prevention of fatal postoperative pulmonary embolism by low doses of heparin. Lancet 2:45, 1975

International Multicentre Trial. Prevention of fatal postoperative pulmonary embolism by low doses of heparin. Lancet 2:567, 1977

Johnson R, Green JR, Charnley J. Pulmonary embolism and its prophylaxis following the Charnley total hip replacement. Clin Orthop 127: 123, 1977

Just-Vierra JO, Yeager GH, Jurf A, Lewers DT, Scanlan E. Massive lethal pulmonary emboli. Surgery 53:109, 1963

Kakkar VV, Lawrence C. Hemodynamic and clinical assessment after therapy for deep vein thrombosis: A prospective study. Am J Surg 150: 54, 1985

Kakkar VV, Howe CT, Flanc C, Clarke MB. Natural history of postoperative deep-vein thrombosis. Lancet 2:230, 1969

Kistner RL, Ball JJ, Nordyke RA, Freeman GC. Incidence of pulmonary embolism in the course of thrombophlebitis of the lower extremities. Am J Surg 124: 169, 1972

Lagerstedt CI, Olsson CG, Fagher BO et al. Need for longterm anticoagulant treatment in symptomatic calf vein thrombosis. Lancet 2:515, 1985

Lohr JM, Kerr TM, Lutter KS et al. Lower extremity calf thrombosis: To treat or not to treat? J Vasc Surg 14:618, 1991

Markel A, Manzo RA, Bergelin RO, Strandness DE. Venous reflux after DVT. Incidence and time occurrence. J Vasc Surg 15:377, 1992

Miller GA, Hall RJ, Paneth M. Pulmonary embolectomy, heparin and streptokinase: Their place in the treatment of acute massive pulmonary embolism. Am Heart J 93: 568, 1977

Modan B, Sharon E, Jelin N. Factors contributing to the incorrect diagnosis of pulmonary embolic disease. Chest 62: 388, 1972

Moreno-Cabral R, Kistner RL, Nordyke RA. Importance of calf vein thrombophlebitis. Surgery 80:735, 1976

Moser KM, LeMoine JR. Is embolic risk conditioned by location of deep venous thrombosis. Ann Intern Med 94:439, 1981

O'Donnell TF, Browse NL, Burnand KG, Thomas ML. The socioeconomic effects of iliofemoral venous thrombosis. J Surg Res 22:483, 1977

Philbrick JT, Becker DM. Calf deep venous thrombosis: A wolf in sheep's clothing. Arch Intern Med 148:2131, 1988

PIOPED Investigators. Value of the ventilation/perfusion scan in acute pulmonary embolism. JAMA 263:2753, 1990

Plate G, Ohlin P, Eklöf B. Pulmonary embolism in acute iliofemoral venous thrombosis. Br J Surg 72:912, 1985

Sandler DA. Autopsy proven pulmonary embolism in hospital patients: are we detecting enough deep vein thrombosis? J Roy Soc Med 82:203, 1989

Schulman S, Granqvist S, Juhlin-Dannfelt A, Lockner D. Long-term sequelae of calf vein thrombosis treated with heparin or low-dose streptokinase. Acta Med Scand 219:349, 1986

Strandness DE, Longlois Y, Cramer M, Randlett A, Thiele BL. Long-term sequelae of acute venous thrombosis. JAMA 250:1289, 1983

Tow DE, Wagner HN. Recovery of pulmonary arterial blood flow in patients with pulmonary embolism. N Engl J Med 2765: 1053, 1969

Urokinase pulmonary embolism trial: Phase I Results. JAMA 214:2163, 1970

Urokinase-streptokinase embolism trial: Phase 2 Results. JAMA 229:1606, 1974

Widmer LK, Zemp E, Widmer MT et al. Late results in deep vein thrombosis of the lower extremity. VASA 14:265, 1985

Virchow, R. Cellular Pathology. Churchill, London, 1860

PART II

# Methods of Primary Prevention

CHAPTER 11

# The current practice of prevention

Ernest D Cooke

To provide some idea of the current practice in the prophylaxis of venous thromboembolism, a random sample of 1,920 surgeons, general, vascular and orthopaedic, in Western Europe and the USA were sent a questionnaire between March and September of 1991.

The questionnaire asked the following details: the respondents' speciality; whether or not they use prophylaxis against DVT; which of the available methods were used, either alone or in combination; when did they start prophylaxis and when did they stop; to whom was protection provided, i.e., all or selected high risk patients; and the risk factors considered important. Those that did not provide prophylaxis were asked to give their reasons for not doing so; whether their belief was that DVT was not a problem, that prophylaxis was ineffective, too risky, too expensive or difficult to organise.

The countries involved (Fig. 11.1) were the UK, Germany, Switzerland and the USA. The individual number and response rates were: UK 340 (56.6%), Western Germany 31 (25.4%), Switzerland 163 (40.75%) and the USA 332 (41.5%).

Seventy percent of the respondents were general or vascular surgeons, and the remainder orthopaedic surgeons, mainly from the USA. Orthopaedic surgeons in the UK were not circulated, as this has been done recently, and the results published (Laverick et al, 1991).

Overall 113 (13%) used no form of prophylaxis, 9% in the USA. All the German respondents, and 99.7% of those from the UK did use prophylaxis. Of those who did not, more than half (55%) believed postoperative thromboembolism was not a problem in their practice, 15% thought prophylaxis ineffective, 11.5% thought it too risky. Half of the US non-users thought it to be too expensive, an observation not made by practitioners from the other countries. Organisational problems were not a reason for non-usage in Germany or Switzerland, but were given as a reason by 10% of US and 20% of UK non-users.

Subcutaneous heparins were used by more than 90% of respondents in the UK and Switzerland and by all in Germany, in contrast to only 65% of respondents from the US. Warfarin was used most commonly in the US (35%) which may reflect the greater

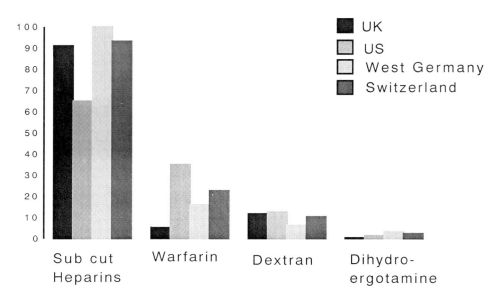

Fig. 11.1 The use of anticoagulants in the four countries surveyed

preponderance of orthopaedic surgeons in the sample; in fact, combining the anticoagulant users in the US gives 100%. If these figures are taken as reflecting orthopaedic usage, then taking the figures of Haverick and his colleagues (Haverick et al, 1991) for British orthopaedic surgeons (subcutaneous heparins 71%, warfarin 33%), there is little difference between orthopaedic practice in the UK and USA (Fig. 11.1).

Considering other countries studied, warfarin is little used other than in orthopaedic practice, 5.3% in the UK, 16% in Germany and 22.7% in Switzerland. These may reflect difficulties encountered in control and organisation.

Elastic stockings are patently the simplest form of prophylaxis. However, only in West Germany are they in universal usage (93%) but only by just over half of the surgeons in Switzerland (52.1%) and the US (60%). About three-quarters of British surgeons use elastic stockings. Intermittent calf compression is unpopular in West Germany (9.6%) and scarcely used in Switzerland (3.0%). US (59%) and UK (32.6%) surgeons appear to use it more frequently. Calf stimulation on the other hand, is used only rarely (Fig. 11.2).

Presently, dextrans are not in common use. Of the four countries studied, dextrans are used by only one surgeon in ten, while the use of dihydroergotamine is negligible.

Use of combined methods is not popular (Fig. 11.3). Their use is greatest in the UK where they are used by one-third of surgeons and by one-fifth in the US and Switzerland, but only by 6.4% in West Germany, which may seem surprising considering that all the German respondents claimed to use subcutaneous heparins.

Although more than 15% of respondents in the UK, USA and West Germany did not specify when prophylaxis was started, it was evident that, except in the US — where prophylaxis often starts after surgery (again, a reflection of the orthopaedic practice and use of warfarin), prophylaxis is started just before or, less commonly, during surgery. However, in West Germany, almost one-fifth of surgeons start protection, presumably including

# THE CURRENT PRACTICE OF PREVENTION

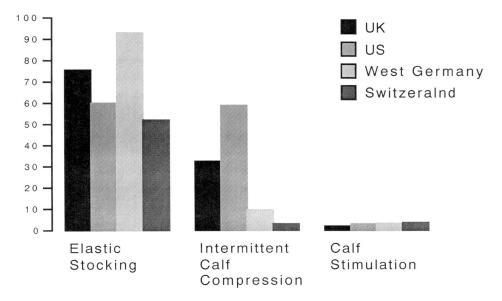

Fig. 11.2  The use of mechanical methods in the four countries surveyed

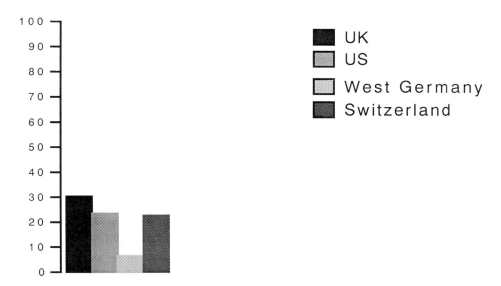

Fig. 11.3  The low usage of combined methods of prophylaxis against thromboembolism in all countries surveyed

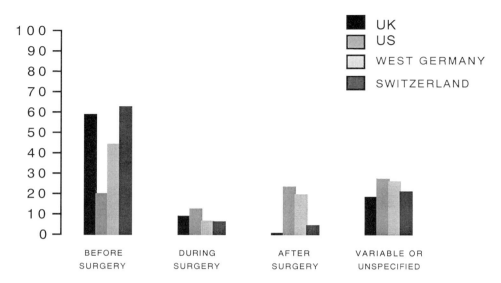

Fig. 11.4 Time of commencement of prophylaxis against venous thromboembolism

subcutaneous heparins, after surgery (Fig. 11.4). Further, it is evident that some surgeons, about 10% in each country studied, do not have a fixed regimen, but change this according to the clinical situation. Similarly, while mobilisation is by far the commonest endpoint for prevention, 15% of British and 22.1% of Swiss surgeons stop prevention before one week, apparently irrespective of patients' mobility (Fig. 11.5).

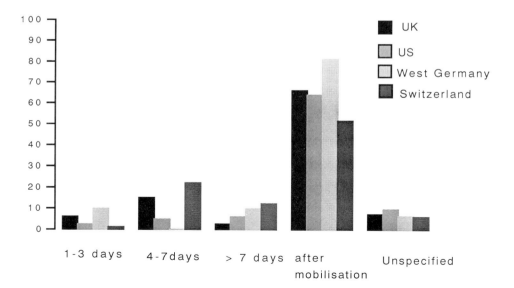

Fig. 11.5 Post-operative day when prohylaxis against venous thromboembolism was stropped

# THE CURRENT PRACTICE OF PREVENTION

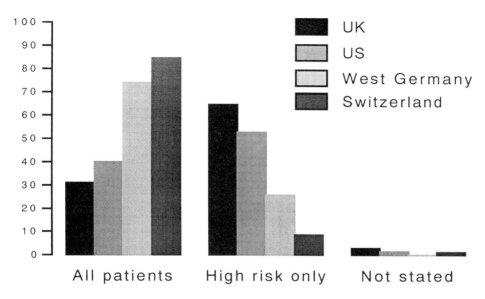

Fig. 11.6 Type of patient (percentage) offered prophylaxis against thromboembolism

Surgeons in the UK are much more selective than elsewhere, only one-third giving some form of prevention to all. This is in sharp contrast to Switzerland where it appears prophylaxis is offered to almost all surgical patients. Only one-quarter of West German surgeons attempt to identify patients at high risk of DVT. As far as selection is concerned, practice in the US is closest to that in the UK (Fig. 11.6).

When asked to list risk factors (Fig. 11.7), most surgeons mentioned those commonly recognised; however interesting differences have emerged. Surgeons in the UK consider age, a previous history of DVT, the type of surgery and carcinoma, of almost equal importance, obesity less so and immobility even less. In contrast, in the US, a previous history of DVT, immobility, obesity and the type of surgery are important while age and carcinoma are considered less so. Obesity was considered a priority risk factor for DVT in Germany and Switzerland, as was age in Germany, but not in Switzerland. Carcinoma does not appear to be considered a risk factor for DVT in either Germany or Switzerland. Venous surgery, varicose veins or a previous history of thrombophlebitis were not generally considered to be high risk factors. The hypercoagulable state, particularly that related to oral contraceptives, cigarette smoking, the general physical state of the patient or the length of surgery were either not mentioned or given a low priority.

These results, allowing for the differences already discussed, are in general agreement with the recent survey from Belfast by R.A.B. Mollan and his group (Laverick et al, 1991). They indicate a general awareness that venous thromboembolism is presently considered to be a frequent and possibly serious complication of orthopaedic and general surgery and against which most surgeons take active measures. Moreover, they reflect a considerable change in perception and practice when compared to the findings of Morris (Morris, 1980) (Fig. 11.8). Then, 28% of general surgeons did nothing, or depended on early ambulation

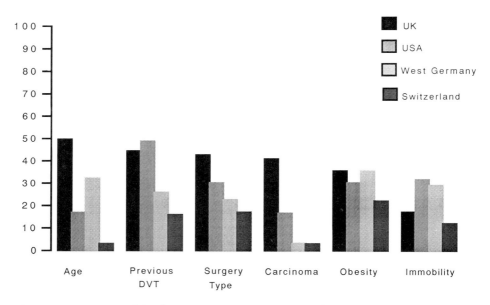

Fig. 11.7 Importance of risk factors as perceived by surgeons from the four countries surveyed (percentages)

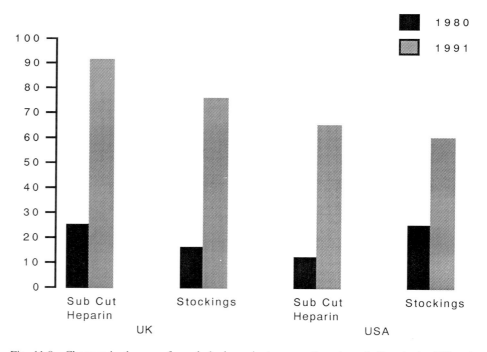

Fig. 11.8 Changes in the use of prophylaxis against venous thromboembolism in the UK and USA over the past decade

and physiotherapy, 25% used heparin routinely, 16% used stockings and 25% used gaiters (undefined). Thus, in the UK only half of the surgeons were using prophylaxis. A similar state of affairs was found in Sweden (Bergqvist, 1980). Around the same time (Conti and Daschbach, 1982), prophylaxis was used by only 25% of surgeons in the US as well.

Despite the limitations of this survey and the apparent low use of combined therapy, the results are encouraging and indicate that the message is getting through.

## References

Bergqvist D. Prevention of postoperative deep venous thrombosis in Sweden. World J Surg 4:489, 1980

Clagett P, Beiusch JS. Prevention of venous thromboembolism in general surgical patients. Ann Surg 208:227, 1988

Colditz G, Tuden R, Oster G. Rates of venous thrombosis after general surgery: combined results of randomised clinical trial. Lancet ii:143, 1986

Conti S, Daschbach B. Venous thromboembolism prophylaxis: a survey of its use in the United States. Aich Surg 117:1036, 1982

Laverick MD, Croal SA, Mollan RAB. Orthopaedic surgeons and thromboprophylaxis. Br Med J 303:549, 1991

Morris GK. Prevention of venous thromboembolism. Lancet ii:572, 1980

## Acknowledgement

The author expresses his appreciation to all members of staff of the Unit at St Bartholomews Hospital, London, especially Clare Fleming and Juliana Elusade, without whom this survey would not have been possible.

CHAPTER 12

# Low dose heparin with and without dihydroergotamine

Vijay V Kakkar    Alexander T Cohen

## Introduction

Venous thrombi are generally regarded as an expression of blood coagulation and fibrin formation in the presence of venous stasis. So many factors contribute to the formation of a thrombus that it is, perhaps, impossible to expect a precise dividing line between the patient who is at high risk of developing a thrombus and one in whom actual deposition of fibrin has already occurred within major veins. Some degree of stimulation of intravascular coagulation is probably a common event in many diseases. The stimulus might come directly from damaged vessel wall or indirectly from entry into the blood of potentially coagulant material from inflamed tissue. While blood flow continues, the active coagulation enzymes will be carried away from the site of a local stimulus to be cleared by the cells of the reticulo-endothelial system (Wessler et al, 1967) and while in transit their effect will be held in check by inhibitors in the plasma, which are capable of neutralising more of the enzyme than can possibly be generated from the unit volume of blood in which they are contained. These important inhibitors include antithrombin III, which has been shown to have inhibitory power particularly against activated factor X (factor Xa) (Wessler et al, 1967) and thrombin; and also protein C, protein S and plasminogen activator inhibitor (PAI-1). Thrombosis is likely when these compensating mechanisms are overwhelmed, particularly so in areas of reduced blood flow. The postoperative changes which predispose to thrombosis are a result of three parallel, different but closely related, processes; pre- and postoperative stress, consumption of clotting factors — most probably in the wound — and metabolic changes affecting plasma proteins in general and acute phase reactants in particular.

## Low dose heparin

Ideally, any agent used for prophylaxis of deep vein thrombosis should be well tolerated by the patients, have no side effects, require no special monitoring, and produce no bleeding in a clinical situation in which the patient is subjected to major tissue trauma. One established approach is the use of low dose heparin, given subcutaneously, which prevents thrombosis without markedly increasing the risk of bleeding.

### Rationale of low dose heparin prophylaxis

The rationale for low dose heparin prophylaxis was first put forward nearly 45 years ago by de Takats (1950), who showed that small amounts of heparin will effectively block the coagulation process if given at an early stage. Its prophylactic use was introduced by Sharnoff (1966), who found accelerated blood coagulation during and after surgery and thought this might be related to thrombus formation.

During the activation of intravascular coagulation, thrombin is produced from its precursor, prothrombin, by the concentrated action of factor Va and activated factor X (factor Xa) in the presence of a surface lipid and calcium ions. Thrombin thus formed initiates the development of fibrin clot. The anticoagulant effect of heparin has been shown to occur only in the presence of the plasma cofactor antithrombin III. Antithrombin III binds to heparin and this accelerates the inhibition of thrombin and factor Xa by up to 10,000 fold. Another cofactor, heparin cofactor II may also contribute but only inhibits thrombin. The activity of these cofactors is enhanced by only trace amounts of heparin.

The interaction between antithrombin III (AT-III), heparin and thrombin has been extensively investigated by several workers. The structure of the antithrombin molecule has now been defined. It is a single-chain glycoprotein with a molecular weight of approximately 68,000. It is composed of 425 amino acids containing three disulphide bridges (cys 3-cys 127, cys 21-cys 95, cys 238-cys 420). Four oligosaccharide side chains are attached to amino acids 96, 134, 154 and 191 (Peterson and Zucker, 1970). The secondary structure comprises approximately 8 percent β-helix, 30 percent ß-structure and 62 percent random coil (Villanueva and Danishefsky, 1977). Rosenberg and Damus (1973) postulated that heparin binds primarily to the lysyl residues of AT-III, thereby inducing a conformational change which renders the arginine reactive of AT-III more accessible to the active serine of thrombine. AT-III neutralises thrombin and factor Xa by forming a 1:1 stoichiometric complex which is enzymatically inactive. They have suggested that via this specific interaction other serine proteases might be neutralised in a similar manner. Heparin was thought to act merely as an accelerator of this reaction. However, Holme, Soderstrom and Anderson (1979) have proposed that heparin first binds to AT-III, which indicates a conformational change in the thrombin receptor site by which the AT-III reactive site is made more susceptible to the enzyme. Thereafter, thrombin binds to another segment of the heparin molecule. The complex formation between AT-III and thrombin probably results in a conformational change in the heparin-binding sites of both proteins, by which heparin dissociates from the AT-III-thrombin complex and again may interact with other available AT-III molecules.

## Results of clinical trials with low dose heparin

Numerous studies have investigated the efficacy of low dose heparin in preventing postoperative deep vein thrombosis (DVT) assessed by the technique of the fibrinogen uptake

**Table 12.1**
Low dose heparin in the prevention of postoperative deep vein thrombosis detected by FUT

|  | Control group |  | Heparin group |  |  |
| --- | --- | --- | --- | --- | --- |
| Study | n | DVT incidence (%) | n | DVT incidence (%) | Statistical significance (p value) |
| Kakkar et al, 1971 | 27 | 26 | 26 | 4 | <0.05 |
| Williams, 1971 | 29 | 41 | 27 | 15 | <0.02 |
| Kakkar et al, 1972 | 39 | 42 | 39 | 8 | <0.001 |
| Gordon-Smith et al, 1972 | 50 | 42 | 48 | 8.3 | <0.001 |
| Nicolaides et al, 1972 | 122 | 24 | 122 | 0.8 | <0.001 |
| Gallus et al, 1973 | 118 | 16 | 108 | 2 | <0.001 |
| Ballard et al, 1973 | 55 | 29 | 55 | 3.6 | <0.001 |
| Corrigan et al, 1974 | 434 | 27.8 | 320 | 7.1 | <0.005 |
| Scottish study, 1974 | 128 | 37 | 128 | 12 | <0.001 |
| Rosenberg et al, 1974 | 71 | 42 | 46 | 6.5 | <0.001 |
| Gallus et al, 1976 | 412 | 16 | 408 | 4.2 | <0.005 |
| International Multi-centre Trial, 1975 | 667 | 24.6 | 625 | 7.7 | <0.001 |
| Lahnberg et al, 1974 | 54 | 56 | 58 | 19 | <0.001 |
| Rem et al, 1975 |  | 35.8 |  | 13.3 | — |
| Geloven, 1975 | 80 | 25 | 79 | 5.9 | <0.001 |
| Abernethy, 1974 |  | 4.8 |  | 6.3 | <0.05 |
| Covey, 1975 | 52 | 9.6 | 53 | 7.5 | <0.05 |

test (FUT), non-fatal pulmonary embolism detected by ventilation-perfusion lung scanning, and fatal pulmonary emboli demonstrated at autopsy.

**Prevention of deep vein thrombosis**
The largest experience has been acquired in patients undergoing general abdominal operations (Table 12.1) and orthopaedic surgery (Table 12.2). In almost all trials there was a significant reduction in the incidence of DVT in patients receiving heparin. Few physicians would deny that venous thrombosis, although very common, is most likely a benign disease. Using the FUT and venography, it has been shown that in surgical patients the majority of thrombi form in the calf veins; a surprisingly high proportion of these undergo spontaneous lysis and only in something like 20 percent of patients do these thrombi extend more proximally from the calf into the popliteal, femoral and iliac veins. In this group with extending thrombosis, pulmonary embolism occurs in almost 50 percent, but only a very small proportion prove fatal (Kakkar, 1969). The effect of low dose heparin prophylaxis on the extension of venous thrombosis was evaluated in four of the larger studies of patients undergoing elective abdominal surgery, including more than 3,000 patients (Table 12.3); of 1,631 patients in the control group, thrombi were detected in 380, while extension of thrombus occurred in 99 (6%). In contrast, out of 1,485 patients included in the heparin group, thrombi were detected in 95 and extension occurred in only nine (0.6%). The difference in the frequency of extending thrombi between the two groups was highly

**Table 12.2**
Low dose heparin prophylaxis in patients undergoing total hip replacement

|  | Control Group | | Heparin Group | |
| --- | --- | --- | --- | --- |
|  | n | DVT incidence (%) | n | DVT incidence (%) |
| Morris et al, 1974 | 32 | 50 | 27 | 11 |
| Hampson et al, 1974 | 52 | 54 | 48 | 46 |
| Venous Thrombosis Clinical Study Group, 1975 | 27 | 40 | 25 | 1 |
| Mannucci et al, 1972 | 46 | 39 | 45 | 18 |
| Kakkar et al, 1972 | 18 | 39 | 15 | 27 |
| Evarts and Alfidi, 1973 | — | — | 25 | 32 |
| Dechavanne et al, 1974 | 27 | 48 | 27 | 32 |
| Sagar et al, 1976 | 32 | 69 | 25 | 32 |
| Harris et al, 1974 | — | — | 20 | 55 |
| Hume et al, 1973 | 19 | 42 | 18 | 33 |

significant, not only in the aggregate of these four studies but in each of the individual trials as well.

Patients who have surgery for malignant disease are considered to have a particularly high risk of developing venous thromboembolism and a number of patients having operations for malignancy were included in several trials of heparin prophylaxis in general surgical patients. Analysis of data of such patients indicate that low dose heparin is equally effective in protecting such patients; isotopic deep vein thromboses occur in 49% of patients with malignancy who do not receive prophylaxis, compared to 13 percent in those who receive low dose heparin.

Conflicting results have been reported regarding the efficacy of low dose heparin in patients undergoing urological operations. In a randomly allocated trial involving fairly large numbers of patients, there was a significant reduction in the incidence of deep vein thrombosis in the group receiving low dose heparin; other studies have failed to confirm the protective effects.

**Table 12.3**
Effect of low dose heparin on the proximal extension of thrombi

|  | Control Group | | | Heparin Group | | |
| --- | --- | --- | --- | --- | --- | --- |
|  | n | DVT incidence | Extension Incidence | n | DVT incidence | Extension incidence |
| Corrigan et al, 1974 | 434 | 121 | 29 | 320 | 23 | 1 |
| Nicolaides et al, 1972 | 122 | 29 | 9 | 128 | 11 | 0 |
| Gallus et al, 1973 | 408 | 66 | 12 | 412 | 11 | 3 |
| International Multi-centre Trial, 1975 | 667 | 164 | 49 | 625 | 48 | 5 |
| Total | 1631 | 380 (23.3%) | 99 (6.1%) | 1485 | 93 (6.3%) | 9 (0.6%) |

Another study has also confirmed the efficacy of low dose heparin prophylaxis in patients undergoing neurosurgery. Patients undergoing elective craniotomy, laminectomy or similar operations were included in this trial. Children under the age of 14 years, those having operations under local anaesthesia and those having acute cranial traumatology were excluded. In patients who had operations for vascular lesions, prophylaxis was started after the lesion had been removed. Patients received 5000 units (IU) of calcium heparin every 12 hours; if additional high risk factors were present, heparin was given every eight hours. Nine hundred and eighty-three patients were investigated; one developed wound haematoma and one had clinical evidence of deep vein thrombosis. None developed fatal or non-fatal pulmonary embolisms.

The value of low dose heparin prophylaxis has also been assessed in patients with spinal cord injuries (Flachen, 1974): 44 patients with an acute spinal cord injury received low dose heparin prophylaxis; 29 were paraplegics and 15 tetraplegics. They received 5000 units (IU) of calcium heparin every 12 hours, prophylaxis being started 36 hours after injury and continued for at least three weeks or longer if the patients were confined to bed. Of these patients, 6.8% developed deep vein thrombosis; nine died as a result of fatal pulmonary emboli or developed non-fatal pulmonary emboli, but two patients developed minor bleeding complications. The same authors compared these results with patients who had similar lesions and received oral anticoagulants with prophylaxis again being started 36 hours after injury. The incidence of deep vein thrombosis in this group was 21%, but more important was the incidence of fatal pulmonary embolism, which was 6.5%; 5.3% had bleeding complications.

**Prevention of fatal and non-fatal pulmonary embolism**
The efficacy of low dose heparin prophylaxis against fatal pulmonary embolism was specifically investigated in a large International Multicentre Trial organised from King's College Hospital, London (International Multicentre Trial, 1975). The trial was designed on the assumption that five of every 1000 adults subjected to major surgery will die from massive pulmonary embolism. It was estimated that at least 10,000 patients would be required, equally divided into controls and treatment groups, to give an 80 percent probability of detecting a statistically significant difference at the 5 percent level of confidence. Analysis of the results of the first 2,000 patients indicated a substantially greater benefit from heparin than had been envisaged at the planning stage, and the incidence of fatal pulmonary embolism in the control group was approximately 1% and not 0.5% as was originally thought. The intake to the trial was therefore closed when 4,471 patients were admitted to the study. Three hundred and fifty patients were excluded from the analysis for several reasons (International Multicentre Trial, 1975) leaving 4,121 patients in which the protocol was correctly followed — 2,076 in the control group and 2,045 in the heparin group. The two groups were well matched for age, sex, weight, blood group and other factors which could predispose to the development of venous thromboembolism. One hundred and eighty (4.4%) patients died during the postoperative period, 100 in the control and 80 in the heparin group. Seventy two percent of deaths in the control and 66% in the heparin group had necropsy examinations. Sixteen patients in the control group and two in the heparin group were found at necropsy to have died because of acute massive pulmonary embolism ($p<0.005$). In addition, emboli found at necropsy in six patients in the control group and three in the heparin group were considered either contributory to death or an incidental finding since death in these patients was attributed to other causes (Table 12.4). Taking all pulmonary emboli together, the findings were again significant ($p<0.005$). One of the 350

**Table 12.4**
Low dose heparin and postoperative pulmonary embolism (results of two multicentre trials)

|  | Multicentre Trial (1975) |  | Swiss Scandinavian Trial (1980) |
| --- | --- | --- | --- |
|  | Control group | Heparin group | Heparin group |
| *Patients correctly admitted* | 2076 | 2045 | 1991 |
| Patients died | 100 | 80 | 37 |
| Autopsy rate | 72% | 66% | 86% |
| Fatal pulmonary embolism | 16 | 2 (1)[*] | 3 |
| Contributory pulmonary embolism | 6 | 3 | 3 |

[*] 1 of the 74 patients who received heparin and were excluded from the trial because randomisation was not followed also died due to PE

patients excluded from the trial also died due to pulmonary embolism. This patient had received heparin. Even if this patient is included in the analysis, the results are still highly significant (p<0.005).

**Complications of low dose heparin prophylaxis**
The main limitation for using anticoagulants in the prevention of thromboembolic disease in surgical patients is the risk of haemorrhage. The only definite criterion which one can use to evaluate this risk is the frequency of wound haematoma formation. In two reported studies in which large numbers of patients were investigated, a significant difference was observed in the development of wound haematoma between the number of patients receiving heparin and their control counterparts (Table 12.5). However, a double blind study failed to confirm such a difference (Kiil et al, 1978). The reason for this discrepancy lies in the fact that in the International Multicentre Trial and in the study reported by Gallus and Hirsh (1976), heparin was administered every eight hours while Kiil et al did so every 12 hours.

**Table 12.5**
Low dose heparin prophylaxis and bleeding complications

|  | Control group |  | Heparin group |  |  |
| --- | --- | --- | --- | --- | --- |
|  | n | Haematoma incidence | n | Haematoma incidence | p |
| International Multi-centre Trial, 1975 | 2076 | 117 (5.6%) | 2045 | 158 (7.7%) | 0.01 |
| Gallus and Hirsch, 1976 | 412 | 2 (0.4%) | 408 | 10 (2.5%) | 0.01 |
| Kiil et al, 1978 | 653 | 6 (0.9%) | 643 | 4 (0.6%) | NS |

**Table 12.6**
DVT rates in abdominal thoracic or pelvic surgery

| Study | Regimens | Heparin | Heparin + DHE | Risk reduction (%) | p |
|---|---|---|---|---|---|
| Koppenhagen & Haring, 1981 | H10/HDHE 5 | 14/153 (9.2%) | 12/150 (8.0%) | 12.6 | 0.72 |
| Butterman et al, 1981 | H10/HDHE 5 | 15/161 (9.3%) | 13/162 (8.0%) | 13.9 | 0.68 |
| Ammann & Aebi, 1983 | H10/HDHE 5 | 2/245 (0.8%) | 2/242 (0.8%) | -1.2 | 0.99 |
| Multicentre, 1984 | H10/HDHE 5 | 32/190 (16.8%) | 32/190 (16.8%) | 0.0 | 1.00 |
| Kakkar et al, 1979 | H10/HDHE 7.5 | 2/ 48 (4.2%) | 3/ 49 (6.1%) | -46.9 | 0.66 |
| Hohl et al, 1980 | H15/HDHE 5 | 2/ 64 (3.1%) | 4/ 61 (6.6%) | -109.8 | 0.37 |
| Koppenhagen & Haring, 1981 | H15/HDHE 5 | 12/169 (7.1%) | 17/169 (10.1%) | -41.7 | 0.33 |
| Breddin et al, 1983 | H15/HDHE 7.5 | 20/130 (15.4%) | 17/129 (13.2%) | 14.3 | 0.61 |
| Combined data |  |  |  | -9.1 | 0.84 |

# The combination of dihydroergotamine and heparin

Changes in blood coagulation and stasis in the deep veins of the lower limbs are both considered to be important factors in the pathogenesis of deep vein thrombosis. It is, therefore, logical to propose that prophylaxis might be better achieved by methods which minimise or eliminate both of these factors rather than by methods directed at counteracting either factor alone.

Dihydroergotamine (DHE) is a potent vasoconstrictor in man (Aellig, 1975). Its site of action seems to be the capacitance vessels of the limbs. DHE administered subcutaneously has been shown to increase the velocity of venous flow in the major veins of the lower limbs by constricting the capacitance vessels, while exerting a negligible influence on resistance vessels and capillary filtration (Mellander and Nordenfelt, 1970). A single injection of 0.5 mg of DHE has been shown to increase the mean calf muscle blood flow significantly, an effect which persists for up to five hours (Stamatakis et al, 1978). It has also been shown that DHE enhances the synthesis of prostaglandins and this may affect platelet function (Kakkar et al, 1979). Furthermore, several workers have also shown that the administration of drugs which affect vascular motility lead to increases in the release of plasminogen activator from the vein wall (Aberg et al, 1975, Mannucci et al, 1976). Therefore it is possible that DHE, by its action on $\alpha$-adrenoreceptors of the vein wall producing venoconstriction, may enhance the release of plasminogen activator and thus increase fibrinolytic activity.

Heparin-Dihydergot — a fixed combination of either 5000 or 2500 IU of heparin sodium with 0.5 mg dihydroergotamine mesylate — is available in single-dose vials as sterile, lypholysed mixture. This preparation has been developed to overcome the physico-chemical incompatibility of the available parenteral formulations of both sodium and calcium heparin with that of dihydroergotamine mesylate.

During the last few years, a number of clinical trials (Table 12.6) on low dose heparin prophylaxis have been reported in a variety of patient populations, using objective methods of diagnosis such as the fibrinogen uptake test (FUT) and venography. All those trials were

**Table 12.7**
Incidence of vasospastic reactions to DHE/Heparin

| Number of patients treated | Number of cases | Incidence, %* |
|---|---|---|
| 20,300 | — | — |
| 169,353 | 4 | 0.0024 |
| 295,633 | 2 | 0.0007 |
| 414,000 | 5 | 0.0012 |
| 515,000 | 12 | 0.0023 |
| 679,233 | 45 | 0.0066 |
| 574,000 | 22 | 0.0033 |
| 709,333 | 16 | 0.0022 |
| 360,033 | 1 | 0.0003 |
| 3,736,885 | 107 | 0.0029 |

*Calculated estimates based on (a) number of ampules sold; and (b) average of 21 doses per patient

randomised. In general, the addition of dihydroergotamine had little effect on the already low incidence of deep vein thrombosis detected when heparin was used alone. However, clinical trials in which deep vein thrombosis was detected by the FUT and venography performed in orthopaedic patients demonstrated the superiority of the antithrombotic effect of the combination compared with heparin alone (Sagar et al, 1976; Stamatakis et al, 1977; Westermann et al, 1978; Kakkar et al, 1979). Of the patients admitted to these four trials who received heparin alone, approximately 45% developed a DVT compared with 20% of those receiving the combination. There was no difference in the amount of operative or postoperative blood loss in the two treatment groups, although the heparin concentration in the plasma was significantly higher in the patients receiving the combined treatment (Kakkar et al, 1979).

The most worrisome complication associated with the administration of DHE is vasospasm. Although low doses of this agent given subcutaneously do not seem to affect arteriolar smooth muscle in the normal individual, these low doses may affect arteriolar tone in patients with a high degree of sympathetic activity (severely traumatised patients, septic shock, severe hypovolaemia). In a review of the European experience, a total of 107 vasospastic reactions have been reported. The incidence of these reactions per year is listed in table 12.7. Since 1977 the calculated incidence of annual vasospastic reactions is 0.003%. Most of the patients who suffered a vasospastic complication following the administration of the drug did so in a clinical setting in which the drug was contraindicated. Therefore, if used according to the recommended guidelines, the anticipated frequency of side-effects and complications should be sufficiently low to make its use very safe, which is a prerequisite for any general prophylactic agent.

# The combination of dihydroergotamine and low molecular weight heparin

Three double blind, randomised trials have compared the efficacy and safety of fixed combinations of low molecular weight or unfractionated heparin plus dihydroergotamine in the prevention of postoperative deep vein thrombosis.

In one of these trials (Sasahara et al, 1986), 269 patients undergoing elective major abdominal surgery were randomised into two groups. One hundred and thirtytwo patients received a fixed combination of heparin sodium 5000 units plus dihydroergotamine mesylate 0.5 mg (H/DHE) twice a day and 137 patients received a fixed combination of low molecular weight heparin 1500 units plus dihydroergotamine mesylate 0.5 mg (LMWH/DHE) once a day as well as one injection of placebo per day. Treatment was initiated 2 hours before operation in both groups and continued for 7-10 days. The frequency of DVT determined by the fibrinogen uptake test and venography was 10.3% in patients receiving H/DHE and 10.4% in those receiving LMWH/DHE. DVT of the femoral vein was detected in four patients of the H/DHE group and in none of the LMWH/DHE group. Intra- and postoperative blood loss did not differ significantly between both groups. Also, no difference in the incidence of wound haematoma and injection site haematoma was found. While intraoperative volume substitution was comparable in both groups, significantly more patients under H/DHE prophylaxis received volume substitution during the postoperative phase. These results show that once-daily prophylaxis with the combination of low molecular weight heparin and dihydroergotamine is equally effective and as safe as the twice-daily regimen using a combination of unfractionated heparin and dihydroergotamine in patients undergoing elective, major abdominal surgery. The advantages of the once-daily regimen of LMWH/DHE include greater patient acceptance, less nursing time and greater cost effectiveness, provided the new combination can be sold at a cost which maintains this advantage.

In the second prospective trial (Kakkar et al, 1989), high risk patients undergoing elective major abdominal surgery were studied. Two hundred patients, with a mean age of 66.6 years and almost half with malignancy, were allocated to receive either 5000 IU unfractionated heparin plus 0.5 mg dihydroergotamine mesylate twice daily or 1500 IU low molecular weight heparin plus 0.5 mg dihydroergotamine mesylate once daily together with one placebo injection per day. Treatment was commenced 2 hours before operation and continued for at least 7 days. The incidence of deep vein thrombosis, determined by the fibrinogen uptake test and venography was 11% in the unfractionated heparin plus dihydroergotamine mesylate group, and 11.4% in the low molecular weight heparin and dihydroergotamine mesylate group. Neither these figures nor those for major proximal thrombi proved significantly different. Of the four parameters used to assess haemorrhagic complications, only the decrease in postoperative haemoglobin levels in the low molecular weight and dihydroergotamine mesylate group reached statistical significance. These results indicate that once daily prophylaxis with a combination of low molecular weight heparin and dihydroergotamine is safe, effective and convenient in high risk patients undergoing major abdominal surgery.

In the third prospective randomised double blind trial (Skinner et al, 1994:Unpublished data), the efficacy of once daily, subcutaneous, low molecular weight heparin and the combination of low molecular weight heparin and dihydroergotamine as prophylaxis against venous thrombosis in 200 patients undergoing total hip replacement was assessed. Patients were allocated to receive either 3200 antifactor Xa units of low molecular weight heparin (LMWH) or the combination of 3200 anti- factor Xa units of LMWH and 0.5 mg of dihydroergotamine mesylate (LMWH/DHE), subcutaneously, once a day. Assessment of venous thrombosis was by bilateral ascending venography. The overall incidence of deep vein thrombosis was 23.2%. The incidence of major calf and proximal vein thrombosis which is most likely to give rise to pulmonary emboli, was 11.6%. There was no statistical difference between the incidence of major DVT in those receiving low molecular weight heparin alone (13.7%) and those receiving the combination (9.5%). There were no differences between the groups with regard to operative blood loss, transfusion requirements and post-operative drain loss.

A once-daily subcutaneous injection of low molecular weight heparin is very effective prophylaxis against deep vein thrombosis in hip surgery.

# References

Aberg M, Bergentz SE, Hedner U. The effect of dextran on the lysability of ex vivo thrombi. Ann Surg 181:342, 1975

Abernethy EA and Hartsuck, JM. Postoperative pulmonary embolism. A prospective study utilising low dose heparin. Am J Surg 128:739, 1974

Aellig WH. Untersuchung uber die venekonstringierende wirkung von ergotverbindungen am Menschen. Triangle 14:39, 1975

Ammann JF, Aebi B. Das blutungrisiko der thromboembolis-prophylaxe in der allgemeinchirurgie: vergleich von low-dose heparin mit heparin-dihydergot 2500. Chirug 54:29, 1983

Ballard RM, Bradley-Watson PJ, Johnstone FD. Low doses of subcutaneous heparin in the prevention of deep vein thrombosis after gynaecological surgery. J Obstet Gynae Brit Commonwealth 80:469, 1973

van Berg E, Walterbusch G, Gotzen L, Rumpf KD, Otten B, Frohlich H. Ergotism leading to threatened limb amputation or to death in two patients given heparin-dihydroergotamine prophylaxis. Lancet 1:955, 1982

Bredin K, Horing R, Koppenhagen K. Prevention postoperative thrombotische komplicationen mit heparin und dihydroergotamin. Dtsch Med Wochenschr 8:98, 1983

Butterman G and Haluzzcynski I. Postoperative thromboembolie-prophylaxe mit low-dose heparin-artiel unter dihydroergotamin in fixer thombination. Medizine Wochenschrift 123:1213, 1981

Corrigan TP, Kakkar VV and Fossard DF. Low dose subcutaneous heparin — optional dose regimen. Brit J Surg 61:320, 1974

Covey TH, Sherman L and Baue AE. Low dose heparin in postoperative patients. A prospective coded study. Arch Surg 110:1021, 1975.

Echterhoff HM, Kottman UR, Okoye XR, Rohrer MG. Ergotismus: eine wichtige komplikation in der medikamentosen thromboembolie-prophylaxe. Dtsch Med Wochenschr 106:1717, 1981

Evarts CM, Alfidi S. Low dose heparin prophylaxis. J Am Med Assoc 225:515, 1973

Gallus AS, Hirsh J. Prevention of venous thromboembolism. Sem Thromb Haemost 2:232, 1976

Gallus AS, Hirsh J, O'Brien SE. Prevention of venous thrombosis with small subcutaneous doses of heparin. J Am Med Assoc 235:1980, 1976

Gallus AS, Hirsh J, Tuttle RJ, Trebilcock R and O'Brien SE. Small subcutaneous doses of heparin in the prevention of venous thrombosis. New Eng J Med 288:545, 1973

Gordon-Smith IC, Grundy DJ, Le Quesne LP and Newcombe JF. Controlled trial of two regimens of subcutaneous heparin in prevention of postoperative deep vein thrombosis. Lancet i:1133, 1972

Hampson WG, Harris FC, Lucas HK, Roberts PH, McCall IW, Jackson PC et al. Failure of low dose heparin to prevent venous thrombosis after hip replacement arthroplasty. Lancet ii:795, 1974

Harris WH, Salzman EA, Athanasoulis C. Comparison of warfarin, low molecular weight dextran, aspirin and subcutaneous heparin in prevention of venous thromboembolism following total hip replacement. J Bone Joint Surg 50:1552, 1974

Hohl M, Luscher P, Annaheim M, Fridrich R, Gruber UF. Dihydroergotamine and heparin or heparin alone for the prevention of postoperative thrombosis in gynaecology. Arch Gynecol 230:15, 1960

Hume M, Kuriakose TX, Zuch L. I-125 fibrinogen and the prevention of venous thrombosis. Arch Surg 107:803, 1973

International Multicentre Trial. Prevention of postoperative pulmonary embolism by low doses of heparin. Lancet ii:45, 1975

Kakkar VV, Corrigan TP, Spindler J, Fossard DP, Flute PT, Crellin RQ. Efficacy of low doses of heparin in prevention of deep vein thrombosis after major surgery. Lancet ii:101, 1972

Kakkar VV, Stamatakis JD, Bentley PG, Lawrence D, de Haas H, Ward VP et al. Prophylaxis for postoperative deep vein thormbosis: synergistic effect of heparin and dihydroergotamine. J Amer Med Assoc 241:39, 1979

Kakkar VV. The problems of thrombosis in the deep veins of the leg. Ann Royal Coll Surg 45:257, 1969

Kakkar VV, Stringer MD, Hedges AR, Parker CP, Welzel D, Ward VP, Sanderson RM. Fixed combinations of low molecular weight or unfractionated heparin plus dihydroergotamine in the prevention of postoperative deep vein thrombosis. Amer J Surg 157:413, 1989

Kiil A, Axelsen F, Kiil J, Anderson D. Prophylaxis against postoperative pulmonary embolism and deep vein thrombosis by low dose heparin. Lancet i:1115, 1978

Koppenhagen K and Haring R. Vergleich ende Untarstachung Zurichen Heparin-Dihydroergot 2500 und low-dose heparin. Klinikarzt 10:782, 1981

Krup P, Monka C. Heparin-dihydroergot/peripheral vasospastic reactions. In: Drug monitoring, Basel, Sandoz Ltd, 1985

Lahnborg G, Friman L, Bergstrom K and Lagergren H. Effect of low dose heparin on incidence of post-operative embolism detected by photoscanning. Lancet i:329, 1974

Mannucci PM, Ciherio LE, Panajofapoulos N. Low dose heparin and DVT after total hip replacement. Thromb Diath Haemorrh 36:157, 1976

Mellander S, Nordenfelt I. Comparative effects of dihydroergotamine and noradrenaline on resistance, exchange and capacitance functions in the peripheral circulation. Clin Science 39:183, 1970

Morris GK, Henry APJ, Preston BJ. Prevention of deep vein thrombosis by low dose heparin in patients undergoing hip replacement. Lancet ii:797, 1974

Nicolaides AN, Dupont AN, Desai S. Small doses of subcutaneous sodium heparin in preventing deep venous thrombosis after major surgery. Lancet ii:890, 1972

Peterson J, Zucker MB. The effect of adenosine monophosphate, arcaine and anti-inflammatory agents on thrombosis and platelet function in rabbits. Thromb Diath Haemorrh 23:148, 1970

Rem J, Duckert F, Fridrich R. Subkutane klein heparindosen zur 6th rromboseprophylaxe in der allgerneinen chirugie und urologie. Schweiz Medizine Wochenschrift 105:827, 1975

Rosenberg IL, Evans M and Pollock AV. Prophylaxis of post-operative leg vein thrombosis by low dose subcutaneous heparin or pre-operative calf muscle stimulation: A controlled clinical trial. Brit Med J 1:649, 1975

Sagar S, Nairn D, Stamatakis JD, Maffei FH, Higgins AF, Thomas DP et al. Efficacy of low dose heparin in the prevention of extensive deep vein thrombosis in patients undergoing total hip replacement. Lancet i:1151, 1976

Sasahara AA, Koppenhagen K, Häring, Welzel D, Wolf H. Low molecular weight heparin plus dihydroergotamine for prophylaxis of postoperative deep vein thrombosis. Br J Surg 73:697, 1986

Sharnoff JG. Results on the prophylaxis of postoperative thromboembolism. Surg Gynaecol Obstet 123:303, 1966

Stamatakis JD, Kakkar VV, Lawrence D, Bentley PG, Nairn D, Ward V. Failure of aspirin to prevent postoperative deep vein thrombosis in patients undergoing total hip replacement. Br Med J i:1031, 1978

de Takats G. Anticoagulants in surgery. J Amer Med Assoc 142:527, 1950

Venous Thrombosis Clinical Study Group. Small doses of subcutaneous sodium heparin in the prevention of deep vein thrombosis after elective hip replacement. Br J Surg 62:348, 1975

Wessler S, Yin ET, Gaston LW. A distinction between the role of precursor and activated forms of clotting factors in the genesis of stasis thrombi. Thromb Diath Haemorrh 18:12, 1967

Westerman K, Trentz O, Pretschner P, Mellman J, Reuter T. Use of heparin-dihydergot (5000 IU heparin) in total hip replacement surgery. In: 6th Rotherburger Colloquium 20-21 May 1977. Past HW, Maurer G. (Eds) Schattauer Verlag, Stuttgart, New York, p. 146, 1977

Williams HT. Prevention of postoperative deep vein thrombosis with perioperative subcutaneous heparin. Lancet ii:950, 1971

Yin ET, Wessler S, Stoll PJ. Rabbit plasma inhibitor of the activated species of blood coagulation factor X. J Biol Chem 246:3649, 1971

CHAPTER 13

# Low molecular weight Heparins: mode of action and dosage

Michel M Samama

## Mode of action of heparins

Two different co-factors are required for the anticoagulant activity of heparins: Antithrombin III, which is the most important because it can inhibit Factors Xa and IIa, and Heparin Co-factor II which is specific for thrombin. Heparin derivatives may be found at the surface of the vascular endothelium.

It is generally accepted that Low Molecular Weight Heparins (LMWH) have higher activities by anti-Xa assays than by APTT or anti-IIa assays. In contrast unfractionated heparins (UH) have similar anti-Xa and anti-IIa activities (Samama and Desnoyers, 1991). It has been shown recently that the injection of LMWH or UH induces the release of TFPI (tissue factor pathway inhibitor) or EPI (Extrinsic Pathway Inhibitor) activity. The release of this physiologic coagulation inhibitor plays a role in the anticoagulant activity of these drugs (Sandset et al, 1988; Lindahl et al, 1991). These results demonstrate that the in-vivo effect of heparins is partly different from the in-vitro effect observed after heparin addition to human blood.

The main unanswered question is the respective role of anti-Xa and anti-IIa activity in patients.

In-vitro, there is some evidence that the inhibition of factor Xa does not seem to interfere with the clotting process, except when factor Xa is almost completely neutralised. This can only be achieved by very large doses of heparins. However, it has recently been demonstrated that factor Xa possesses enzymatic activity through factor V activation which is as great as that of thrombin itself (Monkovic and Tracy, 1990). It has also to be noted that the inhibition of factor Xa or IIa added to plasma is not strictly parallel to that seen with the same factors when formed during the clotting process. Moreover, the neutralisation of factor Xa by heparins is easier when factor Xa is in a liquid phase while much higher doses of heparins are required to inhibit factor Xa bound to phospholipids in the prothrombinase complex (Bendetowicz et al, 1990).

In vivo it has been postulated that factor Xa generation is restricted to the phospholipids present in the membrane of activated platelets. The main findings of Hemker et al (1988) and of Beguin et al (1988) are related to the importance of thrombin (factor IIa) inhibition as compared to factor Xa inhibition. Heparins are able to act as scavengers of the first traces of thrombin which are formed at an initial phase of blood coagulation delaying or preventing factor V and factor VIII activation: inhibition of the so-called thrombin feedback loops. These results are in very good agreement with the findings of Ofosu et al (1987). However, none of the clinical trials have shown a correlation between anti-thrombotic activity and anti-IIa activity. In contrast, in haemodialysed patients receiving LMW Heparins, Lane and his coworkers (1984) were able to find a good correlation between anti-Xa activity and the effective prevention of clotting in the circuits. Anti-Xa activity and Fibrinopeptide A plasma levels were in good correlation.

Interestingly, studies with an ultra-low molecular weight heparin (CY 222, mean molecular weight 2,500 daltons) have shown that the dosage required in patients (expressed in anti-Xa units) is about 50% higher than that of conventional LMW Heparins such as CY 216, Fraxiparine[R], the mean molecular weight of which is about 5,000 daltons (Elias et al, 1986). These results are in good agreement with animal studies where it was shown (Walenga et al, 1986) that the doses of pentasaccharide necessary to obtain biological activity (inhibition of thrombin generation) and antithrombotic activity expressed in anti-Xa international units are much higher than those needed for LMW heparins. Pentasaccharide inhibits exclusively factor Xa activity while LMW heparins possess both anti-Xa and anti-IIa activity.

We have been able to demonstrate that at equipotent anti-Xa units, LMW heparins administered subcutaneously in patients are more efficacious than UH, in inhibiting *ex vivo* prothrombin activation. We have measured residual prothrombin in serum in volunteers and in patients who received a subcutaneous injection of LMW heparin or UH. Residual prothrombin concentration in serum was significantly higher in volunteers and in patients who received a LMW heparin as compared to those who received UH (Samama and Bara, 1991; Samama et al, 1991). This difference could be explained by a decreased sensitivity of LMW heparin versus UH to Platelet Factor 4 (PF4) formed during platelet activation (Lane et al, 1984).

In conclusion, as suggested by Barrowcliffe (1991), there is some evidence gained from clinical trials with LMW heparins, that anti-Xa activity "whilst an imperfect expression of their *in-vivo* effects, gives the best correlation with their anti-thrombotic action".

## LMW Heparin dosage

Different preparations are available and different clinical situations are encountered.

It has been suggested that the IVth International Standard for Unfractionated Heparin is not appropriate for the titration of LMW heparins (Barrowcliffe et al, 1985). An international standard for LMW heparin which is to be preferred has been available since 1988 (Barrowcliffe et al, 1988). In a collaborative study, Fraxiparine[R] (CY 216), Fragmine[R] (Kabi 2165) and Lovenox[R] or Clexan[R] (Enoxaparine) were analysed in five different laboratories and the results are indicated in table 13.1 (Dautzenberg et al, 1990).

## Table 13.1
Comparative activity of various low molecular weight heparins

|  | Code | Molecular Wt (daltons) | Activity (according to manufacturer) | Unit package (anti-Xa, International units) | Anti-Xa activity* (mg raw material) Anti-Xa, International units) | Anti-IIa activity (mg raw material) |
|---|---|---|---|---|---|---|
| Enoxaparine (Lovenox^R) (Clexan^R) | PK 10169 | 4500-5000 (3000-8000) | 20 mg | 2000 | 100 | 30 |
| Tedelparine (Fragmin^R) | KABI2165 | 4000-6000 (2000-9000) | 2500 IU Anti-Xa Amidolytic | 2500 | 122 | 60 |
| Nadroparine (Fraxiparine^R) | CY 216 | 4500 (2000-8000) | 7500 U Anti-Xa/IC | 3100 | 97 | 30 |

*Values obtained in a collaborative study performed by five laboratories using the same methods and reagents, versus the first international standard of low molecular weight heparin. Anti-xa activity was determined in a purified system using human antithrombin III (Kabi-Vitrum)

Logiparin^R from Novo prepared by enzymatic depolymerisation has an anti-Xa activity of 72 IU/mg and an APTT activity of 53 U/mg (Siegbahn et al, 1989).

LMW Heparins have been proposed for the prophylaxis and more recently for the treatment of DVT. The doses used in *prophylaxis* vary, an important increase of the dose being recommended in high risk patients as compared to moderate risk patients (Samama and Desnoyers, 1991). The definition of patients according to the thrombotic risk is shown in table 13.2.

The dose of Fraxiparin^R which is recommended in moderate risk patients is 7.500 Anti-Xa Institute Choay Units (= 3,075 Anti-Xa IU) once a day subcutaneously. In high

## Table 13.2
Risk categories for postoperative venous thromboembolism (Hirsh and Hull, 1987)

*Moderate Risk**
General surgery in patients over 40 years lasting 30 minutes or more
Major medical illness including cardiac diseases

*High Risk*
General surgery in patients over 40 years with recent history of DVT or PE
Extensive pelvic or abdominal surgery for malignant disease
Major orthopaedic surgery of lower limbs
Paralysis of lower limb

*Risk is increased by advancing age, malignancy, prolonged immobility, varicose veins, and cardiac failure

risk patients such as in orthopaedic surgery (total hip replacement), the recommended dose for Fraxiparine is 100 Anti-Xa I.C. units per kg of body weight once daily before and after operation on Days 1 to 3, with the dose being increased to 150 Anti-Xa I.C. units per kg of body weight from Day 4 (Leyvraz et al, 1991).

For Fragmin[R] the doses for high risk patients are twice higher (5,000 Anti-Xa IU once a day) than the doses recommended for moderate risk patients, starting 12 hours before operation (2,500 Anti-Xa IU once a day, first injection two hours before surgery).

For Clexan[R] (Enoxaparine) the respective doses for high risk and low risk patients are 40 and 20 mg corresponding to 4,000 and 2,000 Anti-Xa IU respectively. The first dose of 40 mg is given 12 hours before operation whilst the first dose of 20 mg is given two hours before surgery.

For Logiparin in moderate risk patients, a multicentre trial has recently shown that a daily dose of 3,500 Anti-Xa IU is efficacious and safe (Liezorovicz et al, 1991). In patients undergoing total hip replacement (high risk patients), the recommended dose for Logiparin[R] is 50 Anti-Xa IU per kilogram of body weight once daily, the first injection being given two hours before operation (Matzsch et al, 1988).

Prophylactic treatment does not require laboratory monitoring since no correlation has been clearly evidenced between anti-Xa activity and treatment efficacy and safety (Bara et al, 1992; Leizorovicz et al, 1993).

The doses of LMW heparins used for the treatment of patients with established DVT are much higher than the prophylactic doses. Fragmin[R] and Fraxiparin[R] are given at a dose of 100 Anti-Xa IU per kilogram of body weight every 12 hours (2 subcutaneous injections per day) (Samama and Desnoyers, 1991). The recommended dose for Clexan is 1 mg per kilogram of body weight twice daily (Simonneau, 1991).

A recent therapeutic trial has shown that a daily subcutaneous injection of 175 Anti-Xa IU per kilogram of body weight of Logiparin[R] is efficacious and safe in patients with established DVT (Hull et al, 1991).

Finally, one has to consider the problem regarding the relationship between the anti-Xa response and the patient's body weight. A significant correlation between Anti-Xa activity and patient's body weight has been clearly demonstrated (Bara et al, 1987; Vitoux et al, 1988; Bara et al, 1992; Leizorovicz et al, 1993). However, when a standard dose is given to a large number of patients, the relationship between Anti-Xa and patient's body weight accounts for about 20% of the interindividual variation.

These results suggest that laboratory monitoring, using the measurement of anti-Xa activity at the peak level, that is, 3-4 hours after the subcutaneous injection, can be helpful.

In our experience, in moderate risk patients treated with LMW heparins, the Anti-Xa activity varies from 0.1 to 0.3 IU In high risk patients, who receive a higher dose of LMW heparin, it varies from 0.2 to 0.5 IU, and in patients treated for established DVT, the provisional therapeutic range is 0.5 to 1 Anti-Xa IU. Laboratory monitoring is said to be less stringent with LMW heparins than with UH (Handeland et al, 1990; Aiach, 1991).

# Conclusion

The mechanism of the antithrombotic action of LMW heparins is not well understood. The respective role of Anti-Xa , anti-IIa activities and others is not well elucidated.

Dose-finding studies have been able to define three groups of prophylactic doses in moderate risk patients, in high risk patients and doses to be administered in patients with established venous thrombosis.

# References

Aiach M. Should deep venous thrombosis treatment with low molecular weight heparin (Fragmin[R]) be monitored or not? Results of a randomised comparative multicentric French study. Thromb Haemostas, 65:754, abst. 307, 1991

Anastassiades E, Lane DA, Ireland H, Flynn A, Curtis JR. A low molecular weight heparin ("Fragmin") for routine hemodialysis: a crossover trial comparing three dose regimens with a standard regimen of commercial unfractionated heparin. Clinical Nephrol 12:290, 1989

Bara L, Combe-Tamzali S, Conard J, Horellou MH, Samama M. Modifications biologiques induites par trois héparines de bas poids moléculaire PK 10169, Kabi 2165 et CY 216, comparées à l'héparine non fractionée, injectées par voie sous-cutanée chez le volontaire sain en chirurgie générale et chez le sujet âgé en médecine. J Mal Vasc 12:78, 1987

Bara L, Leizorovicz A, Picolet H, Samama M. Correlation between anti-Xa and occurence of thrombosis and haemorrhage in post-surgical patients treated with either logiparin or unfractionated heparin. Thromb Res 65:641, 1992

Barrowcliffe TW, Curtis AD, Tomlinson TP et al. Standardisation of low molecular weight heparins: a collaborative study. Thromb Haemostas 54:675, 1985

Barrowcliffe TW, Curtis AD, Johnson EA et al. An international standard for low molecular weight heparin. Thromb Haemostas 60:1, 1988

Barrowcliffe TW. Relationship between antithrombotic and anticoagulant activities of heparin and LMW heparin. Internat Symp Hep Rel Polysacc, Uppsala, 1991

Beguin S, Lindhout T, Hemker C. The mode of action of heparin in plasma. Thromb Haemostas 60:457, 1988

Bendetowicz AV, Bara L, Samama MM. The inhibition of intrinsic prothrombinase and its generation by heparin and four derivatives in prothrombin poor plasma. Thromb Res 58:445, 1990

Dautzenberg MD, Bara L, Cornu P, Samama M. Specific anti-Xa activity of LMWH (Kabi 2165, CY 216, PK 10169) against the first international standard of LMWH: a collaborative study. Thromb Haemostas 64:490, 1990

Elias A, Legoff G, Bouvier JL, Aillaud MF, Juhan-Vague I, Toulemond F, Serradimigni A. Treatment of deep vein thrombosis by a very low molecular weight heparin fragment (CY 222): a dose range study. Thromb Haemostas 65:251, 1989

Handeland GF, Abildgaard U, Holm HA, Arnesen KE. Dose adjusted heparin treatment of deep venous thrombosis: a comparison of unfractionated and low molecular weight heparin. Eur J Clin Pharmacol 39:107, 1990

Hemker HC, Beguin S, Pieters J, Lindhout T. The ex vivo correlate of the antithrombotic action of heparin. Annals N Y Acad Sci 566:146, 1988

Hirsh J, Hull RD. Venous thromboembolism: natural history, diagnosis, CRC Press Inc., Boca Raton, Florida, 1987

Hull RD, Rasbob GE, Pineo GF, Green D, Trowbridge AA, Elliott CG et al. A randomised double-blind trial of low molecular weight heparin in the initial treatment of proximal vein thrombosis. Thromb Haemostas 62:872, abst 620, 1991

Lane DA, Denton J, Flynn AM et al. Anticoagulant activities of heparin oligosaccharides and their neutralisation by platelet factor 4. Biochem J 218:725, 1984

Leizorovicz A, Bara L, Samama MM, Haugh MC. Factor Xa inhibition: correlation between the plasma levels of anti-Xa activity and occurence of thrombosis and haemorrhage. Haemostasis 23 (suppl. 1):89, 1993

Leizorovicz A, Picolet H, Peyrieux JC, Boissel JP, and HBPM Group: Bara L, Zittoun D, Samama M. Prevention of perioperative deep vein thrombosis in general surgery: a multicentre double blind study comparing two doses ofLogiparin and standard heparin. Br J Surg 78:412, 1991

Leyvraz PF, Bachmann F, Hoek J, Büller HR, Postel M, Samama M, Vandenbroek MD. Prevention of deep vein thrombosis after hip replacement: randomised comparison between unfractionated heparin and low molecular weight heparin. Br Med J 303:543, 1991

Lindahl AK, Abildgaard U, Larsen ML, Aamodt LM, Nordfang O, Beck TC. Extrinsic pathway inhibitor (EPI) and the post-heparin anticoagulant effect in tissue thromboplastin induced coagulation. Thromb Res, suppl. XIV:39, 1991

Matzsch T, Bergqvist D, Fredin H, Hedner U. Safety and efficacy of low molecular weight heparin (Logiparin) versus dextran as prophylaxis against thrombosis after total hip replacement. Acta Chir Scand, suppl. 543:80, 1988

Monkovic DD, Tracy PB. Activation of human factor V by factor Xa and thrombin. Biochemistry 29:1118, 1990

Ofosu FA, Sie P, Modi GJ, Fernandez F, Buchanan MR, Blajchman MA, Boneu G, Hirsh J. The inhibition of thrombin-dependent positive feedback reactions is critical to the expression of the anticoagulant effect of heparin. Biochem J 243:579, 1987

Samama MM, Bara L. The effect of subcutaneous injection of a LMWH and unfractionated heparin on intrinsic prothrombinase in whole blood during coagulation. Thromb Haemostas 6, abst 2190:1299, 1986

Samama M, Desnoyers P. Low molecular weight heparins and related glycosaminoglycans in the prophylaxis and treatment of venous thromboembolism. In: Poller L (ed.) Recent Advances in Blood Coagulation 5:177. Churchill Livingstone, Edinburgh, 1991

Samama MM, Combe S, Horellou MH, Augras D, Truc JB, Conard J, Girard P, Bara L, Poitout PH. Anti-Xa activity and prothrombinase inhibition in patients treated with two different doses of enoxaparin in gynecologic surgery. Thromb Res, suppl. XIV:29, 1991

Sandset PM, Abildgaard U, Larsen ML. Heparin induces release of extrinsic pathway inhibitor (EPI). Thromb Res 50:803, 1988

Seigbahn A, Hassan SY, Boberg J, Bylund H, Neerstrand HS, Ostergaard P, Hedner U. Subcutaneous treatment of deep venous thrombosis with low molecular weight heparin. A dose finding study with LMWH-Novo. Thromb Res 55:767, 1989

Simonneau G. Subcutaneous fixed dose of Enoxaparine (E) versus intravenous adjusted dose of unfractionated heparin (UH) in the treatment of deep venous thrombosis (DVT). TVPENOX Group Study. Thromb Res 65:754, abstract 306, 1991

Vitoux JF, Aiach M, Roncato M, Fiessinger JN. Should thromboprophylactic dosage of low molecular weight heparin be adapted to patient's weight? Thromb Haemostas 59:120, 1988

Walenga J, Fareed J, Petitou M, Samama M, Lormeau J, Choay J. Intravenous antithrombotic activity of a synthetic heparin pentasaccharide in human serum induced stasis thrombosis model. Thromb Res 43:243, 1986

CHAPTER 14

# The efficacy of low molecular weight heparins

Sylvia Haas
Peter Haas

## Introduction

Prophylaxis with low dose heparin (LDH) has significantly contributed to the reduction of thromboembolic complications. Data on more than 70 randomised trials (comprising 16,000 cases) on perioperative subcutaneous heparin prophylaxis were collected and analysed by Collins et al (1988). Their analysis clearly demonstrates that the prophylactic administration of LDH results in a significant reduction of the incidence of deep vein thrombosis (DVT) and pulmonary embolism (PE) in patients undergoing general, elective orthopaedic, urologic or major bone surgery after trauma. The investigators found that perioperative heparin prophylaxis prevents at least 50% of PE and two-thirds of DVT. Colditz et al (1986) studied data from randomised controlled trials by means of meta-analysis in order to determine the extent to which various prophylactic methods reduce the incidence of postoperative DVT. In patients undergoing general surgery, defined as abdominothoracic, gynaecologic or prostatic surgery but excluding patients having operations for malignant diseases, the rate of DVT diagnosed by the fibrinogen uptake test (FUT) was 27% in patients without prophylaxis and 9.5% in those receiving low dose heparin. Similar results were obtained by Clagett and Reisch (1988) in a meta-analysis of trials with patients undergoing general surgery.

At the moment, various heparin fragments and fractions are available for clinical use and the question arises whether these low molecular weight heparins (LMWHs) are equal or even superior to unfractionated heparin (UFH) in preventing thromboembolic complications. This general question implies, however, that all LMWH preparations are comparable with respect to their pharmacological profile and their antithrombotic efficacy and safety. Is each LMWH a distinct and separate drug, or are LMWHs a family of closely-related drugs? On the one side, there are similarities with respect to certain attributes: The currently marketed products have an average molecular weight of between 4,000 and 7,000 Dalton and the proportion of the total amount of polysaccharides between 2,000 and 8,000 Dalton is 60-80%; all products have anti-Xa/anti-IIa activity ratios greater than 1.5; pharmacokinetic studies have shown that the bioavailability of all products is close to 100% and the half life of anti-Xa activity after subcutaneous injection is 3-5 hours. On the other hand, each manufacturer makes a different product using different depolymerisation procedures (Cifonelli, 1976; Casu, 1984). All of these processes result in depolymerisation, but the individual products obtained from each process exhibit marked differences. Chemical modification, charge density differences and degree of desulfation during the manufacturing processes add to the individuality of these products (Hook et al,1976; Bianchini et al, 1980; Ayotte et al, 1981; Hurst et al, 1983; Atha et al, 1984; Kim and Linhardt, 1989). Moreover, most of the LMWH preparations are produced from raw material containing various non-heparin glycosaminoglycans; the presence of these biologically active substances in the final product can significantly influence its action (Robinson et al, 1978; Thomas et al, 1979; Fernandez et al, 1986).

The commercially available LMWHs were found to differ in further biochemical and pharmacological attributes, e.g., differences in AT III and heparin cofactor II profiles are known (Cade et al, 1984; Fareed, 1988; Fareed et al, 1988). The AT III dependent inhibition of serine proteases is an important determinant of the *in-vitro* anticoagulant actions of heparin, but it is unclear whether this property is equally important for the *in vivo* antithrombotic effect. Using various test systems, Stemberger and his colleagues (Stemberger et al, 1991) could demonstrate that chemically modified heparin and LMWHs do not produce alterations of the *ex vivo* plasma clotting profile despite showing an antithrombotic effect.

Therefore, the conclusions derived from the above mentioned variations in the attributes of LMWHs should be to test each LMWH product separately and employ special care in comparing data from different studies. Moreover, since UFH has been tested in large and well designed trials, comparisons of its prophylactic efficacy with that of LMWHs should be done on a very strict basis, i.e., results of trials with LMWHs should only be accepted if these trials do conform to the same strict quality criteria as employed in the trials with UFH.

## Review of studies with LMWH

This section presents a concise summary of selected clinical studies on the antithrombotic efficacy of LMWH in general and major orthopaedic surgery. The selection criteria applied were similar to those used in published meta-analyses, namely adequacy of study design, control of bias, statistical analysis as well as of sensitivity and specificity of methods. The study design had to comply with the following criteria: randomisation, control versus unfractionated heparin either with a fixed combination of 0.5 mg dihydroergotamine or without, and adequate assessment of endpoints. For diagnosis of DVT, the FUT was accepted for patients undergoing general surgery, whereas bilateral venography was required for patients undergoing major bone surgery. Only studies concerning the following drugs were considered: Fragmin[R], Fraxiparin[R], Clexane[R], Embolex[R] NM and Mono-Embolex[R] NM.

More than 60 studies have been assessed according to the criteria mentioned above, yielding a total of 23 trials as qualified to be referenced in this paper. To allow a synoptical

**Table 14.1**
Comparison of the efficacy of Fragmin with UFH (I) in general surgery

| Fragmin: | 2,500 anti-Xa units once daily |
| | start 2 h preop |
| UFH: | 5,000 IU b.i.d. |
| | start 2 h preop |

|  | *Fragmin* | *UFH* |
|---|---|---|
| **Caen, 1988; n = 385** | | |
| DVT | 3.1% | 3.7% |
| PE | 0 | 0 |
| **Hartl et al, 1990; n = 250** | | |
| DVT | 9.0% | 9.0% |
| PE | 1 | 1 |
| **Koller et al, 1986; n = 146** | | |
| DVT | 2.9% | 2.9% |

comparison of the results of these trials, only the most significant data (name of drug, regimen, number of patients, incidence of DVT and number of PE) are presented.

## Prophylaxis of thromboembolism in general surgery
*Studies with Fragmin*
In a French multicentre and double-blind trial the antithrombotic efficacy of Fragmin given in a dose of 2,500 anti-Xa units once a day was assessed against calcium heparin in a dose of 5,000 UI b.i.d. (Caen, 1988). Similar study protocols have been used in an Austrian (Hartl et al, 1990) and a Swiss (Koller et al, 1986) double-blind monocentre study. The results are shown in table 14.1.

In further general surgery studies, Fragmin was compared under double-blind conditions in a dosage of 5,000 anti-Xa U per day with a 5,000 IU b.i.d. administration of UFH (Bergqvist et al, 1986; Onarheim et al, 1986; Bergqvist et al, 1988). The results are summarised in tables 14.2 and 14.3.

**Table 14.2**
Comparison of efficacy of Fragmin with UFH (II) in general surgery

| Fragmin: | 5,000 anti-Xa units once daily |
| | start 2 h preop |
| UFH: | 5,000 IU b.i.d. |
| | start 2 h preop |

|  | *Fragmin* | *UFH* |
|---|---|---|
| **Bergqvist et al, 1986; n = 382** | | |
| DVT | 5.4% | 4.3% |
| PE | 0 | 0 |
| **Onarheim et al, 1986; n = 250** | | |
| DVT | 8.0% | 8.0% |
| PE | 0 | 0 |

## Table 14.3
Comparison of efficacy of Fragmin with UFH (III) in general surgery

**Bergqvist et al, 1988; n = 826**
Fragmin: 5,000 anti-Xa U once daily
start 12 h preop
UFH: 5,000 IU b.i.d.
started 2 h preop

|  | Fragmin | UFH |
|---|---|---|
| DVT | 5.0% | 9.2% |
| PE fatal n | 0 | 1 |
| PE non fatal n | 0 | 4 |

## Table 14.4
Comparison of efficacy of Fragmin with UFH (IV) in general surgery

**Fricker et al, 1988; n = 80**
Fragmin: 2,500 anti-Xa U b.i.d.
op. day, followed by
5,000 anti-Xa U once daily
start 2 h preop
UFH: 5,000 IU t.i.d.
start 2 h preop

|  | Fragmin | UFH |
|---|---|---|
| DVT | 5.0% | 0% |
| PE | 0 | 2 |

## Table 14.5
Comparison of efficacy of Fraxiparin with UFH in general surgery

**Kakkar and Murray, 1985; n = 395**
Fraxiparine: 7500 anti-Xa U IC once daily
start 2 h preop.
UFH: 5,000 IU b.i.d.
start 2 h preop.

|  | Fraxiparin |  | UFH |
|---|---|---|---|
| DVT | 2.5% $p<0.05$ | $p<0.05$ | 4.5% |
| PE fatal n | 0 |  | 1 |

**Encke & Breddin, 1988; n = 1,896**
Fraxiparin: 7,500 anti-Xa U IC b.i.d. op. day, followed by
7,500 anti-Xa IC once daily
start 2 h preop.
UFH: 5,000 IU t.i.d.
start 2 h preop.

|  | Fraxiparin |  | UFH |
|---|---|---|---|
| DVT | 2.8% | $p = 0.034$ | 4.5% |
| PE | 2 |  | 5 |

**Table 14.6**
Comparison of efficacy of Clexane with UFH in general surgery

| | Samama et al, 1988 | |
|---|---|---|
| Clexane: | 20 mg once daily start 2 h preop | |
| UFH: | 5,000 IU t.i.d. start 2 h preop | |
| n = 317 | | |

| | Clexane | UFH |
|---|---|---|
| DVT | 3.8% | 7.6% |
| PE | 0 | 0 |

| Clexane: | 40 mg once daily start 2 h preop | |
|---|---|---|
| UFH: | 5000 IU t.i.d. start 2 h preop | |
| n = 216 | | |

| | Clexane | UFH |
|---|---|---|
| DVT | 2.8% | 2.7% |
| PE | 0 | 0 |

| Clexane: | 60 mg once daily start 2 h preop | |
|---|---|---|
| UFH: | 5,000 IU t.i.d. start 2 h preop | |
| n = 270 | | |

| | Clexane | UFH |
|---|---|---|
| DVT | 2.9% | 3.8% |
| PE | 0 | 1 |

One more trial used a different regimen for Fragmin as well as for UFH (Fricker et al, 1988; Table 14.4).

*Studies with Fraxiparin*
Fraxiparin has been compared with UFH in two trials with patients undergoing general surgery (Kakkar and Murray, 1985; Encke and Breddin, 1988). The dosage regimens were different in both studies (Table 14.5).

*Studies with Clexane*
Samama and his colleagues (Samama et al, 1988) performed three consecutive open randomised studies to determine the optimum dosage of Clexane for the prevention of DVT in general surgery (Table 14.6).

*Studies with Embolex NM*
In two double-blind studies, Sasahara (Sasahara et al, 1986) and Welzel (Welzel et al, 1989) compared the antithrombotic efficacy of a once-daily administration of the fixed combination of 1,500 aPTT-U LMWH with 0.5 mg dihydroergotamine (Embolex NM) with the regimen of a twice-daily injection of 5,000 IU heparin plus 0.5 mg dihydroergotamine (H-DHE). A similar study was performed by Baumgartner (Baumgartner et al, 1989), but

**Table 14.7**
Comparison of efficacy of Embolex NM with H-DHE in generalsurgery

| | | |
|---|---|---|
| Embolex NM: | 1,500 aPTT-U once daily start 2 h preop. | |
| H-DHE: | 5,000 IU b.i.d. start 2 h preop. | |
| | *Embolex* | *NMH-DHE* |
| **Sasahara et al, 1986; n = 260** | | |
| DVT | 10.4% | 10.3% |
| PE | 0 | 2 |
| **Welzel et al, 1989; n = 200** | | |
| DVT | 11.4% | 11.0% |
| Embolex NM: | 1,500 aPTT-U once daily start 2 h preop. | |
| H-DHE: | 2,500 IU b.i.d. start 2 h preop. | |
| | *Embolex* | *NMH-DHE* |
| **Baumgartner et al, 1989; n = 176** | | |
| DVT | 6.9% | 7.9% |
| PE | 1 | 1 |

they compared Embolex NM with a b.i.d. subcutaneous injection of 2,500 IU heparin plus 0.5 mg DHE. The results are summarised in table 14.7.

*Studies with Mono-Embolex NM*
Mono-Embolex NM has been compared with UFH by Adolf and co-workers (Adolf et al, 1989) and Koppenhagen et al (1990) in double-blind studies with patients undergoing general surgery. The results are shown in table 14.8.

**Table 14.8**
Comparison of efficacy of Mono-Embolex NM with UFH in general surgery

| | | |
|---|---|---|
| Mono-Embolex NM: | 1,500 aPTT-U once daily start 2 h preop. | |
| UFH: | 5,000 IU t.i.d. started 2 h preop. | |
| **Adolf et al, 1989; n = 390** | | |
| DVT | 10.8% | 11.4% |
| PE | 0 | 0 |
| **Koppenhagen et al, 1990; n = 104** | | |
| DVT | 7.8% | 13.2% |

**Table 14.9**
Comparison of efficacy of Fragmin with UFH in elective hip replacement

| | | | |
|---|---|---|---|
| Fragmin: | 2,500 anti-Xa U b.i.d. | | |
| | start 2 h preop. | | |
| UFH: | 3,750 IU preop. followed by doses adjusted to TT | | |
| | and aPTT t.i.d. | | |
| | start 2 h preop. | | |

**Barre et al, 1987; n = 80**

| | *Fragmin* | | *UFH* |
|---|---|---|---|
| DVT total | 17.5% | | 10.0% |
| DVT prox. | 5.0% | | 5.0% |
| PE | 0 | | 0 |

| | | |
|---|---|---|
| Fragmin: | 5,000 anti-Xa U once daily | |
| | start 12 h preop. | |
| UFH: | 5,000 IU t.i.d. | |
| | start 2 h preop. | |

**Eriksson et al, 1991; n = 122**

| | *Fragmin* | | *UFH* |
|---|---|---|---|
| DVT total | 30.0% | | 42.0% |
| DVT prox. | 10.0% | $p = 0.011$ | 31.0% |
| PE scintigr. | 12.3% | $p = 0.016$ | 30.6% |

**Prophylaxis of thromboembolism in orthopaedic surgery**
*Studies with Fragmin*
Different administration schemes with a daily dosage of 5,000 anti-Xa U Fragmin were compared with various doses of UFH by Barre et al (1987) as well as by Eriksson et al (1991) in patients with elective hip replacement. The results of these studies are summarised in table 14.9.

Dechavanne and his colleagues (Dechavanne et al, 1989) tested two different dosage regimens of Fragmin against UFH (Table 14.10).

**Table 14.10**
Comparison of efficacy of Fragmin with UFH in elective hip replacement

**Dechavanne et al, 1989; n = 122**

| | |
|---|---|
| Fragmin I: | 2,500 anti-Xa U b.i.d. |
| | start 2 h preop. |
| Fragmin II: | 2,500 anti-Xa U b.i.d. on days 1 and 2, followed by |
| | 5,000 anti-Xa U once daily |
| | start 2 h preop. |
| UFH: | 5,000 IU b.i.d. on days 1 and 2, followed by dose adjust. to aPTT |
| | start 2 h preop. |

| | *Fragmin(I)* | *Fragmin(II)* | *UFH* |
|---|---|---|---|
| DVT total | 4.9% | 7.3% | 10.0% |
| DVT prox. | 2.6% | 2.6% | 7.9% |

## Table 14.11
Comparison of efficacy of Fraxiparin with UFH in elective hip replacement

**Leyvraz and Bachmann, 1990; n = 349**

| | |
|---|---|
| Fraxiparin: | 100 anti-xA U IC/kg once daily on days 1-3, followed by 150 anti-Xa U IC/kg once daily on days 4-10 start 2 h preop. |
| UFH: | 4,000 IU 10-18 hours preop. followed by aPTT-adjusted doses t.i.d. start 10-18 h preop. |

| | Fraxiparin | | UFH |
|---|---|---|---|
| DVT total: | 12.6% | | 16.0% |
| DVT prox.: | 2.9% | p<0.001 | 13.1% |
| PE non fatal n | 1 | | 3 |
| PE fatal n | 0 | | 1 |

## Table 14.12
Comparison of efficacy of Clexane with UFH in elective hip replacement

**Planes et al, 1988; n = 237**

| | |
|---|---|
| Clexane: | 40 mg once daily start 12 h preop. |
| UFH: | 5,000 IU t.i.d. start 2 h preop |

| | Clexane | | | UFH |
|---|---|---|---|---|
| DVT total | 12.5% | p = 0.03 | | 25.0% |
| DVT prox. | 7.5% | p = 0.014 | | 18.5% |
| PE | 2 | | | 3 |

## Table 14.13
Comparison of efficacy of Clexane with UFH in elective hip replacement

**Levine et al, 1991; n = 521**

| | |
|---|---|
| Clexane: | 30 mg b.i.d. start 12-24 h postop. |
| UFH: | 7,500 IU b.i.d. start 12-24 h postop. |

| | Clexane | UFH |
|---|---|---|
| DVT total | 19.4% | 23.2% |
| DVT prox. | 5.4% | 6.5% |

*Studies with Fraxiparin*
Leyvraz and Bachmann (1990) compared single daily injections of Fraxiparin in a dose adapted to body weight with UFH adjusted to daily measurements of aPTT in elective hip replacement. Table 14.11 shows the results of this study.
*Studies with Clexane*
In patients undergoing total elective hip replacement, Planes et al (1988) compared the antithrombotic efficacy of a single daily administration of 40 mg Clexane with that of a dosage of 5,000 IU UFH given t.i.d. The results of this trial are shown in table 14.12.

The prophylactic efficacy of 30 mg Clexane administered b.i.d. and started after operation was compared with a regimen using 7,500 IU UFH twice daily by Levine et al (1991) in elective hip replacement; results are noted in table 14.13.
*Studies with Embolex NM and Mono-Embolex NM*
So far, no clinical trials comparing Embolex NM or Mono-Embolex NM with UFH in patients undergoing major orthopaedic surgery and also complying with the standards set in the above-mentioned criteria catalogue have been performed.

# Discussion

The advent of commercially available LMWHs has fostered the question of whether the antithrombotic efficacy of these drugs is equal or even better when compared with UFH. An answer was sought through a plethora of clinical trials, but only a minor part of them complies with generally acknowledged methodological standards. Furthermore, the selection, assessment and comparative evaluation of trials with LMWHs is hampered by some specific difficulties.

One of these problems is the fact that LMWHs show a greater chemical and biological heterogeneity than UFH (Fareed et al, 1989). This means that data derived from trials with different LMWHs are not directly comparable. This problem should have been solved by the establishment of an International Standard for LMWHs which allows reliable comparisons based on anti-Xa and anti-IIa activities in vitro. However, it cannot be assumed that products with the same activity in vitro would have the same clinical effect.

A further problem is that different dosages of LMWHs and UFH have been used and that there is no general agreement as to whether fixed dosages should be used in all patients or whether the dosage should be adjusted to the patient's body weight or other parameters. In this connection it is important to consider whether the results in some studies were caused by a true property of LMWH since adequate dosage finding studies are not available. Welzel et al (1988) have shown that an increase of dosage does not necessarily lead to an increased bleeding risk but might achieve an improvement in antithrombotic efficacy. They compared a dosage of 2,500 aPTT-U of LMWH-DHE once per day with 5,000 IU Heparin-DHE b.i.d. in general surgery; the incidence of DVT was 14% in the Heparin-DHE-Group versus 4% in the LMWH-DHE-Group without increasing the bleeding risk. It is interesting that in all studies with 1,500 aPTT-U Embolex NM no marked reduction of DVT has been reported when compared with Heparin-DHE. Thus, further dose related studies are required in order to define minimal and maximal doses in patients at moderate and at high risk. The question of dosage does not only apply to the LMWH-group, but is also far from being answered for the control group.

There is also no agreement on the adequate point of time for the administration of the first and the second dose of prophylaxis. A previous study (Haas et al, 1988) has provided evidence that the antithrombotic efficacy might be influenced by the time interval between first injection and onset of surgery. In this trial, two dosage regimens of the same LMWH-preparation (Embolex NM) were tested in high-risk patients undergoing total hip replacement. One group received the first verum injection of 1,500 aPTT-U in the evening of the preoperative day, followed by single daily injections in the evening beginning on the day of operation. The second group was treated with the same dose, however the first verum injection was given two hours pre-operatively, followed by single daily administrations in the morning. By this direct comparison it could be shown that the antithrombotic activity of the drug is fully maintained when prophylaxis is given in the evening, although there is a lag phase of at least 12 hours between first dose and onset of surgery. The frequency of DVT was 11% in the evening group versus 19% in the morning group. In order to give a final answer as to whether prophylaxis should be started before or after operation, it seems to be advisable that this should be studied in another direct comparison having the point of time of first administration again as the only variable.

One of the most interesting and important endpoints is the occurrence of pulmonary embolism (PE). Unfortunately most studies include too small a number of patients to allow scientifically sound comparisons of the incidence of PE. Thus, concerning this endpoint, the data from the trials available and reviewed are far from being sufficient, and particularly, there are no heparin controlled studies available so far. However, the results of a controlled study including approximately 20,000 patients and assessing the incidence of fatal PE in general surgery will be available in the near future.

The comparison of the thromboprophylactic efficacy of LMWH with UFH is furthermore complicated by the fact that thrombogenesis is a multifactorial event which may be influenced by many factors, e.g., the surgeon, the patient population, peri- and post-operative treatment, concomitant disease, etc. Therefore, not only interobserver but also intraobserver variations may occur. This became evident by the three consecutive studies of Samama (Samama et al, 1988), and the two trials of Bergqvist et al (1986 and 1989). The incidence of DVT under UFH varied from 2.7% to 7.6%, and from 4.3% to 9.2% respectively.

Considering all these problems and peculiarities, the authors have chosen a relatively restricted catalogue of criteria to be applied for the selection and assessment of trials with LMWHs. Endpoints have been restricted to DVT and PE, since there is no generally acknowledged and scientifically sound assessment procedure available so far, for example, for bleeding complications. In addition, the data furnished on bleeding, haematoma and transfusions are very inhomogeneous and often incomplete. Therefore, the aspect of safety could not be addressed in this review. Furthermore, types of operation had to be restricted to general surgery and elective hip replacement, since trials including patients undergoing other types of operation did not comply to the criteria set for this study.

On account of the above-mentioned difficulties and restrictions, a general assessment of the antithrombotic efficacy of LMWHs in comparison with UFH cannot be made. But on the basis of the evaluated data it may be concluded that single daily injections of LMWH seem to be at least as efficient as multiple doses of UFH per day, although the results are slightly different for each preparation. The most evident reduction of the relative risk can obviously be achieved in high-risk patients, i.e., in patients who are still at high risk despite UFH-prophylaxis (Planes et al, 1988; Eriksson et al, 1991). A concluding judgment, however, must rest on additional data derived from further trials comparing LMWHs with UFH as well as LMWHs between each other.

# References

Adolf J, Knee H, Roder JD, Van de Flierdt E, Siewert RJ. Thromboembolieprophylaxe mit niedermolekularem Heparin in der Abdominalchirurgie. Dtsch Med Wschr 114:48, 1989

Atha DH, Stephens AW, Rimon A, Rosenberg RD. Sequence variation of heparin octosaccharides with high affinity for antithrombin III. Biochem 23:5801, 1984

Ayotte L, Lormeau JC, Perlin AS. Influence of variations in the chemical structure of heparin on its anticoagulant and anti-factor Xa activities. Thromb Res 22:97, 1981

Barre J, Pfister G, Potron G, Droulle C, Baudrillard JC, Barbier P, Kher A. Efficacité et tolérance comparée du Kabi 2165 et de l'héparine standard dans la prévention des thromboses profondes au cours des prothèses totales de hance. J Mal Vasc 12:90, 1987

Baumgartner A, Jacot N, Moser G, Krähenbuhl B. Prevention of postoperative deep vein thrombosis by one daily injection of low molecular weight heparin and dihydroergotamine. VASA 18:152, 1989

Bergqvist D, Burmark US, Frisell J, Hallböök T, Lindblad B, Risberg B, Törngren S, Wallin G. Low molecular weight heparin once daily compared with conventional low-dose heparin twice daily. A prospective double-blind multicentre trial on prevention of postoperative thrombosis. Br J Surg 73:204, 1986

Bergqvist D, Mätzsch T, Burmark US, Frisell J, Guilbaud O, Hallböök T, Horn A, Lindhagen A, Ljungner H, Ljungström KG, Onarheim H, Risberg B, Törngren S. Örtenwall P. Low molecular weight heparin given the evening before surgery compared with conventional low-dose heparin in prevention of thrombosis. Br J Surg 75:888, 1988

Bianchini P, Nader HB, Takahaski HK, Osima B, Straus AH, Dietrich CP. Fractionation and identification of heparin and other acidic mucopolysaccharides by a new discontinuous electrophoretic method. J Chromat 196:455, 1980

Cade JF, Buchanan MR, Boneu B, Ockelford PA, Carter CJ, Cerskus AL, Hirsh J. A comparison of antithrombotic and haemorrhagic effects of low molecular weight heparin fractions: The influence of the method of preparation. Thromb Res 35:613, 1984

Caen JP. A randomised double-blind study between a low molecular weight heparin (Kabi 2165) and standard heparin in the prevention of deep vein thrombosis in general surgery — a French multicentre trial. Thromb Haemost 52:216, 1988

Casu B. Structure of heparins and their fragments. Nouv Rev Fran Hematol 26:211, 1984

Cifonelli JA. Nitrous acid depolymerisation of glycosaminoglycans. Meth Carbohydr Chem 7:139, 1976

Clagett GP, Reisch JS. Prevention of venous thromboembolism in general surgical patients — results of meta-analysis. Ann Surg 208:227, 1988

Colditz GA, Tuden RL, Oster G. Rates of venous thrombosis after general surgery — combined results of randomised clinical trials. Lancet 2:143, 1986

Collins R, Scrimgeour A, Yusuf S, Petro R. Reduction in fatal pulmonary embolism and venous thrombosis by perioperative administration of subcutaneous heparin. N Engl J Med 318:1162, 1988

Dechavanne M, Ville D, Berruyer M, Trepo F, Dalery F, Clermont N, Lerat JL, Moyen B, Fischer LP, Kher A, Barbier P. Randomised trial of a low-molecular weight heparin (Kabi 2165) versus adjusted dose subcutaneous standard heparin in the prophylaxis of deep vein thrombosis after elective hip surgery. Haemostasis 1:5, 1989

Encke A, Breddin K. Comparison of a low molecular weight heparin and unfractionated heparin for the prevention of deep vein thrombosis in patients undergoing abdominal surgery. Br J Surg 75:1058, 1988

Eriksson BI, Kälebo P, Anthmyr BA, Wadenvik H, Tengborn L, Risberg B. Prevention of deep vein thrombosis and pulmonary embolism after total hip replacement. J Bone Joint Surg 73-A:484, 1991

Fareed J. Comparative preclinical studies on various low molecular weight heparins. Haemostasis 18(3):3, 1988

Fareed J, Walenga JM, Racanelli A, Hoppensteadt D, Huan XQ, Messmore HL. Validity of the newly established low molecular weight heparin standard in cross-referencing low molecular weight heparins. Haemostasis 18 Suppl. 3:33, 1988

Fareed J, Walenga JM, Hoppensteadt D, Racanelli A, Coyne E. Chemical and biological heterogeneity in low molecular weight heparins: implications for clinical use and standardisation. Semin Thromb Hemost 15:440, 1989

Fernandez FA, van Ryn J, Ofosu FA, Hirsh J, Buchanan MR. The haemorrhagic and antithrombotic effects of dermatan sulfate. Br J Haematol 64:309, 1986

Fricker JP, Vergnes Y, Schach R, Heitz A, Eber M, Grunebaum L, Wiesel ML, Kher A, Barbier P, Cazenave HP. Low dose heparin versus low molecular weight heparin (Kabi 2165, Fragmin) in the prophylaxis of thromboembolic complications of abdominal oncological surgery. Eur J Clin Invest 18:561, 1988

Haas S, Fritsche HM, Stemberger A, Otto J, Lechner F, Blümel G. Antithrombotic efficiency of Embolex NM in total hip replacement under various schedules of administration. Haemostasis 18(S2):20, 1988

Hartl P, Brücke P, Dienstl E, Vinazzer H. Prophylaxis of thromboembolism in general surgery: comparison between standard heparin and Fragmin. Thromb Res 57:577, 1990

Hook M, Bjork I, Hopwood J, Lindahl U. Anticoagulant activity of heparin: separation of high activity and low activity heparin species by affinity chromatography on immobilised antithrombin. FEBS Letters, 66:90, 1976

Hurst RE, Poon M, Griffith MJ. Structure-activity relationship of heparin. J Clin Invest 72:1042, 1983

Kakkar VV, Murray WJG. Efficacy and safety of low molecular weight heparin (CY 216) in preventing postoperative venous thromboembolism: a co-operative study. Br J Surg 71:786, 1985

Kim YS, Linhardt RJ. Structural features of heparin and their effect on heparin cofactor II mediated inhibition of thrombosis. Thromb Res 53:55, 1989

Koller M, Schoch U, Buchmann P, Largiadèr F, von Felten A, Frick PG. Low molecular weight heparin (Kabi 2165) as thromboprophylaxis in elective visceral surgery. A randomised double-blind study versus unfractionated heparin. Thromb Haemost 56:243, 1986

Koppenhagen K, Matthes M, Häring R, Tröster E, Wolf H, Welzel D. Thromboembolieprophylaxe in der Abdominalchirurgie. Vergleich der Wirksamkeit und Verträglichkeit von niedermolekularem Heparin und unfraktioniertem Heparin. Münch Med Wschr 132:677, 1990

Levine MN, Hirsh J, Gent M, Turpie AG, Leclerc J, Powers P, Jay RM, Neemeh J. Prevention of deep vein thrombosis after elective hip surgery. A randomised trial comparing low molecular weight heparin with standard unfractionated heparin. Ann Int Med 114:545, 1991

Leyvraz PF, Bachmann F. Prophylaxie thromboembolique sous-coutanée en chirurgie de la hanche (Héparine standard en doses ajustées versus Fraxiparine). Schweiz Med Wschr 120 (Suppl. 32):404, 1990

Onarheim H, Lund T, Heimdal A, Arnesjo B. A low molecular weight heparin (Kabi 2165) for prophylaxis of postoperative deep venous thrombosis. Acta Chir Scand 152:593, 1986

Planes A, Vochelle N, Mazas F, Mansat C, Zucman J, Landais A, Pascariello JC, Weill D, Butel J. Prevention of postoperative venous thrombosis: a randomised trial comparing unfractionated heparin with low molecular weight heparin in patients undergoing total hip replacement. Thromb Haemost 60:407, 1988

Robinson HC, Horner AA, Hook M, Ogren S, Lindahl U. A proteoglycan form of heparin and its degradation to single-chain molecules. J Biol Chem 253:6687, 1978

Samama M, Bernard P, Bonnardot JP, Combe-Tamzali A, Lanson Y, Tissot E. Low molecular weight heparin compared with unfractionated heparin in prevention of postoperative thrombosis. Br J Surg 75:128, 1988

Sasahara AA, Koppenhagen K, Häring R, Welzel D, Wolf H. Low molecular weight heparin plus dihydroergotamine for prophylaxis of postoperative deep vein thrombosis. Br J Surg 73:697, 1986

Stemberger AW, Riedl A, Haas S, Breddin HK, Walenga JW, Blümel G. Action of modified heparins on coagulation: in vitro and in vivo studies. Semin Thromb Hemost 17(1):80, 1991

Thomas DP, Merton RE, Barrowcliffe TW, Mulloy B, Johnson EA. Antifactor Xa activity of heparin sulfate. Thromb Res 14:501, 1979

Welzel D, Wolf H, Koppenhagen K. Antithrombotic defense during the postoperative period. Clinical documentation of low molecular weight heparin. Drug Res 38:120, 1988

Welzel D, Stringer MD, Hedges AR, Parker CJ, Kakkar VV, Ward VP, Sanderson RM, Cooper D, Kakkar S. Fixed combinations of low molecular weight or unfractionated heparin plus dihydroergotamine in the prevention of postoperative deep vein thrombosis. Thromb Haemost 62:523, 1989

CHAPTER 15

# Low molecular weight heparin versus standard heparin in general and orthopaedic surgery: a meta-analysis

Michael T Nurmohamed   Harry R Büller   Evelien Dekker
Daan W Hommes   Jan W ten Cate

## Introduction

Venous thrombosis is common in postoperative patients not receiving prophylaxis with anticoagulants. Approximately 50% of patients undergoing major orthopaedic procedures will develop deep vein thrombosis (DVT), whereas this occurs in about 25% of patients having major general surgery (Carter et al, 1987). Therefore, it is widely acknowledged that thromboprophylaxis is indicated in both these patient categories (National Institute of Health conference, 1986).

Since 1972, several randomised controlled trials as well as three recent meta-analyses have documented the efficacy of perioperative administration of unfractionated heparin in reducing the incidence of deep vein thrombosis (Colditz et al, 1986; Clagett and Reisch, 1988; Collins et al, 1988). As compared to no treatment, prophylactic perioperative subcutaneous heparin (usually 5,000 I.U., twice or thrice daily) reduced the incidence of DVT by approximately 70%, whereas this regimen was associated with an absolute excess of major haemorrhage of about 1 to 2% i.e., from a mean of 3.8% to a mean of 5.9% for general surgery and from a mean of 2.9% to a mean of 3.5% for orthopaedic surgery; relative increases of 55% and 21% respectively (Collins et al, 1988).

Low molecular weight heparins (LMWH) are fractions of heparin with a mean molecular weight below 10 kD. Conventional heparin sensitive clotting assays, such as the

---

ACKNOWLEDGEMENT: Dr HR Büller is a recipient of a fellowship from the Royal Netherlands Academy of Arts and Sciences. We have appreciated the collaboration with our colleagues Drs FR Rosendaal, E Briet and JP Vandenbroucke from the University Hospital, Leiden, in the development of the database of the studies considered.

activated partial thromboplastin time, are hardly influenced by LMWH (Andersson et al, 1976; ten Cate et al, 1984) and as compared to unfractionated heparin these compounds have a significantly reduced inhibitory effect on platelet function (Salzman et al, 1980). Based on these two characteristics, it was hypothesised that LMWH would have an increased benefit to risk ratio, as compared to unfractionated heparin, which was further fueled by the findings in experimental animal models for thrombosis and haemorrhage (Carter et al, 1981; Thomas et al, 1981; Holmer et al, 1982; Cade et al, 1984).

Since 1984, numerous clinical trials with LMWH have been performed in patients undergoing major surgical procedures. To evaluate the efficacy and safety of low molecular weight heparins, we collected all controlled studies in which these new compounds were compared to unfractionated heparin. These analyses were performed separately for studies in general surgery and orthopaedic surgery patients.

The results of the individual trials were pooled in a meta-analysis to obtain more valid and precise estimates of the occurrence of thromboembolic and bleeding complications (Nurmohamed et al, 1992). In addition, we assessed the methodologic quality of each study using predefined standards and repeated the analysis for studies with strong and weak methodology.

## Methods

### Data collection and definitions

We attempted to identify all comparative trials of perioperative prophylaxis against DVT or pulmonary embolism (PE) with LMWH published in medical journals in the English, French or German language. We searched the literature using the Medline database from 1984 to January 1991. Current Contents was used for the period between January 1991 and April 1991; in addition, the citations from the retrieved articles and abstract books of recent conferences were scanned. Authors of abstracts were contacted in order to obtain complete manuscripts. No attempt was made to obtain results from unpublished studies from either investigators or pharmaceutical companies.

From these articles we selected those reporting on patients undergoing general surgery (defined as abdominothoracic or gynaecological surgery) or orthopaedic surgery (defined as elective or traumatic hip surgery). The analysis in this report is limited to the investigations in which LMWH was compared to unfractionated heparin (usually given either every 8 or 12 hours in a dose of 5,000 I.U., starting preoperatively). Studies combining unfractionated heparin or LMWH with dihydroergotamine were also included. In addition, we only considered those studies in which a dose of low molecular weight heparin was used which corresponds to the currently recommended dose for the respective surgical indications.

For the main analysis, we only included here those general surgery trials in which expectant fibrinogen uptake test (FUT) was carried out in all patients and served as the endpoint for the diagnosis of DVT, regardless of whether confirmatory ascending venography was performed. From orthopaedic surgery trials we only included the studies which used routine venography in all patients for establishing the presence or absence of DVT, since in this category of patients the FUT is inappropriate (Büller et al, 1991).

Each article was assessed by two independent investigators who retrieved the following information for each treatment group: a) rate of DVT (defined as a positive leg scan or abnormal venogram in general or orthopaedic patients, respectively); b) rate of fatal and non-fatal pulmonary embolism (the diagnosis was accepted if one or more of the following methods or criteria were applied in both study groups: autopsy, perfusion-ventilation scanning, angiography or clinical diagnosis); c) total mortality; and d) major bleeding (defined as clinically overt with one or more of the following criteria: fall in haemoglobin of more than 1.25 mmol/L, bleeding necessitating re-operation or cessation of prophylaxis or when it was retroperitoneal or intracranial). The definitions of the above mentioned outcomes were agreed upon a priori. In case of disagreement between the two assessors, a third investigator was consulted to reach consensus.

### Assessment of methodological strength

In a secondary analysis all studies, regardless of the screening method for DVT, were scored by two independent investigators on eight predefined items that were considered indicative of methodological strength (Sackett et al, 1985). For each item, either nil (not satisfied) or one point was given. Subsequently, the scores were added to form an eight-point scale of methodological strength. The items were:
1. Type of publication peer-reviewed full paper (included in-press papers)
2. Inclusion and exclusion criteria clearly described
3. Randomisation method clearly specified
4. Clinical characteristics of the study groups adequately described (i.e., at least three of the following characteristics had to be mentioned: age, sex, type of operation, presence of malignancies, duration of operation or type of anaesthesia)
5. Description of bleeding complications
6. Accurate diagnosis of DVT, i.e., venography in orthopaedic surgery patients and FUT in all other patients
7. Blinded end-point assessment
8. Adequate description of patients not completing the study protocol.

A study was considered to have a strong methodology if it satisfied seven or eight of the standards, and to have a weaker methodology if it satisfied less than seven standards. The analysis for efficacy and safety was performed for the studies with a strong and weak methodology separately.

### Statistical analysis

The studies were analysed on an intention-to-treat basis on the information provided in the articles. For each study, the relative risk and the 95% confidence interval were calculated both for the efficacy and safety of LMWH over unfractionated heparin treatment. Subsequently, the data from the 2×2 tables considering treatment and outcomes within each study were combined using the Mantel-Haenszel method. Overall 95% confidence intervals were calculated by the test-based method according to Miettinen (Miettinen, 1976).

# Results

A total of 24 orthopaedic and 34 general surgery studies evaluating various strategies of thromboprophylaxis were identified. In 43 studies LMW heparin was compared to unfractionated heparin (30 general surgery studies and 13 orthopaedic surgery studies). A total of 8 studies, 7 performed in general surgery patients and 1 in orthopaedic surgery patients, used dosages which were higher than currently recommended and these investigations were

**Table 15.1**
Studies comparing unfractionated heparin with LMWH excluded from the meta-analysis because of the use of currently not recommended dosages

| Authors | Type of surgery | LMWH Manufacturer |
| --- | --- | --- |
| Bergqvist et al, 1986 | General | Kabi Pharmacia |
| Bergqvist et al, 1988 | General | Kabi Pharmacia |
| Borstad et al, 1988 | General | Kabi Pharmacia |
| Briel et al, 1988 | General | Kabi Pharmacia |
| Korninger et al, 1989 | Orthopaedic | Sandoz |
| Onarheim et al, 1986 | General | Kabi Pharmacia |
| Schmitz-Heubner et al, 1984 | General | Sandoz |
| Welzel et al, 1988 | General | Sandoz |

not included in the analysis (Table 15.1). For the analysis of efficacy and safety another 12 studies (6 general surgery and 6 orthopaedic surgery trials) were excluded prior to the analysis, because of an inadequate screening method employed for the detection of DVT (Table 15.2). The remaining studies considered for analysis, encompassed a total of 8,172 patients, with 6,878 patients in the general surgery trials (17 studies) and 1,294 patients in the orthopaedic surgery trials (6 studies) (Table 15.3). For the analysis of methodological strength, all 35 heparin controlled studies, which used the presently recommended dosage of LMWH for comparison, were considered.

**Deep vein thrombosis**
The relative risk for DVT of LMWH over standard heparin for all surgical trials combined was 0.74 (95% CI: 0.65-0.86). The relative risks for the general and orthopaedic surgery studies separately were comparable (RR:0.79; 95% CI 0.65-0.96 and RR: 0.68; 95% CI: 0.54-0.86, respectively). The number of patients studied as well as the number of events in

**Table 15.2**
Studies comparing unfractionated heparin with LMWH excluded from the meta-analysis, because of an inadequate screening method for the detection of deep vein thrombosis

| Authors | Type of surgery | LMWH Manufacturer |
| --- | --- | --- |
| Breyer et al, 1987 | Orthopaedic | Kabi Pharmacia |
| Catania et al, 1988 | General | Alfa Farmaceutici |
| Haas et al, 1987 | Orthopaedic | Sandoz |
| Heilmann et al, 1989 | General | Sandoz |
| Hoffmann et al, 1987 | General | Sandoz |
| Lassen et al, 1988 | Orthopaedic | Sandoz |
| Lassen et al, 1989 | Orthopaedic | Sandoz |
| Monreal et al, 1989 | Orthopaedic | Kabi Pharmacia |
| Pini et al, 1989 | Orthopaedic | Alfa Farmaceutici |
| Salcuni et al, 1988 | General | Alfa Farmaceutici |
| Steiner et al, 1989 | General | Sandoz |
| Von Voight et al, 1986 | General | Sandoz |

**Table 15.3**
Studies comparing LMWH with unfractionated heparin included in the meta-analysis*

| Authors | Type of surgery | Total number of patients studied | LMWH Manufacturer |
| --- | --- | --- | --- |
| Adolf et al, 1989 | General | 404 | Sandoz |
| Barre et al, 1987 | Orthopaedic | 80 | Kabi Pharmacia |
| Baumgartner et al, 1989 | General | 201 | Sandoz |
| Blum et al, 1989 | General | 128 | Organon |
| Cade et al, 1989 | General | 516 | Organon |
| Caen et al, 1988 | General | 385 | Kabi Pharmacia |
| Dahan et al, 1989 | General | 100 | Sanofi-Choay |
| Dechavanne et al, 1989 | Orthopaedic | 122 | Kabi Pharmacia |
| Encke and Breddin, 1988 | General | 1,909 | Sanofi-Choay |
| Eriksson et al, 1989 | Orthopaedic | 136 | Kabi Pharmacia |
| Estoppey et al, 1989 | Orthopaedic | 310 | Organon |
| Fricker et al, 1988 | General | 80 | Kabi Pharmacia |
| Hartl et al, 1990 | General | 250 | Kabi Pharmacia |
| Kakkar et al, 1985 | General | 395 | Sanofi Choay |
| Koller et al, 1986 | General | 150 | Kabi Pharmacia |
| Leizorovicz, 1989 | General | 859 | Novo Nordisk |
| Leyvraz et al, 1990 | Orthopaedic | 409 | Sanofi-Choay |
| Planes et al, 1988 | Orthopaedic | 237 | Rhone Poulenc |
| Samama et al, 1988 | General | 334 | Rhone Poulenc |
| Sasahara et al, 1986 | General | 269 | Sandoz |
| Verardi et al, 1988 | General | 610 | Alfa Farmaceutici |
| Verardi et al, 1989 | General | 88 | Alfa Farmaceutici |
| Welzel et al, 1989 | General | 200 | Sandoz |

*The studies included all used dosages of LMWH which are currently recommended and in addition adequate screening techniques for the diagnosis of DVT were employed (see Methods section for definition)

the two surgical groups are given in table 15.4. The absolute mean incidence of DVT clearly differed. In general surgery patients this incidence decreased from 6.7% in those receiving standard heparin to 5.3% in patients given LMWH, while in patients undergoing orthopaedic surgery the absolute mean incidence fell from 21.2% to 13.8%.

**Pulmonary embolism (fatal and non-fatal) and total mortality**
The relative risk for all pulmonary emboli (fatal and non-fatal) in the two surgical groups together was 0.43 (95% C.I.: 0.26-0.72). These relative risks were 0.44 (95% C.I.:0.21-0.95) in those patients undergoing general surgical procedures and 0.43 (95% C.I.: 0.22-0.82) in orthopaedic surgery patients (Table 15.4). The absolute mean incidence of pulmonary embolism (fatal and non-fatal) was again higher in the orthopaedic surgery trials, i.e., 4.1% in the patients receiving heparin, which decreased to 1.7% during LWMH prophylaxis. The corresponding incidences in the general surgery studies were 0.70% and 0.31% respectively.

In all studies combined there were two fatal pulmonary emboli in the patients given LMWH, whereas nine patients receiving standard heparin died as a result of pulmonary

**Table 15.4**
Outcomes in general and orthopaedic surgery studies comparing unfractionated heparin (UFH) with low molecular weight heparin (LMWH)[*]

| Surgical group & studied outcome | Number of patients evaluated LMWH | UFH | Number of patients with outcome LMWH | UFH | Relative risk and 95% confidence interval |
|---|---|---|---|---|---|
| *General Surgery* | | | | | |
| DVT[**] | 3467 | 3411 | 184 | 230 | 0.79 (0.65-0.95) |
| PE[***] | 2888 | 2843 | 9 | 20 | 0.44 (0.21-0.95) |
| Major bleeding | 1977 | 1966 | 52 | 51 | 1.01 (0.70-1.48) |
| *Orthopaedic Surgery* | | | | | |
| DVT[**] | 672 | 622 | 93 | 132 | 0.68 (0.54-0.86) |
| PE[***] | 590 | 582 | 10 | 24 | 0.43 (0.22-0.82) |
| Major bleeding | 672 | 622 | 6 | 8 | 0.75 (0.26-2.14) |

[*] All studies used dosages of LMWH currently recommended and applied adequate screening techniques for the detection of DVT (see Methods section for definition)
[**] DVT denotes deep venous thrombosis
[***] PE denotes pulmonary embolism, and includes both fatal and non-fatal pulmonary embolism

embolism. There was no significant difference in the total number of deaths in all surgical trials combined (20 LMWH treated patients and 24 unfractionated heparin treated patients). No patients died due to haemorrhage.

**Major bleeding**
For all studies combined there was no difference in the incidences of major bleeding (RR: 0.98%; 95% C.I.: 0.69-1.40). Similar relative risks for major bleeding were observed in the general and orthopaedic surgery trials separately (RR: 1.01 95% C.I.: 0.70-1.48 and RR: 0.75; 95% C.I.: 0.26-2.14 respectively). In the general surgery trials the absolute mean incidence of major bleeding was 2.6% in each of the two treatment groups. The absolute mean incidence of major haemorrhage in the orthopaedic studies, although in a much smaller number of patients, was 0.9% during the administration of LWMH and 1.3% in patients receiving unfractionated heparin.

**Methodological strength**
Thirteen studies (8 general surgery studies and 5 orthopaedic surgery trials) were designated to have a strong methodology, while the remaining 22 investigations (15 general surgery and 7 orthopaedic surgery trials) turned out have a less strict design (Table 15.5). This secondary analysis revealed a comparable risk reduction of DVT for the two methodological orthopaedic study groups (RR:0.75; 95% C.I.: 0.56-0.99 for the strong studies and RR: 0.82; 95% C.I.: 0.66-1.02 for the weaker studies, respectively), whereas in the methodologically strong general surgery trials, in contrast to the weaker general surgery studies, almost no risk reduction of DVT was observed (RR: 0.91; 95% C.I.: 0.68-1.23 for the strong studies and RR: 0.67; 95% C.I.: 0.54-0.85 for the less stringent designs, respectively).

With respect to haemorrhage a difference (i.e., increase versus decrease) in the occurrence of major bleeding was only evident in the general surgery trials and not in the

**Table 15.5**
Outcomes in general and orthopaedic surgery studies comparing unfractionated heparin (UFH) with low molecular weight heparin (LMWH) subdivided by methodological strength[*]

| Surgical group & studied outcome | Number of patients evaluated LMWH | UFH | Number of patients with outcome LMWH | UFH | Relative risk and 95% confidence interval |
|---|---|---|---|---|---|
| *General Surgery* | | | | | |
| Strong methodology | | | | | |
| DVT[**] | 1137 | 1127 | 76 | 83 | 0.91 (0.68-1.23) |
| PE[***] | 1137 | 1127 | 5 | 8 | 0.62 (0.21-1.87) |
| Major bleeding | 1137 | 1127 | 20 | 15 | 1.32 (0.69-2.56) |
| Weaker methodology | | | | | |
| DVT[**] | 3092 | 3028 | 117 | 169 | 0.67 (0.54-0.85) |
| PE[***] | 2363 | 2310 | 6 | 16 | 0.37 (0.15-0.90) |
| Major bleeding | 1529 | 1515 | 46 | 53 | 0.86 (0.58-1.26) |
| *Orthopaedic Surgery* | | | | | |
| Strong methodology | | | | | |
| DVT[**] | 387 | 337 | 67 | 85 | 0.75 (0.56-0.99) |
| PE[***] | 305 | 297 | 15 | 20 | 0.76 (0.41-1.41) |
| Major bleeding | 387 | 337 | 6 | 5 | 1.19 (0.36-3.90) |
| Weaker methodology | | | | | |
| DVT[**] | 682 | 686 | 112 | 138 | 0.82 (0.66-1.02) |
| PE[***] | 682 | 686 | 2 | 6 | 0.33 (0.07-1.51) |
| Major bleeding | 622 | 626 | 7 | 5 | 1.40 (0.45-4.36) |

[*] All studies used dosages of LMWH currently recommended and applied adequate screening techniques for the detection of DVT (see Methods section for definition)
[**] DVT denotes deep venous thrombosis
[***] PE denotes pulmonary embolism, and includes both fatal and non-fatal pulmonary embolism

orthopaedic studies, when subdivided for methodological strength. In the general surgery studies, the relative risk for major bleeding in the methodologically stronger studies was 1.32 (95% C.I.: 0.60-2.56) as compared to 0.86 (95% C.I.: 0.61-1.39 in the investigations with a weaker methodology. The corresponding relative risks in the orthopaedic studies, although again a limited number of patients, were 1.19 (95% C.I.: 0.36-3.90) and 1.40 (95%C.I.: 0.45-4.36) respectively.

# Discussion

It is now well recognised that thromboprophylaxis is indicated in all patients undergoing general or orthopaedic surgical procedures. Since low dose heparin administered subcutaneously is the most widely used thromboprophylactic agent, we restricted the present analysis of the efficacy and safety of LMWH to those investigations in which unfractionated heparin was the comparative agent. Moreover, for the primary analysis we only considered the trials with dosages of LMWH currently recommended and with an appropriate screening method for the detection of DVT. Failure to exclude studies which evaluated higher dosages of LMWH than currently used (as was the case in the initial investigations of LMWH as thromboprophylactic agents) would lead to incorrect conclusions about the efficacy and safety of LMWH and thereby to improper advice to clinicians about the potential use of LMWH. It has now been shown beyond any doubt that contrast venography is the only accurate method for the diagnosis of asymptomatic DVT in patients after hip surgery (Cruickshank et al, 1989). Although FUT lacks specificity and has a suboptimal sensitivity, it still can be considered a satisfactory screening method in direct comparative studies in patients undergoing general surgical procedures (Büller et al, 1991).

In the primary meta-analysis, we observed an approximate overall 25-30% reduction in the incidence of DVT in patients given LMWH as compared to unfractionated heparin (Table 15.4) These overall reductions were comparable in both surgical indications investigated. This observation of a similar relative reduction, regardless of the type of surgery, was also noted in an earlier analysis comparing unfractionated heparin to no treatment (Collins et al, 1988). It should, however, be realised that the absolute reduction in the rate of DVT is much larger for patients undergoing orthopaedic surgery. Expressed as the number of patients needed to be treated in order to prevent one event (Laupacis et al, 1988), it can be calculated that approximately 14 hip surgery patients given LMWH are required to prevent one additional episode of DVT, whereas for this effect about 71 general surgery patients should be treated. This contrast becomes even more relevant if one realises that the venous thrombi in hip surgery patients are usually larger and more often located in the proximal veins. Moreover, the diagnosis of DVT in the general surgery studies was based on an abnormal leg scan, whereas the thrombi in the orthopaedic studies were detected by contrast venography.

The greater efficacy of LMWH in the prevention of venous thrombi in the leg is also reflected by the observed reduction in the occurrence of non-fatal pulmonary emboli. Again, this effect is comparable in the two surgical groups. Exclusion of the studies combining LWMH and standard heparin with dihydroergotamine (Sasahara et al, 1986; Baumgartner et al, 1989; Welzel et al, 1989) had no significant effect on the results of the main analysis (data not shown).

In contrast to the expectations, based on previous experimental studies, the use of LMWH (at the dosages used in the studies analysed) is not associated with a lower bleeding risk. In fact, the incidence of major haemorrhage was identical to that observed in patients receiving standard heparin.

Our secondary analysis, in which the various studies were subdivided by methodological strength (using predefined criteria), yielded some interesting observations (Table 15.5). The reductions in venous thromboembolic complications with LMWH in the general surgery trials were much lower in the investigations with a strong study methodology. The explanation for this difference is at present unclear but may suggest an inaccurate assessment of venous thrombosis in the studies with a less stringent design. Furthermore, in this secondary analysis we observed a moderately increased frequency of major bleeding with LMWH in the general surgery studies with a strong methodology. This suggests a difference in the reporting of haemorrhage in the studies with a weaker methodology. In the orthopaedic studies, when subdivided by study methodology, no such differences were observed. It is at present unclear whether this is a true finding or the result of the small number of patients in each category.

In any meta-analysis, publication bias, as a result of under-reporting of smaller trials with no significant effect, must always be considered as a possible explanation of the outcome. However, analysis of the distribution of the various trials by the number of study patients included did not suggest that such a bias was present.

In our meta-analysis we did not differentiate between the various LMWH preparations, since subgroup analysis for each LMWH preparation would not yield enough patients per treatment group to detect clinically relevant differences between the preparations. Direct comparative studies as well as subsequent meta-analyses, including a larger number of studies, may resolve this issue.

In summary, taking both the effects on efficacy and safety of LMWH into account, it is at present unlikely that these compounds induce a clinically relevant improvement in the prophylaxis of venous thrombosis in patients undergoing general surgical procedures. In orthopaedic surgical patients, however, the absolute benefit is much larger and therefore these agents should be considered a better alternative than unfractionated heparin.

# References

Adolf J, Knee H, Roder JD, Van de Flierdt E, Siewert RJ. Thromboembolieprophylaxe mit niedermolekularem Heparin in der Abdominalchirurgie. Dtsch Med Wschr 114:48, 1989

Andersson LO, Barrowcliffe TW, Holmer E, Johnson EA, Sims GEC. Anticoagulant properties of heparin fractionated by affinity chromatography on matrix bound antithrombin III and by gel filtration. Thromb Res 9:575, 1976

Barre J, Pfister G, Potron G, Droulle C, Baudrillard JC, Barbier P, Kher A. Efficacité et tolérance comparée du Kabi 2165 et de l'héparine standard dans la prévention des thromboses profondes au cours des prothèses totales de hance. J Mal Vasc 12:90, 1987

Baumgartner A, Jacot N, Moser G, Krahenbuhl B. Prevention of postoperative deep vein thrombosis by only one daily injection of low molecular weight heparin and dihydroergotamine. VASA 18:152, 1989

Bergqvist D, Burmark US, Frisell J, Hallböök T, Lindblad B, Risberg B, Törngren S, Wallin G. Low molecular weight heparin once daily compared with conventional low-dose heparin twice daily. A prospective double-blind multicentre trial on prevention of postoperative thrombosis. Br J Surg 73:204, 1986

Bergqvist D, Mätzsch T, Burmark US, Frisell J, Guilbaud O, Hallböök T, Horn A, Lindhagen A, Ljungner H, Ljungström KG, Onarheim H, Risberg B, Törngren S. Örtenwall P. Low molecular weight heparin given the evening before surgery compared with conventional low-dose heparin in prevention of thrombosis. Br J Surg 75:888, 1988

Blum A, Desruennes E, Elias A, Lagrange G, Loriferne JF. DVT prophylaxis for digestive tract cancer comparing the LMWH heparinoid ORG 10172 (Lomoparan) with calcium heparin. Thromb Haemost 62:126, abstract, 1989

Borstad E, Urdal K, Handeland G, Abildgaard U. Comparison of low molecular weight heparin vs unfractionated heparin in gynaecological surgery. Acta Obstet Gynecol Scand 67:99, 1988

Breyer HG, Hahn F, Koppenhagen K, Bacher P, Werner B. Prevention of deep vein thrombosis in orthopaedic surgery: Fragmin versus heparin-DHE. Thromb Haemost VII (Suppl.):23, 1987

Briel RC, Doller P, Hermann C, Hermann P. Thromboembolie-Prophylaxe bei Hysterektomien mit dem niedermolekularem Heparin Fragmin. Geburts Frauenheilk 48:160, 1988

Büller HR, Lensing AWA, Hirsh J, ten Cate JW. Deep venous thrombosis: New noninvasive diagnostic tests. Thromb Haemost 66:133, 1991

Cade JF, Buchanan MR, Boneu B, Ockelford PA, Carter CJ, Cerskus AL, Hirsh J. A comparison of antithrombotic and haemorrhagic effects of low molecular weight heparin fractions: The influence of the method of preparation. Thromb Res 35:613, 1984

Cade J, Gallus A, Ockelford P, Magnani H. Org 10172 or heparin for preventing venous thrombosis (VT) after surgery for malignant disease? A double blind multicentre comparison. Thromb Haemost 61(1):42, abstract, 1989

Caen JP. A randomised double-blind study between a low molecular weight heparin (Kabi 2165) and standard heparin in the prevention of deep vein thrombosis in general surgery — a French multicentre trial. Thromb Haemost 52(2):216, 1988

Carter CJ, Kelton JG, Hirsh J, Gent M. Relationship between antithrombotic and anticoagulant effects of low molecular weight heparin. Thromb Rs 21:169, 1981

Carter C, Gent M, Leclerc JR. The epidemiology of venous thrombosis. In: Colman RW, Hirsh J, Marder VJ, Salzman EW (eds). Hemostasis and thrombosis: basic principles and clinical practice, 2nd edn. JB Lippincott Co, Philadelphia, 1185, 1987

Catania G, Salanitri G. Prevention of postoperative deep vein thrombosis by two different heparin types. Int J Clin Pharmacol Ther Toxic 26:304, 1988

Clagett GP, Reisch JS. Prevention of venous thromboembolism in general surgical patients. Ann Surg 208:227, 1988

Colditz G, Tuden R, Oster G. Rates of venous thrombosis after general surgery: combined results of randomised clinical trial. Lancet ii:143, 1986

Collins R, Scrimgeour A, Yusuf S, Petro R. Reduction in fatal pulmonary embolism and venous thrombosis by perioperative administration of subcutaneous heparin. N Engl J Med 318:1162, 1988

Cruickshank MK, Levine MN, Hirsh J et al. An evaluation of impedance plethysmography and $^{125}$I-fibrinogen leg scanning in patients following hip surgery. Thromb Haemostas 62:830, 1989

Dahan M, Levasseur Ph, Bogaty J, Boneu B, Samama M. Prevention of postoperative deep vein thrombosis (DVT) in malignant patients by Fraxiparine (a low molecular weight heparin). A co-operative trial. Thromb Haemost 62(1):519, abstract, 1989

Dechavanne M, Ville D, Berruyer M, Trepo F, Dalery F, Clermont N, Lerat JL, Moyen B, Fischer LP, Kher A, Barbier P. Randomised trial of a low-molecular weight heparin (Kabi 2165) versus adjusted dose subcutaneous standard heparin in the prophylaxis of deep vein thrombosis after elective hip surgery. Haemostasis 1:5, 1989

Encke A, Breddin K. Comparison of a low molecular weight heparin and unfractionated heparin for the prevention of deep vein thrombosis in patients undergoing abdominal surgery. Br J Surg 75:1058, 1988

Eriksson BI, Eriksson E, Wadenvik H, Tengborn L, Risberg B. Comparison of low molecular weight heparin and unfractionated heparin in prophylaxis of deep vein thrombosis and pulmonary embolism in total hip replacement. Thromb Haemost 62(1):470, abstract, 1989

Estoppey D, Hochreiter J, Breyer GH et al. Org 10172 (Lomoparan) versus heparin-DHE in prevention of thromboembolism in total hip replacement — a multicentre trial. Thromb Haemost 62:356, abstract, 1989

Fricker JP, Vergnes Y, Schach R et al. Low dose heparin versus low molecular weight heparin in the prophylaxis of thromboembolic complications of abdominal oncological surgery. Eur J Clin Inv 18:561, 1988

Haas S, Stemberger A, Fritsche HM et al. Prophylaxis of deep vein thrombosis in high risk patients undergoing total hip replacement with low molecular weight heparin plus dihydroergotamine. Arznei Forsch Drug Res 37(II):839, 1987

Hartl P, Brücke P, Dienstl E, Vinazzer H. Prophylaxis of thromboembolism in general surgery: comparison between standard heparin and Fragmin. Thromb Res 57:577, 1990

Heilmann L, Kruck M, Schindler AE. Thromboseprophylaxe in der Gynäkologie: Doppelblindvergleich zwischen niedermolekularem (LMWH) und unfraktioniertem (UFH) Heparin. Geburts Frauenheilk 49:803, 1989

Hoffman R, Largiardèr F, Roethlin M. Perioperative Thromboembolie-Prophylaxe: niedrig dosiertes Heparin oder low molecular Heparin-DHE, Vor- und Nachteile. Helv Chir Acta 54:521, 1987

Holmer E, Mattson C, Nilsson S. Anticoagulant and antithrombotic effects of heparin and low molecular weight heparin fragment in rabbits. Thromb Res 25:475, 1982

Kakkar VV, Murray WJG. Efficacy and safety of low molecular weight heparin (CY 216) in preventing postoperative venous thromboembolism: a co-operative study. Br J Surg 71:786, 1985

Koller M, Schoch U, Buchmann P, Largiadèr F, von Felten A, Frick PG. Low molecular weight heparin (Kabi 2165) as thromboprophylaxis in elective visceral surgery. A randomised double-blind study versus unfractionated heparin. Thromb Haemost 56(3):243, 1986

Korninger C, Schlag G, Poigenfürst J, et al. Randomised trial of low molecular weight heparin (LMWH) versus low dose heparin/acenocoumarin (H/AC) in patients with hip fracture — Thromboprophylactic effect and bleeding complications. Thromb Haemost 62(1):187, abstract, 1989

Lassen MR, Borris LC, Christensen HM, et al. Heparin/dihydroergotamine for venous thrombosis prophylaxis: comparison of low dose heparin and low molecular weight heparin in hip surgery. Br J Surg 75:686, 1988

Lassen MR, Borris LC, Christensen HM et al. Prevention of thromboembolism in hip fracture patients. Arch Orthop Trauma Surg 108:10, 1989

Laupacis A, Sackett DL, Roberts RS. An assessment of clinically useful measures of the consequences of treatment. N Engl J Med 318:1728, 1988

Leizorovicz A. Comparison of two doses of low molecular weight heparin in the prevention of postoperative vein thrombosis (DVT). Thromb Haemost 62:521 (abstract) 1989

Leyvraz PF, Postel M, Bachmann F, Hoek JA, Samama M, Vandenbroek D. Prevention of deep vein thrombosis after total hip replacement: Randomised comparison between adjusted dose unfractionated heparin and low molecular weight heparin (CY216) In: Hoek JA, Deep vein thrombosis following total hip replacement, PhD thesis, Amsterdam, The Netherlands, 105, 1990

Miettinen OS. Estimability and estimation in case-referent studies. Am J Epidemiol 103:226, 1976

Monreal M, Lafoz E, Navarro A et al. A prospective double blind trial of a low molecular weight heparin once daily compared with conventional low dose heparin three times daily to prevent pulmonary embolism and venous thrombosis in patients with hip fracture. J Trauma 29(6):873, 1989

National Institute of Health Consensus Development Conference, JAMA 256:744, 1986

Nurmohamed MT, Rosendaal FR, Büller HR, Dekker E, Hommes DW, Vandenbroucke DP, Briet F. Low molecular weight heparin versus standard heparin in general and orthopaedic surgery: a meta-analysis. Lancet 340:152, 1992

Onarheim H, Lund T, Heimdal A, Arnesjo B. A low molecular weight heparin (Kabi 2165) for prophylaxis of postoperative deep venous thrombosis. Acta Chir Scand 152:593, 1986

Pini M, Talgiaferri A, Manotti C, Lasagni F, Rinaldi E, Dettori AG. Low molecular weight heparin (Alfa LMWH) compared with unfractionated heparin in prevention of deep vein thrombosis after hip fractures. Inter Angio 8:134, 1989

Planes A, Vochelle N, Mazas F et al. Prevention of postoperative venous thrombosis: A randomised trial comparing unfractionated heparin with low molecular weight heparin in patients undergoing total hip replacement. Thromb Haemost 60:407, 1988

Sackett DL, Haynes RB, Tugwell P, eds: Clinical Epidemiology, a basic science for clinical medicine; Little Brown and Company, Boston, Toronto, 300, 1985

Salcuni PF, Azzarone M, Palazinni E. A new low molecular weight heparin for deep vein thrombosis prevention: effectiveness in postoperative patients. Curr Ther Res 43:824, 1988

Salzman EW, Rosenberg RD, Smith MH, Lindon JN, Favreau L. Effect of heparin and heparin fractions on platelet aggregation. J Clin Invest 65:64, 1980

Samama M, Bernard P, Bonnardot JP, Combe-Tamzali A, Lanson Y, Tissot E. Low molecular weight heparin compared with unfractionated heparin in prevention of postoperative thrombosis. Br J Surg 75:128, 1988

Sasahara AA, Koppenhagen K, Häring R, Welzel D, Wolf H. Low molecular weight heparin plus dihydroergotamine for prophylaxis of postoperative deep vein thrombosis. Br J Surg 73:697, 1986

Schmitz-Heubner U, Bünte H, Freise G et al. Clinical efficacy of low molecular weight heparin in postoperative thrombosis prophylaxis. Klin Wochenschr 62:349, 1984

Steiner RA, Keller K, Lüscher T, Schreiner WE. A prospective randomised trial of low molecular weight heparin-DHE and conventional heparin-DHE (with anecocoumarol) in patients undergoing gynaecological surgery. Arch Gynecol Obstet 244:141, 1989

Ten Cate H, Lamping RJ, Henny ChP, Prins A, ten Cate JW. Automated amidolytic method for determining heparin, a heparinoid, and a low-MW heparin fragment, based on their anti-Xa activity. Clin Chem 30:860, 1984

Thomas DP, Merton RE, Lewis WE, Barrowclifee TW. Studies in man and experimental animals of a low molecular weight heparin fraction. Thromb Res 45:214, 1981

Verardi S, Casciani CU, Nicora E et al. A multicentre study on LMW-heparin effectiveness in preventing postsurgical thrombosis. Inter Angio 7 (Suppl. 3):19, 1988

Verardi S, Cortese F, Baroni B, Boffo V, Casciani CU, Palazinni E. Deep vein thrombosis prevention in surgical patients: effectiveness and safety of a new low molecular weight heparin. Curr Ther Res 46:366, 1989

Von Voigt J, Hamelmann H, Hedderich J, Seifert J, Buchhammer T, Köhler A. Wirksamheit und unerwünschte Wirkungen von niedermolekularem Heparin-dihydroergotamin zur Thromboembolieprophylaxe in der Abdominalchirurgie. Zent Bl Chir 111:1296, 1986

Welzel D, Wolf H, Koppenhagen K. Antithrombotic defense during the postoperative period. Clinical documentation of low molecular weight heparin. Drug Res 38(I):120, 1988

Welzel D, Stringer MD, Hedges AR, Parker CJ, Kakkar VV, Ward VP, Sanderson RM, Cooper D, Kakkar S. Fixed combinations of low molecular weight or unfractionated heparin plus hihydro-ergotamine in the prevention of postoperative deep vein thrombosis. Thromb Haemost 62:523, 1989

Chapter 16

# Orgaran (ORG 10172): A low molecular weight heparinoid

Alexander G G Turpie

## Introduction

Orgaran (ORG 10172), a new antithrombotic agent, is a mixture of low molecular weight glycosaminoglycuronans, comprising mainly of heparan sulphate, some dermatan sulphate and a small amount of chondroitin sulphate. Orgaran is chemically distinct from standard heparin and low molecular weight heparins (LMWH).

Orgaran has been shown in studies of animal models of thrombosis to effectively inhibit the formation of thrombi (Meuleman, 1989); to be more efficacious than heparin and LMWH in preventing the extension of established thrombi (Boneau et al, 1985); and to produce less bleeding than standard heparin (Meuleman, 1989). Orgaran does not affect normal blood platelet function (Meuleman et al 1982). Based on these early experimental and pharmacological data, it was suggested that Orgaran may have a significantly better benefit to risk profile than heparin (Hirsh et al, 1987).

The safety and efficacy of Orgaran in the prevention of deep vein thrombosis has been investigated in several large scale studies in patients at high risk of venous thromboembolism and bleeding, such as patients undergoing orthopaedic surgery, cancer surgery or those with non-haemorrhagic stroke. The results of these studies are summarised in table 16.1.

## Elective hip surgery

Orgaran has been evaluated for the prevention of DVT in patients undergoing total hip replacement in two studies, one compared with placebo and one with heparin in combination with dihydroergotamine. In the placebo study (Hoek et al, 1992) Orgaran was given in a dose of 750 anti-Xa units twice daily subcutaneously starting before operation and its efficacy was assessed by bilateral venography at Day 10, interpreted by an independent

**Table 16.1**
Randomised trials of orgaran in the prevention of deep vein thrombosis in high risk patients

| Study | Treatment | n | TOTAL DVT rate | Risk reduction | PROXIMAL DVT rate | Risk reduction |
|---|---|---|---|---|---|---|
| *Elective Hip Surgery* | | | | | | |
| Hoek et al, 1992 | Orgaran | 97 | 15% | | 8% | |
| | | | | 74% | | 68% |
| | Placebo | 99 | 57% | | 25% | |
| Estoppey et al, 1989 | Orgaran | 146 | 17% | | 4.8% | |
| | | | | 47% | | 41% |
| | Heparin-DHE | 149 | 32% | | 8.1% | |
| *Fractured Hip Surgery* | | | | | | |
| Gerhart et al, 1991 | Orgaran | 132 | 7% | | 2.2% | |
| | | | | 67% | | 58% |
| | Warfarin | 131 | 21% | | 5.3% | |
| Bergvistt et al, 1991 | Orgaran | 107 | 13% | | 4.7% | |
| | | | | 63% | | 46% |
| | Dextran | 115 | 35% | | 8.7% | |
| *Stroke* | | | | | | |
| Turpie et al, 1987 | Orgaran | 50 | 4% | | 0.0% | |
| | | | | 86% | | 100% |
| | Placebo | 25 | 20% | | 16% | |
| Turpie et al, 1992 | Orgaran | 45 | 9% | | 4.4% | |
| | | | | 71% | | 63% |
| | Heparin | 42 | 31% | | 11.9% | |
| *Major Cancer Surgery* | | | | | | |
| Blum et al, 1989 | Orgaran | 63 | 11% | | 1.6% | |
| | | | | −10% | | 6% |
| | Heparin | 58 | 10% | | 1.7% | |
| Gallus et al, 1992 | Orgaran | 219 | 9% | | 0.5% | |
| | | | | 37% | | 62% |
| | Control | 227 | 15% | | 1.3% | |

panel unaware of the treatment groups. In this study, the incidence of DVT was reduced from 57 (56%) of 99 placebo-treated patients to 15 (15.5%) of 97 Orgaran-treated patients ($p<0.001$). The corresponding rates for proximal DVT were 25% and 8.2% respectively ($p<0.005$). No major bleeding complications were observed in either group but six patients (6.2%) in the Orgaran group developed wound haematomas, none of which required surgical intervention. In a second multicentre study in patients undergoing total hip replacement, (Estoppey et al, 1989) Orgaran, given in a dose of 750 anti-Xa units twice daily, subcutaneously, was compared with heparin-DHE (5000 units + 0.5 mg DHE, twice daily, subcutaneously). In this study, which was randomised and assessor-blind, prophylaxis was started two hours prior to surgery and continued for up to ten days; DVT was assessed by mandatory bilateral venography at day 10, interpreted by a panel of radiologists blinded to treatment. The incidence of DVT was reduced from 48 (32%) of 149 patients in the heparin-DHE group to 25 (17%) of 146 patients in the Orgaran group (risk reduction 47%; $p<0.05$). Major bleeding occurred in one patient in each group and there was no difference in the incidence of minor bleeding between the groups.

The results of these studies indicate that Orgaran is effective and safe in the prevention of DVT in patients undergoing total hip replacement.

## Fractured Hip Surgery

Orgaran has been investigated in two studies for the prevention of DVT in patients with hip fractures. In the first study (Bergqvist et al, 1991), Orgaran 750 anti-Xa units twice daily subcutaneously was compared with Dextran in a randomised, assessor-blind study. In this study, DVT was detected by mandatory bilateral venography at the end of the study or by screening with fibrinogen leg scanning. Prophylaxis was started on admission to hospital and was continued for 10 days. DVT occurred in 14 (13.1%) of 107 patients receiving Orgaran compared with 40 (34.8%) of 115 patients given Dextran ($p<0.001$). Proximal DVT occurred in 4.7% of the patients on Orgaran and in 7.8% of the patients on Dextran and the incidence of PE was 3.1% and 0% in the Dextran and Orgaran groups respectively. No major bleeding events occurred in either group and there was no difference in perioperative and total blood loss in the two groups. In the second study (Gerhart et al, 1991), Orgaran, 750 anti-Xa units, was given twice daily subcutaneously on admission and continued until the 9th postoperative day and on the 7th postoperative day, warfarin was started and continued until discharge on Day 14. This regimen was compared with warfarin alone started on admission and given for 14 days or until discharge. DVT was assessed by fibrinogen leg scanning and impedance plethysmography and verified by ultrasound or venography, whenever possible. DVT was reduced from 28 (21%) of 131 patients treated with warfarin alone to 9 (7%) of 132 patients receiving Orgaran ($p<0.001$). Major bleeding occurred in eight patients in the Orgaran group (four during the period that Orgaran was given, and four during the warfarin follow-up period) compared with five patients in the warfarin alone group. There was no difference in intra-operative blood loss or transfusion requirements between the two treatment groups.

These studies indicate that Orgaran is effective in the prevention of DVT in patients undergoing surgery for fracture of the hip.

## Abdominal/thoracic cancer surgery

In a prospective, single-blind randomised study of 121 patients undergoing surgery for gastrointestinal tract cancer (Blum et al, 1989), Orgaran in a dose of 750 anti-Xa units twice daily subcutaneously was shown to be equally as effective as heparin 5000 units twice daily subcutaneously in the prevention of DVT. In this study, venographically proven DVT was found in 11% of the Orgaran treated patients and 10% of the heparin treated patients with no significant difference in bleeding complications between the two groups.

In a randomised, double-blind multicentre DVT prevention trial of 516 patients having elective surgery for malignant abdominal or thoracic disease (Gallus et al, 1992), the incidence of DVT in patients who received correct prophylaxis was reduced from 14.5% in the heparin treated patients (5000 units twice daily subcutaneously) to 9.1% in the patients treated with Orgaran (750 anti-Xa units twice daily subcutaneously) ($p>0.1$). The results of

**Table 16.2**
Comparative cross-reactivity of the heparin-dependent antibody with orgaran and LMW heparins

|  | Orgaran | Incidence of Cross-Reactivity Fraxiparine | Fragmin | Enoxaparin |
|---|---|---|---|---|
| Leroy et al, 1985 | — | 7/16 (44%) | — | — |
| Borg et al, 1986 | — | 28/33 (85%) | 28/33 (85%) | 28/33 (85%) |
| Goualt-Heilman et al, 1987 | — | 1/ 3 (33%) | — | 1/ 5 (20%) |
| Makhoul et al, 1986 | 0/13 (0%) | 11/14 (79%) | 12/14 (85%) | — |
| Chong et al, 1989 | 3/17 (18%) | 16/17 (94%) | — | 3/ 3 (67%) |
| Magnani, 1992 | 11/92 (12%) | 16/17 (94%) | 18/19 (95%) | 2/ 3 (67%) |

these studies suggest that Orgaran is at least as effective as standard low dose heparin in high-risk patients undergoing elective surgery for malignant disease.

## Non-haemorrhagic stroke

Orgaran, given in doses of 750 anti-Xa units twice daily subcutaneously has been compared in two double-blind randomised studies, one with placebo and the second with low dose heparin, for the prevention of DVT in patients with acute non-haemorrhagic stroke resulting in lower limb paralysis.

In the placebo-controlled study (Turpie et al, 1987), patients were monitored by fibrinogen leg scanning and impedance plethysmography and when either test was positive the occurrence of DVT was confirmed by venography. In this study, the incidence of DVT was reduced from 7 (28%) of 25 patients in the placebo group to 2 (4%) of 50 patients in the Orgaran treated group ($p<0.005$). The corresponding rates of proximal DVT were 16% and 0% respectively ($p=0.01$). One major and one minor haemorrhage occurred in the Orgaran group and in the placebo treated patients respectively. In the second study (Turpie et al, 1992) in which Orgaran was compared with standard heparin, the occurrence of DVT (assessed by fibrinogen leg scanning plus confirmatory venography) was reduced from 13 (31.0%) of 42 patients in the heparin treated group to 4 (8.9%) of 45 in the Orgaran treated group ($p<0.012$); the corresponding reduction in proximal DVT was from 11.9% to 4.4% ($p=0.255$). There was no significant difference in the frequency of haemorrhagic complications in the two groups. The results of these two studies demonstrate that Orgaran is effective for DVT prevention in patients with acute thrombotic stroke without causing increased bleeding. When compared directly, Orgaran was shown to be more effective than heparin.

## Heparin induced thrombocytopenia

Heparin induced thrombocytopenia (HIT) is an uncommon complication of heparin treatment which can give rise to a significant morbidity and mortality (Chong et al, 1989, Makhoul et al, 1986). HIT is associated with the presence of a platelet activating antibody but its mechanism of action is poorly understood.

**Table 16.3**
Clinical evaluation of Orgaran treatment in patients with heparin induced thrombocytopenia (HIT)

| Indication | Number of treatment episodes | EVALUATION Success | Failure | Not evaluable |
|---|---|---|---|---|
| Treatment/Prophylaxis of Thromboembolism | 93 | 94 | 5 | 13 |
| Haemofiltration/Haemodialysis | 34 | 27 | 2 | 5 |
| Cardiovascular Surgery | 35 | 29 | 3 | 3 |
| Pregnancy (Prophylaxis of TE) | 3 | 2 | 0 | 1 |
| Other | 4 | 2 | 0 | 2 |
| TOTAL | 169 | 134 | 11 | 24 |

In comparison with heparins and low molecular weight heparins, Orgaran has low cross-reactivity against this antibody in the platelet aggregation test (12% versus approximately 80% for LMWHs; Table 16.2) which suggests that Orgaran has potential as an antithrombotic agent for the treatment of HIT patients. This is supported by favourable clinical results (improved thrombocytopenia, prevention of DVT or exacerbation of existing thrombosis) in a compassionate use programme involving 161 patients (Magnani 1992). The clinical outcomes of HIT patients treated with Orgaran are summarised in table 16.3. The low cross-reactivity of Orgaran and its safe and effective use in HIT patients may be attributed to its distinct composition, which is different from heparin.

# Conclusion

It is concluded that Orgaran is an effective anti-thrombotic agent for the prevention of deep vein thrombosis in high risk patients. Orgaran has the potential advantage over unfractionated heparin and low molecular weight heparins that it does not cross react with antibodies to heparin or low molecular weight heparin.

# References

Bergqvist D, Kettunen K, Fredin H Fauno P, Suomalainen O, Solmakallio S et al. Thromboprophylaxis in patients with hip fractures; A prospective randomised comparative study between ORG 10172 and dextran 70. Surgery 109:617, 1991

Blum A, Desruennes E, Elias A, Lagrange G, Loriferne JF. DVT prophylaxis in surgery for digestive tract cancer comparing the LMW heparinoid ORG 10172 (Lomoparan) with calcium heparin. Thromb Haemost 62:126, 1989 (Abstract)

Boneau B, Buchanan MR, Cade JF, Van Ryn J, Fernandez FF, Ofosu FA, Hirsh J. Effects of heparin, its low molecular weight fractions and other glycosaminoglycans on thrombus growth in vivo. Thromb Res 40: 81, 1985

Borg JY, Flechet B, Cegendre F, Toulemonde F, Piquet H, Moncondult M. Severe heparin and pentosan polysulfate-induced thrombocytopenias: Clinical aspects-in vitro effects of pentosan polysulfate, low molecular weight (LMW) heparins and oligosaccharides. Thromb Res Suppl V:96, 1986

Chong BH, Ismail F, Cade J, Gallus AS, Gordon S, Chesterman CN. Heparin-induced thrombocytopenia: studies with a new low molecular weight heparinoid, ORG 10172. Blood 73:1592, 1989

Estoppey D, Hochreiter J, Breyer HG, Jakubek H, Leyvraz PF, Haas S, Stiekema JCJ. ORG 10172 (Lomoparan) versus heparin-DHE in prevention of thromboembolism in total hip replacement. A multicentre trial. Thromb Haemost 62:356, 1989 (Abstract)

Gallus et al 1992

Gerhart RN, Yett HS, Robertson LK, Lee MA, Smith M, Salzman EW. Low-molecular weight heparinoid compared with warfarin for prophylaxis of deep vein thrombosis in patients who are operated on for fracture of the hip. A prospective, randomised trial. J Bone Joint Surg (Am) 73:494, 1991

Goualt-Heilmann M, Huet Y, Adnot S, Contant G, Bonnet F, Intrator L, Payen D, Levent M. Low molecular weight heparin fractions as an alternative therapy in heparin-induced thrombocytopenia. Haemost 17:134, 1987

Hirsh J, Ofosu FA, Levine M. The development of low molecular weight heparins for clinical use. In: Vetstraete M, Vermylen J, Lijnen R, Arnout J (eds). Thrombosis and Haemostasis. Leuven, pp.325-348, 1987

Hoek AJ, Nurmohamed MT, ten Cate H, ten Cate JW, Buller HR. Prevention of deep vein thrombosis following total hip replacement by low molecular weight heparinoid. Thromb Haemost 67:28, 1992

Leroy J, Leclerc MH, Delahousse B et al. Treatment of heparin-associated thrombocytopenia and thrombosis with low molecular weight heparin (CY 216). Semin Thromb Hemostasis 11:326, 1985

Magnani HN. Personal Communication 1992

Makhoul RG, Greenberg CS, McCann RL. Heparin-associated thrombocytopenia and thrombosis: a serious clinical problem and potential solution. J Vasc Surg 4:522, 1986

Meuleman DG. Synopsis of the anticogulant and antithrombotic profile of the low molecular weight heparinoid Org 10172 in experimental models. Semin Thromb Haemost 15:370, 1989

Meuleman DG, Hobbelen PM, van Dedem G, Moelker HCT. A novel anti-thrombotic heparinoid (Org 10172) devoid of bleeding inducing capacity: a survey of its pharmacological properties in experimental animal models. Thromb Res 27:353, 1982

Turpie AGG, Levine MN, Hirsh J, Carter CJ, Jay RM, Powers PJ, Andrew M, Magnani HN, Hull RD, Gent M: Double-blind randomised trial of ORG 10172 low-molecular-weight heparinoid in prevention of deep-vein thrombosis in thrombotic stroke. Lancet I;523, 1987

Turpie AGG, Gent M, Cote R, Levine MN, Ginsberg JS, Powers P, et al. A low-molecular-weight heparinoid compared with unfractionated heparin in the prevention of deep vein thrombosis in patients with acute ischaemic stroke. Ann Intern Med 117:353, 1992.

CHAPTER 17

# Dextran

David Bergqvist

## Introduction

The polysaccharide 'dextran' was first described in the 1870's as a by-product of beet sugar refining. Its use as a plasma substitute was first conceived during World War II by Ingelman and Grönwall in Sweden. Two fortunate findings secured dextran's place in the history of medicine — it failed to provoke immunological response on infusion into animals when used in the molecular weight range suitable for plasma expansion, and it proved to be completely metabolised by the body. Dextran also offered positive advantages over blood and plasma — it eliminated the risk of transfusion transmitted diseases, was stable, required no crossmatching and was considerably cheaper.

Dextran is a polymer composed of repeating glucose units. It was thus possible to hydrolyse and fractionate very high molecular weight 'raw' dextran to clinically useful fractions such as dextran 70 (70,000 daltons) which has a molecular weight similar to albumin and is composed of about 450 glucose units.

Although various crude fractions of 'clinical dextran' were well tolerated as volume expanders in shock, high molecular weight preparations caused red cell aggregation and tissue damage. In 1947 the first dextran preparation was launched as a 6% solution. Around 1953 dextran production was improved, whereby average molecular weight was lowered and the molecular weight distribution narrowed. In the beginning of the 1960's dextran 40 was introduced. The antithrombotic effect of dextran was first demonstrated experimentally in rabbits by Borgström et al (1959) and for the first time in patients by Koekenberg (1961). This observation started an intensive research activity to establish the mechanisms of action.

Dextran is formed by the enzyme dextran sucrase when the bacterium Leuconostoc mesenteroides B 512 acts on saccharose. It is a neutral high molecular weight substance composed of glucose molecules bound to each other by α-1-6-glucosidic bonds, forming a chain, side chains being formed through 1-3 glucose bonds. The number of side chains depends on the bacterial strain used. With partial acid hydrolysis a fragment of desired molecular weight can be produced. In clinical practice, the most frequently used preparations have the average molecular weights of 1,000, 40,000, 60,000 and 70,000.

Molecules with molecular weights below 40-50,000 are rapidly excreted via the kidneys, the rate being molecular weight dependent. After 6 hours about 60% of dextran 40 and 30% of dextran 70 have been excreted, and after 40 hours 75% and 55% respectively.

Dextran is temporarily taken up by various organs. Dextran, which is not excreted via the kidneys, is degraded to carbon dioxide and water. This degradation is achieved by dextranase, dextran 1-6-glucosidase, which is present in various animal tissues, e.g., the reticuloendothelial system.

The clinical indications for dextran are:
1. Plasma volume expansion (Thorén, 1978)
2. Improvement of arterial circulation during ischaemia (Bergqvist and Bergentz, 1983)
3. Prophylaxis against declamping hypotension in aortic surgery (Bergqvist and Bergentz, 1983)
4. Prophylaxis against early arterial graft failure (Bergentz et al, 1963; Bergqvist and Bergentz, 1983; Rutherford et al, 1984)
5. Prophylaxis against postoperative venous thromboembolism.

## Mechanisms of action
*A. Colloid osmotic (oncotic) effect*
This property is vital for the waterbinding capacity and plasma volume expansion and is dependent on the number of molecules present. The waterbinding capacity is 20-25 ml water/g dextran, which may be compared with 18 ml/g for albumin. The water not available in the circulatory system is absorbed from the extracellular volume. An approximately 2.5% solution of dextran 40 and 3.5% solution of dextran 70 are nearly iso-oncotic with blood in vitro.

*B. Effect on erythrocyte aggregation*
In situations with an increased intravascular cellular aggregation dextran below 60,000 in molecular weight can be used because of its desaggregating effect. Above 60,000 molecular weight in vitro (80,000 in vivo), dextran induces a successive increase in red cell aggregation causing increased peripheral resistance and impaired nutritive flow.

*C. Coating of the vessel wall*
Endothelium and blood corpuscles are coated with a thin dextran film.

*D. Influence on the haemostatic system*
Infusion of dextran in doses up to 1.5g/kg body weight does not affect the number of platelets, but the platelet adhesiveness decreases with a maximum 2-6 hours after the infusion (Bennett et al, 1966; Bygdeman et al, 1966; Åberg, 1978). Platelet aggregation induced by ADP, collagen, ristocetin or heparin is inhibited by dextran.

With the exception of factor VIII, the different coagulation factors are not influenced by dextran more than what can be explained by the haemodilution, factor VIII decreasing considerably more (Bergentz et al, 1961; Cronberg et al, 1966). More specifically this is due to an effect on the von Willebrand factor (VIII R:Ag).

The fibrinolytic system is not influenced by dextran (Bergentz et al, 1961; Cronberg et al 1966), but the coarser fibrin network formed provides better protection for plasmin against fibrinolysis inhibitors (Carlin, 1980). Clots formed in vitro in the presence of dextran are more easily lysed by plasmin than control clots (Tangen et al, 1972). The lysability of ex vivo thrombi in a dextran milieu increases, reaching a maximum 2-4 hours after the dextran infusion, while dextran added in vitro does not induce any increase in lysability

(Åberg et al, 1975). The dextran effect on platelet adhesiveness as well as lysability appears to be mediated by its influences on factor VIII R:Ag (Åberg, 1978). Concurrently with the increased lysability, the platelets become more evenly distributed throughout the thrombus instead of being localised to its head (Åberg and Rausing, 1978). Experimental venous thrombi in vivo are counteracted by dextran (Borgström et al, 1959; Gruber and Bergentz, 1966; Ah-See et al, 1974; Bergqvist et al, 1985b), and data indicate an increased thrombus fragility and lysability (Ah-See et al, 1974; Wieslander et al, 1986).

Already in 1954 it was noted that dextran could prolong bleeding time in patients (Carbone et al, 1954; Bronwell et al, 1954). The molecular weight and the dose of dextran are of vital importance for the effect on haemostatic plug formation (Bergqvist 1985). The relatively more frequent reports of bleeding complications in the early history of dextran might be explained by the presence of a greater proportion of large molecules in clinical dextran at that time compared with clinical dextran today.

*E. Influence on haemodynamics*

This effect is probably due to a combination of:
1. Interaction with cell surfaces, reducing or preventing red blood cell aggregation, platelet adhesiveness, leucocyte plugging etc
2. Haemodilution with decreased viscosity
3. Passive dilatation of microvessels due to the colloid osmotic effect

## Prevention of deep vein thrombosis

### Comparison with untreated controls

The first clinical study was reported by Koekenberg in 1961. He replaced intraoperative blood loss with either bank blood or dextran in a randomised trial and found that the frequency of clinically detected deep vein thrombosis decreased from 21% to 4% in the dextran group. In a double-blind investigation Jansen (1972) confirmed the reduction in frequency of clinically diagnosed thrombi. Thereafter, it has become obvious that when studying thromboprophylactic effects, it is important to use objective methods to diagnose deep vein thrombosis.

Table 17.1 summarises the randomised studies where dextran has been compared with no prophylaxis and where venography has been used for diagnosis. All patients are orthopaedic and in all dextran is the better alternative. Although venography is used for diagnosis, there are great variations in the interval between surgery and time for venography. Bilateral venography has not been performed in all studies, which tends to underestimate the frequency of DVT.

Table 17.2 summarises the studies in which the diagnosis has been based on the fibrinogen uptake test (FUT). Three of them deal with hip surgery and here the fibrinogen uptake test is certainly not optimal, but as the studies are randomised they are included in the table. The beneficial effect of dextran is not as obvious, but overall there is a reduction in the frequency of DVT. In most studies dextran 70 has been used but there are no data indicating a difference between dextran 40 and 70 from a thromboprophylactic point of view. In a meta-analysis, Clagett and Reisch (1988) found a significant effect of dextran on the frequency of postoperative DVT diagnosed by FUT (from 24.2% to 15.6%, odds ratio 0.58; 95% confidence interval 0.45-0.75). The conclusion is that dextran moderately reduces the frequency of postoperative DVT.

## Table 17.1
Deep vein thrombosis (DVT) in studies where dextran is compared with no prophylaxis in orthopaedic surgery. Venography was used for diagnosis in all. Evarts and Feil used dextran 40, the remaining dextran 70.

|  | Dextran groups Patients n | DVT n | Control groups Patients n | DVT n | Type of surgery |
|---|---|---|---|---|---|
| Ahlberg et al, 1968 | 39 | 5 | 45 | 16 | Hip fracture |
| Andersen et al, 1986 | 29 | 5 | 31 | 14 | Hip fracture |
| Evarts & Feil, 1971 | 50 | 7 | 56 | 30 | Total hip replacement |
| Harper et al, 1973 | 12 | 1 | 15 | 10 | Amputation |
| Johnson et al, 1968 | 27 | 1 | 25 | 13 | Hip fracture |
| Myhre and Holen, 1969 | 55 | 11 | 55 | 22 | Hip fracture |
| Nillius et al, 1979 | 28 | 12 | 29 | 19 | Total hip replacement |
| TOTAL | 240 | 42 (17.5%) | 256 | 124 (48.4%) | |

## Table 17.2
Deep vein thrombosis (DVT) in studies comparing dextran with no prophylaxis. Fibrinogen uptake test was used for diagnosis.

|  | Dextran groups Patients n | DVT n | Control groups Patients n | DVT n | Type of surgery |
|---|---|---|---|---|---|
| Becker & Schampi, 1973 | 42 | 13 | 35 | 11 | General surgery |
| Bergman et al, 1975 | 30 | 0 | 30 | 0 | Cholecystectomy |
| Bergqvist & Hallböök, 1980 | 52 | 15 | 51 | 14 | General surgery |
| Bergqvist et al, 1979 | 27 | 13 | 22 | 20 | Hip fracture |
| Bergqvist et al, 1979 | 70 | 40 | 71 | 45 | Total hip replacement |
| Bowman, 1953 | 130 | 1 | 140 | 15 | Gynaecology |
| Carter & Eban, 1973 | 64 | 0 | 65 | 4 | General surgery |
| Daniel et al, 1972[*] | 35 | 21 | 31 | 19 | Hip fracture |
| Gruber et al, 1973[*] | 37 | 9 | 38 | 18 | General surgery |
| Hedlund, 1975 | 37 | 10 | 40 | 18 | Urology |
| v. Hospenthal et al, 1977 | 39 | 3 | 47 | 2 | Urology |
| Hutter et al, 1976[*] | 92 | 20 | 100 | 36 | General surgery |
| Huttunen et al, 1977 | 150 | 52 | 75 | 25 | General surgery |
| Lindström et al, 1982[*] | 35 | 7 | 40 | 12 | General surgery |
| Ruckley, 1976 | 130 | 33 | 128 | 47 | General surgery |
| Stephenson et al, 1973 | 34 | 10 | 46 | 16 | General surgery |
| Total | 872 | 173 (19.8%) | 835 | 218 (26.1%) | |

[*] Dextran 40

**Table 17.3**
Deep vein thrombosis (DVT) in studies where dextran is compared with prophylaxis with anticoagulants. Venography was used for diagnosis. Overall frequency (%) within brackets

|  | Dextran groups | | Anticoagulation groups | | | |
| --- | --- | --- | --- | --- | --- | --- |
|  | Patients n | DVT n | Patients n | DVT n | Type of surgery | Type of anticoagulation |
| Andersen et al, 1986 | 29 | 5 | 36 | 7 | HF | Heparin DHE/TED |
| Bergqvist et al, 1972 | 75 | 25 | 63 | 19 | HF | Dicoumarol |
| Bergqvist et al, 1991 | 138 | 43 | 139 | 14 | HF | Org 10172 |
| Bronge et al, 1971 | 74 | 31 | 61 | 21 | THR | Dicoumarol |
| Francis et al, 1989[*] | 51 | 12 | 52 | 2 | THR | Heparin & ATIII |
| Francis et al, 1983[*] | 43 | 19 | 57 | 11 | THR | Warfarin |
| Francis et al, 1990[*] | 38 | 31 | 39 | 14 | TKR | Heparin & ATIII |
| Fredin et al, 1984a | 58 | 27 | 58 | 29 | THR | Heparin DHE |
| Fredin et al, 1984b | 46 | 25 | 50 | 21 | THR | Heparin DHE |
| Fredin et al, 1983 | 114 | 49 | 93 | 41 | THR | Heparin DHE |
| Harris et al, 1974[*] | 61 | 14 | 55 | 10 | THR | Warfarin |
| Myhre and Holen, 1969 | 55 | 11 | 50 | 9 | HF | Warfarin |
| Heparin | 474 | 192 (40.5%) | 467 | 128 (27.4%) | | |
| Oral Anticoagulation | 308 | 100 (32.5%) | 286 | 70 (24.5%) | | |
| Total | 782 | 292 (35.4%) | 753 | 198 (23.8%) | | |

[*]Dextran 40   DHE: dihydroergotamine   TED: Thromboembolic deterrent stocking
LMWH: Low molecular weight heparin   AT III: Antithrombin III   HF: Hip fracture
THR: Total hip replacement   TKN: Total knee replacement

**Comparison with other prophylactic methods**

In tables 17.3-7.5, randomised studies comparing dextran with anticoagulant prophylaxis are shown. In the investigations in table 17.3, venography was used for diagnosis, all in hip surgery patients. In table 17.4, FUT was used, positive tests being confirmed with venography, also only in hip surgery patients. In table 17.5, only FUT was used, most of the studies being in non-orthopaedic surgical patients. In all types of surgery, prophylaxis with anticoagulants (oral anticoagulants, low dose heparin or low molecular weight heparins), is more efficient than dextran. This is especially true for low molecular weight heparins. In the study by Lambie et al (1970), the frequency of DVT is significantly higher in the warfarin group, but warfarin was not instituted until 36 hours after operation. At least in comparison with oral anticoagulants given prior to operation, the risk for haemorrhage is less for dextran prophylaxis (Bergqvist, 1983).

**Table 17.4**
Deep vein thrombosis (DVT) in studies where dextran is compared with prophylaxis with anticoagulants. Fibrinogen uptake test was used for surveillance with venographic verification

|  | Dextran groups Patients n | Dextran groups DVT n | Anticoagulation groups Patients n | Anticoagulation groups DVT n | Type of surgery | Type of anticoagulation |
|---|---|---|---|---|---|---|
| Eriksson et al, 1988 | 49 | 22 | 49 | 10 | THR | LMWH (Kabi) |
| Fredin et al, 1982 | 41 | 8 | 27 | 6 | HF | PZ 68 |
| Myrvold et al, 1973 | 55 | 20 | 39 | 16 | HF | Heparin |
| Mätsch et al, 1990 | 49 | 18 | 47 | 9 | THR | LMWH (Novo) |
| Mätsch et al, 1991 | 123 | 36 | 120 | 22 | THR | LMWH (Novo) |
| Total | 317 | 104 (32.8%) | 282 | 63 (22.3%) |  |  |

HF: Hip fracture    THR: Total hip replacement    PZ68: Sodium pentosanpolysulphate. Low molecular weight glycosaminoglycan, MW ≈ 2000 Dalton

**Combination prophylaxis**
Combination of dextran and oral anticoagulants slightly reduces the frequency of DVT but significantly increases bleeding problems (Korvald et al, 1973; Swierstra et al, 1984) and can hardly be recommended. The combination of low dose heparin or low molecular weight heparin fragments with dextran is insufficiently documented both from the point of view of thromboprophylactic effect and side effects.

Dextran, combined with mechanical methods shows an additive effect and is therefore of potential clinical interest, especially with graded compression stockings (Smith et al, 1978; Bergqvist and Lindblad, 1984; Harris et al, 1985; Andersen et al, 1986; Bostrom et al, 1986; Fredin et al, 1989). In a study in total hip replacement the combination of elastic stockings and dextran moreover significantly decreased perioperative blood loss compared with that in a group given only dextran (Fredin et al, 1989).

Acetylsalicyclic acid in combination with dextran 40 compared with low dose heparin/dihydroergotamine in hip fracture patients did not influence the frequency of thrombosis, but the combination of ASA and dextran gave significantly more post-operative bleeding problems (Pini et al, 1985).

# Prevention of pulmonary embolism

Very few studies exist which are large enough in themselves and data therefore have mostly been obtained by compiling studies in various ways. Kline et al (1975) noted a significant reduction in the number of fatal pulmonary emboli following 1 litre dextran 70 during surgery in a double-blind study including 831 patients. The study by Ljungström (1983a) is historical but its strength lies in the total coverage within a hospital and that the periods with and without dextran alternated in 2 year sequences (totally 4). To summarise the

**Table 17.5**
Deep vein thrombosis (DVT) in studies where dextran is compared with prophylaxis with anticoagulants (except Lindström: electric stimulation). Fibrinogen uptake test was used for diagnosis

|  | Dextran groups Patients n | Dextran groups DVT n | Anticoagulation groups Patients n | Anticoagulation groups DVT n | Type of surgery | Type of anticoagulation |
|---|---|---|---|---|---|---|
| Barber et al, 1977 | 51 | 26 (20.5%) | 58 | 34 (20.5%) | THR | Warfarin |
| Bergqvist & Dahlgren, 1973 | 43 | 19 (20.5%) | 32 | 16 (20.5%) | HF | Dicoumarol |
| Bergqvist et al, 1979 | 27 | 13 (20.5%) | 28 | 18 (20.5%) | HF | Heparin |
| Bergqvist et al, 1979 | 70 | 40 (20.5%) | 72 | 35 (20.5%) | THR | Heparin |
| Bergqvist & Hallböök, 1980 | 52 | 15 (20.5%) | 46 | 6 (20.5%) | General | Heparin |
| Bergqvist et al, 1980 | 56 | 39 (20.5%) | 59 | 10 (20.5%) | THR | Heparin DHE |
| Bergqvist et al, 1980 | 29 | 21 (20.5%) | 25 | 20 (20.5%) | HF | Heparin DHE |
| Bergqvist & Ljungnér, 1981 | 52 | 10 (20.5%) | 34 | 1 (20.5%) | General | PZ 68 |
| Davidson et al, 1972 | 30 | 3 (20.5%) | 30 | 4 (20.5%) | Gynaecology | Warfarin |
| Gruber et al, 1973[*] | 37 | 9 (20.5%) | 33 | 3 (20.5%) | General | Heparin |
| Hedlund, 1975 | 37 | 10 (20.5%) | 38 | 13 (20.5%) | Urology | Heparin |
| Hohl et al, 1970 | 117 | 17 (20.5%) | 115 | 2 (20.5%) | Gynaecology | Heparin |
| Lambie et al, 1970 | 40 | 4 (20.5%) | 40 | 12 (20.5%) | Gynaecology | Warfarin |
| Lindström et al, 1982 | 35 | 7 (20.5%) | 37 | 5 (20.5%) | General | El. Stimulation |
| McCarthy et al, 1974 | 61 | 11 (20.5%) | 64 | 7 (20.5%) | Gynaecology | Heparin |
| Rosell Pradas and Vara-Thorbeck, 1988[*] | 56 | 6 (20.5%) | 57 | 5 (20.5%) | General | Heparin |
| Ruckley, 1976 | 130 | 33 (20.5%) | 128 | 15 (20.5%) | General | Heparin |
| Total heparin | 542 | 111 (20.5%) | 515 | 52 (10.1%) |  |  |

[*] Dextran 40   HF: Hip fracture   THR: Total hip replacement   DHE: Dihydroergotamine

findings in this study, the frequency of FPE during non-dextran periods was 0.69% (35/5094) and during dextran periods 0.20% (10/4881), a significant reduction.

In table 17.6, the available dextran studies are pooled to give an idea on prevention of fatal pulmonary embolism, comparison being made with and without prophylaxis. This

**Table 17.6**
Data on fatal pulmonary embolism (FPE) and total mortality in studies on dextran vs. control

|  | Dextran groups |  |  | Anticoagulation groups |  |  |
|---|---|---|---|---|---|---|
|  | Patients n | Deaths n | FPE n | Patients n | Deaths n | FPE n |
| Ahlberg et al, 1968 | 39 | 6 | 0 | 45 | 14 | 2 |
| Atik et al, 1970 | 49 | 7 | 1 | 77 | 14 | 8 |
| Becker & Schampi, 1973 | 42 | 1 | 0 | 35 | 1 | 0 |
| Bergman et al, 1975 | 30 | 0 | 0 | 30 | 0 | 0 |
| Bergqvist et al, 1979 | 27 | 2 | 0 | 30 | 0 | 0 |
| Bergqvist et al, 1979 | 70 | 1 | 0 | 71 | 2 | 2 |
| Bergqvist & Hall-böök, 1980 | 52 | 2 | 0 | 51 | 7 | 0 |
| Brisman et al, 1971 | 89 | 8 | 0 | 90 | 5 | 0 |
| Carter & Eban, 1973 | 106 | 0 | 0 (0.34%) | 101 | 0 | 0 |
| Edwards et al, 1975 | 31 | 3 | 2 | 31 | 7 | 6 |
| Elsner-Mackey et al, 1969 | 391 | 0 | 0 | 50 | 0 | 0 |
| Evarts & Feil, 1971[*] | 50 | 0 | 0 | 427 | 0 | 0 |
| Gruber et al, 1973[*] | 37 | 4 | 1 | 38 | 6 | 2 |
| Hedlund, 1975 | 37 | 0 | 0 | 40 | 0 | 0 |
| v. Hospenthal et al, 1977 | 39 | 0 | 0 | 47 | 0 | 0 |
| Hurson et al, 1979 | 55 | 1 | 0 | 51 | 0 | 0 |
| Hutter et al, 1976[*] | 92 | 0 | 0 | 100 | 6 | 4 |
| Huttunen et al, 1977 | 150 | 4 | 1 | 75 | 0 | 0 |
| Huttunen et al, 1971 | 100 | 1 | 1 | 100 | 6 | 4 |
| Jansen, 1972 | 304 | 13 | 1 | 301 | 19 | 4 |
| Johnsson et al, 1968 | 27 | 0 | 0 | 25 | 0 | 0 |
| Kline et al, 1975 | 396 | 27 | 1 | 435 | 35 | 7 |
| Myhre & Holen, 1969 | 55 | 3 | 0 | 55 | 6 | 2 |
| Nillius et al, 1979 | 28 | 0 | 0 | 29 | 1 | 1 |
| Rothermel et al, 1973[*] | 60 | 1 | 1 | 60 | 1 | 0 |
| Ruckley, 1976 | 130 | 0 | 0 | 128 | 1 | 1 |
| Stadil, 1970 | 424 | 21 | 1 | 397 | 22 | 5 |
| Stephenson et al, 1973 | 34 | 0 | 0 | 46 | 0 | 0 |
| Welin-Berger et al, 1982 | 20 | 0 | 0 | 20 | 0 | 0 |
| Total | 2964 | 107 (3.6%) | 10 (0.34%) | 2981 | 148 (5.0%) | 44 (1.5%) |

[*] Dextran 40

compilation showed a reduction of FPE from 1.5% to 0.3% with dextran prophylaxis. In their meta-analysis Clagett and Reisch (1988) arrived at the same conclusion. The frequency in the control group was 1.5% and in the dextran group 0.27% with an odds ratio of 0.18 (95% confidence interval 0.05-0.68).

Another statistical method was used by Ljungström, where each study is regarded as a separate test with three possible outcomes concerning FPE: fewer deaths in the control group, fewer deaths in the dextran group, or an equal number of deaths in the two groups. Significantly, more dextran groups have a lower frequency of FPE than control groups. Other causes of death do not differ.

To conclude, although no prospective randomised study comparing dextran and no prophylaxis has been performed with FPE as an end point, there is strong evidence that dextran does prevent FPE.

The compilation in table 17.7 is similar to that in table 17.6 but anticoagulants are used for comparison. Although there are several types of anticoagulants, this group of substances appears to be as effective as dextran in preventing FPE. This is in keeping with a large randomised prospective study from Tübingen (Lüders et al, 1973) where dextran 60 (2,945 patients) was compared with heparin and oral anticoagulants (3,014 patients). The incidence of fatal pulmonary embolism was 0.36% in the anticoagulant group, and 0.30% in the dextran group. Haemorrhagic complications were noted in 1.12% of the anticoagulant group and in 0.61% of the subjects treated with dextran ($p<0.05$).

**Table 17.7**

Data on fatal pulmonary embolism (FPE) and total mortality in studies on dextran vs. anti-coagulants

|  | Dextran groups | | | Anticoagulation groups | | | |
| --- | --- | --- | --- | --- | --- | --- | --- |
|  | Patients n | Deaths n | FPE n | Patients n | Deaths | FPE n | Type of anticoagulation |
| Barber et al, 1979 | 51 | 1 | 1 | 58 | 0 | 0 | Warfarin |
| Bergqvist et al, 1972 | 75 | 9 | 0 | 63 | 12 | 1 | Dicoumarol |
| Bergqvist et al, 1979 | 27 | 2 | 0 | 28 | 4 | 1 | Heparin |
| Bergqvist et al, 1979 | 70 | 1 | 0 | 72 | 0 | 0 | Heparin |
| Bergqvist & Hallböök, 1980 | 52 | 2 | 0 | 46 | 2 | 0 | Heparin |
| Bergqvist et al, 1980 | 56 | 0 | 0 | 59 | 0 | 0 | Heparin DHE |
| Bergqvist et al, 1980 | 29 | 1 | 0 | 25 | 3 | 1 | Heparin DHE |
| Bergqvist & Ljungnér, 1981 | 52 | 1 | 0 | 34 | 0 | 0 | PZ 68 |
| Bergqvist et al, 1991 | 138 | 8 | 3 | 139 | 9 | 0 | Org 10172 |
| Eriksson et al, 1988 | 49 | 0 | 0 | 49 | 0 | 0 | LMWH |
| Francis et al, 1989[*] | 51 | 0 | 0 | 52 | 0 | 0 | Heparin + AT III |
| Francis et al, 1983[*] | 43 | 0 | 0 | 57 | 0 | 0 | Warfarin |
| Francis et al, 1990[*] | 38 | 0 | 0 | 39 | 0 | 0 | Heparin + AT III |
| Fredin et al, 1982 | 41 | 4 | 0 | 27 | 0 | 0 | PZ 68 |
| Fredin et al, 1984a | 58 | 0 | 0 | 58 | 2 | 0 | Heparin DHE |
| Fredin et al, 1984a | 46 | 0 | 0 | 50 | 0 | 0 | Heparin DHE |
| Fredin et al, 1983 | 114 | 0 | 0 | 93 | 0 | 0 | Heparin DHE |
| Gruber et al, 1973[*] | 37 | 4 | 1 | 33 | 2 | 1 | Heparin |
| Gruber et al, 1980 | 2159 | 38 | 5 | 2193 | 3 | 3 | Heparin |

|  | Dextran groups | | | Anticoagulation groups | | | |
|---|---|---|---|---|---|---|---|
|  | Patients n | Deaths n | FPE n | Patients n | Deaths | FPE n | Type of anticoagulation |
| Gruber, 1982 | 3715 | 27 | 9 | 3698 | 28 | 6 | Heparin DHE |
| Harris et al, 1972[*] | 113 | 0 | 0 | 114 | 0 | 0 | Warfarin |
| Harris et al, 1974[*] | 61 | 0 | 0 | 55 | 0 | 0 | Warfarin |
| Hedlund, 1975 | 37 | 0 | 0 | 38 | 0 | 0 | Heparin |
| Hohl et al, 1980 | 117 | 0 | 0 | 115 | 0 | 0 | Heparin |
| Lambie et al, 1980 | 40 | 0 | 0 | 40 | 0 | 0 | Warfarin |
| McCarthy et al, 1974 | 68 | 0 | 0 | 64 | 0 | 0 | Heparin |
| Myhre & Holen, 1969 | 55 | 3 | 0 | 50 | 4 | 1 | Warfarin |
| Myrvold et al, 1973 | 55 | 2 | 0 | 39 | 2 | 2 | Heparin |
| Mätzsch et al, 1990 | 49 | 0 | 0 | 47 | 0 | 0 | LMWH |
| Mätzsch et al, 1991 | 123 | 1 | 0 | 120 | 1 | 0 | LMWH |
| Rosell Pradas & Vara-Thorbeck, 1988[*] | 56 | 0 | 0 | 40 | 0 | 0 | Heparin |
| Ruckley, 1976 | 130 | 0 | 0 | 128 | 0 | 0 | Heparin |
| Welin-Berger et al, 1982 | 20 | 0 | 0 | 20 | 0 | 0 | Heparin |
| Heparin, LMWH | 7837 | 91 (1.2%) | 20 (0.3%) | 7306 | 93 (1.3%) | 15 (0.2%) |  |
| Oral anticoagulation | 438 | 13 (3%) | 1 (0.2%) | 437 | 17 (3.9%) | 2 (0.5%) |  |
| Total | 7825 | 104 (1.3%) | 21 (0.27%) | 7743 | 110 (1.4%) | 17 (0.22%) |  |

[*]Dextran 40    DHE = dihydroergotamine    LMWH = low molecular weight heparin
AT III = antithrombin III    PZ, see table 17.4

## Dosage and timing aspects

There are considerable variations in dosage and dose interval in the various studies. The optimal dose remains to be established. There seems to be no certain correlation between dose and effect. Concerning timing the most important infusion seems to be that given intra-operatively.

On the basis of the studies performed so far, it is reasonable to recommend infusion of dextran with 500 ml intraoperatively and 500ml after the operation, i.e., 1,000 ml during the day of surgery. An additional 500 ml should then be administered at least on the first postoperative day. In hip surgery, it has been suggested that additional infusions, for instance, on days 3 and 5, would be of prophylactic value, especially if the patients are still immobilised.

Recently, 3% dextran 60 has been introduced as a plasma substitute in blood component therapy and for volume expansion. Three percent colloid seems optimal for perioperative volume treatment. In doses not exceeding 1.5 g per kg body weight, it can be safely used as judged from an investigation on haemostatic factors in patients undergoing orthopaedic surgery (Bergman et al, 1990). Three percent dextran 60 is more effective than Ringer's acetate to maintain haemodynamic stability and carries a lower risk of cardiac overloading than 6% dextran (Schött et al, 1988). One litre of the 3% solution gives the same amount of dextran as 500 ml of the 6% solution, thus there is no reason to expect any difference in thromboprophylactic effect.

A number of aspects remain to be studied with regard to dextran administration, such as optimal dose, dose interval, duration, and time of the first infusion.

# Side effects

### Cardiac Overload
Owing to the volume expanding effect, there is a small risk of cardiac overload especially in elderly patients with latent cardiac failure. However, this side effect is unusual and can mostly be avoided by slow infusion. Rutherford et al (1984) found no increase in cardiac complications in a series where dextran 40 was compared with heparin in connection with femorodistal arterial surgery, although this patient group is old with a high frequency of concomitant cardiovascular disease.

### Haemorrhagic complications
Several observations, especially from the United States, have reported a prolonged bleeding time in association with dextran infusion. However, both clinically (Cronberg et al, 1966) and experimentally (Arfors and Bergqvist, 1975; Bergqvist, 1985) it has been shown that dextran doses of 1 g/kg body weight or less do not induce a defect in haemostasis.

In most prophylactic studies increased blood loss has not been reported in association with dextran prophylaxis, although the exact quantity of the haemorrhage has not always been stated. In some studies more blood was transfused to dextran-treated patients, which might be that the lowered haematocrit in dextran haemodiluted patients guided the need for blood transfusions. If the haemodilution effect of dextran is used, it would in fact be possible to save donor blood.

Under certain circumstances an increased diffuse oozing has been reported in association with dextran administration, but this is difficult to assess in objective terms, and is probably related to the improved capillary perfusion. This could possibly cause difficulties, e.g., in neurosurgery. In patients with haemostatic defects, dextran should be admininstered with caution.

### Anaphylactoid reactions (DIAR, dextran induced anaphylactoid reactions)
Clinical hypersensitivity to dextran has been known ever since dextran became available for patient use (Bauer and Östling, 1970; Hedin et al, 1976; Furhoff, 1977; Hedin, 1977; Ring, 1978). The symptomatology of dextran reaction is variable, the clinical stages being:
1. Skin symptoms and/or slight fever
2. Measurable, but not life threatening, cardiovascular reaction (hypotension, tachycardia). Respiratory disturbances, nausea, vomiting
3. Severe hypotension ($\leq$ 40-60 mm Hg); Life threatening bronchospasm
4. Cardiac and/or respiratory arrest
5. Death.

Most probably specific large immune complexes are involved in the serious reactions. The complement system, platelets, leucocytes and the coagulation cascade are activated and vasoactive substances released (Hedin, 1977; Hedin and Smedegård, 1979; Hedin and Richter, 1982). Metabolic acidosis is always present in severe cases (Ljungström and Renck,

1987) and circulation is not normalised until the acidosis has been corrected. Dextran-reactive antibodies (DRA) arise in response to immunisation with bacterial polysaccharides and are widespread among normal humans.

It is possible to counteract dextran reactions by interfering with the immune complex formation (hapten inhibition) (Richter, 1971; 1973). Using low molecular weight dextran (dextran 1, molecular weight 1,000 daltons), the binding sites on the antibody are blocked, and aggregate formation is prevented. Clinical data, including a multicentre trial with over 130,000 patients, provide strong evidence that the hapten inhibition principle works clinically, reducing the frequency of severe anaphylactoid reactions by at least 20-fold (Messmer et al, 1980; Renck et al, 1983). In practice, 20 ml of dextran 1 are given intravenously immediately before the first infusion of dextran 40 or 70. Renewed injection of dextran 1 is necessary when the interval of dextran infusions exceeds 48 hours.

In patients who react to dextran despite hapten inhibition, exceptionally high titres of IgG-DRA have been recorded. Although the risk for DIAR has not been completely eliminated, the risk has been substantially reduced.

Should a serious reaction develop, the dextran infusion must be stopped immediately. Theophylline or $\beta_2$-antagonists have been recommended in cases of bronchospasm. Epinephrine has been discussed as a possibility but Ljungström (1983b) found no improvement and extremely high levels of catecholamines during the anaphylactoid reaction have been reported. The metabolic acidosis must be corrected. Large doses of corticosteroids and crystalloid infusions seem beneficial.

### Renal dysfunction

Since the dextran solution is hyperoncotic, concurrent fluid administration is required, which is particularly important in dehydrated patients. Renal dysfunction may occur when large quantities of dextran are administered to dehydrated patients or patients with underlying renal disease (Fournier et al, 1968; Matheson and Diomi, 1970). Large quantities of dextran 40 induce a pronounced but reversible morphological vacuolisation (osmotic nephrosis) of the cytoplasma of the proximal tubular cells, but their function is not influenced (Engberg, 1969).

## Concluding remarks

In Sweden, dextran has been the dominating thromboprophylaxis for many years (Bergqvist, 1990). Its efficacy in preventing deep vein thrombosis is controversial, at least in general surgery. In orthopaedic surgery, however, and perhaps also in gynaecologic surgery, its efficacy is well established. Dextran's ability to reduce fatal pulmonary embolism is clear. In the conclusions of the 1986 Consensus conference, dextran infusion was one of the recommended regimens for prevention of deep vein thrombosis and pulmonary embolism. Thus, dextran is a prophylactic alternative with simultaneous volume expansion.

## References

Åberg M, Bergentz S-E, Hedner U. The effect of dextran on the lysability of ex vivo thrombi. Ann Surg 181:342, 1975

Åberg M. On the effect of dextran on lysability and structure of ex vivo thrombi, platelet function and factor VIII. Thesis, Lund University, 1978

Åberg M, Rausing A. The effect of dextran 70 on the structure of ex vivo thrombi. Thromb Res 12:1113, 1978

Ahlberg Å, Nylander G, Robertson B, Cronberg S, Nilsson IM. Dextran in prophylaxis of thrombosis in fractures of the hip. Acta Chir Scand Supply 387:83, 1968

Ah-See, A-K, Árfors K-E, Bergqvist D, Tangen O. Effect of dextran on experimental venous thrombosis in rabbits. Thromb Diath Haemorrh 32:284, 1974

Andersen P, Kjaersgaard E, Beyer-Holgersen R, Fredericksen E. DHEH and Dextran 70 in thrombo-prophylaxis after hip fracture. Acta Orthop Scand 57:469, 1986

Arfors K-E, Bergqvist D. Microvascular haemostatic plug formation in the rabbit mesentery. Effect of blood flow velocity, thrombocytopenia and dextran treatment. Bibl Haematol 41:84, 1975

Atik M, Harkness JW, Wichman H. Prevention of fatal pulmonary embolism. Surg Gynecol Obstet 130:403, 1970

Barber HM, Feil EJ, Galasko CSB, Edwards DH, Sutton RA, Haynes DW, Bentley GA. A comparative study of dextran 70, warfarin and low-dose heparin for the prophylaxis of thromboembolism following total hip replacement. Postgrad Med J 53:130, 1977

Bauer Å, Östling G. Dextran-induced anaphylactic reactions in connection with surgery. Acta Anaesth Scand Suppl 37:182, 1970

Becker J, Schampi B. The incidence of postoperative venous thrombosis of the legs. A comparative study on the prophylactic effect of dextran 70 and electrical calf-muscle stimulation. Acta Chir Scand 139:357, 1973

Bennett PN, Dhall DP, McKenzie FN, Matheson NA. Effects of dextran infusion on the adhesiveness of human blood-platelets. Lancet II:1001, 1966

Bergentz S-E, Eiken O, Gelin LE. Rheomacrodex in vascular Surgery. J Cardiovasc Res 4:388, 1963

Bergentz S-E Eiken O, Nilsson IM. The effect of dextran of various molecular weight on the coagulation in dogs. Thromb Diath Haemorrh 6:15, 1961

Bergman A, Andreen M, Blombäck M. Plasma substitution with 3% dextran 60 in orthopaedic surgery: influence on plasma colloid osmotic pressure, coagulation parameters, immunoglobulin and other plasma constitutents. Acta Anaesthesiol Scand 34:21, 1990

Bergman B, Bergqvist D, Dahlgren S. The incidence of venous thrombosis in the lower limbs following elective gall-bladder surgery. A study with the $^{125}$I-Fibrinogen test. Ups J Med Sci 80:41, 1975

Bergquist E, Bergqvist D, Bronge A, Dahlgren S, Lindquist B. An evaluation of early thrombosis prophylaxis following fracture of the femoral neck. A comparison between dextran and dicoumarol. Acta Chir Scand 138:689, 1972

Bergqvist D. Postoperative thromboembolism. Frequency, etiology, prophylaxis. Springer-Verlag, Berlin Heidelberg New York, 1983

Bergqvist D. The influence of plasma volume expanders on initial haemostasis in the rabbit mesentery. Acta Anaesthesiol Scand 29:607, 1985

Bergqvist D. Prophylaxis against postoperative venous thromboembolism — a survey of surveys. Thromb Haemorrh Disorders 2:69, 1990

Bergqvist D, Bergentz S-E. The role of dextran in severe ischaemic extremity disease and arterial reconstructive surgery. A review. VASA, 12:213, 1983

Bergqvist D, Dahlgren S. Leg vein thrombosis diagnosed by $^{125}$I-Fibrinogen test in patients with fracture of the hip: a study of the effect of early prophylaxis with dicoumarol or dextran 70. VASA 2:121, 1973

Bergqvist D, Hallböök T. Prophylaxis of postoperative venous thrombosis in a controlled trial comparing dextran 70 and low- dose heparin. A study with the $^{125}$I-Fibrinogen test. World J Surg 4:239, 1980

Bergqvist D, Lindblad B. The thromboprophylactic effect of graded elastic compression stockings in combination with dextran 70. Arch Surg 119:1329, 1984

Bergqvist D, Ljungnér H. A comparative study of dextran 70 and a sulphated polysaccharide in the prevention of postoperative thromboembolic complications in patients undergoing abdominal surgery. Br J Surg 68:449, 1981

Bergqvist D, Efsing HO, Hallböök T, Hedlund T. Thromboembolism after elective and post-traumatic hip surgery — a controlled prophylactic trial with dextran and low dose heparin. Acta Chir Scand 145, 1979

Bergqvist D, Efsing HO, Hallböök T, Lindblad B. Prevention of postoperative thromboembolic complications. A prospective comparison between dextran 70, dihydroergotamine heparin and a sulfated polysaccharide. Acta Chir Scand 146:559, 1980

Bergqvist D, Björck C-G, Esquivel C, Nilsson B. Effect of platelet inhibition on experimental venous thrombosis in the rabbit. Acta Chir Scand 151:249, 1985

Bergqvist D, Kettunen K, Fredin H, Faun P, Suomalainen O, Soimakallio S, Karjalainen P, Cederholm C, Jensen LJ, Justesen T, Stiekema JCJ. Thromboprophylaxis in hip fracture patients — a prospective randomised comparative study between Org 10172 and dextran 70. Surgery 109:617, 1991

Borgström S, Gelin L-E, Zederfeldt B. The formation of vein thrombi following tissue injury. Acta Chir Scand Supply 247, 1959

Boström S, Holmgren E, Johsson O, Lindberg S, Lindström B, Winsö I, Zachrisson B. Post-operative thromboembolism in neurosurgery. A study on the prophylactic effect of calf muscle stimulation plus dextran compared to low-dose heparin. Acta Neurochir 80:83, 1986

Bowman HW. Clinical evaluation of dextran as a plasma volume expander. JAMA 153:373, 1953

Brisman R, Parks L, Haller A. Dextran prophylaxis in surgery. Ann Surg 174:137, 1971

Bronge A, Dahlgren S, Lindquist B. Prophylaxis against thrombosis in femoral neck fractures — a comparison between dextran 70 and dicumarol. Acta Chir Scand 137:29, 1971

Bronwell A, Artz C, Sako Y. Evaluation of blood loss from a standardised wound after dextran. Surg Forum 5:809, 1954

Bygdeman S, Eliasson R, Gullbring B. Effect of dextran infusion on the adenosine diphosphate induced adhesiveness and the spreading capacity of human blood platelets. Thromb Diath Haemorrh 15:451, 1966

Carbone JV, Furth FW, Scott R, Crosby WH. A haemostatic defect associated with dextran infusion. Proc Soc Exp Biol Med 85:101, 1954

Carlin G. Effect of dextran on fibrinolysis. Acta Univ Ups Abstr Ups Diss Fac Med 365, 1980

Carter AE, Eban R. The prevention of postoperative deep venous thrombosis with dextran 70. Br J Surg 60:681, 1973

Clagett GP, Reisch JS. Prevention of venous thromboembolism in general surgical patients. Ann Surg 208:227, 1988

Consensus Conference: Prevention of venous thrombosis and pulmonary embolism. JAMA 256:744, 1986

Cronberg S, Robertson B, Nilsson IM, Niléhn J-E. Suppressive effect of dextran on platelet adhesiveness. Thromb Diat Haemorrh 16:384, 1966

Daniel WJ, Moore AR, Flanc C. Prophylaxis of deep vein thrombosis (DVT) with dextran 70 in patients with a fractured neck of the femur. Aust NZ J Surg 41:289, 1972

Davidson AI, Brunt ME, Matheson NA. A further trial comparing dextran 70 with warfarin in the prophylaxis of postoperative venous thrombosis. Br J Surg 59:314, 1972

Edwards DH, Steel WM, Bentley G. Prophylaxis with dextran 70 against thrombosis in patients with fractures of the upper end of the femur. Injury 6:250, 1975

Elsner-Mackey P, Ledermair O, Schastok H, Vinazzer H. Zur Wirkung von Macrodex auf die postoperative Thromboembolic-Frequenz. Wien Med Wochenschr 119:149, 1969

Engberg A. Proximal renal tubule structure and function with special reference to the effect of dextran 40. Acta Univ Ups Diss Med 77, 1969

Eriksson BI, Zachrisson BE, Teger-Nilsson A-C, Risberg B. Thrombosis prophylaxis with low molecular weight heparin in total hip replacement. Br J Surg 75:1053, 1988

Evarts CM, Feil EJ. Prevention of thromboembolic disease after elective surgery of the hip. J Bone Joint Surg (Am) 53:1271, 1971

Fournier A, Watchi JM, Réveillaud RJ. Les nephroses dits osmotiques en vacuolication hydropiques diffuses des tubes proximaux. Actual Nephrol Hop Necker 23, 1968

Francis CW, Marder V, Evarts M, Yaukoolbodi S. Two-step warfarin therapy. Prevention of postoperative venous thrombosis without excessive bleeding. JAMA 249:374, 1983

Francis CW, Pellegrini VD, Marder VJ, Harris CM, Totterman S, Gabriel KR, Baughman DJ, Roemer S, Burke J, Goodman TL, Evarts C McC. Prevention of venous thrombosis after total hip arthroplasty. J Bone J Surg 71-A:327, 1989

Francis CW, Pelligrini V, Stulberg B, Millar M, Totterman S, Marder V. Prevention of venous thrombosis after total knee arthoplasty. Comparison of antithrombin III and low dose heparin with dextran. J Bone Joint Surg 72-A:976, 1990

Fredin HO, Nillius SA, Bergqvist D. Prophylaxis of deep vein thrombosis in patients with fracture of the femoral neck. Acta Orthop Scand 53:413, 1982

Fredin HO, Nilsson B, Rosberg B, Tengborn L. Pre- and postoperative levels of antithrombin III with special reference to thromboembolism after total hip replacement. Thromb Haemostas 49:158, 1983

Fredin H, Gustafson C, Rosberg B. Hypotensive anaesthesia, thromboprophylaxis and postoperative thromboembolism in total hip arthroplasty. Acta Anaesthesiol Scand 28:503, 1984a

Fredin H, Rosberg B, Arborelius M, Nylander G. On thromboembolism after total hip replacement in epidural analgesia: a controlled study of dextran 70 and low-dose heparin combined with dihydroergotamine. Br J Surg 71:58, 1984b

Fredin HO, Bergqvist D, Cederholm C, Lindblad B, Nyman U. Thromboprophylaxis in hip arthroplasty. Dextran with graded compression or preoperative dextran compared in 150 patients. Acta Orthop Scand 60:678, 1989

Furhoff A-K. Anaphylactoid reaction to dextran — a report of 133 cases. Acta Anaesthesiol Scand 21; 161, 1977

Gruber UF, Bergentz S-E. The antithrombotic effect of dextran. J Surg Res 6:379, 1966

Gruber UF, Rem J, Altorfer R, Schaub N, Fredie KE, Fridrich R, Duckert F. Efficacy of dextran 40 or heparin in the prevention of deep vein thrombosis after major surgery. Eur Surg Res 5:15, 1973

Gruber UF, Alleman U, Wettler H. Erster direkter Verglech der allergischen Nebemwirkungen des Dextrans mit und ohne Hapten. Schweiz Med Wochenschr 112:605, 1982

Gruber UF, Saldeen T, Brokop T, Eklöf B, Eriksson I, Goldie I, Gran L, Hohl M, Jonsson T, Kristersson S, Ljungström KG, Lund T, Maartman Moe H, Svensjö E, Thomson D, Torhorst J, Trippestad A, Ulstein A. Incidences of fatal postoperative pulmonary embolism with dextran 70 and low-dose heparin. An International Multicentre Study. Br Med J 280:69, 1980

Harper DR, Dhall DP, Woodruff WH. Prophylaxis in iliofemoral venous thrombosis. The major amputee as a clinical research model. Br J Surg 60:831, 1973

Harris WH, Salzman EW, De Sanctis RW, Coutts RD. Prevention of venous thromboembolism following total hip replacement. Warfarin vs Dextran 40. JAMA 220:1319, 1972

Harris WH, Salzman EW, Athanasoulis C. Comparison of warfarin, low molecular weight dextran, aspirin and subcutaneous heparin in prevention of venous thromboembolism following total hip replacement. J Bone Joint Surg Am 56:1552, 1974

Harris WH, Athanasoulis CA, Waltman AC, Salzman EW. Prophylaxis of deep-vein thrombosis after total hip replacement. J Bone Joint Surg Am 67A:57, 1985

Hedin H. Dextran-induced anaphylactoid reactions in man. Immunological in vitro and in vivo studies. Acta Univ Ups Abst Ups Diss Fac Med 432, 1977

Hedin H, Smedegård G. Complement profiles in monkeys subjected to aggreparticulate polysaccharides. Int Arch Allergy Appl Immunol 60:286, 1979

Hedin H, Richter W. Pathomechanisms of dextran-induced anaphylactoid/anaphylactic reactions in vein. Internat Arch Allerg Apply Immunol 62:122, 1982

Hedin H, Richter W, Ring J. Dextran-induced anaphylactoid reactions in man. Role of dextran reactive antibodies. Int Arch Allergy Appl Immunol 52:145, 1976

Hedlund PO. Postoperative venous thrombosis in benign prostatic disease. A study of 316 patients with the $^{125}$I-Fibrinogen uptake test. Scand J Urol Nephrol Suppl 27:1, 1975

Hohl MK, Lüscher KP, Tichy J, Stiner M, Fridrich R, Gruber UF, Käser O. Prevention of postoperative thromboembolism by dextran 70 or low-dose heparin. Obstet Gynecol 55:497, 1980

Hurson B, Ennis JT, Corrigan TP, Macauley P. Dextran prophylaxis in total hip replacement: a scintigraphic evaluation of the incidence of deep vein thrombosis and pulmonary embolus. Ir J Med Sci 148:140, 1979

Hutter O, Duckert F, Fridrich R, Gruber UF. Dextran 40 zur prophylaxe tiefer Venenthrombosen in der Chirurgie. Dtsch Med Wochenschr 101:1834, 1976

Huttunen H, Mattila MAK, Hakalehto J, Kettunen K, Rehnberg V, Babinski M. Single infusion of dextran 70 in the prophylaxis of postoperative deep venous thrombosis. Ann Chir Gynecol Fenn 60:119, 1971

Huttunen H, Mattila MAK, Alhava EM, Kuttunen K, Karjalainen P, Huttunen K. Preoperative infusion of dextran 70 and dextran 40 in the prevention of postoperative deep venous thrombosis as confirmed by the $^{125}$I-Fibrinogen uptake method. Ann Chir Gynecol Fenn 66:79, 1977

Jansen H. Postoperative thromboembolism and its prevention with 500 ml dextran given during operation. With a special study of the venous flow pattern in the lower extremities. Acta Chir Scand Supply 427, 1972

Johnsson SR, Bygdeman S, Eliasson R. Effect of dextran on postoperative thrombosis. Acta Chir Scand, Suppl 387:80, 1968

Kline A, Hughes LE, Campbell H, Williams A, Zlosnick J, Leach KG. Dextran 70 in prophylaxis of thromboembolic disease after surgery: a clinically oriented randomised double-blind trial. Br Med J 2:109, 1975

Koekenberg LJL. Experimental use of macrodex as a prophylaxis against postoperative thromboembolism. Exp Med Amst 40:123, 1961

Korvald E, Støren E, Ongre A. Simultaneous use of warfarin-sodium and dextran 70 to prevent post-operative venous thrombosis in patients with hip fractures. J Oslo City Hosp 23:25, 1973

Lambie JM, Barber DC, Dhall DP, Matheson NA. Dextran 70 in prophylaxis of postoperative venous thrombosis. A controlled trial. Br Med J 2:144, 1970

Lindström B, Holmdahl D, Jonsson O, Korsan-Bengtsen K, Lindberg S, Petrusson B, Pettersson S, Wikstrand J, Wojciechowski J. Prediction and prophylaxis of postoperative thromboembolism — a comparative calf muscle stimulation with groups of impulses and dextran 40. Br J Surg 69:633, 1982

Ljungström K-G. Dextran prophylaxis of fatal pulmonary embolism. World J Surg 7:767, 1983a

Ljungström K-G. Prophylaxis of postoperative thromboembolism with dextran 70: Improvements of efficacy and safety. Acta Chir Scand Suppl 1:514, 1983b

Ljungström K-G. The antithrombotic efficacy of dextran. Acta Chir Scand Supply, 543:26, 1988

Ljungström K-G, Renck H. Metabolic acidosis in dextran-induced anaphylactic reactions. Acta Anaesthesiol Scand 31:157, 1987

Lüders K, Konold P, Otten GL, Koslowski L. Postoperative Thromboseprophylaxe. Randomisierte, prospektive Untersuchung zum Vergleich einer Thromboemboliprophylaxe mit Antikoagulatien (Heparin-Marcumar) and Dextran 60 (Macrodex). Chirurgie 44:563, 1973

Messmer K, Lungström K-G, Gruber U, Richter W, Hedin H. Prevention of dextran-ionduced anaphylactoid reactions by hapten inhibition. Lancet I:975, 1980

Matheson NA, Diomi P. Renal failure after the administration of dextran 40. Surg Gynecol Obstet 131:661, 1970

McCarthy TG, McQueen J, Johnstone FD, Weston J, Campbell S. A comparison of low-dose subcutaneous heparin and intravenous dextran 70 in the prophylaxis of deep venous thrombosis after gynaecological surgery. J Obstet Gynaecol 81:486, 1974

Myhre H, Holen A. Thrombosis prophylaxis. Dextran or sodium warfarin? A controlled clinical study (In Norwegian). Nord Med 82:1534, 1969

Myrvold HE, Persson J-E, Svensson B, Wallensten S, Vikterlöf KJ. Prevention of thromboembolism with dextran 70 and heparin in patients with femoral neck fractures. Acta Chir Scand 139:609, 1973

Mätzsch T, Bergqvist D, Fredin H, Hedner U. Low molecular weight heparin compared with Dextran as prophylaxis against thrombosis after total hip replacement. Acta Chir Scand, 156:445, 1990

Mätzsch T, Bergqvist D, Fredin H, Hedner U, Lindhagen A, Nistor L. Comparison of the thromboprophylactic effect of a low molecular weight heparin versus dextran in total hip replacement. Thromb Haemorrh Disorders 3:25, 1991

Nillius SA, Ahlberg Å, Arborelius Jr M, Rosberg B. Preoperative normovolemic haemodilution with dextran 70 as a thromboembolic prophylaxis in total hip replacement. Int Orthop 3:197, 1979

Pini M, Spadini E, Carluccio L, Giovanardi C, Magnani E, Ugolotti U, Uggeri E. Dextran/aspirin versus heparin/dihydroergotamine in preventing thrombosis after hip fractures. J Bone Joint Surg Br 67B:305, 1985

Renck H, Ljungström K-G, Hedin H, Richter W. Prevention of dextran induced anaphylactic reactions by hapten inhibition III. A Scandinvavian multicentre study on the effects of 20 ml dextran 1 15%, administered before dextran 70 or dextran 40. Acta Chir Scand 149:355, 1983

Richter W. Hapten inhibition of passive antidextran anaphylaxis in guinea pigs. Role of molecular size in anaphylacticogenecity and precipitability of dextran fraction. Int Arch Allergy Appl Immunol 41:826, 1971

Richter W. Built-in hapten inhibition of anaphylaxis by the low molecular weight subfractions of a B512 dextran fraction of $M_W$ 3400. Int Arch Allergy Appl Immunol 45:930, 1973

Ring J. Anaphylaktoide Reaktionen nach infusion natürlicher und künstlicher Kolloide. Springer, Berlin Heidelberg New York, 1978

Rosell Pradas J, Vara-Thorbeck R. Dextran versus heparin subcutánea en la profilaxis de la trombosis venosa profunda (TVP) postcirugía biliar. Rev Esp Enf Ap Digest, 74:521, 1988

Rothermel JE, Wessinger JB, Stinchfield FE. Dextran 40 and thromboembolism in total hip replacement surgery. Arch Surg 105:135, 1973

Ruckley CV. A multi-unit controlled trial of heparin and dextran in the prevention of venous thromboembolic disease. In: Kakkar VV, Thomas DP (eds). Heparin. Chemistry and clinical usage, Academic Press, London, 1976

Rutherford R, Jones D, Bergentz S-E, Bergqvist D, Karmody AM, Dardik H, Moore WS, Goldstone J, Flinn WR, Comerota AJ et al. The efficacy of dextran 40 in preventing early postoperative thrombosis following difficult lower-extremity by-pass. J Vasc Surg 1:765, 1984

Schött U, Lindbom L-O, Sjöstrand J. Hemodynamic effects of colloid concentration in experimental haemorrhage: a comparison of Ringer's acetate, 3% dextran-60 and 6% dextran-70. Crit Care Med 16:346, 1988

Smith RC, Elton RA, Orr JD, Hart AJL, Graham DF, Fuller GAG, Rundle JSH, Macpherson AIS, Ruckley CV. Dextran and intermittent pneumatic cmpression in prevention of postoprative deep vein thrombosis. Multi-unit trial. Br Med J 1:952, 1978

Stadil F. Prevention of postoperative vein thrombosis with dextran 70 (In Danish). Ugeskr Laeg 132:1817, 1970

Stephenson CBS, Wallace JG, Vaughan JV. Dextran 70 in the prevention of deep vein thrombosis with observations on pulmonary embolism. Report on a pilot study. N Z Med J 77:302, 1973

Swierstra BA, van Oosterhout FJ, Ausema B, Bakker WH, van der Pompe WB, Schouten JHA. Oral anticoagulants and dextran for prevention of venous thrombosis in orthopaedics. Acta Orthop Scand 55:251, 1984

Tangen O, Wik KO, Almqvist IAM, Arfors K-E, Hint HC. Effects of dextran on the structure and plasmin induced lysis of human fibrin. Thromb Res 1:487, 1972

Thorén L. Dextran as a plasma volume substitute. In: Alan R (ed) Blood substitutes and plasma expanders, Liss Inc, News York, 1978

van Hospenthal J, Frey C, Rutishauser G, Gruber UF. Thromboseprophylaxe bei transurethraler Prostataresektion. Urologe (A), 16:88, 1977

Welin-Berger T, Bygdeman S, Mebius C. Deep vein thrombosis following hip surgery. Relation to activated factor X inhibitor activity: effect of heparin and dextran. Acta Orthop Scand 53:937, 1982

Wieslander JB, Dougan P, Stjernquist U, Åberg M, Bergentz S-E. The influence of dextran and saline solution upon platelet behaviour after microarterial anastomosis. Surg Gynecol Obstet 163:256, 1986

Chapter 18

# Oral anticoagulants and antiplatelet drugs

Alexander G G Turpie

## Oral Anticoagulants

Anticoagulant drugs are the mainstay in the prevention and treatment of venous thromboembolic disease. The landmark observation by Sevitt and Gallagher (1959) that oral anticoagulant therapy (Phenindione) reduced the frequency of deep vein thrombosis and fatal pulmonary embolism in patients with fractured neck of femur stimulated interest in the prophylaxis of postoperative venous thrombosis. However, despite the impressive reduction in venous thromboembolism observed in that study, oral anticoagulants have not been used widely, mainly because of fear of bleeding.

More than twenty studies have been performed to evaluate the effectiveness of oral anticoagulants in preventing venous thrombosis in high risk patients, but less than one half had concurrent control patients and objective endpoints to diagnose venous thromboembolism (Hull and Hirsh, 1981). In general or gynaecological surgery patients, oral anticoagulants have been shown in a number of controlled studies to significantly reduce the frequency of venous thromboembolism. The frequency of side effects varied; several authors reported an increase in major bleeding, particularly in those patients in whom prophylaxis began before operation (Salzman and Davies, 1980). Very low doses of warfarin (1 mg) have been reported to be effective in the prevention of venous thrombosis in one small study in patients having gynaecologic surgery (Poller et al, 1987). In a larger study one mg of warfarin per day was effective in preventing subclavian vein thrombosis in patients with chronic subclavian catheters (Bern et al, 1990).

Oral anticoagulants have been shown to be effective in preventing venous thrombosis after hip surgery when used at a targeted INR of 1.5-3.0 (PT ratio of 1.2-1.6). Effectiveness has been demonstrated when treatment is commenced a number of days before surgery, the evening before surgery or on the first postoperative day (Salzman and Davies, 1980). The risk of clinically important bleeding with a moderate intensity regimen (INR 1.5-3.0) is

**Table 18.1**
Efficacy of Oral Anticoagulant Prophylaxis for the prevention of venous thrombosis

| Author | Type of surgery | Endpoint | n | Control DVT (%) | Fatal PE (%) | n | Oral anticoagulants DVT (%) | Fatal PE (%) |
|---|---|---|---|---|---|---|---|---|
| Sevitt & Gallagher, 1959 | Fracture hip | Autopsy | 150 | 83 | 10.0 | 150 | 14 | 1.3 |
| Eskeland et al, 1966 | Fracture hip | Autopsy | 100 | | 7.0 | 100 | | 1.0 |
| Borgstrom et al, 1965 | Fracture hip | Venography | 29 | 56.5 | | 29 | 9.5 | |
| Hamilton et al, 1970 | Fracture hip | Venography | 38 | 49 | | 38 | 26 | |
| Pinto, 1970 | Fracture hip | Leg scan | 25 | 32 | | 25 | 36 | |
| Hume et al, 1973 | Elective hip | Leg scan | 19 | 42 | | 17 | 59 | |
| Morris & Mitchell, 1976 | Fracture hip | Autopsy | 74 | 68 | 8.0 | 75 | 31 | 0 |
| Taberner et al, 1978 | Gynaecologic | Leg scan | 48 | 23 | | 48 | 6 | |
| Francis et al, 1983 | Elective hip or knee | Venography | 57 | 51 | | 53 | 21 | |

small. The demonstration of the effectiveness of warfarin when commenced after operation in patients having hip surgery suggests that contrary to popular opinion, the majority of important thrombi form some time after surgery (Powers et al, 1989). A more recent study demonstrated that a very low dose of warfarin (1 mg) was ineffective in preventing postoperative venous thrombosis in patients having hip surgery (Fordyce et al, 1991). Thus, although attractive because of its safety and simplicity, it would be premature and inappropriate to use the one mg dose for any condition except for the prevention of subclavian vein thrombosis.

One approach to reducing the risk of bleeding is the use of lower doses during the preoperative and early postoperative periods increasing to more conventional doses when the risk of haemorrhage has subsided. The efficacy and safety of such a warfarin regimen has been compared with dextran 40 in the prevention of venous thrombosis in high-risk patients undergoing elective total hip or knee replacement (Francis et al, 1983). A low dose of warfarin was started ten to fourteen days before operation, and the prothrombin time was adjusted to between 1.5 to 3 seconds longer than the control value at the time of surgery; immediately after surgery, the dose was increased to prolong the prothrombim time to 1.5 times the control value. Thus, warfarin was administered in a two-step regimen with the intention of avoiding bleeding complications in the perioperative period while retaining effectiveness in preventing venous thrombosis. The overall frequency of venous thrombosis by venography was reduced significantly, as was the frequency of thrombi in the femoral and popliteal veins. The incidence of excessive postoperative bleeding was similar and was low (4%) in both treatment groups. These findings indicate that by decreasing the intensity of the anticoagulant effect of warfarin, the risk of bleeding can be substantially reduced while effectiveness in preventing venous thromboembolism is retained.

Table 18.1 shows the results of the main clinical trials of oral anticoagulant prophylaxis.

## Antiplatelet Agents

Venous thrombosis occurs as a result of fibrin formation and deposition, but the presence of platelet aggregates at sites of some early venous thrombi suggests platelets play a role in initiating the process (Turpie and Hirsh, 1984; Turpie, 1988). Therefore, drugs that suppress platelet function may help prevent venous thrombosis in some high risk patients. Of the antiplatelet drugs evaluated in prospective clinical trials for the prevention of deep vein thrombosis, only aspirin has been used extensively in practice. The results of the aspirin studies, however, have been inconsistent. Early reports of the use of aspirin to prevent venous thrombosis after general abdominothoracic operations indicated no benefit (MRC Report, 1972). Most reports of its effectiveness after surgery for fractured hip or elective hip replacement have yielded negative results. In some studies, aspirin showed some benefit, but did not decrease the frequency of deep vein thrombosis to a clinically acceptable level (Salzman and Davies, 1980; Hull and Hirsh, 1981).

Because of the confusion regarding venous thromboembolism prophylaxis with aspirin, the Antiplatelet Trialist Group (Antiplatelet Trialists Collaboration, 1993) have carried out a systematic overview of more than 50 trials of 8,000 patients which demonstrated that antiplatelet therapy reduced the risk of deep vein thrombosis by 37% and of pulmonary embolism by 63%. The apparent effects of treatment were similar and significant for non-fatal emboli and for fatal pulmonary emboli. There was a slight non-significant excess of deaths from other causes so that although the difference in total mortality was favourable, it was not statistically significant. Antiplatelet therapy appeared to reduce the risk of deep vein thrombosis and of pulmonary embolism to a similar extent among patients undergoing general, traumatic, orthopaedic and elective orthopaedic surgery, as well as among other patients at elevated risk of thromboembolism. The data available on the effects of adding antiplatelet therapy to other forms of thromboprophylaxis (such as subcutaneous heparin) were limited, but suggested that the effects may be additive. The conclusion of the Antiplatelet Trialist Group was that antiplatelet drugs should be considered for patients at sufficient risk of thromboembolic events, or that further confirmatory studies of antiplatelet thromboprophylaxis be conducted.

The conclusions reached in the overview have been challenged by Lensing and Hirsh (1991) who divided the studies into those that were free from bias and those that assurance that bias in the outcome assessment was not excluded and found that the risk reduction with aspirin was significantly lower in the studies in which bias was excluded. This raises the question that aspirin may not be as effective as previously suggested and the role of aspirin for venous thrombosis prophylaxis remains uncertain.

## References

Antiplatelet Trialists Collaboration. Brit Med J, 1993 (in press)

Bern MM, Lokich JJ, Wallach SR, Bothe A et al. Very low doses of warfarin can prevent thrombosis in central venous catheters. A randomized prospective trial. Ann of Intern Med 112:423, 1990

Borgstrom S, Greitz T, Vander Linden W et al. Anticoagulant prophylaxis of venous thrombosis in patients with fractured neck of the femur: A controlled clinical trial using venous phlebography. Acta Chir Scand 129:500 1965

Eskeland G, Solheim K, Skorten F. Anticoagulant prophylaxis, thromboembolism and mortality in elderly patients with hip fractures. A controlled clinical trial. Acta Chir Scand 131:16, 1966

Fordyce MJF, Baker AS, Staddon GE. Efficacy of fixed minidose warfarin prophylaxis in total hip replacement. BMJ 303:219, 1991

Francis CW, Evarts CM, Yaukoolbodi S. Two-step warfarin therapy. Prevention of postoperative venous thrombosis without excessive bleeding. JAMA 249:374, 1983

Hamilton HW, Crawford JS, Gardiner JH, Wiley AM. Venous thrombosis in patients with fracture of the upper end of the femur. J Bone Joint Surg 52B:258, 1970

Hull R, Hirsh J. Advances and controversies in the diagnosis, prevention and treatment of venous thromboembolism. Prog Hematol 12:73, 1981

Hume M, Kuriakose T, Xavier ZL, Turner RH. $^{125}$I-fibrinogen and the prevention of venous thrombosis. Arch Surg 107:803, 1973

Lensing AWA and Hirsh J 1993 (personal communication)

Medical Research Council Report on the Steering Committee: Effect of aspirin on postoperative venous thrombosis. Lancet 2:441, 1972

Morris CK, Mitchell JR. Warfarin sodium in the prevention of deep venous thrombosis and pulmonary embolism in patients with fractured neck of femur. Lancet 2:869, 1976

Pinto DJ. Controlled trial of an anticoagulant (warfarin sodium) in the prevention of venous thrombosis following hip surgery. Br J Surg 57:349, 1970

Poller L, McKernan A, Thomson JM, Elstein M et al. Fixed minidose warfarin: a new approach to prophylaxis against venous thrombosis after major surgery. BMJ 295:1309, 1987

Powers PJ, Gent M, Jay RM, Julian DH, Turpie AGG et al. A randomized trial of less intense postoperative warfarin or aspirin therapy in the prevention of venous thromboembolism after surgery for fractured hip. Arch Intern Med 149:771,1989

Salzman EW, Davies GC. Prophylaxis of venous thromboembolism. Analysis of cost-effectiveness. Ann Surg 191:207, 1980

Sevitt S, Gallagher NG. Prevention of venous thrombosis and pulmonary embolism in injured patients. The Lancet ii: 981, 1959

Taberner DA, Poller L, Burslem RW, Jones JG. Oral anticoagulants controlled by the British comparative thromboplastin versus low-dose heparin in prophylaxis of deep vein thrombosis. Br Med J 1:272, 1978

Turpie AGG, Hirsh J: Venous thromboembolism. Current concepts. Part I. Hospital Medicine Oct pp 151-166; Part II Hospital Medicine Nov. pp-13-41, 1984

Turpie AGG: Clinical studies. Evidence of intervention with specific antiplatelet drugs in arterial thromboembolism. Semin Thromb Hemost 14:41, 1988

# CHAPTER 19

# Graduated compression stockings for the prevention of venous thromboembolism

John H Scurr

Graduated compression (TED) has been evaluated in many clinical studies and its efficacy in the prevention of deep vein thrombosis is well established (Table 19.1). Using the fibrinogen uptake test to make the initial diagnosis of deep vein thrombosis in general surgical patients, the incidence of deep vein thrombosis in the untreated group ranges from 49% to 4%, with a mean of 32%, and from 23% to 3.6% in the treated group, with a mean of 9%. One early study addressed the incidence of pulmonary embolism in a postmortem study, and again showed that patients wearing graduated compression stockings have a reduced incidence of fatal pulmonary emboli (Wilkins et al, 1952).

Without exception, all studies using graduated compression stockings, have shown a beneficial effect in reducing the incidence of deep vein thrombosis. The stockings are simple, safe and effective, and in a previous consensus document, have already been recommended for use in low risk patients, and in combination with other prophylactic modalities, for moderate to high risk patients.

Our understanding of the mechanism by which graduated compression stockings prevent deep vein thrombosis is incomplete. Original work by Sigel et al (1973), established a compression profile which significantly increased blood velocity measured in the femoral vein by a Doppler flow probe. By increasing and decreasing the amount of graduated compression, it was possible to establish the maximum possible percentage increase in femoral vein blood velocity, and this profile was used to develop the graduated compression stocking. The prevention of venous stasis and increase of blood flow, through the deeper veins, is thought to be important in the prevention of deep vein thrombosis (Stanton et al, 1949; Wright and Osborn, 1952; Makin, 1969; Rosengarten et al, 1970; Lewis, 1976; Lawrence, 1980; Borow and Goldson, 1981; Allan et al, 1983).

**Table 19.1**
Graduated compression stockings in the prevention of venous thromboembolism: a summary of trials

| Authors | Patient group | Endpoint | Untreated | Treated | Other agents |
|---|---|---|---|---|---|
| Wilkins et al, 1952 | Medical | Post-mortem PE | 6/2395 | 1/2346 | |
| | Surgical obstetrics | | | | |
| Tsapogas et al, 1971 | Gen. Surgical | FUT | 6/44 (14%) | 2/51 (4%) | |
| Scurr et al, 1977 | Gen. Surgical (alternate leg) | FUT | 26/70 (37%) | 8/70 (11%) | |
| Holford, 1976 | Major Surgical | FUT | 23/47 (49%) | 11/48 (23%) | |
| Borow and Goldson, 1981 | Various Surgical | FUT | 32/89 (36%) | 14/91 (15.4%) | |
| Inada et al, 1983 | Gen. Surgical (alternate leg) | FUT | 16/110 (14.5%) | 4/110 (3.6%) | |
| Allan et al, 1983 | Gen. Surgical | FUT | 37/103 (35.9%) | 15/97 (15.5%) | |
| | Benign | | 16/51 (31.4%) | 5/49 (10.2%) | |
| | Malignant | | 21/52 (40.4%) | 10/48 (20.8%) | |
| Fasting et al, 1983 | Major Surgery | 99m-Tc plasmin test | 6/54 (11%) | 6/46N (13%) | L.D. Heparin |
| Caprini et al, 1983 | Various Surg. | FUT | 20/96 (21%) retrospective | 4/39 (10.2%) | |
| Turner et al, 1984 | Gynae. Surgery | FUT | 16/150 (11%) | 2/150 (1.4%) | |
| Barnes et al, 1978 | Hip Surgery | FUT | 5/10 (50%) | 0/8 (0%) | |
| Ishak & Morley, 1981 | Hip Surgery | FUT | 22/41 (54%) | 7/35 (20%) | |
| Turner et al, 1984 | Gynae. Surgery | FUT | 4/92 (4%) | 0/104 (0%) | |

By producing graduated compression stockings of differing sizes, it is possible to fit 95% of the population with a stocking offering the correct compression profile. Changes in limb size, when the patient is recumbent, may alter the compression profile and significantly adjust the amount of flow through the deep veins.

In a chance observation when looking at the effectiveness of intermittent pneumatic compression on the leg, when used in combination with a graduated compression stocking (Scurr et al, 1987), it was noted that the presence of a TED stocking increased the effectiveness of external pneumatic compression. The graduated compression stocking prevented venous distension during the relaxation phase of the pneumatic compression cycle. This led to further work, looking at venous distension during surgical procedures (Coleridge-Smith and Scurr, 1991). Comerota (Comerota et al, 1985; Chapter 3) found that venous distension in patients undergoing surgery was associated with an increased incidence of deep vein thrombosis. In his studies, venous distension of greater than 20% measured in the forearm veins by duplex ultrasound, was associated with a high incidence

**Table 19.2**
Graduated compression stockings in combination with other methods of prophylaxis: a summary of trials

| Authors | Patient group | Endpoint | **LD Heparin** | **LD Heparin & graduated compression** |
|---|---|---|---|---|
| Torngren, 1980 | Gen. Surgical (alternate leg) | FUT | 12/98 (12%) | 4/98 (4%) |
| Willie-Jorgensen, 1985 | Gen. Surgical | FUT | 12/102 (12%) | 2/94 (2%) |
| Borow and Goldson, 1983 | Surgical | FUT | 23/86 (26.7%) retrospective | 2/63 (3%) |
| | | | **Intermittent calf compression** | **Intermittent calf compression and graduated compression** |
| Scurr et al, 1987 | Gen. Surgery | FUT | 7/78 (11%) | 1/78 (1%) |
| | | | **Dextran** | **Dextran & stocking** |
| Bergqvist and Lindblad, 1984 | Gen. Surgery | FUT | 8/80 (10%) | 0/80 (0%) |

of deep vein thrombosis in the legs. Patients who did not demonstrate venous distension did not develop deep vein thrombosis.

Patients undergoing surgery demonstrate venous distension, particularly in the posterior tibial veins, gastrocnemius veins, and soleal veins. These veins are important as they are thought to be the site of origin of many deep vein thromboses. In patients placed supine on the operating theatre table, venous diameters increase during the surgical procedure. With the legs dependent, venous distension increases at the end of an operation, compared to at the beginning. Using the graduated compression stocking during surgery this change can be reversed.

It is probable that the graduated compression stocking exerts at least some of its effect, by the prevention of venous distension. The significance of venous distension relates in part to venous pooling, but also in part to an alteration in the nature of the vein wall. As the veins are stretched, gaps appear between the endothelial cells, collagen is exposed, and a site for thrombosis started (Stewart et al, 1980). Whether it is necessary to compress the whole leg, or just calf, has never been established. Further studies addressing this point need to be conducted (Rasmussen et al, 1988; Porteous et al, 1989; Coleridge-Smith and Scurr, 1991).

More recently, clinical studies have looked at the effect of combining modalities (Table 19.2). Graduated compression stockings have been combined with low-dose heparin, and with intermittent pneumatic compression. Torngren (1980), using a graduated compression stocking on alternate legs, demonstrated a 12% incidence of deep vein thrombosis in the non-stockinged leg, compared to a 4% incidence of deep vein thrombosis in the stocking leg. Willie-Jorgensen et al (1989) in a controlled study, demonstrated an incidence of 12% in patients receiving subcutaneous heparin alone, compared to 2% in those patients receiving both subcutaneous heparin and graduated compression stockings. Our team demonstrated an enhanced efficacy of intermittent pneumatic compression, when combined with stockings (Scurr et al, 1987).

## Conclusions

There is now good evidence that graduated compression stockings are effective in the prevention of deep venous thrombosis. The mechanism by which these stockings exert their effect is uncertain, it may be by promoting blood flow, it may be by preventing venous distension.

Until we understand the mechanism fully, it is important that stockings with a proven clinical efficacy are used.

Graduated compression stockings used alone are effective in the prevention of deep vein thrombosis in low-risk patients. In combination with intermittent pneumatic compression or subcutaneous heparin, they are effective in moderate and high- risk patients.

Graduated compression stockings are relatively free of complications, although care should be taken if using these stockings on patients with peripheral vascular disease.

## References

Atkins P, Hawkins LA. Detection of venous thrombosis in the legs. Lancet ii:1217, 1965

Allan A, Williams JT, Bolton JP, Le Quesne LP. The use of graduated compression stockings in the prevention of postoperative deep vein thrombosis. Br J Surg 70:172, 1983

Barnes RW, Brand RA, Clarke W, Hartley N, Hoak JC. Efficacy of graded compression antiembolism stockings in patients undergoing total hip arthroplasty. Clin Orthop 132:61, 1978

Bergqvist D, Lindblad B. The thromboprophylactic effect of graded elastic compression stockings in combination with dextran 70. Arch Surg 119:1329, 1984

Borow M, Goldson H. Prevention of postoperative deep venous thrombosis and pulmonary emboli with combined modalities. Amer Surgeon 49:599, 1983

Borow M, Goldson H. Postoperative venous thrombosis: evaluation of five methods of treatment. Amer J Surg 141:245, 1981

Browse NL, Jackson BT, Mayo ME. The value of mechanical methods of preventing postoperative calf vein thrombosis. Br J Surg 61:219, 1974

Caprini JA, Scurr JH, Hasty JH. Role of compression modalities in a prophylactic program for deep vein thrombosis. Semin Thromb Hemost 14:77, 1988

Clagett GP, Reisch JS. Prevention of venous thromboembolism in general surgical patients. Results of meta-analysis. Ann Surg 208:227, 1988

Colditz GA, Tunden RL, Oster G. Rates of venous thrombosis after general surgery: combined results of randomised clinical trials. Lancet ii:143, 1986

Coleridge-Smith PD, Scurr JH. Deep vein thrombosis: effect of graduated compression stockings on distension of the deep veins of the calf. Br J Surg 78:724, 1981

Comerota A, Stewart GH, White JV. Combined dihydroergotamine and heparin prophylaxis of postoperative deep vein thrombosis: proposed mechanism of action. Am J Surg 150:39, 1985

Fasting H, Koopmann HD, Nielsen HK, Husted SE, Andersen K, Hansen HH. The efficacy of graduated compression stockings compared with low-dose heparin in the prevention of deep vein thrombosis. Thromb Hemostas 50:247, 1983

Fasting H, Andersen K, Kraemmer Nielsen H, Husted SE, Koopmann HD, Simonsen O, Husegaard HC, Vestergaard Madsen J, Pedersen TK. Prevention of postoperative deep venous thrombosis. Low dose heparin versus graded pressure stockings. Acta Chir Scand 151 (3):245, 1985

Flanc C, Kakkar VV, Clarke MB. Postoperative deep vein thrombosis. Effect of intensive prophylaxis. Lancet i:477, 1969

Gold EW. Prophylaxis of deep venous thromboembolism. Literature review. Orthopedics (USA) 11:1197, 1988

Holford CP. Graded compression for preventing deep venous thrombosis. Br Med J 2:969, 1976

Hunter WC, Sneeden VB, Robertson TD, Snyder GAC. Thrombosis of the deep veins of the leg. Arch Int Med 68:1, 1941

Inada K, Shirai N, Hazashi M, Matsumoto K, Hirose M. Postoperative deep venous thrombosis in Japan: Incidence and Prophylaxis. Amer J Surg 145:775, 1983

Ishak MA, Morley KD. Deep venous thrombosis after total hip arthroplasty; a prospective controlled study to determine the prophylactic effect of graded elastic pressure stockings. Br J Surg 68:429, 1981

Jeffery PC, Nicolaides AN. Graduated compression stockings in the prevention of postoperative deep vein thrombosis. Br J Surg 77:380, 1990

Lawrence D, Kakkar VV. Graduated compression stockings in the prevention of postoperative deep vein thrombosis. Br J Surg 67:119, 1980

Lewis CE, Antoine J, Mueller C. Talbot WA, Swaroop R, Edwards WS. Elastic compression in the prevention of venous stasis. A critical re-evaluation. Am J Surg 132:739, 1976

Makin GS, A clinical trial of "Tubigrip" to prevent deep venous thrombosis. Br J Surg 56:373, 1969

Mellbring G, Palmer K. Prophylaxis of deep vein thrombosis after major abdominal surgery. Comparison between dihydroergotamine- heparin and intermittent pneumatic calf compression and evaluation of added graduated static compression. Acta Chir Scand 152:597, 1986

Meyerowitz RB, Nelson R. Measurement of the velocity of blood in lower limb veins with and without compression. Surgery 56:481, 1964

Nicolaides AN, Miles C, Hoare M. et al. Intermittent sequential pneumatic compression of the legs and thromboembolism-deterrent stockings in the prevention of postoperative deep venous thrombosis. Surgery (USA) 94:21, 1983

Nicolaides AN, Irving D. Clinical factors and the risk of deep venous thrombosis. In: Nicolaides AN (ed). Thromboembolism: Aetiology, advances in prevention and management. Lancaster: MTP Medical and Technical Publishing, 1975

Porteous MJ, Nicholson EA, Morris LT, James R, Negus D. Thigh length versus knee length stockings in the prevention of deep vein thrombosis. Br J Surg 76:296, 1989a

Rasmussen A, Hansen PT, Linholt J, Poulsen TD, Toftdahl DB, Gram J, Toftgaard C, Jespersen J. Venous thrombosis after abdominal surgery. A comparison between subcutaneous heparin and antithrombotic stockings, or both. J Med 19:193, 1988

Rosengarten DS, Laird J, Jeyasingh K et al. The failure of compression stockings (Tubigrip) to prevent deep vein thrombosis after surgery. Br J Surg 57:296, 1970

Rosengarten DS. Thromboembolism. Henry Simpson Newland Prize Essay. Royal Australasian College of Surgeons, 1974

Scurr JH, Coleridge-Smith PD, Hasty JH. Regime for improved effectiveness of intermittent pneumatic compression in deep venous thrombosis prophylaxis. Surgery 102:816, 1987

Scurr JH, Ibrahim SZ, Faber RG. LeQuesne LP. The efficacy of graduated compression stockings in the prevention of vein thrombosis. Br J Surg 64:371, 1977

Sigel B, Edelstein AL, Felix WR, Memhardt CR. Compression of the deep venous system of the lower leg during inactive recumbency. Arch Surg 106:38, 1973

Stanton JR, Freis ED, Wilkins RW. The acceleration of linear flow in the deep veins of the lower extermity of man by local compression. J Clin Invest 28:553, 1949

Stewart GJ, Schaub RG, Niewiarowski S. Products of tissue injury. Arch Pathol Lab Med 104:409, 1980

Torngren S. Low dose heparin and compression stockings in the prevention of postoperative deep venous thrombosis. Br J Surg 67:482, 1980

Tsapogas MJ, Groussous H, Peabody RA, Karmody AM, Eckert C. Postoperative venous thrombosis and the effectiveness of prophylactic measures. Arch Surg 103:561, 1971

Turner GM, Cole SE, Brooks JH. The efficacy of graduated compression stockings in the prevention of deep vein thrombosis after major gynaecological surgery. Br J Obst Gyn 91:588, 1984

Turpie AG, Hirsh J, Gent M, Julian D, Johnson J. Prevention of deep vein thrombosis in potential neurosurgical patients. A randomised trial comparing graduated compression stockings alone or graduated compression stockings plus intermittent pneumatic compression with control. Arch Intern Med 149:679, 1989

Wilkins RW, Mixter Jr G, Stanton JR, Litter J. Elastic stockings in the prevention of pulmonary embolism: a preliminary report. NEJM 246:360, 1952

Wille-Jorgensen P, Hauch O, Dimo B, Christensen SW, Jense R, Hansen B. Prophylaxis of deep venous thrombosis after acute abdominal operation. Surg Gynecol Obstet 172 (1):44, 1991

Wille-Jorgensen P, Christensen SW, Bjerg-Nielsen A, Stadeager C, Kjaer L. Prevention of thromboembolism following elective hip surgery. The value of regional anesthesia and graded compression stockings. Clin Orthop (US) 247:163, 1989

Williams JT, Palfrey SM. Cost-effectiveness and efficacy of below knee against above knee graduated compression stockings in the prevention of deep vein thrombosis. Phlebologie (France) 41:809, 1988

Williamson M, Thomas S, Edwards A, Johnson R, Riggs J, Lewis MH. Graduated compression stockings in the prevention of post-operative deep vein thrombosis: a comparative study of pressure profiles and patient compliance. Phlebology (UK) 5:135, 1990

Wright HP, Osborn SB. Effect of posture on venous velocity measured with 24NaCl. Br Heart J 14:325, 1952

CHAPTER 20

# Intermittent pneumatic compression

Joseph A Caprini   Clara I Traverso
Juan I Arcelus

## Introduction

Among the physical methods for preventing deep vein thrombosis (DVT), intermittent pneumatic compression (IPC) has been the most extensively studied, and some noteworthy reviews concur that IPC appears to be the most effective of those (Consensus Conference, 1986; Clagett and Reisch, 1988).

Since IPC was proposed, major interest has been focused on its lack of bleeding complications; thus, it appears to be one of the safest prophylactic modalities. Nevertheless, prior to the newer designs and the incorporation of sequential devices, both the routine employment of this method and its effectiveness were questioned. The uncomfortable, old-fashioned machines were not well-accepted, many patients rejected their use and, if used, the prophylactic period had to be shorter (Turpie et al, 1977; Coe et al, 1978). The currently available enhanced devices have minimised the adverse effects, and cessation of IPC because of discomfort or irritation is uncommon (Caprini et al, 1983; Turpie et al, 1989; Hull et al, 1990), although patient acceptance is always variable (Muhe, 1984; Bartle, 1988). Patient compliance is better because mobility of the knee joint is conserved; thus, the application may be maintained for several postoperative days according to physicians' criteria (Nicolaides et al, 1983). Finally, they are simple to fit and easy to manage by patients and nursing staff, which allows clinicians to set the convenient prophylactic period (Caprini et al, 1988). The inclusion of sequential devices increased the number of advocates of this method, following some evidence that sequential devices were better than non-sequential from an haemodynamic viewpoint. Sequential IPC did not trap blood distally in the vein as uniform IPC did, emptied the thigh veins significantly more rapidly, and was more effective (Nicolaides et al, 1980; Kamn, 1982; Mittelman et al, 1982; Olson et al, 1982; Salzman et al, 1987).

With these modifications, and following numerous studies in several surgical procedures, IPC has become more accepted in the United States during the last five years. In contrast, the newer pharmacological methods, especially low molecular weight heparin, have been the centre of most European studies.

## Thrombogenic factors influenced by IPC

Individuals at risk of developing DVT include hospitalised medical patients, postoperative patients, and medical patients recovering at home from serious illnesses, particularly cancer. Venous stasis and hypercoagulability are commonly seen in these patients and the significant role of both factors in the occurrence of DVT is well known.

Mechanical methods were proposed primarily to avoid venous stasis by supplying the muscle tone that is lacking during the surgical procedure because of the anaesthesia and the leg's position. Venous dilatation during certain surgical procedures has been shown by Coleridge-Smith et al (1990). A close relation between vein wall distension and the development of DVT was found in certain orthopaedic surgical patients at high risk (Comerota et al, 1989). We are now carrying out a study in volunteers to analyse, by real-time B-mode ultrasound scanning, the degree of venous dilatation in the deep venous system that may be provoked by the reverse Trendelenburg position, which is used during laparoscopic cholecystectomy. In addition, we are evaluating how graduated compression stockings may address venous dilatation in such a position.

Increased vein diameter has also been demonstrated in medical patients confined to bed for extended periods (Kierkegaard et al, 1989), suggesting that the venous pump function is compromised in this population.

### Venous stasis
It has been confirmed that IPC maintains venous capacitance and venous outflow (Blackshear et al, 1987) and creates a high flow pulsatility (Roberts et al, 1972). In addition, several studies show that IPC significantly improves flow velocity, volume flow rate, and shear stress, as well as blood clearance from the venous system (Sigel et al, 1983; Muhe, 1984). It is evident that IPC inhibits stasis, therefore, IPC could also influence another aspect of Virchow's triad, the endothelial damage, which has been reported to follow overdistension of the limb veins (Comerota et al, 1985).

### Fibrinolysis
It has been suggested that IPC also addresses the hypercoagulable state by stimulating fibrinolytic activity (FA) (Allenby et al, 1973; Summaria et al, 1985; Weitz et al, 1985). Testing by different techniques, increased levels of prostacyclin (Guyton et al, 1985), B-Beta 15-42 levels (Inada et al, 1988), free protease activity, t-PA levels, and diminished plasminogen concentration (Summaria et al, 1988) have been reported. Accordingly, starting IPC before the surgical procedure avoids the postoperative fibrinolytic shut-down, which is a remarkable advantage of this prophylactic modality (Hartman et al, 1983; Caprini et al, 1983).

An adequate fibrinolytic response to IPC has been related to a decreased incidence of DVT (Summaria et al, 1988). A group of "non-responder" patients to the stimulation of the fibrinolytic system has been identified. Accordingly, the employment of IPC in such a group could be limited (Tarnay et al, 1980; Salzman et al, 1987; Summaria et al, 1988). It has also been shown "*in vitro*" by experimental models involving cultured endothelial cells, that the levels of prostacyclin production are greater under pulsatile flow conditions than under continuous flow conditions, and that continuous flow conditions produce greater levels than stationary conditions (Frangos et al, 1985). In addition, a greater improvement of the FA followed by a diminished incidence of DVT has been reported when sequential devices were used (Salzman et al, 1987). It has been also demonstrated by Tarnay et al (1980) in volunteers, that a larger area of compressed tissue produces a greater fibrinolytic effect as measured by the euglobulin lysis time (ELT). Therefore, the authors point out the superiority of thigh-length sleeves when compared with knee-length sleeves. Inada et al (1988), however, reported that the ELT was not a suitable test for measuring the influences of IPC on the FA. On the other hand, haemodynamic studies have demonstrated that the thigh acts as a reservoir for venous blood; so, compression or elevation of the thigh for venous drainage appears to be necessary (von Schroeder et al, 1991).

# Rationale for its use

**Safety**
As shown above, IPC appears to favourably influence all components of Virchow's triad by its two-fold mechanism of action against venous stasis and the postoperative fibrinolytic shut-down, and these haemostatic changes do not appear to be sufficient to cause haemorrhage (Tarnay et al, 1980). Actually, there have been no reported bleeding complications with IPC utilisation. Accordingly, IPC might be selected in patients who have a high risk of bleeding and whenever pharmacological methods are contraindicated (Consensus Conference, 1986). In neurological patients, no one pharmacological modality has been widely accepted by clinicians (Moskopp and Popoc-Cenic, 1990). Any bleeding complication in neurosurgical or neurological patients could potentially be fatal (Turpie et al, 1979; Krolick et al, 1991). Surgical patients in whom an occult haemostatic defect exists or is strongly suspected are also excellent candidates for this mechanical modality (Caprini and Natanson, 1989), as are those who have procedures which involve major dissection, such as extensive pelvic surgery for malignancies (Nicolaides et al, 1983; Clarke-Pearson et al, 1984) and open urological operations (Coe et al, 1978).

**Factors influencing the effectiveness of IPC**
In reviewing the literature, IPC appears to have well-defined indications (Salzman and Davis, 1980; Borow and Goldson, 1981; Consensus Conference, 1986; Caprini et al, 1988; Clagett and Reisch, 1988). Nevertheless, the effectiveness of IPC for preventing both distal and proximal DVT in certain surgical populations at high risk needs to be established (Gallus et al, 1983; Haas et al, 1990; Paiement et al, 1990; Boniske, 1991). Some results are inconclusive (Consensus Conference, 1986; Clagett and Reisch, 1988) or quite controversial (O'Meara, 1991; Lyne, 1991); so, interpretation should be done carefully.

To analyse the effectiveness of IPC by compiling the entire accessible experience is not feasible due to the fact that devices, sets of pressure utilised, and periods of application, all varied from one study to another. Obviously, results also depend on the type of surgery performed, patient risk factors, and end-points used for the diagnosis. Consequently, prior to reaching any conclusion about the effectiveness of IPC for preventing postoperative DVT, it would be appropriate to consider such factors.

*a. Influence of the pressure selected*
When IPC is used, two important points to be considered are how much compression is applied, and the profile of compression required (Caprini et al, 1988). These issues have been analysed when using different devices.

Initial investigations were carried out on single chamber below-knee devices. A maximum pressure pulse of 40 mmHg for five seconds was applied, and followed by one minute of no pressure for venous refilling (Sabri et al, 1971). Subsequent experiments confirmed that such a profile was adequate for obtaining optimal flow pulsatility (Roberts et al, 1972).

Alternate approaches to IPC have used much slower cycles for development of the pressure applied (Hills et al, 1972). The more remarkable advantage provided by this modification, when compared with earlier investigations, was the prolonged time required to attain the maximum pressure, and consequently, a more complete emptying of the deep veins was achieved.

The optimal pressure for sequential compression devices was settled in volunteers by Nicolaides et al (1980), following a haemodynamic study in which the authors measured the modifications induced on blood velocity of the femoral vein by five different sets of pressures. The optimal pressure set was 35-30-20 mmHg, and higher pressures were not followed by more effective increases of flow velocity. However, these authors contemplated the possibility of employing pressures slightly higher because they found considerable individual variations. With another haemodynamic study that was carried out in general abdominal surgery, Muhe (1984) concluded that 55 mmHg appeared to be too low a pressure to generate a high venous flow velocity, as analysed by Xe-133. This is in disagreement with results reported by von Schroeder et al (1991), who showed in volunteers that the aforementioned pressure increases the femoral venous flow, as measured by a thermodilution technique. In any case, Muhe also recommends ruling out large thrombi before applying pressure higher than 55 mmHg, because such pressures could provoke an occasional, yet hazardous proximal migration of a calf vein thrombus.

Apart from these haemodynamic studies, maximum pressures applied by different authors range from 35 mmHg to 50 mmHg when below-knee devices are used, and from 35 mmHg to 55 mmHg with thigh-length sleeves. On the other hand, inflation periods vary from 10 to 25 seconds with below-knee devices and from 10 to 35 seconds when thigh-length sleeves are utilised (Caprini et al, 1991). The devices are designed to cycle once every minute, which is approximately the time requried for veins to refill (Sabri et al, 1971; Nicolaides et al, 1980).

*b. Influence of the prophylactic period utilised*
One of the most important criteria for assessing the effectiveness of IPC is the period during which this method is applied. Actually, the period of application is an essential topic to consider whenever any prophylactic modality is evaluated.

Generically, the reported results have been superior when IPC was begun just before the operation, which is used by most authors (Table 20.1). Other authors recommend starting the night before surgery (Bartle, 1988). In fact, some reported cases of fatal pulmonary embolism following orthopaedic procedures have been related to the lack of application of IPC prior to the operation (Hartman et al, 1982; Hull et al, 1990). In addition, Wuh et al (1989) observed in four out of five patients studied, that IPC was able to intraoperatively maintain the femoral flow through the twisted veins during total hip replacement, as measured by Doppler. This suggests that prophylaxis should be started preoperatively and continued intraoperatively rather than following operations. Today, this is possible since

## Table 20.1
Incidence of DVT in several surgical populations related to the prophylactic period in which IPC was applied

| Surgical population | Authors | Modality | Pre | Io | Po | Days Mn-Mx | DVT (%) |
|---|---|---|---|---|---|---|---|
| General | Smith et al, 1978 | Below | N | Y | N | — | 38# |
| | Nicolaides et al, 1980 | Thigh | N | Y | Y | 1-1 | 19.9# |
| | Nicolaides et al, 1983 | Thigh | Y | Y | Y (GEC) | 3-14 | 4# |
| | Inada et al, 1988 | Thigh | N | Y | Y | 2-2 | 6.2#~ |
| Gynaecological | Clarke-P. et al, 1984 | Below | N | Y | Y | 5-5 | 9.1#~[x] |
| Neurosurgical | Skillman et al, 1978 | Below | N | Y | Y | A-5 | 8.5#~ |
| | Turpie et al, 1979 | Below | N | N | Y | D-14 | 7.8#~[x] |
| Orthopaedic | Hull et al, 1979 | Below | N | N | Y | D-17 | 6.3[+] |
| | McKenna et al, 1980 | Thigh | N | N | Y | D-D | 10[+] |
| | Hartman et al, 1982 | Thigh | Y | Y | Y (GEC) | A-D | 1#~[d] |
| | Gallus et al, 1983 | Below | N | Y | Y | 7-7 | 3[+] |
| | Balley et al, 1990 | Thigh | N | N | Y (GEC) | 5-7 | 4.5[+] |
| | Hull et al, 1990 | Thigh | N | N | Y | A-14 | 24#[x+] |
| | Haas et al, 1990 | Thigh | Y | Y | Y | 7-D | 48[+] |
| | Woolson and Watt, 1991 | Thigh | N | Y | Y (GEC) | D-D | 8[+] |
| Urological | Coe et al, 1978 | Below | N | Y | Y | D-D | 7# |
| Various | Borow and Goldson, 1983 | Below | Y | Y | Y | A-D | 11.5#~[xd] |
| | Caprini et al, 1983 | Thigh | Y | Y | Y (GEC) | 3-D | 10.2#~[xd] |

Pre: Preoperative   Io: Intraoperative   Po: Postoperative
GEC: Graduated elastic compression stockings were also fitted
Mn: Minimum   Mx: Maximum   N: No   Y: Yes
A: Ambulation   D: Discharge   #: Fibrinogen uptake test (FUT)
~: Venography confirms   *: $p<0.05$   [x]: Impedance plethysmography
[d]: Doppler   [+]: Venography as end-point

there are sterile sleeves that can be applied intraoperatively on the operated leg (Woolson and Wats, 1991).

When IPC was only applied during the surgical procedure (Smith et al, 1978), the results were not conclusive. Some authors support restricting the use of IPC to the time of surgery as adequate (Bynke et al, 1987; Nolan, 1988); others do not (Smith et al, 1978). Salzman et al (1980) did not find any statistically significant difference when comparing the use of intraoperative IPC with a longer, three-day period of application. In contrast, Colditz et al (1986) established in a review of the literature involving general surgical patients a relationship between shorter prophylactic periods and IPC failures.

When IPC was begun after surgery, the results were favourable (Table 20.1). However, it is interesting to note that, in these cases, there was a trend to prolong the prophylactic period.

As shown above, the optimal period of application for IPC remains to be established definitively, but most authors agree that it should be maintained until the patient is fully ambulatory (Skillman et al, 1978; Salzman et al, 1980; Clarke-Pearson et al, 1984). Such a time is defined as the day on which the patient is able to ambulate unaided (Scurr et al, 1984). Prior to selecting IPC, the patient's risk should be established, which is a comon practice with other prophylactic modalities (Nicolaides and Irving, 1975; Consensus Conference, 1986). If IPC is considered appropriate, it should be continued for the entire risk period (Turpie et al, 1979; Caprini et al, 1983).

All the considerations made above are independent of the anatomical coverage provided by IPC, i.e., they are applicable to both below-knee and thigh-length devices. Although results are still not conclusive, thigh-length sleeves are considered superior to below-knee devices by some authors because they trigger a greater fibrinolytic response (Tarnay et al, 1980). Likewise, it has been documented that the thigh would act as a reservoir for venous blood, and it should be compressed itself (von Schroeder et al, 1991). In any case, a trend toward using full-length devices during the last several years is noted (Table 20.1).

*Graduated elastic compression combined with IPC*
Enhanced results have been reported when thigh-length devices were combined with graduated elastic compression (GEC) (Nicolaides et al, 1983; Scurr et al, 1987). In most of these cases, prophylaxis was maintained until discharge (Table 20.1). This has been attributed to the fact that GEC would offer protection in those periods in which IPC is not operating, i.e., between pneumatic compression cycles as well as when the sleeves are disconnected, during clinical or nursing procedures (Borow and Goldson, 1983; Scurr et al, 1987). In total hip replacement, the application of IPC plus GEC intra- and post-operatively until discharge was as effective as such a combination plus acetylsalicylic acid or low-dose warfarin, as screened by venography and/or duplex scan (Woolson and Watt, 1991) In contrast, IPC-GEC was only effective for reducing distal DVT in orthopaedic populations; however, the incidence of proximal DVT was lower in the treated group than in the control group, but without a statistically significant difference (Hartman et al, 1982). On the other hand, GEC alone was as effective as GEC plus thigh-length IPC in neurology; therefore, adding IPC to GEC is only suggested as an option in these patients (Turpie et al, 1989).

*IPC combined with some pharmacologic modalities*
Apart from the aforementioned physical association, IPC has also been combined with several prophylactic drugs in orthopaedic populations. In total hip replacement, Harris et al (1985) reported a diminished incidence of both distal and proximal DVT when thigh-length IPC was combined with a three-day course of dextran 40. However, in the same group of patients, a combination of below-knee devices and coumadin failed to prevent the development of pulmonary embolism in one patient, which happened 42 days after surgery (Borow and Goldson, 1983). In total knee arthroplasty, an association of rehabilitation exercises (one day preoperatively and the morning of surgery) plus below-knee IPC (intra- and post-operatively until discharge) plus ASA (in the recovery room and also until discharge) was very effective (Clayton and Thompson, 1987); however, objective diagnostic end-points were not utilised.

## Table 20.2
Incidence of DVT in several surgical populations: IPC versus no prophylaxis

| Authors | Patient group | Prophylactic modalities | Patients n | DVT |
|---|---|---|---|---|
| Skillman et al, 1978 | Neurosurgical | B-IPC | 47 | 8.5#~ |
|  |  | Control | 48 | 25[*] |
| Turpie et al, 1979 | Neurosurgical | B-IPC | 65 | 7.8#~[x] |
|  |  | Control | 64 | 21[*] |
| Turpie et al, 1989 | Neurological | T-IPC (GEC) | 78 | 9#~ |
|  |  | Control | 81 | 19.8[*] |
| Hull et al, 1979 | Orthopaedic | B-IPC | 32 | 6.3[+] |
|  |  | Control | 29 | 65[*] |
| Hartman et al, 1982 | Orthopaedic | T-IPC (GEC) | 53 | 1#~[d] |
|  |  | Control | 52 | 19[*] |
| Gallus et al, 1983 | Orthopaedic | B-IPC | 152 | 24#~[x] |
|  |  | Control | 158 | 49[*] |
| Coe et al, 1978 | Open Urological | B-IPC | 29 | 7# |
|  |  | Control | 24 | 25[*] |
| Borow & Goldson, 1983 | Various | B-IPC | 95 | 11.5#~[xd] |
|  |  | Control | 95 | 35.6[*] |
| Caprini et al, 1983 | Various | T-IPC (GEC) | 39 | 10.2~#[xd] |
|  |  | Control | 96 (retrospective) | 20.8[*] |
| Clarke-Pearson et al, 1984 | Gynaecological | B-IPC | 55 | 9.1~#[x] |
|  |  | Control | 52 | 33[*] |

B: Below-knee devices   T: Thigh length devices   GEC: This method was also fitted
Characters that symbolise the different diagnostic methods are defined in Table 20.1
[*]: $p<0.05$

### Effectiveness of IPC versus a non-treated group

Table 20.2 compiles data about the reported incidence of distal DVT in several surgical populations when the employment of IPC is compared with a group that did not receive prophylaxis (control group). Different diagnostic tests were used, and are specified there. These and some other studies (which are listed in parentheses) indicate that IPC is effective in reducing distal DVT versus a non-treated group in general surgery: — cancer (Clagett and Reisch, 1988; Inada et al, 1988) and non-malignant diseases (Hills et al, 1972; Clark et al, 1974; Roberts and Cotton, 1974; Nolan, 1988); gynaecologic malignancy interventions; open urological operations (Salzman et al, 1980); neurological patients — operated (Bynke et al, 1987; Salzman et al, 1987) and non-operated patients (Black et al, 1986; Editorial, 1987), and orthopaedic (McKenna et al, 1980; Caprini et al, 1987) and trauma surgical procedures.

Regarding proximal DVT, results are not conclusive. In 1988, available results were found not to be sufficient for appraising this issue, according to the meta-analysis carried out by Clagett and Reisch in urological, gynaecological and general surgical populations. Since then, although newer data have been collected, diagnostic end-points in these surgical procedures appear not to be suitable for definitely reaching conclusions. In total hip

**Table 20.3**
Effectiveness of IPC compared with other pharmacological modalities

| Authors | Patient group | Prophylactic modalities | Patients n | DVT (%) |
|---|---|---|---|---|
| Paiement et al, 1987 | Orthopaedic | IPC | 66 | 19#+ |
|  |  | LDW | 73 | 16 (ns) |
| Balley et al, 1990 | Orthopaedic | T-IPC (GEC) | 44 | 4.5+ |
|  |  | LDW (GEC) | 38 | 28.9* |
| Haas et al, 1990 | Orthopaedic | T-IPC | 36 | 22+ |
|  |  | ASA | 36 | 47* |
| Coe et al, 1978 | Urological | B-IPC | 29 | 7#~ |
|  |  | LDH | 28 | 21* |
| Hansberry et al, 1991 | Urological | IPC | 25 | 12.5$^{spt}$ |
|  |  | HDHE | 24 | 8** (ns) |
| Smith et al, 1978 | General | B-IPC | 95 | 38# |
|  |  | Dextran 70 | 97 | 22** (ns) |
| Nicolaides et al, 1983 | Abdominal | T-IPC (GEC) | 50 | 4# |
|  |  | LDH | 50 | 9 (ns) |
| Borow & Goldson, 1983 | Various | B-IPC | 95 | 11.5#~$^{xd}$ |
|  |  | LDH | 94 | 25.5* |
|  |  | Dextran 40 | 85 | 18.5 (ns) |
|  |  | ASA | 87 | 19.2 (ns) |

B: Below knee devices   T: Thigh length sleeves   GEC: This method was also fitted
LDW: Low dose warfarin   ASA: Acetylsalicylic acid   LDH: Unfractionated heparin
HDHE: Heparin-Dihydroergotamine   spt: 111In-labelled platelet scan
Characters that symbolise the different diagnostic methods are defined in Table 20.1
* IPC was superior to the other prophylactic modality ($p<0.05$)
** The other prophylactic modality was superior to IPC
(ns): There was no statistically significant difference between both modalities

arthroplasty, venography is commonly used. IPC appears not to reduce proximal DVT (Gallus et al, 1983; Paiement et al, 1990; Boniske, 1991). This is in disagreement with results reported by Hull et al (1990) who did demonstrate such a decrease in a comprehensive study, involving 310 patients; venography was also used as the diagnostic end-point.

Data related to how IPC prevents both pulmonary embolism and the development of late onset DVT are also considered insufficient.

### Effectiveness of IPC versus other pharmacologic methods
Table 20.3 is a collection of data regarding the effectiveness of IPC when it is compared with some pharmacologic methods of prophylaxis. Table 20.4 is a complement to it, and shows similar information but involves patients whose risk of developing DVT was high, and in comparison with control groups in some cases.

In total hip replacement, when IPC is compared to low-dose warfarin, results are dissimilar, using venography for the diagnosis (Table 20.3). Such a difference may be explained because of GEC.

In total knee arthroplasty, Lynch et al (1990) have reported that mechanical methods, including IPC, were equal to or more effective than pharmacological modalities. When IPC

**Table 20.4**
Effectiveness of IPC versus both the control group and other pharmacological modalities in several surgical populations at high risk of developing DVT

| Surgical population | Authors | Prophylactic modalities | Diagnostic methods | Results |
|---|---|---|---|---|
| Orthopaedic: Total Knee Replacement | Hull et al, 1979 | B-IPC vs C | FUT Venography | ns |
| Miscellaneous | Hartman et al, 1982 | T-IPC vs C | FUT Doppler X(V) | ns |
| Total Hip Arthroplasty | Gallus et al, 1983 | B-IPC vs C | Venography | ns |
| Total Hip Arthroplasty | Balley et al, 1990 | T-IPC (GEC) vs C | Venography | ns |
| Total Hip Arthroplasty | Hull et al, 1990 | T-IPC vs C | FUT IPG Venography | ns |
| Total Hip Arthroplasty | Paiement et al, 1990 | IPC vs LDW | FUT Venography | ns |
| Unilateral Total Knee Replacement | Haas et al, 1990 | T-IPC vs ASA | Venography | ns |
| Bilateral Total Knee Replacement | Haas et al, 1990 | T-IPC vs ASA | Venography | ns |
| Open Urological | Coe et al, 1978 | B-IPC vs C | FUT | ns |
| Cancer | Hansberry et al, 1991 | IPC vs HDHE | SPT | ns |
| Gynaecological cancer | Clarke-P. et al, 1984 | B-IPC vs C | FUT IPC X(V) | ns |
| General (cancer) | Smith et al, 1978 | B-IPC vs Dex 70 | FUT | ns |

B: Below knee device   T: Thigh length device   GEC: This method was also fitted
C: Control   LDW: Low dose warfarin   ASA: Acetylsalicylic acid
HDHE: Heparin-Dihydroergotamine   FUT: Fibrinogen uptake test
IPG: Impedance plethysmography   X(V): Venography confirms if the other tests were positive
ss: There was a statistically significant difference   ns: There was no statistically significant difference
Note: The number of patients is specified in Tables 2 and 3, except for Smith et al, 1978 who studied 28 patients at high risk in the dextran group and 20 in the IPC group (%DVT Dext 60 = 32 vs ICP = 45), and Haas et al, 1990, who analysed 32 patients in ASA group vs 35 in the IPC group (%DVT : ASA = 68% vs IPC = 48%)

was compared with ASA (Haas et al, 1990), IPC was superior to ASA in both uni- and bilateral knee arthroplasty (Tables 20.3, 20.4), as diagnosed by venography, although the only statistically significant difference was in the unilateral operation. In addition, IPC was only considered effective on the ipsilateral leg in the unilateral procedure, yet it was not effective on the operated leg, nor was it effective in bilateral knee arthroplasty. These results are in disagreement with those reported previously by McKenna et al (1980) in patients undergoing unilateral total knee replacement. T-IPC was as effective as dosages of ASA equal to 3.9 g per day, and the two methods were significantly more effective than much lower dosages of ASA (0.995 g/day), as assessed by venography. In addition, proximal DVT was abolished by using both high doses of ASA and T-IPC, while in patients taking low doses of ASA, 43 percent of the total number of DVT were proximal. The difference is also significant.

In open oncologic urological procedures, heparin plus dihydroergotamine (HDHE) was superior to IPC, although without a statistically significant difference, as measured by an objective diagnostic test (Hansberry et al, 1991). In general surgery indicated because of cancer, dextran-70 was superior to IPC, but there was not a statistically significant difference, and the diagnostic method appears to be insufficient (Table 20.4). In total hip replacement, both methods were only considered effective for distal DVT, as assessed by venography (Paiement et al, 1990). Finally, IPC has been demonstrated to be equal or more effective than low-dose heparin in several non-orthopaedic types of surgery, using different non-invasive diagnostic methods (Table 20.3).

**Limitations**
Major orthopaedic surgical procedures could be a limitation for employing IPC, and both the type of surgery and the risk of bleeding in an individual patient appear to be the main factors for selecting the prophylactic methods to be used (Hull and Raskob, 1986). To date, the data are very controversial. Moreover, there is a need to reach a consensus on which pharmacological method is more suitable for orthopaedic populations (Boniske, 1991). In any case, there is an agreement that in patients at high risk of developing DVT, as in total hip replacement, a combined prophylaxis might be essential (Consensus Conference, 1986; Coon et al, 1987; Goldhaber, 1988; Moser, 1990; Caprini et al, 1991). On the other hand, it is surprising to know that at present, in many institutions, only two-thirds of patients at high risk of developing DVT receive prophylaxis, as recently surveyed by Wheeler and Anderson (1991).

Confirmed or suspected DVT is another limitation for applying IPC. Because such a thrombus could become detached and cause pulmonary embolism, ruling out DVT before using IPC is recommended, especially in patients with prior immobilisation (Muhe, 1984; Moser, 1990). For the same reason, diagnostic screening should be performed prior to reapplying compression if it had to be discontinued during some time for any cause.

IPC should not be applied to patients with significant leg oedema secondary to severe congestive heart failure. In some of these patients, the mobilisation of a considerable volume of fluid from the extracellular to the intravascular compartment might worsen the patient's heart failure. In our experience, compression should be avoided in patients with cellulitis of the legs.

As mentioned above, patients whose fibrinolytic system does not respond to the stimulation would be considered a group in which the use of IPC could be supplemented with a pharmacologic regimen (Tarnay et al, 1980; Salzman et al, 1987; Summaria et al, 1988).

The availability of IPC in each hospital could be another limitation, although it is considered a non-expensive method. Its cost ranges from US$10-$20 per day (Clayton and Thompson, 1987; Bartle, 1988). In the analysis carried out by Oster et al (1987), IPC was a very cost-effective prophylactic method in orthopaedic surgery.

**Table 20.5**
Indications of IPC firmly established by compiling the available experience

---

Groups at high risk of bleeding complications
* With haemostatic defects — proved or strongly suspected
* Neurological patients — operated and non-operated
* Operations involving major dissection
    — Extensive pelvic surgery
    — Open urological operations

Contraindications for pharmacological modalities
* General surgical patients at moderate risk of DVT
* Gynaecological surgery at moderate and high risk of DVT
* Traumatic patients
    — Hip fracture in elderly patients
    — Severe musculoskeletal trauma in young people

---

# Final remarks

Apart from the generally accepted role of IPC in patients at high risk of clinically significant bleeding complications, there are currently other indications for the prophylactic use of this modality (Table 20.5).

The value of IPC in the prevention of pulmonary embolism needs to be further documented with appropriate endpoints. Does IPC prevent fatal pulmonary embolism? More studies are required to evaluate the role of IPC in preventing proximal deep vein thrombosis. Finally, the advantages of combining pharmacological agents and IPC should be definitely explored.

# References

Allenby F, Boardman L, Pflug JJ, Calnan J. Effects of external pneumatic intermittent compression on fibrinolysis in man. Lancet 2:1412, 1973

Balley JP, Kruger MP, Solano FX, Zajko AB, Rubash HE. A prospective randomised trial of sequential compression devices versus low dose warfarin for deep venous thrombosis prophylaxis in total hip arthroplasty (Abs) Proceeding of the 57th Annual Meeting of the Am Acad Orthop Surg, 1990

Bartle E. Pneumatic compression stockings to prevent deep vein thrombosis. Am J Surg 156:16, 1988

Black PMcL, Baker MF and Snook CP. Experience with external pneumatic calf compression in neurology and neurosurgery. Neurosurgery 18:440, 1986

Blackshear WM, Prescott C, LePain F, Benoit S, Dickstein R, Seifert B. Influence of sequential pneumatic compression on postoperative venous function. J Vasc Surg 5:432, 1987

Boniske ChH. Joint replacement surgery. N Engl J Med 324, 1367, 1991

Borow M, Goldson HJ. Postoperative venous thrombosis. Evaluation of five methods of treatment. Am J Surg 141:245, 1981

Borow M, Goldson HJ. Prevention of postoperative deep vein thrombosis and pulmonary emboli with combined modalities. The American Surgeon 49:599, 1983

Bynke O, Hillman J, Lassvik C. Does perioperative external pneumatic leg muscle compression prevent postoperative venous thrombosis in neurosurgery? Acta Neurochir 88:46, 1987

Caprini JA, Arcelus JI, Traverso CI, Hasty JH. Low molecular weight heparins and external pneumatic compression as options for venous thromboembolism prophylaxis. A surgeon's perspective. Semin Thromb Hemost 17:356, 1991

Caprini JA, Chucker JL, Zuckerman L, Vagher JP, Franck CA, Cullen JE. Thrombosis prophylaxis using external compression. Surg Gynecol Obstet 156:599, 1983

Caprini JC, Kudrna JC, Mitchell AS. Thrombosis prophylaxis in total hip arthroplasty patients using a combination of physical methods (Abs) Thromb Haemost 58:385, 1987

Caprini JA, Natanson RA. Postoperative deep vein thrombosis: Current clinical considerations. Sem Thromb Haemostas 15:8, 1989

Clagett GP, Reisch JS. Prevention of venous thromboembolism in general surgical patients. Ann Surg 208:227, 1988

Clark WB, McGregor AB, Prescott RJ, Ruckley CV. Pneumatic compression on the calf and postoperative deep vein thrombosis. Lancet 2:5, 1974

Clarke-Pearson D, Synan IS, Hinshaw WM, Coleman RE, Creasman WT. Prevention of postoperative venous thromboembolism by external pneumatic calf compression in patients with gynecologic malignancy. Surg Gynecol Obstet 63:92, 1984

Clayton ML, Thompson TR. Activity, air boots, and aspirin as thromboembolism prophylaxis in knee arthroplasty. A multiple regimen approach. Orthopaedics 10:1525, 1987

Coe NP, Collins REC, Klein LA, Bettmann MA, Skillman JJ, Shapiro RM, Salzman EW. Prevention of deep vein thrombosis in urological patients: a controlled, randomised trial of low dose heparin and external pneumatic compression boots. Surgery 83:230, 1978

Colditz GA, Tuden RL, Oster G. Rates of venous thrombosis after general surgery: combined results of randomised clinical trials. Lancet 2:143, 1986

Coleridge-Smith PD, Hasty J, Scurr JH. Venous stasis and vein lumen changes during surgery. Br J Surg 77:1055, 1990

Comerota AJ, Stewart GJ, Alburger PD, Smalley K, White JV. Operative venodilation: A previously unsuspected factor in the cause of postoperative deep vein thrombosis. Surgery 106:301, 1989

Comerota AJ, Stewart GJ, White JV. Combined dihydroergotamine and heparin prophylaxis of postoperative deep vein thrombosis: proposed mechanism of action. Am J Surg 150:39, 1985

Coon WW, Hirsh J, Rubin LJ. Preventing deep venous thrombosis. Patient Care 21:82, 1987

Editorial. Preventing venous thrombosis and pulmonary embolism. AFP 35:95, 1987

Frangos JA, McIntire LV, Ives CL. Flow effects on prostacyclin production by cultured human endothelial cells. Science 227:1477, 1985

Gallus A, Raman K, Darby T. Venous thrombosis after elective hip replacement — the influence of preventive intermittent calf compression and of surgical technique. Br J Surg 70:17, 1983

Goldhaber SZ. Venous thromboembolism: How to prevent a tragedy. Hosp Pract 23:164, 1988

Guyton DP, Khayat A, Schreiber H. Pneumatic compression stockings and prostaglandin synthesis — a pathway of fibrinolysis? Critical Care Medicine 13:266, 1985

Haas SB, Insall JN, Scuderi GR, Windsor RE, Ghelman B. Pneumatic sequential compression boots compared with aspirin prophylaxis of deep vein thrombosis after total knee arthroplasty. J Bone Joint Surg 72:27, 1990

Hansberry KL, Thompson IM Jr, Bauman J, Deppe S, Rodriguez FR. A prospective comparison of thromboembolic stockings, external pneumatic compression stockings and heparin sodium/dihydroergotamine mesylate for the prevention of thromboembolic complications in urological surgery. J Urol 145:1205, 1991

Harris WH, Athanasoulis CA, Waltman AC, Salzman EW. Prophylaxis of deep vein thrombosis after total hip replacement. Dextran and external pneumatic compression compared with 1.2 or 0.3 gram of aspirin daily. J Bone Joint Surg 67-A:57, 1985

Hartman JT, Pugh JL, Smith RD, Robertson WW, Yost RP, Janssen HF. Cyclic sequential compression of the lower limb in prevention of deep venous thrombosis. J Bone Joint Surg 64:1059, 1982

Hills N, Pflug J, Jeyesingh K. Prevention of deep vein thrombosis in intermittent pneumatic compression of calf. Br Med J 1:131, 1972

Holford CP. Graded compression for preventing deep venous thrombosis. Br Med J 2:969, 1976

Houghton GR, Papadakis EG, Rizza CR. Changes in blood coagulation during total hip replacement. Lancet 1:1336, 1978

Hull RD, Delmore TJ, Hirsh H et al. Effectiveness of intermittent pulsatile elastic stockings for the prevention of calf and thigh vein thrombosis in patients undergoing elective knee surgery. Thromb Res 16:367, 1979

Hull RD, Raskob GE. Prophylaxis of venous thromboembolic disease following hip and knee surgery. J Bone Joint Surg 68-A:146, 1986

Hull RD, Raskob GE, Gent M et al. Effectiveness of intermittent pneumatic leg compression for preventing deep vein thrombosis after total hip replacement. JAMA 263:2313, 1990

Inada K, Koike S, Shirai N, Matsumoto K, Hirose M. Effects of intermittent pneumatic compression for prevention of postoperative deep venous thrombosis with special reference to fibrinolytic activity. Am J Surg 155:602, 1988

Kamn RD. Bioengineering studies of periodic external compression as prophylaxis against deep vein thrombosis — I: Numerical studies. J Biochem Eng 104:87, 1982

Kierkegaard A, Norgren L, Thilen U. Venous function of the leg in patients with acute myocardial infarction. Phlebology 4:83, 1989

Knight MLN, Dawson R. Effect of intermittent compression of the arms on deep venous thrombosis in the legs. Lancet 2:1265, 1976

Krolick MA, Cintron GB. Spinal epidural haematoma causing cord compression after tissue plasminogen activator and heparin therapy. Southern Med J 84:670, 1991

Lynch JA, Baker PL, Polly RE et al. Mechanical measures in the prophylaxis of postoperative thromboembolism in total knee arthroplasty. Cli Orthop & Rel Res 260:24, 1990

Lyne E. Prophylaxis for venous thromboembolism in total hip arthroplasty (letter). Orthopedics 14:226, 1991

McKenna R, Galante J, Bachmann F, Wallace DL, Kaushal SP, Meredith P. Prevention of venous thromboembolism after total knee replacement by high dose aspirin or intermittent calf and thigh compression. Br Med J 280:514, 1980

Mittelman JS, Edwards WS, McDonald JB. Effectiveness of leg compression in preventing venous stasis. Am J Surg 144:611, 1982

Moser KM. Venous thromboembolism. Am Rev Resp Dis 141:235, 1990

Moskopp D, Popov-Cenic S. Perioperative prevention of thromboembolism in neurosurgery. Neurochirurgia 33:137, 1990

Muhe F. Intermittent sequential high pressure compression of the leg. A new method of preventing deep vein thrombosis. Am J Surg 147:781, 1984

National Institutes of Health: Consensus Conference on prevention of venous thrombosis and pulmonary embolism. JAMA 256:744, 1986

Nicolaides AN, Fernandes e Fernandes J, Pollock AV. Intermittent sequential pneumatic compression of the legs in the prevention of venous stasis and postoperative deep venous thrombosis. Surgery 87:69, 1980

Nicolaides AN, Irving D. Clinical factors and the risk of deep venous thrombosis. In: Nicolaides AN (ed), Thromboembolism: Aetiology, advances in prevention and management, MTP, Lancaster, 193, 1975

Nicolaides AN, Miles C, Hoare M, Jury P, Helmis E, Venniker R. Intermittent sequential pneumatic compression of the legs and thromboembolism-deterrent stockings in the prevention of postoperative deep venous thrombosis. Surgery 94:21, 1983

Nolan TR. Prevention of postoperative thrombophlebitis. South Med J 81:937, 1988

Olson DA, Kamn RD, Shapiro AH. Bioengineering studies of periodic external compression as prophylaxis against deep vein thrombosis — part II: Experimental studies on a stimulated leg. J Biomech Eng 104:96, 1982

O'Meara PM. Prophylaxis for venous thromboembolism in total hip arthroplasty (reply). Orthopaedics 14:227, 1991

Oster G, Tuden RL, Colditz GA. A cost-effectiveness analysis of prophylaxis against deep-vein thrombosis in major orthopedic surgery. JAMA 257:203, 1987

Paiement GD, Desautels C. Deep vein thrombosis: Prophylaxis, diagnosis and treatment — lessons from orthopedic studies. Clin Cardiol 13:19, 1990

Paiement GD, Wessinger SJ, Waltman AC, Harris WH. Low dose warfarin versus external pneumatic compression against venous thromboembolism following total hip replacement. J Arthroplasty 2:23, 1987

Roberts VC, Cotton LT. Prevention of postoperative deep vein thrombosis in patients with malignant disease. Br J Surg 1:358, 1974

Roberts VC, Sabri S, Beely AH, Cotton LT. The effect of intermittently applied external pressure on the haemodynamics of the lower limb in man. Br J Surg 59:223, 1972

Sabri S, Roberts VC, Cotton LT. Effects of externally applied pressure on the haemodynamics of the lower limb. Br Med J 3:503, 1971

Salzman EW, Davis GC. Prophylaxis of venous thromboembolism. Ann Surg 191:207, 1980

Salzman EW, McManama GP, Shapiro AH et al. Effect of optimisation of hemodynamics on fibrinolytic activity and antithrombotic efficacy of external pneumatic calf compression. Ann Surg 206:636, 1987

Salzman EW, Ploetz J, Bettmann M, Skillman J, Klein L. Intraoperative external pneumatic calf compression to afford long term prophylaxis against deep vein thrombosis in urological patients. Surgery 87:239, 1980

Scurr JH, Coleridge-Smith PD, Hasty JH. Regimen for improved effectiveness of intermittent pneumatic compression in deep venous thrombosis prophylaxis. Surgery 102:816, 1987

Sigel B, Edelstein AL, Felix WR. Compression of the deep venous system of the lower leg during inactive recumbency. Arch Surg 106:38, 1973

Skillman JJ, Collins REC, Coe NP et al. Prevention of deep vein thrombosis in neurosurgical patients: A controlled randomised trial of external pneumatic compression boots. Surgery 83:354, 1978

Smith RC, Elton RA, Orr JD et al. Dextran and intermittent pneumatic compression in prevention of postoperative deep vein thrombosis: Multiunit trial. Br Med J 1:952, 1978

Summaria L, Caprini JA, McMillan R et al. Relationship between postsurgical fibrinolytic parameters and deep vein thrombosis in surgical patients treated with compression devices. Am Surg 54:156, 1988

Summaria L, Sandesara J, Vagher JP. Coagulation, fibrinolytic and antithrombin III profiles monitored in surgical patients treated with sequential compression devices. Thromb Haemost 54:98, 1985

Tarnay TJ, Rohr PR, Davidson AG, Stevenson MM, Byars EF, Hopkins GR. Pneumatic calf compression, fibrinolysis and the prevention of deep venous thrombosis. Surgery 88:489, 1980

Turpie AGG, Delmore T, Hirsh J, Hull R, Genton E, Hiscoe C, Gent M. Prevention of venous thrombosis by intermittent sequential calf compression in patients with intracranial disease. Thromb Res 15:611, 1979

Turpie AGG, Gallus AS, Beattie WS, Hirsh J. Prevention of venous thrombosis in patients with intracranial disease by intermittent pneumatic compression of the calf. Neurology 27:435, 1977

Turpie AGG, Hirsch J, Gent M, Julian D, Johnson J. Prevention of deep vein thrombosis in potential neurosurgical patients. A randomised trial comparing graduated compression stockings alone or graduated compression stockings plus intermittent pneumatic compression with control. Arch Intern Med 149:679, 1989

Von Schroeder HP, Coutts RD, Billings E, Mai MT, Aratow M. The changes in intramuscular pressure and femoral vein flow with continuous passive motion, pneumatic compressive stocking, and leg manipulations. Clin Orthop & Related Res 266:218, 1991

Weitz J, Michelson J, Gold K. Effects of intermittent calf compression on postoperative thrombin and plasmin action. Thromb Hamost 54:98, 1985

Wheeler HB, Anderson FA Jr. Prophylaxis against venous thromboembolism in surgical patients. Am J Surg 161:507, 1991

Wilson NV, Das SK, Maurice H, Smibert G, Thomas EM, Kakkar V. Thrombosis prophylaxis in total knee replacement. A new mechanical device. XIII Congress of Thrombosis and Haemostasis, Amsterdam, The Netherlands, 1991

Woolson ST, Watt JM. Intermittent pneumatic compression to prevent proximal deep venous thrombosis during and after total hip replacement. A prospective, randomised study of compression alone, compression and aspirin, and compression and low dose warfarin. J Bone Joint Surg 73-A:507, 1991

CHAPTER 21

# Combined methods

Andrew N Nicolaides

## Introduction

In the early 1970s it was realised that the hypercoagulable state produced by tissue trauma and venous stasis were the most important factors responsible for the initiation of deep vein thrombosis (DVT). Thrombosis is the result of activated coagulation factors in an area of stasis. Activation of coagulation factors or stasis on their own do not produce thrombosis (Wessler and Yin, 1968). In the 1980s, it became recognised that the endothelium also plays an important role. During anaesthesia there is progressive dilatation of the venous wall, due to relaxation of the smooth muscle (Chapter 3). This leads to tearing of the endothelium and exposure of collagen to the blood constituents. It is now believed that, in the majority of surgical patients, all three factors play an important role, and in high risk groups, a combination of methods, which act on more than one of these factors (hypercoagulable state, stasis and endothelial damage), is more effective than one prophylactic modality on its own.

Prophylaxis is based on the concept that prevention of DVT will, in the majority of patients, prevent pulmonary embolism (PE) and the post-thrombotic syndrome (PTS). This has been the rationale for the extensive clinical trials to determine the risk of DVT and PE and to establish the efficacy of various prophylactic methods.

In general surgical patients the overall incidence of post-operative DVT is 27% (Colditz et al, 1986). The majority of these thrombi start in the calf (Nicolaides et al, 1972). In approximately 80% of patients the thrombosis remains confined to the calf and only in 20% the thrombus propagates into the popliteal, femoral and iliac veins (Kakkar et al, 1969). Whenever there is a major clinical PE, the thrombus extends above the knee. Patients with thrombosis confined to the calf do not develop major clinical PE. In fact, the most clinically significant PE originate in the most proximal deep veins and, in turn, they are often extensions of thrombi which originated in the calf.

Graduated elastic compression (GEC), intermittent pneumatic compression (IPC) and low dose heparin (LDH) are three established methods that are effective in reducing

**Table 21.1**
Overall reduction in postoperative DVT by different prophylactic methods in general surgical and gynaecological patients

| Method | Number of randomised controlled trials using objective criteria for DVT | Reduction in DVT |
| --- | --- | --- |
| Graduated elastic compression (Table 21.3) | 9 | 63% |
| Intermittent pneumatic compression (Table 21.4) | 7 | 73% |
| Low dose Heparin (Collins et al, 1988) | 30 | 67% |

**Table 21.2**
Overall reduction in postoperative DVT by different prophylactic methods in orthopaedic surgery

| Method | Number of studies | Reduction in DVT |
| --- | --- | --- |
| Graduated elastic compression (Ishak & Morley, 1981) | 1 | 63% |
| Intermittent pneumatic compression (Table 21.5) | 3 | 90% |
| Low dose Heparin (Collins et al, 1988) | 10 hip fractures<br>10 elective hip replacement | 68% |

**Table 21.3**
The effect of graduated elastic compression on the incidence of DVT in general surgical and gynaecological patients

| Author | Control group n | Control group DVT | Treatment group n | Treatment group DVT |
| --- | --- | --- | --- | --- |
| Tsapogas et al, 1971 | 44 | 6 (14%) | 51 | 2 (4%) |
| Holford, 1976 | 47 | 23 (49%) | 48 | 11 (23%) |
| Scurr et al, 1977 (alternate leg) | 70 | 26 (37%) | 70 | 8 (11%) |
| Borow et al, 1981 | 89 | 32 (36%) | 91 | 14 (15%) |
| Inada et al, 1983 | 103 | 37 (36%) | 97 | 15 (15%) |
| Turner et al, 1984 | 92 | 4 (4.3%) | 104 | 0 |
| Turpie et al, 1989 | 81 | 16 (20%) | 80 | 7 (8.8%) |
| Total | 526 | 144 (27%) | 541 | 57 (10.25) |
| 95% CI |  | (23.5% - 31.2%) |  | (7.9% - 13.1%)* |

(Overall reduction of DVT: 61%)   *$p<0.05$

## Table 21.4
The effect of intermittent sequential compression on the incidence of DVT in general surgical and gynaecological patients

| Author | Control group n | DVT | Treatment group n | DVT |
|---|---|---|---|---|
| Sabri et al, 1971 | 39 | 12 (31%) | 39 | 2 (5%) |
| Hills et al, 1972 | 70 | 23 (33%) | 70 | 7 (10%) |
| Roberts & Cotton, 1974 | 104 | 27 (27%) | 94 | 6 (6%) |
| Clark et al, 1974 | 36 | 7 (19%) | 36 | 0 |
| Coe et al, 1978 (Urological) | 24 | 6 (25%) | 29 | 2 (7%) |
| Clarke-Pearson et al, 1984 | 52 | 18 (35%) | 55 | 7 (13%) |
| Total | 325 | 93 (29%) | 323 | 24 (7.4%) |
| 95% CI | | (23.7% - 33.5%) | | (4.6% - 10.3%)* |

(Overall reduction of DVT: 73%)  *$p<0.05$

postoperative DVT in both patients having abdominal and orthopaedic operations (Tables 21.1-21.5). However, they do not abolish DVT. There is a high risk resistant group of patients (10-20%) particularly in orthopaedic surgery that develops DVT despite prophylaxis with one of these methods. One of the questions posed in the early 1970s has been whether a combination of methods that act on different aspects of Virchow's triad would be more effective than each individual method used on its own.

The aim of this chapter is to summarise the studies that have attempted to answer the above question and indicate the efficacy and place of prophylactic methods used in combination.

## Table 21.5
The effect of intermittent sequential compression on the incidence of DVT in patients having orthopaedic operations

| Author | Control group n | DVT | Treatment group n | DVT |
|---|---|---|---|---|
| Hull et al, 1979 (elective knee) | 29 | 19 (66%) | 32 | 2 (6%) |
| McKenna et al, 1980 (elective knee) | 12 | 9 (75%) | 10 | 1 (10%) |
| Hartman et al, 1982 (hip operations) | 52 | 10 (19%) | 52 | 1 (2%) |
| Total | 93 | 38 (41%) | 94 | 4 (4.2%) |
| 95% CI | | (31.% - 51%) | | (0.2% - 8.3%)* |

(Overall reduction of DVT: 90%)  *$p<0.01$

**Table 21.6**
The effect of adding DHE to LDH on the incidence of DVT in patients having abdominal and pelvic operations

| Author | LDH n | LDH DVT | LDH + DHE n | LDH + DHE DVT |
|---|---|---|---|---|
| Kakkar et al, 1979 | 50 | 2 (4%) | 50 | 3 (6%) |
| Multicenter Trial, 1975 | 222 | 32 (14%) | 214 | 18 (8%) |
| Hohl et al, 1980 | 64 | 2 (3%) | 61 | 4 (7%) |
| Veth et al, 1985 | 114 | 14 (12%) | 115 | 10 (9%) |
| DiSerio and Sasahara, 1985 | 190 | 32 (17%) | 118 | 17 (9%) |
| Pedersen and Christiansen, 1983 | 50 | 9 (19%) | 50 | 6 (12%) |
| Brücke et al, 1983 | 86 | 26 (30%) | 91 | 13 (14%) |
| Total | 776 | 117 (15%) | 699 | 71 (10.2%) |
| 95% CI |  | (12.6% - 17.6%) |  | (7.9% - 12.4%)* |

(32% further reduction in DVT by the addition of DHE to LDH)   *$p<0.05$

## Combined prophylaxis

The addition of dihydroergotamine (DHE) to LDH produced a further reduction of 32% in patients having abdominal and pelvic operations (Table 21.6) and of 39% in patients having hip operations (Table 21.7).

In patients having general surgery the addition of GEC to LDH produced a further reduction of 73% (Table 21.8). The overall incidence of 16% in the LDH groups was reduced to 4.4% in the LDH and GEC groups.

The addition of GEC to IPC in a study involving 38 general surgical patients reduced the incidence of DVT from 9% (IPC alone) to 1% (Scurr et al, 1987). Finally, the addition

**Table 21.7**
The effect of adding DHE to LDH on the incidence of DVT in patients having hip operations

| Author | LDH n | LDH DVT | LDH + DHE n | LDH + DHE DVT |
|---|---|---|---|---|
| Schöndorf and Weber, 1980 (hip replacement) | 54 | 8 (14%) | 53 | 2 (4%) |
| Lahnborg, 1980 (fractured hip) | 70 | 15 (21%) | 71 | 12 (17%) |
| Total | 124 | 23 (18.5%) | 124 | 14 (11.2%) |
| 95% CI |  | (11.7% - 25.4%) |  | (5.7% - 16.8%)* |

(39% further reduction in DVT by the addition of DHE to LDH)   *Results not significant $p>0.05$

**Table 21.8**
The effect of adding GEC to LDH on the incidence of DVT

| Author | LDH n | DVT | LDH + GEC n | DVT |
|---|---|---|---|---|
| Torngren, 1980 (General surgery, alternate leg) | 98 | 12 (12%) | 98 | 4 (4%) |
| Willie-Jorgensen et al, 1990 (General Surgery) | 90 | 12 (13%) | 86 | 5 (6%) |
| Borow and Goldson, 1983 | 56 | 15 (27%) | 63 | 2 (3%) |
| Total | 244 | 39 (16%) | 247 | 11 (4.4%) |
| 95% CI | | (11.4% - 20.5) | (1.8% - 7.0%)* | |

(73% further reduction in DVT by the addition of GEC to LDH)   *$p<0.05$

of IPC to LDH in another study reduced the incidence of DVT from 27% to 1.5% (Borow and Goldson, 1983).

It appears that the combination of prophylactic methods is more effective than the use of each one on its own, particularly in high risk groups.

On the basis of the above, 480 consecutive patients having general surgery were classified into three groups according to risk: 163 as low risk (age 40-60 having minor operations), 250 as moderate risk (age 40-60 having major operations without additional risk factors and patients over 60 having any operation), and 67 as high risk (as in moderate risk but with the additional risk factors). GEC was the only method of prophylaxis used in the low risk group. GEC & LDH or GEC & SCD if extensive dissection was contemplated was used in the moderate risk group. All three methods were combined (GEC + LDH + SCD) in the high risk group. Patients in the moderate and high risk group were scanned with the fibrinogen uptake test. DVT occurred in 5 (2%) in the moderate risk group and 3 (4.5%) in the high risk group (Nicolaides, unpublished data). These results suggest that there is a place for combined methods in moderate and high risk groups in surgical practice.

# References

Allan et al. The use of graduated compression stockings in the prevention of postoperative deep vein thrombosis. Br J Surg 70:172, 1983

Borow M, Goldson H. Postoperative venous thrombosis: Evaluation of five methods of treatment. Am J Surg 141:245, 1981

Borow M, Goldson HJ. Prevention of postoperative deep venous thrombosis and pulmonary embolism with combined modalities. Am J Surg 49:599, 1983

Brücke P et al. Prophylaxis of postoperative thromboembolism: Low dose heparin plus dihydroergotamine. Thromb. Res 29:377, 1983

Clark WB, MacGregor AB, Prescott RJ, Ruckley CV. Pneumatic compression of the calf and postoperative deep vein thrombosis. Lancet ii:5, 1974

Coe et al. Prevention of deep vein thrombosis in urological patients: A controlled randomised trial of low-dose heparin and external pneumatic compression boots. Surgery 83:230, 1978

Colditz GA, Tuden RL, Oster G. Rates of venous thrombosis after general surgery: combined results of randomised clinical trials. Lancet ii:143, 1986

Collins R et al. Reduction in fatal pulmonary embolism and venous thrombosis by perioperative administration of subcutaneous heparin. N Engl J Med 318:1162, 1988

DiSeri EJ, Sasahara AA. United States trial of dihydroergotamine and heparin prophylaxis of deep vein thrombosis. Am J Surg 150:25, 1985

Hartman JT et al. Cyclic sequential compression of the lower limb in prevention of deep venous thrombosis. J Bone Joint Surg 64A:1059, 1982

Hills et al. Prevention of deep venous thrombosis by intermittent pneumatic compression of calf. Br Med J 1:131, 1972

Hohl et al. Dihydroergotamine and heparin or heparin alone for the prevention of postoperative thromboembolism in gynaecology. Arch Gynaecol 230:15, 1980

Holford CP. Graded compression for preventing deep venous thrombosis. Br Med J 2:969, 1976

Hull et al. Effectiveness of intermittent pulsatile elastic stockings for the prevention of calf and thigh vein thrombosis in patients undergoing knee surgery. Thromb Haemost 16:37, 1979

Inada et al. Postoperative deep venous thrombosis in Japan: Incidence and prophylaxis. Am J Surg 145:775, 1983

Ishak MA, Morley KD. Deep venous thrombosis after total hip arthroplasty: A prospective controlled study to determine the prophylactic effect of graded pressure stockings. Br J Surg 68:429, 1981

Kakkar VV, Howe CT, Flanc C, Clarke MB. Natural history of deep vein thrombosis. Lancet ii:230, 1969

Kakkar VV et al. Prophylaxis for postoperative deep vein thrombosis. Synergistic effect of heparin and dihydroergotamine. JAMA 241:39, 1979

Lahnborg G. Effect of low dose heparin and dihydroergotamine on frequency of postoperative deep vein thrombosis in patients undergoing post-traumatic hip surgery. Acta Chir Scand 146:319, 1980

McKenna et al. Prevention of venous thromboembolism after total knee replacement by high doses of aspirin or intermittent calf and thigh compression. Br Med J 66:514, 1980

Multicentre trial. Prevention of fatal postoperative pulmonary embolism by low doses of heparin. Lancet ii:45, 1975

Nicolaides AN, Kakkar VV, Field ES, Fish P. Venous stasis and deep vein thrombosis. Br J Surg 59:51, 1972

Pedersen B, Christiansen J. Thromboembolic prophylaxis with dihydroergotamine-heparin in abdominal surgery. Am J Surg 145:788, 1983

Roberts VC, Cotton LT. Prevention of postoperative deep vein thrombosis in patients with malignant disease. Br Med J. 1:358, 1974

Sabri S, Roberts VC, Cotton LT. Prevention of early postoperative deep vein thrombosis by intermittent compression of the leg during surgery. Br Med J 4:394, 1971

Schöndorf TH, Weber U. Prevention of deep vein thrombosis in orthopaedic surgery with the combination of low dose heparin plus either dihydroergotamine or dextran. Scand J Haematol 25:126, 1980

Scurr JH et al. The efficacy of graduated compression stockings in prevention of deep vein thrombosis. Br J Surg 64:371, 1977

Scurr JH et al. Regimen for improved effectiveness of intermittent pneumatic compression in deep venous thrombosis prophylaxis. Surgery 102:816, 1987

Torngren S. Low dose heparin and compression stockings in the prevention of postoperative deep venous thrombosis. Br J Surg 57:481, 1980

Tsapogas MJ et al. Postoperative venous thrombosis and the effectiveness of prophylactic measures. Arch Surg 103:561, 1971

Turner GM, Cole SE, Brooks JH. The efficacy of graduated compression stockings in the prevention of deep vein thrombosis after major gynaecological surgery. Br J Obstet Gyn 91:588, 1984

Turpie AG et al. Prevention of deep vein thrombosis in potential neurosurgical patients; A randomized trial comparing graduated compression stockings alone or graduated compression stockings plus intermittent pneumatic compression with control. Arch Intern Med 149:679, 1989

Veth G et al. Prevention of postoperative deep vein thrombosis by a combination of subcutaneous heparin with subcutaneous dihydroergotamine or oral sulphinpyrazone. Thromb Haemost. 54:570, 1985

Wessler S, Yin ET. On the mechanism of thrombosis. Prog Hemat 6:201, 1968

Willie-Jorgensen P, Thorup J, Fischer A, Holst-Christensen J, Flamsholt. Heparin with and without graded compression stockings in the prevention of thromboembolic complications of major abdominal surgery: A randomized trial. Br J Surg 72:577, 1985

Part III

# Prevention in Individual Patient Groups

CHAPTER 22

# Preoperative risk factors in the prediction of postoperative venous thromboembolism

Daan W Hommes   Harry R Büller
Desiderius PM Brandjes   Jan W ten Cate

## Introduction

Many studies have demonstrated that surgical patients are at risk of developing venous thromboembolism in the postoperative phase. The risk attributable to surgery is associated with the magnitude and duration of the surgical procedure and with the immobilisation following surgery. Other clinical circumstances contributing to the risk of thromboembolism, include age, obesity, malignancy and other underlying diseases.

The incidence of postoperative deep vein thrombosis (DVT) varies considerably according to the type of surgery (Hampson et al, 1974; Hume et al, 1976; Todd et al, 1976; Bergqvist, 1983; Becker, 1986; Collins et al, 1988). DVT develops in approximately 20-30% of patients after major abdominal surgery without anticoagulant prophylaxis, while for urological and gynaecological patients this risk is 10-35% and 5-35%, respectively. Following major elective orthopaedic surgery, more than 50% of the unprotected patients will develop deep vein thrombosis. In most studies, those thromboses which are detected by the fibrinogen uptake test (FUT), remain subclinical and most thrombi resolve completely when mobility is restored. Occasionally, some thrombi do produce permanent valvular damage and chronic venous insufficiency, or cause nonfatal pulmonary embolism (Kakkar et al, 1969). Excluding major orthopaedic and extensive pelvic surgery, both with a high prevalence of postoperative thrombosis, only a small proportion of general surgery patients will develop postoperative venous thrombosis. At present, the majority of patients undergoing surgery, receive prophylactic antithrombotic therapy to protect the small proportion of patients that will actually develop venous thromboembolism which in particular applies to patients undergoing general surgery. To increase the safety and cost-effectiveness of thrombosis prophylaxis, attention has been focused on the pre-surgical identification of the patient at risk of developing postoperative venous thromboembolism. If this could be achieved, selective prophylaxis would become feasible and the morbidity and mortality from thromboembolic disease could be prevented in that proportion of patients who really are in need of prophylaxis. As a further consequence, morbidity due to anticoagulant induced haemorrhagic complications could be prevented in patients receiving prophylaxis unnecessarily.

Over the last decade, considerable efforts have been undertaken to investigate the predictive value of various patient characteristics: coagulation and fibrinolytic parameters in order to identify the population requiring prophylaxis. Mathematical formulae were computed, utilising the risk factors derived from group comparative studies (Kakkar et al, 1970; Clayton et al, 1976; Rokoczi et al, 1978; Low et al, 1982; Sue Ling et al, 1986). These formulae (risk factor indices) were, however, constructed retrospectively and therefore prospective studies evaluating the clinical validity of these indices in surgical patients were undertaken (Clayton et al, 1976; Lowe et al, 1982; Sue Ling et al, 1986).

In this chapter we will discuss each of these items separately, thereby actualising our previously published review (Brandjes et al, 1990).

## Risk factors

Group comparison type of investigations have revealed risk factors for postoperative thrombosis from the patient's history, from the findings at physical examination and from blood coagulation assays. Kakkar and colleagues (1970) studied a group of 203 consecutive patients undergoing elective surgery. The incidence of DVT, using the fibrinogen uptake test (FUT), was 30.5%. A significant higher incidence of DVT was found in patients aged over sixty, and in obese patients. However, the most important risk factor was a history of previous DVT (68% compared to 26% of patients without such a history). Less important risk factors were varicose veins, type of operation and the presence of malignant disease.

## Coagulation and fibrinolysis tests

Blood tests have been under investigation for almost 20 years in an attempt to identify a patient population at higher risk of developing postoperative thromboembolism. The aim was to select a test allowing to detect coagulation and/or fibrinolysis changes at an early stage. A major prerequisite of such a test is a high sensitivity and specificity in order to be able to screen patient populations.

In 1972, Becker investigated the relation of platelet adhesiveness and the incidence of postoperative DVT (Becker, 1986). A total of 100 patients, undergoing surgery, were studied of whom 22% developed DVT as detected by venography or FUT. Pre-operative platelet adhesiveness measurements were of no predictive value; on the other hand, postoperative platelet adhesiveness measurements were correlated with a higher incidence of postoperative DVT. However, this test lacked the sensitivity and specificity to be applied as a screening method for the prediction of postoperative DVT (positive predictive value (PPV) = 40%; negative predictive value (NPV) = 83%).

Gallus and colleagues were the first to detect an association between pre- and postoperative coagulation test results and the occurrence of postoperative DVT (Gallus et al, 1973).

In 73 patients undergoing major elective surgery, the FUT revealed postoperative DVT in 37% of the patients. In this proportion of patients, statistically significant shorter activated partial thromboplastin times and higher fibrin degradation products (FDP) were found before and immediately after operation.

The assay of thrombin-antithrombin III complex (TAT) levels in plasma has subsequently been suggested as a sensitive parameter for the detection of thrombotic events (Hoek et al, 1989; Venous Thrombosis Group, 1989; Jorgensen et al, 1990; De Prost et al, 1990) and was applied in several studies to assess its predictive power for postoperative DVT. In 48 patients undergoing total hip arthroplasty, significantly higher TAT levels were found before operation in patients with postoperative DVT compared with patients without DVT, suggesting that preoperative plasma TAT levels may represent a valuable predictive marker for postoperative DVT (PPV = 18.5%; NPV = 100% for a cutoff point of 2.9 ng/ml) (Jorgensen et al, 1990). These findings were, however, not confirmed by Hoek and colleagues (1989), who set out to investigate the clinical utility of pre-operative TAT complex measurements in the prediction of postoperative DVT (revealed by venography which was performed on all patients). On the contrary, in 196 consecutive patients who underwent elective total hip surgery, pre-operative TAT plasma levels were similar in patients with and without thrombosis. In this study, patients were randomised to receive either low molecular weight heparin or placebo, as prophylaxis for the development of postoperative DVT. The investigators used ROC curve analysis at days one and four in the placebo-treated patients to identify those with enhanced risk for DVT. However, their analysis revealed no satisfactory discriminitive power for the diagnosis of DVT at any of the studied cut-off values for TAT complex. Further evidence for the limited value of TAT levels as a valid screening method, came from the study by the Venous Thrombosis Group (1989) in 64 patients undergoing total hip surgery, and from a study in 11 total knee replacement patients (De Prost et al, 1990) (Table 22.1).

The preoperative value of D-Dimer, a cleavage product specific for fibrin, as a predictor of postoperative DVT was investigated in subsequent studies (Haugh et al, 1988; De Prost et al, 1990; Jorgensen et al, 1990; Olt et al, 1990). In the study by Olt et al (1990), the incidence of postoperative DVT in the 89 study patients was 7%, none of whom had preoperative abnormal plasma levels of fragment D-dimer (PPV = 0%; NPV = 93%). Moreover, increased preoperative D-dimer levels were noted in patients with cancer, none of whom had a positive FUT. The limited significance of D-dimer as a valid screening procedure was confirmed in 18 patients undergoing elective abdominal surgery (Haugh et al, 1990), in 11 patients undergoing total knee replacement (De Prost et al, 1990) and in 48 patients undergoing total hip arthroplasty (Jorgensen et al, 1990). A significant rise in D-dimer levels immediately after operation is observed in these studies with no apparent difference between patients with and without postoperative DVT.

Increased plasma levels of plasminogen activator inhibitor (PAI) have also been associated with the development of postoperative DVT, in particular after total hip replacement surgery (Paramo et al, 1985; Rocha et al, 1988; Grimaudo et al, 1989; Sorensen et al, 1990a). Three investigations, involving a total number of 274 patients undergoing total hip surgery, showed that patients with postoperative DVT had significantly higher PAI plasma levels compared to those patients without DVT. However, Sorensen and colleagues (1990) could not confirm these findings in a similar study comprising 114 patients, who were randomised to receive either heparin or Dextran as prophylaxis. These authors were unable to show any significant differences of either PAI or tissue plasminogen activator antigen

**Table 22.1**
Results of the preoperative coagulation and fibrinolytic tests, i.e., D-dimer, thrombin antithrombin III complex (TAT), fibrinogen degradation products (FDP), plasminogen activator inhibitor (PAI), tissue plasminogen activator (tPA), fibrin monomers (FM) and euglobulin lysis time (ELT), in the prediction of postoperative thrombosis.

| Investigator | Type of surgery | Patients n postoperative thromboembolism (%) | Preoperative test | Preoperative differences between patients with and without postoperative DVT |
|---|---|---|---|---|
| Macintyre et al, 1976 | Major abdominal | 23 7 (30%) | ELT | No difference |
| Mellbring et al, 1985 | Major abdominal | 50 13 (26%) | tPA | No difference |
| Paramo et al, 1985 | Total hip replacement | 60 13 (22%) | PAI tPA ELT | Significant difference No difference No difference |
| Kluft et al, 1986 | Major abdominal | 24 9 (38%) | tPA | No difference |
| Sue Ling et al, 1987 | Major abdominal | 128 37 (29%) | tPA ELT | No difference No difference |
| Rocha et al, 1988 | Total hip replacement | 111 16 (14%) | tPA PAI FDP FM | Significant difference Significant difference Significant difference No difference |
| Hauch et al, 1988 | Major abdominal | 18 1 (6%) | D-Dimer | No difference |
| Grimaudo, 1989 | Total hip replacement | 103 16 (16%) | PAI | Significant difference |
| Hoek et al, 1989 | Elective total hip replacement | 196 71 (36%) | TAT | No difference |
| Jorgensen et al, 1990 | Total hip arthroplasty | 48 5 (10%) | D-dimer TAT FDP | Significant difference Significant difference No difference |
| Sorensen et al, 1990 | Total hip replacement | 40 22 (55%) | tPA tPA-antigen | Significant difference No difference |
| Sorensen et al, 1990a | Total hip replacement | 107 22 (21%) | tPA PAI | No difference No difference |
| Olt et al, 1990 | Gynaecologic oncologic | 89 6 (7%) | D-dimer | No difference |
| De Prost et al, 1990 | Total knee replacement | 11 6 (55%) | D-dimer TAT | No difference No difference |

(tPA) levels, before as well as after operation, between patients with and without postoperative DVT.

As can be appreciated from table 22.1, euglobulin lysis time (ELT), fibrin monomers (FM) or tPA, did not prove to have predictive power for postoperative DVT. The data presented in the studies discussed herein, did not allow for further analysis of predictive values for the development of DVT.

## Prognostic indices

In order to achieve selective prophylaxis, several attempts have been undertaken to identify high risk patients before surgery by means of predictive indices. These risk factor indices were developed by combining preoperative data on the patient's history, physical examination and coagulation or fibrinolysis test results. Subsequently, the predictive power of these indices for postoperative deep vein thrombosis has been investigated retrospectively.

The studies of Clayton et al (1976), Lowe et al (1982), and Sue Ling et al (1986) were followed by investigations in which their indices were also evaluted prospectively. Clayton et al (1976) investigated 124 patients undergoing gynaecological surgery. The thrombosis incidence was 16% as assessed by leg scanning followed by venography in all patients with a positive FUT. They concluded that, of all the preoperatively collected clinical and laboratory data, the euglobulin clot lysis test result expressed in minutes (a) was the best predictor for postoperative thrombosis. Other variables that added to the prediction power, as identified by a stepwide logistic discriminant analysis were (b) age, (c) presence of varicose veins, (d) FDP levels, and (e) weight:height ratio. The Clayton risk factor formula is as follows:

$$I = 11.3 + 0.0090a + 0.22d + 0.085b + 0.043e + 2.19c$$

In order to use a risk factor index (I) to decide whether a patient should receive thrombosis prophylaxis, an index which correctly identifies all patients with thrombosis would be sufficient. Therefore, the original Clayton data were reanalysed and it was calculated that, with an index of -5, all patients with DVT were correctly identified. However, at this cutoff point of -5, 77 patients who did not develop post-operative DVT were also included. The total number of patients without DVT was 104. This indicates that using the Clayton index with a cutoff point of -5, prophylaxis could be safely withheld in 27 of the 124 gynaecological surgery patients, which is equal to 21% of the total patient group.

Lowe et al (1982) developed an index from a group of 63 patients undergoing major abdominal surgery. The thrombosis incidence, as assessed by leg scanning, was 33%. In this study they discarded all the pre-operatively collected laboratory data, because of their low predictive power. Therefore, the index (I) was simple and considered age and body weight [expressed in percent of the mean body weight (w) for a given age, sex and height].

$$I = \text{age in years} + 1.3 \times w$$

From the data of Lowe et al, it was calculated that all DVT patients were correctly identified at an index of ≥165. Using a similar analysis, it was concluded that, at this cutoff point, 60% of all patients without DVT were included. Hence prophylaxis could be safely withheld in 17 of the total of 63 patients (26%).

Sue-Ling et al (1986) computed a risk factor index from a group of 85 patients who underwent major abdominal and vascular surgery in which an incidence of thrombosis of

27% was observed, using fibrinogen leg scanning only. After analysing the pre-operative data in comparison with the thrombosis incidence, they produced the following formula:

$$I = -8.08 + 0.185a + 0.008b - 2.24c + 2.02d - 0.054e - 0.118f - 0.006g$$

where a = age (years), b = ELT (min), c = previous abdominal surgery (yes = 1, no = 0), d = varicose veins (0 = absent, 1 = present), e = antithrombin III (%), f = cigarettes smoked per day and g = platelet count. All deep vein thrombosis patients were correctly predicted if a cutoff point of -4 was used. Using the discriminant, 30 out of the 62 patients without DVT were also included. Therefore, applying this index, 35% of the total number of patients could be safely spared from prophylaxis.

Likewise, a predictive index was computed by Rocha and colleagues (1988) in a study involving 111 patients undergoing total hip replacement, in order to identify patients at risk for developing DVT after operation. Using stepwise discriminant analysis, the authors showed that the following preoperative variables were most useful in predicting postoperative thrombosis: (a) FDP, (b) PAI, (c) tPA. The following equation was generated, based on 111 patients:

$$I = -2.09 + 0.46a + 1.39b - 0.24c$$

When the cutoff point was taken at I = +2, the predictive index had correctly identified 100% of all patients who developed postoperative DVT (sensitivity 100%) and wrongly allocated 1 patient without postoperative DVT to the high risk group (specificity 99%).

As can be appreciated from the retrospective studies, selective prophylaxis is potentially feasible. Prospective validation of the risk factor indices was performed in only a small number of studies with a limited number of patients (Grandon et al, 1980; Grandon et al, 1980a; Lowe et al, 1982; Sue Ling et al, 1986; Rocha et al, 1988). If these studies are reanalysed, with the cutoff point which identified the patients developing a postoperative thrombosis in the retrospective studies, then it appears that the Clayton index identifies all patients with DVT correctly in two independent studies (Grandon et al, 1980; Grandon et al, 1980a). In these studies, prophylaxis could have been withheld from 40% and 30% of all patients, respectively. Using the same analysis, the Lowe et al (1982), and Sue Ling et al (1986), indices would miss approximately 10% of patients with thrombosis, in cases where prophylaxis is only given to patients with an abnormal index, but research shows that 15-56% of all patients can be spared prophylaxis without a risk of developing venous thrombosis. Finally, as discussed above, when using the predictive index of Rocha et al (1988) in total hip replacement surgery, almost all patients who did not develop DVT after operation could have been identified before operation. This would have enabled highly selective prophylaxis. Future prospective investigations are required to confirm these observations, preferably also in other types of surgery.

## Conclusion

Several laboratory tests, i.e., global coagulation and fibrinolysis assays or more specific assays for coagulation activation and fibrin degradation products, have been applied in the immediate pre- and post-operative phase to discriminate patients at high risk for developing venous thromboembolism. With a few exceptions, most studies were not successful in this respect. Those studies revealing a potentially applicable methodology, urgently require confirmation of their favourable results in prospective studies.

Several risk factor indices, combining physical and laboratory test results, have been developed to predict before operation which patient will develop venous thrombosis. Most of these indices use information which can be simply obtained by pre-operative investigation. It should, however, be realised that with a few exceptions, surgeons do not use these indices to decide whether a patient should receive perioperative thrombosis prophylaxis. Instead, most surgical patients receive routine prophylaxis with low dose heparin or oral anticoagulants. Are these indices useless? From the current literature, it can be concluded that these indices may be useful, though further collaborative studies are needed to precisely determine their usefulness in selective prophylaxis. It would particularly be useful to identify those patients in whom prophylaxis can be safely withheld. This may be very cost-effective in those patients undergoing surgical procedures that have a low absolute risk of postoperative venous thrombosis.

# References

Becker D. Venous thromboembolism: epidemiology, diagnosis, prevention. J Gen Int Med I:402, 1986

Bergqvist D. Frequency of thromboembolic complications. In: Postoperative thromboembolism: frequency, etiology and prophylaxis. Berlin, Springer: 8, 1983

Brandjes DPM, ten Cate JW, Büller HR. Pre-surgical identification of the patient at risk for developing venous thromboembolism post-operatively. Acta Chir Scand Suppl, 556:18, 1990

Clayton JK, Anderson JA, McNicol GP. Preoperative prediction of postoperative deep vein thrombosis. Br Med J II:910, 1976

Collins R, Scrimgeour A, Yusuf S, Peto R. Reduction in fatal pulmonary embolism and venous thrombosis by perioperative administration of subcutaneous heparin. N Engl J Med 318:1162, 1988

De Prost D, Ollivier V, Vie P et al. D-dimer and thrombin-antithrombin III complex levels uncorrelated with phlebographic findings in 11 total knee replacement patients. Ann Biol Clin 40:235, 1990

Gallus AS, Hirsh J, Gent M. Relevance of preoperative and post-operative blood tests to detect postoperative leg-vein thrombosis. Lancet 13:805, 1973

Grandon AJ, Peel KR, Anderson JA, Thompson V, McNicol GP. Prophylaxis of postoperative deep vein thrombosis: selective use of low dose heparin in high risk patients. Br Med J 281:345, 1980

Grandon AJ, Peel KR, Anderson JA, Thompson V, McNicol GP. Postoperative deep vein thrombosis: identifying high risk patients. Br Med J 281:343, 1980a

Grimaudo V, Kruithof EKO, Stiekema JCJ, Bachmann F. High pre-operative plasminogen activator inhibitor levels are correlated with post-operative deep vein thrombosis in total hip replacement. Thromb Hemost (Abstract), 96, 1989

Hampson WJG, Harris FC, Lucas HK et al. Failure of low dose heparin to prevent deep vein thrombosis after hip replacement arthroplasty. Lancet ii:795, 1974

Haugh O, Jorgensen LN, Kolle TR et al. Plasma crosslinked fibrin degradation products fraction D in patients undergoing elective abdominal surgery. Thromb Res 51:385, 1988.

Hoek JA, Nurmohamed MT, Ten Cate JW, Buller HR, Knipscheer HC, Hamelynch KJ, Marti RK, Sturk A. Thrombin-antithrombin III complexes in the prediction of deep vein thrombosis following total hip replacement. Thromb Haemost 62:1050, 1989

Hume M, Turner RH, Kuriakose TA, Suprenant J. Venous thrombosis after total hip replacement J Bone J Surg 58A:933, 1976

Jorgensen LN, Lind B, Hauch O, et al. Thrombin-antithrombin III complex fibrin degradation products in plasma: surgery and postoperative deep venous thrombosis. Thromb Res 59:69, 1990

Kakkar VV, Howe C, Flanc C, Clarke M. Natural history of postoperative deep vein thrombosis. Lancet ii:230, 1969

Kakkar V, Howe C, Nicolaides AN, Renney JTC, Clarke MB. Deep vein thrombosis of the leg: is there a high risk group? Am J Surg 20:527, 1970

Lowe GDO, Osborne DM, McArdle BM et al. Prediction and selective prophylaxis of venous thrombosis in elective gastrointestinal surgery. Lancet i:409, 1982

Macintyre IMC, Webber RG, Crispin JR et al. Plasma fibrinolysis and postoperative deep vein thrombosis. Br J Surg 63:694, 1976

Olt GJ, Greenberg Ch, Synan I et al. Preoperative assessment of fragment D-dimer as a predictor of postoperative venous thrombosis. Am J Obstet Gynecol 162:772, 1990

Paramo JA, Alfaro MJ, Rocha E. Postoperative changes in the plasmatic levels of tissue-type plasminogen activator and its fast-acting inhibitor-relationship to deep vein thrombosis and influence of prophylaxis. Thromb Haemost 54 (3):713, 1985

Rakoczi I, Chamone D, Collen D et al. Prediction of postoperative leg vein thrombosis in gynaecological patients. Lancet i:509, 1978

Rocha E, Alfaro MJ, Paramo JA, Canadell JM. Preoperative indentification of patients at high risk of deep venous thrombosis despite prophylaxis in total hip replacement. Thromb Haemost 59(1):93, 1988

Sorensen JV, Lassen MR, Borris LC et al. Postoperative deep vein thrombosis and plasma levels of tissue plasminogen activator inhibitor. Thromb Res 60:247, 1990

Sorensen JV, Borris LC, Lassen MR et al. Association between plasma levels of tissue plasminogen activator and postoperative deep vein thrombosis — influence of prophylaxis with a low molecular weight heparin. Thromb Res 59:131, 1990a

Sue Ling HM, Johnston D, McMakon MJ, Philips PR, Davies JA. Preoperative identification of patients at high risk of deep venous thrombosis after elective major abdominal surgery. Lancet i:1173, 1986

The Venous Thrombosis Group. The value of the enzymatic TAT test in the diagnosis of postoperative deep vein thrombosis after hip surgery. Thromb Res 54:505, 1989

Todd JW, Frisbie JM, Rossier AB et al. Deep venous thrombosis in acute spinal cord injury a comparison of 125I fibrinogen scanning, impedance plethysmography and venography. Paraplegia 14:50, 1976

# CHAPTER 23

# General surgery

**David Bergqvist**

## Introduction

Most patients undergoing general surgical procedures, mostly abdominal, can be considered as belonging to a low or intermediate risk group concerning the development of venous thromboembolism. Hip and knee surgery are considered to be a high risk. Most studies on prophylactic methods have been performed using the fibrinogen uptake test (FUT) for thrombosis diagnosis, which is adequate in general surgery. In most instances patients undergoing general surgery also belong to an intermediate or low risk group concerning bleeding complications and usually this is not a problem. Table 23.1 summarises the prophylactic methods which are of interest to consider in patients undergoing general surgery. Most of the documentation has been obtained with low dose heparin and more recently with low molecular weight heparin.

Although the majority of thrombi after general surgery develop in the calf veins and lyse spontaneously, some 10-20% will progress and become potentially dangerous because

**Table 23.1**
Prophylactic methods used in general surgery

| Prophylactic methods used in general surgery |
|---|
| Mechanical methods |
| Oral anticoagulation |
| Dextran |
| Low dose heparin with or without dihydroergotamine |
| Low molecular weight heparin and heparin analogues |
| Combination of methods, especially graduated compression stockings with pharmacological agents |

**Table 23.2**
The incidence of DVT in groups of patients having different prophylactic regimens

| Author | Patients n | Control | LDH | DHE/LDH | DHE/LDH red | GCS | IC | Dextran | LMWH |
|---|---|---|---|---|---|---|---|---|---|
| Lindblad, 1988 | 5993 | 24 | 10 | | | | | | |
| Lindblad, 1988 | 4059 | | 17 | 7 | | | | | |
| Lindblad, 1988 | 1927 | | 11 | | 11 | | | | |
| Colditz, 1986 | 7345 | 27 | 10 | 10 | | 11 | 18 | | |
| Clagett and Reisch, 1988 | 4310 | 25 | | | | | | | |
| Clagett and Reisch, 1988 | 6647 | 25 | 9 | | | | | | |
| Clagett and Reisch, 1988 | 1537 | 24 | | | | | | 16 | |
| Clagett and Reisch, 1988 | 899 | | 10 | | | | | 21 | |
| Clagett and Reisch, 1988 | 1684 | | 15 | 9 | | | | | |
| Collins, 1988 | 7362 | 22 | 9 | | | | | | |
| Bergqvist, 1991 | 8024 | | 7 | | | | | | 5 |
| Bergqvist, 1991 | 1707 | 26 | | | | | | 20 | |
| Bergqvist, 1991 | 1057 | | 10 | | | | | 21 | |
| Jeffery and Nicolaides, 1990 | 999 | 31 | | | | 11 | | | |

red: reduced dose; GCS: graduated compression stockings; IC: intermittent compression

of embolisation. As there are no methods sensitive enough to identify the patietns at risk of developing fatal pulmonary embolism a fairly general prophylaxis must be adopted, and there is evidence that methods which prevent calf vein thrombosis will prevent pulmonary embolism also. From a practical point of view prophylaxis should be given to patients above 40 to 45 years of age who undergo surgery with a duration of one hour or more. In the presence of other risk factors prophylaxis should be given irrespective of the patient's age.

# Effectiveness of various prophylactic methods to prevent deep vein thrombosis

The number of studies is great and recently there have been various types of compilations and meta-analyses to try to make an overall evaluation of present day knowledge (Bergqvist 1983; Colditz et al, 1986; Clagett and Reisch, 1988; Lindblad, 1988; Bergqvist, 1988; Ljungstrom, 1988; Levine and Hirsh, 1988; Collins et al, 1988; Jeffery and Nicolaides, 1990; Nenci and Agnelli, 1990; Bergqvist, 1998; Hirsh, 1990). Because the different methods are evaluated on their own merits in other chapters in this volume, table 23.2 shows pooled results from the various compilations. There is some overlapping between the compilations. Concerning low molecular weight heparin there is now one study in general surgery where comparison has been made versus placebo (Ockelford et al, 1989), while most of the other investigations have been performed with standard low dose heparin in the control group. Although every low molecular weight heparin should be considered a unique pharmacological substance and evaluated as such, data hitherto published indicate that it will be extremely difficult to show any clinically relevant difference between them. Therefore they are pooled together in the table.

Low molecular weight heparin is at least as effective as standard low dose heparin and has the advantage of having a better subcutaneous availability and a longer biological half life, necessitating only one daily injection. Low molecular weight heparin is also effective in surgery for malignant disease (Bergqvist et al, 1990).

The time for the first heparin injection has traditionally been 1-2 hours before operation. However, in reality this means a fairly wide range because of difficulties to exactly foresee when an operation is to be performed (Bergqvist et al, 1988). Recently, it has been shown that at least low molecular weight heparin is effective also when given in the evening before surgery and every evening thereafter (Bergqvist et al, 1988; Planes et al, 1988). In two studies on elective hip surgery, low molecular weight heparin with the first dose 12-24 hours after operation was also more effective than placebo (Turpie et al, 1986; Levine et al, 1991), but this concept has so far not been analysed in general surgery. Obviously, the approach is practically attractive but has to be confirmed by further studies.

In recent years various low molecular weight heparin analogues have been evaluated, and at least Org 10172 has been shown to be highly effective, also in high risk groups such as orthopaedic surgery (Chapter 16).

Data on oral anticoagulants in general surgery are rare, most studies having been made in gynaecology, but there is no reason to believe that they are not effective (Bergqvist, 1988). The idea of mini-dose warfarin, introduced by Poller et al (1987), turned out to be effective in gynaecological surgery but has to be verified in further studies. The commencement 20 days preoperatively certainly is impractical. Dextran is effective but not nearly to the same extent as mechanical methods, low dose heparin, or low molecular weight heparin (Chapter 17). It is possible to further reduce the frequency by combining pharmacological methods and graduated elastic compression (Jeffrey and Nicolaides, 1990; Chapter 21).

# Effectiveness of various prophylactic methods to prevent fatal pulmonary embolism

The problem with fatal pulmonary embolism is its rarity and studies showing a preventive effect must therefore be large, often with several thousands of patients. Again, pooling of data and meta-analyses have been made and those are summarised in table 23.3. Data on the effect of fatal pulmonary emobolism of mechanical methods are largely lacking. Although all methods have not been compared with each other, there seems to be no doubt that it is possible to significantly reduce the frequency of pulmonary embolism with pharmacological methods. In studies made so far it also seems fair to suggest that low molecular weight heparins are at least as effective as the other methods. Whether the reduced frequency of fatal pulmonary embolism will influence total mortality is still a controversial issue, the problem being that even larger studies are needed to show an effect. However, it seems important to prevent every isolated cause of death. In one study where low molecular weight heparin (Cy 216) was compared with placebo, in fact total mortality was reduced in the treatment group in addition to the reduction in fatal pulmonary embolism (Pezzuoli et al, 1989). A great problem in analysing the frequency of fatal pulmonary embolism is the autopsy rate.

**Table 23.3**
The incidence of PE in patients having different prophylactic regimens

|  | Patients n | Control | LDH | LDH/DHE | Dextran | LMWH |
|---|---|---|---|---|---|---|
| Int Multicent Trial, 1975 | 4121 | 0.77 | 0.10 | | | |
| Kline et al, 1975 | 831 | 1.6 | | | 0.25 | |
| Gruber et al, 1980 | 3984 | | 0.10 | | 0.25 | |
| Gruber, 1982 | 7413 | | | 0.16 | 0.24 | |
| Clagett and Reisch, 1988 | 1535 | 1.5 | | | 0.27 | |
| Clagett and Reisch, 1988 | 9471 | 0.71 | 0.21 | | | |
| Bergqvist, 1992 | 55545 | | | | | 0.04 |
| Bergqvist, 1992 | 12179 | | 0.13 | | | 0.02 |
| Bergqvist, (Chapter 1) | 5945 | 1.5 | | | 0.34 | |
| Bergqvist, (Chapter 1) | 15568 | | 0.22 | | 0.27 | |
| Lindblad, 1988 | 8091 | | 0.29 | 0.12 | | |
| | 13340 | 0.78 | 0.21 | | | |
| Collins, 1988 | 14084 | 0.81 | 0.26 | | | |

## Side effects

General surgery belongs to an intermediate group as far as the risk of bleeding is concerned and there is no reason for exceptional precautions. Some of the earliest studies with low molecular weight heparin used a somewhat too high dose based on *in vitro* and experimental data with an increased frequency of haemorrhagic complications. Later on it has been possible to define an effective dose which was also safe. Except for conventional doses of oral anticoagulants with an effect during surgery, bleeding is rarely a clinical problem. Bleeding is, however, also somewhat increased after low dose heparin. Dihydroergotamine may in rare cases cause arterial spasm with poor prognosis concerning the extremity and it seems to be on the way out from the prophylactic arsenal (Mattsson et al, 1991).

## Emergency general surgery

Patients undergoing emergency general surgery belong to a group which is difficult to study, partly because of their irregular arrival at hospital and partly because of the general turbulence in connection with their treatment. The frequency of venous thromboembolism without prophylaxis is not known, although there is reason to believe it to be at least as high as in patients undergoing elective general surgery (Torngren and Engstrom, 1991). The few available studies indicate that it is possible to reduce the frequency by prophylactic means (Bergqvist et al, 1984; Wille-Jorgensen et al, 1991).

## Conclusion

There are several prophylactic options in general surgery, but today one of the low molecular weight heparins seems to be both efficient, safe and practical. Both deep vein thrombosis and fatal pulmonary embolism can be significantly prevented. Low dose heparin is also effective and has hitherto been the dominating method worldwide (Bergqvist, 1990). The frequency of deep vein thrombosis seems to be further reduced when a graduated elastic compression stocking is also applied. From a purely economical point of view prophylaxis is cost-effective in groups of patients where the frequency of thrombosis exceeds 8% (Bergqvist et al, 1990). The need for prophylaxis in groups with lower frequencies is not known, graduated compression being recommended by some.

# References

Bergqvist D. Postoperative thromboembolism. Frequency, etiology, prophylaxis. Springer Verlag, Berlin, Heidelberg, New York, 1983

Bergqvist D. Oral anticoagulants for prophylaxis against postoperative thromboembolism. Acta Chir Scand Suppl 543:43, 1988

Bergqvist D. Prophylaxis against postoperative venous thromboembolism — a survey of surveys. Thromb Haemorrh Disorders 2:69, 1990

Bergqvist D. Review of clinical trials of low molecular weight heparins. Clinical review. Acta Schir Scand 158:67, 1992

Bergqvist D, Lindblad B, Ljungstrom K-G, Persson NH, Hallbook T. Does dihydroergotamine potentiate the thromboprophylactic effect of dextran 70? A controlled prospective study in general and hip surgery. Br J Surg 71:516, 1984

Bergqvist D, Mätzsch T, Burmark US et al. Low molecular weight heparin given the evening before surgery compared with conventional low dose heparin in prevention of thromboembolism. Br J Surg 75:888, 1988

Bergqvist D, Mätzsch T, Jendteg S, Lindgren B, Persson U. The cost-effectiveness of prevention of postoperative thromboembolism. Acta Chir Scand, Suppl 556:36, 1990

Clagett GP, Reisch JS. Prevention of venous thromboembolism in general surgical patients. Results of meta-analysis. Ann Surg 208:227, 1988

Colditz GA, Tuden RL. Oster G. Rates of venous thrombosis after general surgery: combined results of randomised clinical trials. Lancet 2:143, 1986

Collins R, Scrimgeour A, Yusuf S, Phil D, Peto R. Reduction in fatal pulmonary embolism and venous thrombosis by perioperative administration of subcutaneous heparin. N Engl J Med 318:1162, 1988

Gruber UF. Prevention of fatal postoperative pulmonary embolism by heparin dihydroergotamine or dextran 70. Br J Surg 69:554, 1982

Gruber UF, Saldeen T, Brokop T, et al. Incidences of fatal postoperative pulmonary embolism with dextran 70 and low-dose heparin. An international multicentre study. Br Med J 280:69, 1980

Hirsh J. From unfractionated heparins to low molecular weight heparins. Acta Chir Scand, Suppl 556:42, 1990

Jeffery PC, Nicolaides AN. Graduated compression stockings in the prevention of postoperative deep vein thrombosis. Br J Surg 77:380, 1990

Kline A, Hughes LE, Campbell H, et al. Dextran 70 in prophylaxis of thromboembolic disease after surgery: a clinically oriented randomized double-blind trial. Br Med J 2:109, 1975

Levine MN, Hirsh J. An overview of clinical trials of low molecular weight heparin fractions. Acta Chir Scand, Supply 543:73, 1988

Levine MN, Hirsch J, Gent M, et al. Prevention of deep vein thrombosis after elective hip surgery. A randomized trial comparing low molecular weight heparin with standard unfractionated heparin. Ann Intern Med 114:545, 1991

Lindblad B. Prophylaxis of postoperative thromboembolism with low dose heparin alone or in combination with dihydroergotamine. A review. Acta Chir Scand 543:31, 1988

Ljungstrom K-G. The antithrombotic efficacy of dextran. Acta Chir Scand, Suppl 543:26, 1988

Mattsson E, Ohlin A, Fredin H, Nilsson P, Bergqvist D. Lower limb vasospasm and renal failure during postoperative thromboprophylaxis. Eur J Surg 157:289, 1991

Nenci GG, Agnelli G. Clinical experience with low molecular weight heparins. Thromb Res, Suppl XI:69, 1990

Ockelford PA, Patterson J, Johns AS. A double blind randomised placebo controlled trial of thromboprophylaxis in major elective general surgery using once daily injections of a low molecular weight heparin fragment (Fragmin). Thromb Haemost 62:1046, 1989

Pezzuoli G, Neri Serneri GG, Settembrini P et al. Prophylaxis of fatal pulmonary embolism in general surgery using low molecular weight heparin Cy 216: a multicentre double-blind randomised controlled clinical trial versus placebo (STEP). Int Surg 74:205, 1989

Planes A, Vochelle N, Mazas F et al. Prevention of postoperative venous thrombosis: a randomised trial comparing unfractionated heparin with low molecular weight heparin in patients undergoing total hip replacement. Thromb Haemost 60:407, 1988

Poller L, McKernan A, Thomson JM, Elstein M, Hirsh PJ, Jones JB. Mixed mini-dose warfarin: a new approach to prophylaxis against venous thrombosis after major surgery. Br Med J 295:1309, 1987

Turpie AGG, Levine MN, Hirsh J et al. A randomised controlled trial of a low molecular weight heparin (Enoxaparin) to prevent deep vein thrombosis in patients undergoing elective hip surgery. N Engl J Med 315:925, 1986

Torngren S, Engstrom L. Deep venous thrombosis after emergency gastrointestinal operations: a pilot study. Eur J Surg 157:389, 1991

Wille-Jorgensen P, Hauch O, Dimo B, Christensen SW, Jensen R, Hansen B. Prophylaxis of deep venous thrombosis after acute abdominal operation. Surg Gynecol Obstet 172:44, 1991

CHAPTER 24

# Obstetrics and gynaecology

Daniel L Clarke-Pearson

## Introduction

Deep vein thrombosis and pulmonary embolism, though largely preventable, are significant complications occurring in obstetric and gynaecologic patients. In the specialty of obstetrics and gynaecology, 40% of all deaths following gynaecologic surgery are attributed to pulmonary emboli (Jeffcoate and Tindall, 1965). Pulmonary embolism is also the second leading cause of death in women who undergo a legally induced abortion (Kimball et al, 1978). In high risk patients with uterine or cervical carcinoma, PE is the leading cause of postoperative death (Clarke-Pearson et al, 1983; Creasman and Weed, 1981).

The incidence of postoperative DVT, when detected by the fibrinogen uptake test (FUT), varies widely, based in large part on the risk factors of the particular group of gynaecologic surgery patients. Patients with benign conditions have DVT detected in from 29-4% (Ballard et al, 1973; Taberner et al, 1978). Patients with gynaecologic malignancies have an increased risk of between 45-17% (Walsh et al, 1974; Crandon and Koutts, 1983; Clarke-Pearson et al, 1987).

Pulmonary embolism is also one of the commonest causes of maternal mortality (Rutherford and Phelan, 1988; Kaunitz et al, 1985; Sachs et al, 1987). Estimates of the incidence of venous thromboembolism in obstetrics vary with the method of diagnosis and the reporting institution (Bolan, 1983; Bergqvist et al, 1983; Kierkegaard, 1983). Although older studies suggest DVT occurs in 2 to 5/1,000 pregnant patients, these estimates are based on clinical diagnosis. Using objective diagnostic techniques, the best current studies report an incidence of DVT from 0.13 to 0.5/1,000 in antepartum and 0.61 to 1.5/1,000 in postpartum patients (Bergqvist et al, 1983; Kierkegaard, 1983). The incidence of calf vein thrombosis as diagnosed by FUT is 3% (Friend and Kakkar, 1970). Pulmonary embolism occurs in approximately 0.01/1,000 antepartum and 0.5/1,000 postpartum patients (Kierkegaard, 1983). This paper will review the information currently available (in the English

**Table 24.1**
Variables associated with postoperative deep vein thrombosis (Clarke-Pearson et al, 1987)

| Overall incidence of DVT in 411 gynaecologic surgery patients = 17.5% | | |
|---|---|---|
| Diagnosis | % DVT | p value |
| Benign | 6 | |
| Cancer | 17.7 | |
| Recurrent cancer | 39 | (<0.001) |
| Past history of DVT | 56 | (<0.001)* |
| Prior radiation therapy | 36 | (<0.001)* |
| Nonwhite race | 25 | (0.03)* |
| Ankle oedema | 40 | (0.005)* |
| Leg stasis changes | 45 | (0.002) |
| Severe varicose veins | 86 | (0.001)* |
| Radical vulvectomy | 32 | (0.001)* |
| Pelvic exenteration | 88 | (0.001)* |
| Duration of surgery (min) | | |
| <120 | 5 | |
| 120-300 | 14 | |
| >300 | 32 | (0.001)* |
| Estimated blood loss (ml) | | |
| <200 | 17.7 | |
| 200-600 | 12 | |
| >600 | 23.5 | (0.01) |
| Weight | | (0.02) |
| Age | | (<0.001)* |

*Factors significant in logistic regression model

language literature) as it relates to the identification of risk factors and prevention of deep vein thrombosis and pulmonary embolism in gynaecology and obstetrics.

# Risk factors

Two prospective studies have evaluated risk factors associated with the postoperative occurrence of FUT detected DVT in gynaecologic surgery patients (Clayton et al, 1976; Clarke-Pearson et al, 1987). Clayton and associates (1976) studied the risk factors of 125 patients undergoing vaginal and abdominal surgery for gynaecologic disease. Most of the patients had benign gynaecologic conditions. Using logistic regression analysis, they identified five factors associated with postoperative DVT: age, varicose veins, percentage overweight, euglobulin lysis time, and serum fibrin-related antigen. A prognostic index score, which was created on the basis of these five variables, was applied in a subsequent study to select high risk patients who might most benefit from intensive perioperative thromboembolism prophylaxis (Crandon et al, 1980). The results of that study confirmed the usefulness of these criteria in the selection of patients most likely to benefit from the application of prophylactic methods.

The clinical factors associated with venous thromboembolic complications have also been assessed by Clarke-Pearson and associates (1987) in 411 patients undergoing major abdominal and pelvic gynaecologic surgery. Eighty-four percent of these patients had gynaecologic malignancies. Risk factors associated with postoperative DVT identified in this study included age, nonwhite patients, increasing stage of malignancy, a past history of DVT, lower extremity oedema or venous stasis changes, varicose veins, excessive weight, and a past history of radiation therapy. Intraoperative factors associated with postoperative DVT included increased anaesthesia time, increased blood loss, and transfusion requirements in the operating room. When all of these factors were evaluated in a stepwise logistic regression model, the type of surgical procedure, age, ankle oedema, nonwhite patients, varicose veins, prior radiation therapy, a past history of DVT, and duration of surgery were found to be the most important variables associated with postoperative thromboembolic complications. The relative risk of these factors are shown in table 24.1.

Patients taking oral contraceptives or oestrogen replacement therapy immediately prior to surgery are also believed to be at higher risk to develop postoperative DVT (Vessey, 1973).

Pregnancy also alters many of the parameters of Virchow's triad (Virchow, 1858), resulting in an increased risk of DVT or PE in the pregnant patient. Hypercoagulability is recognised in pregnancy with increasing levels of fibrinogen, factors VII, VIII, IX and X, and fibrin split products. This hypercoagulable state is compounded by decreased fibrinolysis and diminished factors XI and XII as well as antithrombin III activity, especially in those patients with the hereditary deficiency. Enhanced coagulation and diminished fibrinolytic activity shift the balance in favour of thrombosis (Gerbasi et al, 1990).

Venous stasis is a well-recognised component of normal pregnancy. Venous distensibility, increased blood volume, vena caval occlusion by the gravid uterus, lower extremity oedema, and worsening varicose veins are all evidence of the venous stasis associated with advancing gestation. Venous trauma from unpadded or poorly positioned stirrups in the lithotomy position should not be overlooked. Vessel wall injury is increased by difficult operative deliveries, caesarean section, and endometritis or pelvic cellulitis. Although physiologic events of normal pregnancy and the puerperium potentially fulfill all of Virchow's classic triad, clinical DVT and PE are fortunately rare complications.

The single most important clinical risk factor associated with the development of DVT/PE in pregnancy is a history of prior DVT or PE. Previous venous thromboembolism may have occurred during a prior pregnancy, as a result of oral contraceptive use, or after leg trauma or surgery. A survey of 72 women who became pregnant after a prior pulmonary embolus revealed that 17 of their subsequent 87 pregnancies were complicated by venous thromboembolism (20%) (Tengborn et al, 1989). Others have estimated the risk of recurrent thromboembolism as between 4-12% (Badaracco and Vessey, 1974; Lao et al, 1985). Other variables thought to increase the risk of venous thromboembolism include: pre-eclampsia, caesarean section, prolonged bed rest, obesity, diabetes, cardiac disease, high parity, advanced maternal age or severe varicosities (Laros and Alger, 1979; Weiner, 1985). Patients at risk are those who relate a family history of hypercoagulable syndromes that can exacerbate the thrombotic tendency of normal pregnancy, namely, antithrombin III deficiency, pregnancy-specific protein PAPP-A, protein C or S, or prostacyclin deficiency (Bergqvist and Hedner, 1983; Nelson et al, 1985; Brenner et al, 1987; Comp, 1985; Lanham et al, 1986).

**Table 24.2**
Variables associated with thromboembolism in pregnancy

---

Past history of DVT or PE
Caesarean section
Obesity
Pre-eclampsia
Severe varicosities
Advanced maternal age
Prolonged bedrest
Cardiac disease
High parity
Antithrombin III deficiency
Protein C, S or prostacyclin deficiency
Elevated lupus anticoagulant levels

---

The identification of the lupus anticoagulant (LAC) in patients who have suffered recurrent abortion has been labelled the LAC syndrome. Patients with significantly elevated LAC levels appear to experience thrombosis of the placental villi or abruption causing recurrent abortion or stillbirth. Even with treatment and successful pregnancy, intrauterine growth retardation and pre-eclampsia are frequently noted (Branch et al, 1985). These patients suffer additional thrombotic complications during pregnancy or in the puerperium that may have the same underlying pathophysiology: disruption of the normal balance between thrombosis and fibrinolysis (Feinstein, 1985).

The incidence of thrombosis in patients with elevated LAC levels is alarmingly high. Gastineau et al (1985) found that of 219 patients who had elevated LAC levels, the incidence of thrombotic events in one year was 25%. Venous thrombosis accounted for 75% of all thrombotic events in the non-SLE group who had elevated LAC levels, and arterial thromboses accounted for 50% of all events in the SLE patients. Prevention of recurrent thrombosis required prolonged anticoagulant or antiplatelet therapy. Aspirin had efficacy for both arterial and venous thrombosis, although sodium warfarin was also used. Several patients suffered recurrent thrombosis at cessation of such therapy. Prednisone did not seem to decrease the occurrence of thrombotic events. Branch et al (1985) report a cohort of eight obstetric patients with elevated LAC levels who were treated with prednisone (40mg/day) and low-dose aspirin (81 mg/day) during pregnancy. Four patients had suffered DVT or PE in the past. Three of these eight patients developed DVT in the immediate postpartum period, one of whom progressed to PE. Harris and associates reported on the predictive value of antiphospholipid antibody testing for thrombosis, recurrent fetal loss, and thrombocytopenia in 121 patients. Twenty-nine percent suffered venous thrombosis, whereas an additional 20% suffered arterial thrombosis during a 1-year period. Patients who have SLE and elevated LAC levels are at the greatest risk for antenatal arterial and venous thrombotic events. For the majority of patients with elevated LAC levels the major venous thrombotic risk appears to be during puerperium, with an anticipated rate of DVT of approximately 25%. Variables associated with venous thromboembolism in pregnancy are listed in table 24.2.

The recognition of the factors associated with venous thromboembolism in the gynaecologic surgery and obstetric patients should allow the clinician to stratify patients into low- and high-risk groups and thereby apply appropriate prophylactic methods while at the same time not exposing a low-risk group of patients to the potential complications and expense of some prophylactic treatment regimens.

## Prevention of deep venous thrombosis

An awareness of the risk factors associated with venous thromboembolic complications as well as the natural history of these complications allow us to develop strategies for the prevention of thromboembolic complications. Over the past two decades a number of prophylactic methods have undergone clinical trials and many have been shown to significantly reduce the incidence of postoperative deep vein thrombosis. There are no studies in the obstetrics and gynaecology patient which have demonstrated a reduction in fatal pulmonary emboli. Of the methods reported, each has its advantages and disadvantages. The ideal prophylactic method would be effective, free of significant side effects to the patient or fetus, well accepted by the patient and nursing staff, applicable to most patient groups, and inexpensive.

Information as to the benefits of prophylaxis in pregnancy is lacking. For most methods we assume a benefit similar to that of the surgical patient, although randomised clinical trials are needed.

## Low dose heparin (LDH)

Small doses of subcutaneously administered heparin for the prevention of DVT and PE is the most widely studied of all prophylactic methods. More than 80 controlled trials in 16,000 patients have demonstrated that heparin given subcutaneously 2 hours before operation and every 8 to 12 hours after operation is effective in reducing the incidence of postoperative venous thrombi (Collins et al, 1988; Clagett and Reisch, 1988). Studies performed in gynaecologic surgery are listed in table 24.3.

### Benign gynaecologic surgery

There are two controlled randomised trials in the English literature of low dose heparin used in surgery predominantly for benign gynaecologic conditions (Ballard et al, 1973; Taberner et al, 1978). Both studies used the same regimen of low dose heparin administration: 5,000 units subcutaneously 2 hours before operation and every 12 hours for 7 days after operation. The fibrinogen uptake test (FUT) for the detection of thrombosis was used for the final diagnosis. All patients were more than 40 years of age, and follow up was discontinued at the time of discharge from the hospital.

The results of the trial by Taberner et al (1978) of 97 patients showed a 23% incidence of DVT in the control group compared with a 6% incidence of DVT in the patients treated with low dose heparin. This difference was statistically significant ($p<0.05$). Unfortunately, although this was a randomised trial, the control group contained a larger number of patients with malignancy. When the cancer patients were excluded from the trial analysis, there remained no significant value in the use of low dose heparin in patients with benign conditions (Table 24.3). In the second study, Ballard and associates (1973) evaluated a group of 110 patients who also had a predominance of benign gynaecologic diseases. The nontreated control group had a 29% incidence of DVT compared with a 3.6% incidence in

**Table 24.3**
Summary of studies evaluating low dose heparin prophylaxis in gynaecologic surgery

| Study | Treatment regimen | Diagnostic method | Control n/DVT (%)/ n PE | Treatment n/DVT (%)/ n PE | p value |
|---|---|---|---|---|---|
| Ballard et al, 1973 | LDH 5000u 12h | FUT | 55/15(29%)/0 | 55/2(3.6%)/0 | <0.001 |
| Taberner et al, 1978 (all patients) | LDH 5000 u 12h | FUT | 48/11(23%)/0 | 49/3(6%)/1 | <0.05 |
| (benign patients only) | | | 44/9(20%)/0 | 47/3(6%)/0 | 0.10 |
| McCarthy et al, 1974 | LDH 5000u 12h | FUT | NONE | 64/7(6%)/1 | N/A |
| Borow and Goldson, 1981 | LDH 5000u 12h | FUT | ?/?(16%)/1 | ?/?(9.1%)/? | |
| Clarke-Pearson et al, 1983 | LDH 5000u 12h | FUT | 97/12(12.4%)/1* | 88/13(14.8%)/4 | NS |
| Clarke-Pearson et al, 1990 | LDH 5000u 8h | FUT | 103/19(18.4%)/0 | 104/9(8.7%)/1 | 0.04 |
| | LDH 5000u 3× pre-op 8h postop | FUT | 103/19(18/4%)/0 | 97/4(4.1%)/1 | 0.001 |
| Hohl et al, 1980 | LDH 8h | FUT | NONE | 115/2(1.7%)/0 | N/A |

*patient died of PE   LDH = Low dose heparin   FUT = Fibrinogen uptake test

the group treated with low dose heparin (p<0.001). In this trial, none of the patients developed DVT proximal to the calf, and none developed a pulmonary embolus.

**Gynaecologic oncology**
Despite the apparent benefit of low dose heparin (LDH) prophylaxis in gynaecologic surgery patients, LDH given every 12 hours after operation to patients with a gynaecologic cancer has been found to be ineffective (Clarke-Pearson et al, 1983). In a randomised controlled trial of 185 patients undergoing major abdominal and pelvic surgery for gynaecologic malignancy, there was no difference in the incidence of thromboembolic complications between the control group (12.4%) and the group treated with low dose heparin (14.8%). When analysis of thromboembolic complications was confined to the first 7 postoperative days, the incidence of DVT was 12.4% for the control group compared with 6.8% in the group treated with low dose heparin. This difference was not statistically significant (p=0.2), but it does suggest that low dose heparin may be effective while the patient is receiving heparin prophylaxis but that the beneficial effect is lost when the drug is discontinued. Patients with malignancy or decreased capacity due to age or extent of surgery may remain at risk longer and may require a longer duration of low dose heparin prophylaxis to truly benefit from this regimen.

In a more recent controlled trial of gynaecologic oncology patients, a more intense low dose heparin regimen (5,000 units subcutaneously every 8 hours after operation or in three doses before operation at 8 hour intervals and every 8 hours after operation) reduced the incidence of DVT significantly (Clarke Pearson et al, 1990). The incidence of FUT DVT was 18.4% for the control group, 8.7% for those receiving heparin as a single dose and 4.1%

for those receiving at least three doses of heparin before operation. Although not statistically significant when compared with patients receiving the other heparin regimen, the group receiving three preoperative doses appeared to have the best outcome.

Weiner and associates (1985) have evaluated the circulating levels of heparin when administered subcutaneously to gynaecologic cancer patients (especially with advanced stage malignancy) and found that the latter were able to neutralise heparin, thus making heparin prophylaxis ineffective. This finding may explain why low dose heparin was of benefit to gynaecologic cancer patients only when given in larger than usual doses.

# Obstetrics

As previously noted, PE is a common cause of maternal mortality. Recognising that up to 12% of patients with a prior history of DVT or PE will develop DVT in a subsequent pregnancy, many authors have recommended prophylaxis with low dose heparin in high risk pregnant women. The benefit of low dose heparin in pregnancy has not been adequately demonstrated in clinical trials. Recommended regimens of LDH prophylaxis (Table 24.4) are extrapolated from experience with LDH in surgical patients, and some take into consideration increased risk of DVT and PE during labour and delivery and postpartum (Gerbasi et al, 1990), as well as the risks of osteoporosis associated with prolonged heparin use (Wise and Hall, 1980; Griffiths and Liu, 1984; Ginsberg and Hirsh, 1989).

Howell and colleagues (1983) have reported the only randomised controlled trial in high risk pregnant patients. Twenty patients served as untreated antepartum controls and twenty were randomly assigned to receive 10,000 units of heparin subcutaneously every 12 hours throughout their antenatal course (average of 25 weeks). Both groups received LDH 8,000 units subcutaneously every 12 hours for 6 weeks postpartum. Heparin doses were adjusted to keep the heparin level <4.1 u/ml. One patient in the control group developed DVT at 28 weeks gestation. None of the LDH patients developed DVT. Bleeding complications and premature delivery were similar in both groups although one LDH patient developed severe osteoporosis (Wise and Hall, 1980). Although the number of patients was small, Howell questioned the wisdom of LDH prophylaxis, given the potential complications as well as the required avoidance of epidural anaesthesia in LDH treated patients. Finally, a retrospective analysis of 72 patients was unable to demonstrate a reduced incidence of DVT in patients treated with LDH (Tengborn et al, 1989).

Lao and colleagues (1985) felt that antepartum DVT was so infrequent, even in high risk patients, that they proposed a prophylactic regimen aimed at labour, delivery, and postpartum when DVT was considered to be more frequent. Their regimen used IV Dextran during labour, then LDH or warfarin postpartum. Dextran was chosen for use during labour since epidural anaesthesia could be used safely. In this report of 26 pregnancies treated with this regimen, none developed DVT or PE postpartum. Only one patient developed DVT in the antepartum period. The authors concluded that antenatal DVT is very infrequent and prophylaxis is probably not warranted until labour and postpartum.

The risk of osteoporosis and fractures have been reported to be increased in pregnancies treated with heparin. DeSwiet (1983) reported that radiographic evidence of bone loss associated with the use of heparin (10,000 u BID) was increased proportionately to the duration of therapy and patients receiving heparin for more than 20 weeks were at significantly higher risk ($p<0.1$). Other reports have also suggested that a daily dose of

**Table 24.4**
Recommended thrombosis prophylaxis in high risk pregnant women

---

**Ginsberg and Hirsch (1989)**
*1st 28-36 weeks of pregnancy:*
Heparin 5000 u sc 12 h
*36 weeks to delivery:*
Increase heparin dose to have aPTT approximately 1.5 × control
*Postpartum:*
Warfarin p.o.

---

**Weiner (1985)**
*1-13 weeks:*
Heparin 5000u sc 12 h
*14-29 weeks:*
Heparin 7500u sc 12 h
*30 weeks - labour:*
Heparin 10,000u sc 12 h
*Postpartum:*
Heparin 5000u sc 12 h

---

**Lao et al (1985)**
*Conception to labour:*
None
*Labour:*
Dextran 70 iv (500-1000 ml) over 8-12 hours
*Postpartum:*
Heparin 8000u sc 12 h × 6 weeks

---

**Dahlman et al (1989)**
*Conception through labour:*
Heparin sc q 12 h
Adjust heparin dose to achieve a plasma heparin level of 0.1 IU/ml (range 0.08-0.15 IU/ml)
*Postpartum:*
Heparin 10,000 - 15,000 u sc 12 h × 6 weeks

---

sc = subcutaneous    aPTT = activate partial thromboplastin time

heparin in excess of 15,000 u/day was associated with an increased risk of osteopenia and fractures (Wise and Hall, 1980; Griffiths and Liu, 1984; Ginsberg and Hirsh, 1989).

Dahlman and colleagues (1989) attempted to minimise the dose of heparin administered for prophylaxis by measuring heparin levels with an aim of keeping heparin peak level at 0.1 iu/ml (range of 0.08 to 0.15 iu/ml). An increased need for heparin was noted later in pregnancy. None of the 26 high risk women studied developed DVT, PE or osteoporosis. Others have recommended empirically increasing heparin doses late in pregnancy to allow for increased plasma volume, increased renal clearance, and placental heparinase (Weiner, 1985; Ginsberg and Hirsh, 1989).

In summary, it appears that a high risk group of pregnant patients (past history of DVT or PE) can be identified. Low dose heparin prophylaxis is recommended by many authorities although prospective data is lacking. Further, suggested heparin regimens vary considerably

(Table 24.4), and because of the risks of prolonged heparin use in pregnancy, (osteoporosis, thrombocytopenia and bleeding) some authors do not recommend prophylaxis or only recommend prophylaxis during labour and postpartum. Clearly, well designed multicentre clinical trials are needed to clearly evaluate these many issues.

**Low dose heparin complications**
Complications associated with bleeding induced by low dose heparin must also be considered in evaluating the risks of this prophylactic regimen. In a study of 182 patients undergoing major surgery for gynaecologic malignancy, low dose heparin complications were evaluated from both a clinical viewpoint as well as alteration in common laboratory parameters. That study found a trend toward increased intraoperative blood loss, transfusion requirements, and wound haematomas associated with the use of low dose heparin (Clarke-Pearson et al, 1984).

Low dose heparin has been shown to alter the aPTT in 10% to 15% of patients given 5,000 units of sodium heparin subcutaneously (Gurewich et al, 1978; Clarke-Pearson et al, 1984). In patients who had prolongation of the aPTT greater than 1.5 times the control value, haemorrhagic complications were significantly increased. This alteration of aPTT by low dose heparin occurred in approximately 15% of patients being treated for gynaecologic malignancy (Clarke-Pearson et al, 1984). Thrombocytopenia has also been associated with the use of low dose heparin, although it is much more frequently noted during the use of therapeutic anticoagulant doses of heparin (Galle et al, 1978).

Of particular relevance to the gynaecologic surgeon performing pelvic, para-aortic, and inguinal lymphadenectomy for treatment or staging of malignancy are three reports of increased lymphocyst formation and increased lymph fluid drainage attributed to the use of low dose heparin (Clagett and Collins, 1978; Catalona et al, 1979; Piver et al, 1983). Although our prospective randomised study did not find an increased incidence of lymphocysts, the volume of suction drainage from the retroperitoneal surgical site was increased nearly twofold (Clarke-Pearson et al, 1984).

Heparin use in the pregnant patient also carries a risk of inducing osteoporosis, although it has only been reported once at heparin doses of less than 16,000 units/day (Wise and Hall, 1980; DeSwiet et al, 1983; Griffiths and Liu, 1984). Osteoporosis is much more likely to occur in the pregnant patient who is receiving full doses of heparin as treatment for a major venous thromboembolism.

# Dextran

Intravenous dextran has been found to be effective in the prevention of venous thromboembolism in general surgery and gynaecologic surgery patients in several trials (Table 24.5). Controlled clinical trials of patients undergoing general surgical procedures have shown that dextran is effective in preventing DVT and fatal pulmonary emboli to a magnitude similar to that achieved with low dose heparin therapy. Bonnar et al (1973) demonstrated that dextran 70 reduced the incidence of FUT detected DVT in patients undergoing surgery for benign gynaecologic conditions as well as malignancy. In uncontrolled studies comparing low dose heparin with IV dextran, the results are more variable. McCarthy et al (1974) showed no significant difference in the incidence of FUT detected DVT between a group of patients treated with low dose heparin and those treated with dextran 70. On the other hand, Hohl et al (1980) and Borow and Goldson (1981) found a significant decrease in the

**Table 24.5**
Summary of studies evaluating the efficacy of dextran prophylaxis in gynaecologic surgery

| Study | Treatment regimen | Diagnostic method | Control n/DVT(%)/PE | Treatment n/DVT(%)/PE | p value |
|---|---|---|---|---|---|
| McCarthy et al, 1974 | IV Dextran 70 500 ml in OR 500 ml 1st 24 hrs | FUT | None | 68/11(16.2%)/1 | N/A |
| Borow and Goldson, 1981 | Dextran | FUT | ?/?(16.6%)/1 | ?/0(0%)/0 | ? |
| Bonnar et al, 1973 | Dextran 70 500 ml in OR 500 ml 6 hrs p/op | FUT | 140/15(10.7%)/0 | 120/1(0.8%)/0 | <0.001 |
| Hohl et al, 1980 | Dextran | FUT | None | 117/17(14.5%)/0 | N/A |

incidence of DVT in patients treated with IV dextran compared with a group treated with low dose heparin.

Complications associated with dextran therapy include the potential for fluid overload in patients with limited cardiovascular and renal reserve, and (rarely) an anaphylactic reaction has been noted. Bleeding complications associated with dextran therapy are considered to be significantly less frequent than those associated with the use of low dose heparin (Gruber et al, 1977).

Dextran has been used infrequently in pregnancy since it may only be used in the labour and postpartum period when intravenous fluids are given. Lao (1985) used dextran prophylaxis during labour in 26 pregnancies and reported no postpartum DVT or PE. When compared to heparin, the use of dextran during labour has the added advantage that epidural anaesthesia may be used safely.

# Other pharmacologic methods of prophylaxis

Several other pharmacologic methods of DVT prophylaxis have been evaluated in gynaecologic surgery patients (Table 24.6) The drugs evaluated include low molecular weight heparin, dihydroergotamine, defibrotide, warfarin, aspirin, dipyridamole, and naproxen. Unfortunately, only two of these studies had contemporary randomised control groups and used prospective objective DVT surveillance by the FUT.

One controlled trial comparing nicomalone therapy with low dose heparin in gynaecologic surgery showed both treatments to be beneficial when compared with the untreated control group. Although both the nicomalone and the low dose heparin treatment groups had approximately the same incidence of DVT, Taberner et al (1978) concluded that in moderate risk patients such as those undergoing surgery for benign gynaecologic conditions, low dose heparin appears to be a more convenient mode of therapy, because it does not require 5 days of preoperative adjustment of PT or continued laboratory monitoring of the PT. Nicomalone, although an effective method for prevention of postoperative DVT

**Table 24.6**
Summary of studies evaluating other pharmacologic methods of DVT prophylaxis in gynaecologic surgery

| Study | Treatment regimen | Diagnostic method | Control n/DVT(%)/PE | Treatment n/DVT(%)/PE | p value |
|---|---|---|---|---|---|
| Steiner et al, 1989 | LMWH[1] + DHE[2] | Clinical, confirmed by Doppler | None | 92/1(1%)/1 | NS |
|  | LDH[3] + DHE/A[4] | Clinical, confirmed by Doppler | None | 99/1(1%)/0 |  |
| Ciavarella et al, 1986 | Defibrotide 200 mg IV qid | FUT[5] | 45/13(28.8%)/0 | 44/4(9%)/0 | <0.05 |
| Ferrari et al, 1990 | Defibrotide 400 mg IM bid | IPG[6] | None | 80/0(0%)/0 | <0.05 |
| Hunter et al, 1990 | Warfarin[8] | Clinical PE | (historical) 41/?(12%)/5 | 84/0(0%)/0 | <0.001 |
| Borow et al, 1981 | Aspirin[10] | Clinical PE | ?/?(16.6%)/? | ?/?(15.4%)/0 | ? |
| Taberner et al, 1978 | Nicomalone[9] | Clinical PE | 48/11(22.9%)/0 | 48/3(6.3%)/0 | <0.05 |
| Kajanoja and Forss, 1981 | po Dipyridamole[7] and po Naproxen[7] | FUT | None | 30/1(3%)/0 |  |
|  | LDH 5000u 12h | FUT | None | 35/0(0%)/0 |  |

1. LMWH = 1500 IU low molecular weight heparin
2. DHE = Dihydroergatamine 0.5 mg
3. LDH = low dose heparin
   2,500 UI subcutaneously 2 hours preop
   2,500 IU subcutaneously 12 hours postop
4. A = Acenocoumarol beginning at 48 hours postop
5. FUT = Fibrinogen uptake test
6. IPG = impedance plethysmography
7. Dipyridamole (persantine[R]): D
   Naproxen (Naprosyn[R]): N
   D75mg po, N 500 mg po evening before surgery
   D10mg IV at beginning of surgery
   D75mg po, N 250mg po evening of surgery
   D75mg po, tid, N 250mg po bid for 7 days
8. Warfarin: 10mg po morning of surgery. Adjusted dose postop, then 2.5 mg po q d × 4 weeks
9. Nicoumalone: 6mg q d beginning 5 days before surgery. Adjusted by PT ratio (2.0-4.0) BCT. Continued for 14 days
10. Aspirin: 600mg suppository preop and every 12 hours postop

and PE, might be reserved for the very high risk patient such as some patients with gynaecologic malignancies or those patients who have demonstrated repeated bouts of

DVT. The value of oral anticoagulant prophylaxis has not been tested in very high risk gynaecologic surgery patients.

Defibrotide, a polydeoxyribonucleotide extracted from mammalian organs, an antithrombic compound without anticoagulant activity, has been evaluated in a randomised controlled trial reported by Ciavarella (1986). In this study the incidence of FUT detected DVT was significantly lower ($p<0.05$) in the defibrotide treated patients (9%) when compared with the control patients (28.8%). There were no apparent side effects or complications of defibrotide when given intravenously.

Sodium warfarin should not be used during pregnancy due to its embryopathic and haemorrhagic complications (Laros and Alger, 1979; Weiner, 1985).

## Mechanical methods of prophylaxis

Stasis in the veins of the legs has been clearly demonstrated on the operating table, after operation, and in the pregnant patient. Many authors believe that the combination of stasis occurring in the capacitance veins of the calf during surgery or pregnancy plus the hypercoagulable state induced by surgery and pregnancy are the prime factors contributing to the development of acute DVT. Prospective studies of the natural history of postoperative venous thrombosis show that the calf veins are the predominant site of thrombi and that most thrombi develop within 72 hours of surgery. Although reduction of venous stasis in the perioperative period by various methods has been less extensively investigated (when compared to pharmacologic methods), a growing body of literature supports the important role that these mechanical prophylactic methods may play in the prevention of postoperative DVT.

Although probably of only modest benefit, reduction of stasis by short preoperative hospital stays, early postoperative ambulation and elevation of the foot of the bed should be encouraged in all patients. In the third trimester of pregnancy, the lateral recumbent position should be encouraged to reduce venous occlusion by the gravid uterus. More active forms of mechanical prophylaxis which have been evaluated in the gynaecologic surgery patient include graded elastic compression stockings, and intermittent pneumatic leg compression (IPC).

### Graded compression stockings

In a survey of general surgeons in the United States, graded compression elastic stockings were second only to low dose heparin as the prophylactic method of choice in high risk and moderately high risk surgical patients (Conti and Daschback, 1982). The simplicity of elastic stockings and the absence of significant side effects are probably the two most important reasons that they are part of the routine postoperative orders of many surgeons. To be effective, the stockings must be designed and used properly. Early studies of static uniform compression stockings demonstrated no benefit from this style of stocking (Rosengarten et al, 1970; Browse et al, 1974). Further evaluation of venous flow dynamics found better venous emptying and increased venous flow from stockings that had a gradient of pressure higher at the ankle and diminishing at the thigh (Sigel et al, 1975; Lawrence and Kakkar, 1980).

Turner and associates (1984) have evaluated the benefits of graded compression stockings in a randomised controlled trial of patients with benign gynaecologic conditions (Table 24.7). This group was at relatively low risk of developing DVT (mean age 45 years;

**Table 24.7**
Summary of studies evaluating mechanical (antistasis) prophylactic methods in gynaecologic surgery

| Study | Treatment regimen | Diagnostic method | Control n/DVT(%)/PE | Treatment n/DVT(%)/PE | p value |
|---|---|---|---|---|---|
| Turner et al, 1984 | TEDS[1] periop | FUT | 92/4(4.3%)/0 | 104/0(0%)/0 | 0.048 |
| Clarke-Pearson et al, 1984 | IPC[2] intraop and 5 days | FUT | 52/18(34.6%)/1 | 55/7(12.7%)/2 | <0.005 |
| Clarke-Pearson et al, 1984a | IPC[2] intraop and 24 hours | FUT | 97/12(12.4%)/1 | 97/18(18.6%)/4 | NS |
| Borow et al, 1981 | IPC[2] intraop and ?duration postop | FUT | ?/?(16.6%)/? | ?/?(7.6%)/? | ? |

1. TEDS = gradient compression stockings
2. IPC = intermittent pneumatic compression

cancer patients, diabetics and patients with a history of DVT or PE were excluded from the study). When evaluated by FUT, none of the 104 patients in the compression stocking group developed DVT, while 4 of the 92 patients (4.3%) in the control group developed calf vein DVT (p=0.48). Although compression stockings lowered the incidence of DVT, the authors questioned whether this prophylaxis was cost effective in low risk groups of patients.

Ensuring a proper fit of the compression stockings may be a major stumbling block and may make the stockings hazardous to some patients who develop a tourniquet effect at the knee or midthigh by poorly fitted stockings. Variations in human anatomy do not allow perfect fit of all patients to stocking sizes manufactured. As an example of this problem, a retrospective study of 281 patients undergoing radical hysterectomy or total abdominal hysterectomy found a fourfold increase in the incidence of clinically significant postoperative DVT and PE in patients weighing more than 90 kg who wore thigh length elastic stockings perioperatively. It was suggested that a tourniquet effect of these stockings may have led to increased stasis in this group of patients already at high risk due to obesity, age, malignancy and major surgery (Clarke-Pearson et al, 1983).

Graded compression stockings may also be of some benefit to the pregnant patient in compressing varicose veins and reducing venous stasis and oedema. The value of compression stockings in preventing DVT in the pregnant patient has not been studied in controlled trials.

# Intermittent pneumatic compression (IPC)

The largest body of literature evaluating the benefit of the reduction of postoperative venous stasis deals with intermittent compression of the leg by pneumatically inflated sleeves placed around the calf, or leg, during the high risk intraoperative and postoperative periods. Clagett and Reisch (1988) have reviewed the results of IPC trials through 1988. Various pneumatic compression devices and leg sleeve designs are available, but the current literature has not demonstrated superiority of one system over another. The single-chambered compression device has been studied the most extensively and appears to significantly reduce the incidence of DVT on a par with that of low dose heparin. In addition to increasing venous flow and pulsatile emptying of the calf veins, IPC also appears to augment endogenous fibrinolysis (Allenby et al, 1976; Knight and Dawson, 1976; Guyton et al, 1985). Activation of the fibrinolytic system might lead to lysis of very early thrombi before they become clinically significant.

The duration of postoperative IPC has been different in various trials. Our understanding that the onset of most DVT occurs intraoperatively and in the first 48 hours after operation suggests that this time interval should be a minimum length for IPC. Several investigators have found IPC to be effective when used only in the operating room or for the first 24 hours after operation (Roberts and Cotton, 1974; Nicolaides et al, 1980; Salzman et al, 1980). Salzman and associates (1980) reported that intraoperative IPC was as beneficial as IPC applied for longer periods of time in patients after urologic surgical procedures. On the other hand, Turpie et al (1977; 1979) found continuing benefit in the use of IPC for up to 14 days postoperatively.

Intermittent pneumatic compression has not been evaluated in a controlled trial of patients undergoing surgery for benign gynaecologic disease. In patients with gynaecologic malignancy IPC has been found to reduce the incidence of postoperative venous thromboembolic complications by nearly threefold (Table 24.6) (Clarke-Pearson et al, 1984). Calf compression was applied intraoperatively and for the first 5 postoperative days. The maximum benefit was realised during the first 5 postoperative days of compression and diminished after IPC was discontinued. In a subsequent trial designed to evaluate whether IPC might achieve similar benefits when used only intraoperatively and for the first 24 hours after operation, there was no reduction of DVT compared with the control group (Clarke-Pearson et al, 1984). It appears that patients with gynaecologic malignancies remain at risk because of stasis and hypercoagulable states for a longer period of time than the general surgical or urology patients, and if compression is to be effective, it must be used for at least five days after operation.

Two studies have directly compared IPC and low dose heparin in gynaecology. Jobson et al (1983) reported (in an abstract) IPC to be superior to LDH in a randomised trial of 330 patients undergoing major gynaecologic surgery procedures. In this uncontrolled randomised trial, the clinical endpoint was the diagnosis of symptomatic pulmonary emboli. Of 164 patients in the low dose heparin group, 7 developed postoperative PE, including 2 that were fatal. None of the 139 patients with IPC prophylaxis developed PE ($p=0.006$). This large trial would have been more significant had a prospective method been used to screen all patients for postoperative DVT or pulmonary emboli. Further, a full length manuscript of this abstract has never been published. Without such prospective screening, one might argue that bias in the clinical detection of pulmonary emboli may have occurred. Borow and Goldson (1981) in a smaller group of gynaecologic surgery patients also found the incidence of FUT detected thrombi to be lower in an IPC treatment group (7.6%) compared with a low dose heparin treated group (9.1%) and in the untreated control group (16.6%). There was no statistically significant difference in the incidence of DVT between the IPC and low dose heparin treated groups. The true significance of this trial is questioned because details as to the number and characteristics of patients in the groups has not been published.

To date there are no studies of IPC in the pregnant patient at risk of developing DVT. Since most pregnant patients are ambulatory, pneumatic compression would be of limited utility. On the other hand, IPC might be of benefit to the gravid patient confined to bed rest or for the postpartum period.

Intermittent pneumatic leg compression has no significant side effects or risks, although patient tolerance has been cited as a drawback to the use of this equipment. However, we have had only 6 patients of nearly 800 treated with IPC request removal because of discomfort. The equipment is easily managed by the nursing staff, and although initial capital outlay for intermittent pneumatic compressors may seem large, Salzman and Davies (1980) calculated that the cost per patient of this prophylactic method is slightly less than that of low dose heparin given for 7 days after operation.

## Inferior vena caval interruption

Interruption of the vena cava, while not preventing DVT, is effectve in preventing fatal pulmonary emboli (Fullen et al, 1973). Heaps and Lagasse (1990) reported the successful prophylactic clipping of the vena cava of 16 patients during laparotomy for gynaecological cancer. All patients had a past history of DVT at the time of surgery. None of these patients developed postoperative pulmonary emboli. Similar results have been reported by Morley (1976) in 66 consecutive patients undergoing pelvic exenteration. A vena caval filter or umbrella appears more attractive when compared with caval ligation, plication, or clipping because of relative ease of application and the lower incidence of sequelae. This invasive prophylactic technique should be reserved only for very high risk patients and has been used successfully in pregnancy (Banfield et al, 1990).

## Surveillance

Under selected circumstances, it may be deemed that prophylaxis is inappropriate, even though a patient is considered to be at high risk of developing a venous thromboembolic complication. This may be due to evidence that suggests that any prophylaxis is ineffective under specific circumstances, that the risk of bleeding cannot be tolerated, or that a specific prophylactic method is not available in a particular institution. Although DVT might not be prevented, recognition (diagnosis) and treatment of occult thrombi may prevent the more devastating sequelae of PE. Early detection of symptomatic DVT in the leg is most appropriately performed by the FUT initiated immediately after surgery and continued throughout the postoperative period while the patient remains at risk. Surveillance with the FUT and the prevention of fatal PE is supported by nine studies in which 1,373 patients were screened with FUT. Of these patients, none suffered a fatal pulmonary embolus (Salzman and Davies, 1980). There are no studies of gynaecology patients undergoing surveillance alone.

$^{125}$Iodine fibrinogen should be avoided in the pregnant woman or in the breast-feeding mother because $^{125}$I crosses the placenta and is present in breast milk.

Surveillance of the patient at risk for pelvic venous thrombosis is a more difficult problem. From prospective studies of gynaecologic patients, it appears that approximately 40% of pulmonary emboli must arise from the veins in the pelvis (Clarke-Pearson et al, 1984). Further, of 12 PE reported in four low dose heparin trials, nine patients (75%) had normal FUT scans (McCarthy et al, 1974; Clarke-Pearson et al, 1983; 1984; 1985, 1990). We presume that these PE must have arisen from the pelvis. Although we have assumed that a prophylactic method which reduces leg DVT will also reduce pelvic vein thrombosis, this presumption may not be correct for gynaecologic surgery patients. The pelvic veins are not accessible to the FUT or any other noninvasive diagnostic method thus making prospective studies impossible. Preliminiary studies using [111]I-labelled platelet imaging as a diagnostic method for the detection of pelvic vein thrombosis remains to be fully investigated as to its sensitivity and specificity as well as the true incidence and significance of pelvic vein thrombosis.

## Pelvic vein thrombosis

Although it is generally believed that most pulmonary emboli arise from venous thrombi in the lower extremities and that most significant thrombi initially originate in the calf veins and then propagate proximally, the occurrence of pelvic and ovarian vein thrombosis is recognised as a complication unique to obstetrics and gynaecology. The surgical and pathologic description of septic pelvic vein thrombosis, often associated with PE, is typified by the clinical findings of a hectic fever curve unresponsive to antibiotics and persisting despite exclusion of other sources of infection. Collins (1971) described the surgical approach to this disease process; more recently IV heparin has been used to successfully treat presumed septic pelvic vein thrombosis. The diagnosis of septic pelvic vein thrombosis, however, continues to rest on the clinical course of the patient and is usually a presumptive diagnosis based on a clinical response to heparin therapy. Unfortunately, the natural history and incidence of this disease process suffer from the lack of an accurate diagnostic technique. None of the noninvasive techniques previously described in the monograph can diagnose thrombi in the internal iliac or ovarian veins. Case reports have demonstrated the potential usefulness of MRI, computed tomography, duplex Doppler ultrasound, and [111]I-labelled platelet imaging in the diagnosis of pelvic vein thrombosis (Clarke-Pearson et al, 1984; Brown et al, 1986; Martin et al, 1986; Baran and Frisch, 1987; Isada et al, 1987; Mintz et al, 1987). The diagnostic sensitivity and specificity of these techniques have not yet been fully evaluated.

## References

Allenby F, Boardman L, Pflug JJ et al. Effects of external pneumatic intermittent compression on fibrinolysis in man. Lancet 2:1412, 1976

Badaracco MA, Vessey MP. Recurrence of venous thromboembolic disease and use of oral contraceptives. Brit Med J i:215, 1974

Ballard M, Bradley-Watson PJ, Johnstone ED et al. Low doses of subcutaneous heparin in the prevention of deep venous thrombosis after gynaecologic surgery. J Obstet Gynaecol Br Commonw 80:469, 1973

Banfield PJ, Pittman M, Marwood R. Recurrent pulmonary embolism in pregnancy managed with the Greenfield vena cava filter. Int J Obstet Gynecol 33:275, 1990

Baran GW, Frisch KM. Duplex Doppler evaluation of puerperal ovarian vein thrombosis. AJR 149:321, 1987

Bergqvist D, Hedner U. Pregnancy and venous thromboembolism. Acta Obstet Gynecol Scand 62:449, 1983

Bergqvist A, Bergqvist D, Hallbook T. Deep venous thrombosis during pregnancy: a prospective study. Acta Obstet Gynecol Scand 62:443, 1983

Bolan JC. Thromboembolic complications of pregnancy. Clin Obstet Gynecol 26:913, 1983

Bonnar J, Walsh JJ, Haddon M et al. Coagulation system changes induced by pelvic surgery and the effect of dextran 70. Bibl Anat 12:351, 1973

Borow M, Goldson H. Postoperative venous thrombosis: evaluation of five methods of treatment. Am J Surg 141:245, 1981

Branch DA, Scott JR, Kochenour KN, et al. Obstetric complications associated with the lupus anticoagulant. N Engl J Med 313:1322, 1985

Brenner B, Shapira A, Bahari C et al. Hereditary protein C deficiency during pregnancy. Am J Obstet Gynecol 157:1160, 1987

Brown CEL, Lowe TW, Cunningham G et al. Puerperal pelvic thrombophlebitis: impact on diagnosis and treatment using x-ray computed tomography and magnetic resonance imaging. Obstet Gynecol 68:789, 1986

Browse NL, Jackson BT, Maye ME et al. The value of mechanical methods of preventing postoperative calf vein thrombosis. Br J Surg 60:319, 1974

Catalona WJ, Kadmon D, Crane DB. Effect of minidose heparin on lymphocele formation following extraperitoneal pelvic lymphadenectomy. J Urol 123:890, 1979

Ciavarella N, Ettorre C, Schiavone M, Schonauer S, Cicinelli E, Cagnozzo G. Effectiveness of defibrotide for prophylaxis of deep venous thrombosis in gynecological surgery: a double-blind placebo controlled clinical trial. Haemostasis 16:39, 1986

Clagett GP, Collins GJ. Platelets, thromboembolism and the clinical utility of antiplatelet drugs. Surg Gynecol Obstet 142:357, 1978

Clagett GP, Reisch JS. Prevention of venous thromboembolism in general surgical patients. Ann Surg 208:227, 1988

Clarke-Pearson DL, Coleman RE, Synan IS et al. Venous thromboembolism prophylaxis in gynecologic oncology: a prospective controlled trial of low dose heparin. Am J Obstet Gynecol 145:606, 1983

Clarke-Pearson DL, Jelovsek FR, Creasman WT. Thromboembolism complicating surgery for cervical and uterine malignancy: incidence, risk factors and prophylaxis. Obstet Gynecol 61:87, 1983

Clarke-Pearson DL, Coleman RE, Petry N et al. Postoperative pelvic vein thrombosis and pulmonary embolism detected by indium-111-labelled platelet imaging: a case report. Am J Obstet Gynecol 149:796, 1984

Clarke-Pearson DL, Creasman WT, Coleman RE et al. Perioperative external pneumatic calf compression as thromboembolism prophylaxis in gynecologic oncology: report of a randomised controlled trial. Gynecol Oncol 18:226, 1984

Clarke-Pearson DL, DeLong ER, Synan IS, et al. Complications of low dose heparin prophylaxis in gynecologic oncology surgery. Obstet Gynecol 64:689, 1984

Clarke-Pearson DL, Synan IS, Coleman RE, Hinshaw W, Creasman WT. The natural history of postoperative venous thromboembolism in gynecologic surgery: a prospective study of 382 patients. Am J Obstet Gynecol 148:1051, 1984

Clarke-Pearson D, Synan IS, Hinshaw WM, Coleman RE, Creasman WT. Prevention of postoperative venous thromboembolism by external pneumatic calf compression in patients with gynecologic malignancy. Surg Gynecol Obstet 63:92, 1984

Clarke-Pearson DL, Coleman RL, Siegel R et al. [111]Indium-labelled platelet imaging for the detection of deep venous thrombosis and pulmonary embolism in patients without symptoms after surgery. Surgery 98:98, 1985

Clarke-Pearson DL, DeLong ER, Synan IS, et al. Variables associated with postoperative deep venous thrombosis: a propsective study of 411 gynecology patients and creation of a prognostic model. Obstet Gynecol 69:146, 1987

Clarke-Pearson DL, DeLong ER, Synan IS et al. A controlled trial of two low dose heparin regimens for the prevention of deep vein thrombosis. Obstet Gynecol 75:684, 1990

Clayton JK, Anderson JA, McNicol GP. Preoperative prediction of postoperative deep venous thrombosis. Br Med J 2:910, 1976

Collins CG. Suppurative pelvic thrombophlebitis. Am J Obstet Gynecol 108:681, 1971

Collins R, Scrimbeour A, Yusuf S et al. Reduction in fatal pulmonary embolism and venous thrombosis by perioperative administration of subcutaneous heparin. N Engl J Med 318:1162, 1988

Comp P. Clinical implications of the protein c/s system. Ann NY Acad Sci 68:149, 1985

Conti S, Daschback M. Venous thromboembolism prophylaxis: a survey of its use in the United States. Arch Surg 117:1036, 1982

Crandon AJ, Koutts. Incidence of post-operative deep vein thrombosis in gynecologic oncology. Aust NZ J Obstet Gynecol 23:216, 1983

Crandon AJ, Peel KR, Anderson JA et al. Prophylaxis of postoperative deep venous thrombosis: selective use of low dose heparin in high risk patients. Br Med J 2:345, 1980

Creasman WT, Weed JC Jr. Radical hysterectomy. In: Schaefer G, Graber EA (eds): Complications in Obstetrics and Gynecologic Surgery. Hagerstown MD, Harper & Row, p389, 1981

Dahlman TC, Hellgren MSE, Blombeck M. Thrombosis prophylaxis in pregnancy with use of subcutaneous heparin adjusted by monitoring heparin concentration in plasma. Am J Obstet Gynecol 161:420, 1989

DeSwiet M, Ward PD, Fidler J ET AL. Prolonged heparin therapy in pregnancy causes bone demineralisation. Br J Obstet Gynaecol 90:1129, 1983

Feinstein DI. Lupus anticoagulant, thrombosis and fetal loss. N Engl J Med 313:1348, 1985

Ferrari A, Dindelli M, Sellaroli CM. Preventing postoperative deep venous thrombosis in gynecological surgery with defibrotide. Int Surg 75:184, 1990

Friend JR, Kakkar VV. The diagnosis of deep vein thrombosis in the puerperium. J Obstet Gynaecol Br Commonw 77:820, 1970

Fullen WD, Miller DH et al. Prophylactic vena caval interruption in hip fractures. J Trauma 13:403, 1973

Galle PC, Muss HB, McGrath KM et al. Thrombocytopenia in two patients treated with low dose heparin. Obstet Gynecol 52:95, 1978

Gastineau DA, Kazmier FJ, Nichols WL et al. Lupus anticoagulant: an analysis of the clinical and laboratory features of 219 cases. Am J Hematol 19:265, 1985

Gerbasi FR, Bottoms S, Farag A, Mammen EF. Changes in hemostasis activity during delivery and the immediate postpartum period. Am J Obstet Gynecol 162:1158, 1990

Ginsberg JS, Hirsh J. Use of anticoagulants during pregnancy. Chest 95:156S, 1989

Griffiths HT, Liu DYT. Severe heparin osteoporosis in pregnancy. Postgrad Med J 60:424, 1984

Gruber UF, Duckert F, Fridrich R et al. Prevention of postoperative thromboembolism by dextran-40, low doses of heparin, or xanthinol nicotinate. Lancet 1:207, 1977

Gruber VF, Saldeen T, Brokop T et al. Incidences of fatal postoperative pulmonary embolism after prophylaxis with dextran-70. Br Med J 1:83, 1980

Gurewich V, Numm T, Thazhathekudyil T et al. Hemostatic effect of uniform, low dose subcutaneous heparin in surgical patients. Arch Intern Med 138:41, 1978

Guyton DP, Khayat A, Schreiber H. Pneumatic compression stockings and prostaglandin synthesis — a pathway of fibrinolysis. Crit Care Med 13:266, 1985

Heaps J, Lagasse LD. Use of the inferior vena cava clip in patients at high risk of pulmonary emoblism. Gynecol Oncol 39:227, 1990

Hohl MK, Luscher KJP, Tichy J et al. Prevention of postoperative thromboembolism by dextran-70 or low dose heaprin. Obstet Gynecol 55:497, 1980

Howell R, Fidler J, Letsky E. The risks of antenatal subcutaneous heparin prophylaxis: a controlled trial. Br J Obstet Gynaecol 90:1124, 1983

Hunter GR, Barney MF, Crapo RO, Broadbent TR, Reilly WF, Jensen RL. Perioperative warfarin therapy in combined abdominal lipectomy and intra-abdominal gynecological surgical procedures. Ann Plast Surg 25:37, 1990

Isada NB, Landy HJ, Larsen JW. Postabortal septic pelvic thrombophlebitis diagnosed with computer tomography. J Reprod Med 32:866, 1987

Jeffcoate TNA, Tindall VR. Venous thrombosis and embolism in obstetrics and gynaecology. Aust NZ J Obstet Gynaecol 5:119, 1965

Jobson VW, Homesley HD, Welander CE. Comparison of heparin and intermittent calf compression for prevention of pulmonary embolism. Gynecol Oncol 15:143, 1983

Kajanoja P, Forss M. Prevention of venous thrombosis by dipyridamole-naproxen and low dose heparin in patients undergoing hysterectomy. Ann Clin Res 13:392, 1981

Kaunitz AM, Hughes JM, Grimes DA, Smith JC, Rochat RW, Kafrissen ME. Causes of maternal mortality in the United States. Obstet Gynecol 65:605, 1985

Kierkegaard A. Incidence and diagnosis of deep vein thrombosis associated with pregnancy. Acta Obstet Gynecol Scand 62:239, 1983

Kimball AM, Hallum AV, Cates W. Deaths caused by pulmonary thromboembolism after legally induced abortion. Am J Obstet Gynecol 132:169, 1978

Knight MTN, Dawson R. Effect of intermittent compression of the arms on deep venous thrombosis in the legs. Lancet 2:1265, 1976

Lanham JG, Levin M, Brown Z et al. Prostacyclin deficiency in a young woman with recurrent venous thrombosis. Br Med J 292:435, 1986

Lao TT, DeSwiet M, Letsky E, Walters BNJ. Prophylaxis of thromboembolism in pregnancy: an alternative. Br J Obs Gyn 92:202, 1985

Laros RK, Alger LS, Thromboembolism and pregnancy. Clin Obstet Gynecol 22:871, 1979

Lawrence D, Kakkar VV. Graduated, static, external compression of the lower limb: a physiological assessment. Br J Surg 67:119, 1980

Martin B, Mulopulos GP, Bryan PJ. MRI of puerperal ovarian vein thrombosis. AJR 147:291, 1986

McCarthy TG, McQueen J, Johnstone FD et al. A comparison of low dose subcutaneous heparin and intravenous dextran-70 in the prophylaxis of deep venous thrombosis after gynaecologic surgery. J Obst Gynae Br Commonw 81:486, 1974

Mintz MC, Levy DW, Axel L et al. Puerperal ovarian vein thrombosis: MR diagnosis. AJR 149:1273, 1987

Morley GW, Lindenauer SM. Pelvic exenterative therapy for gynaecologic malignancy. Cancer 38:581, 1976

Nelson DM, Stempel LE, Brandt JT. Hereditary antithrombin III deficiency and pregnancy: report of two cases and review of the literature. Obstet Gynecol 65:848, 1985

Nicolaides AN, Fernandes e Fernandes J et al. Intermittent sequential pneumatic compression of the legs in the prevention of venous stasis and postoperative deep venous thrombosis. Surgery 87:69, 1980

Piver MS, Malfetano JH, Lele SB et al. Prophylactic anticoagulation as a possible cause of inguinal lymphocyst after radical vulvectomy and inguinal lymphadenectomy. Obstet Gynecol 62:17, 1983

Roberts VC, Cotton LT. Prevention of postoperative deep venous thrombosis in patients with malignant disease. Br Med J 1:358, 1974

Rosengarten DS, Laird Jeyasingh K et al. The failure of compression stocking (Tubigrip) to prevent deep venous thrombosis after operation. Br J Surg 57:296, 1970

Rutherford SE, Phelan JP. Deep venous thrombosis and pulmonary embolus. In: Clark SL, Phelan JP, Cotton DB (eds): Critical care obstetrics. Oradell NJ, Medical Economics Books, 1987

Sachs BP, Brown DAJ, Driscoll SG, Schulman E, Acker D, Ransil BJ, Jewett JF. Maternal mortality in Massachusetts: trends and prevention. N Engl J Med 316:667, 1987

Salzman W, Davies GC. Prophylaxis of venous thromboembolism: analysis of cost effectiveness. Ann Surg 191:207, 1980

Salzman EW, Ploet J, Bettlemann M et al. Intraoperative external pneumatic calf compression to afford longterm prophylaxis against deep vein thrombosis in urological patients. Surgery 87:239, 1980

Sigel B, Edelstein AL, Savitch L et al. Type of compression for reducing venous stasis. Arch Surg 110:171, 1975

Steiner RA, Kellerk, Luscher T, Schreiner WE. A prospective randomised trial of low molecular weight heparin-DHE and conventional heparin-DHE (with acenocoumarol) in patients undergoing gynecologic surgery. Arch Gynecol Obstet 244:141, 1989

Taberner DA, Poller L, Burnstein RW et al. Oral anticoagulants controlled by the British comparative thromboplastin versus low dose heparin in prophylaxis of deep venous thrombosis. Br Med J 1:272, 1978

Tengborn L, Bergqvist D, Matzsch T, Bergqvist A, Hedner U. Recurrent thromboembolism in pregnancy and puerperium: is there a need for thrombo-prophylaxis? Am J Obstet Gynecol 160:90, 1989

Turner GM, Cole SE, Brooks JH. The efficacy of graduated compression stockings in the prevention of postoperative deep venous thrombosis after major gynecologic surgery. Br J Obstet Gynaecol 91:588, 1984

Turpie AGG, Gallus AS, Beattie WS et al. Prevention of venous thrombosis in patients with intracranial disease by intermittent pneumatic compression of the calf. Neurology 27:435, 1977

Turpie AGG, Delmore T, Hirsh J et al. Prevention of venous thrombosis by intermittent sequential calf compression in patients with intracranial disease. Thromb Res 15:611, 1979

Vessey MP. The epidemiology of venous thromboembolism. In: Poller L (ed). Recent advances in thrombosis. London, Churchill Livingston, p 39, 1973

Virchow R. Die cellularpathologie in ihrer begrundung auf physioliche und pathologiche gewebslehre. Berlin, A Hirschwald, 1858

Walsh JJ, Bonnar J, Wright FW. A study of pulmonary embolism and deep leg thrombosis after major gynaecologic surgery using labelled fibrinogen phlebography and lung scanning. J Obstet Gynaecol Br Commonw 81:311, 1974

Weiner CP. Diagnosis and management of thromboembolic disease in pregnancy. Clin Obstet Gynecol 28:107, 1985

Wise PH, Hall AJ. Heparin induced osteopenia in pregnancy. Br Med J 281:110, 1980

CHAPTER 25

# Elective hip surgery

Andre Planes   Marc Silsiguen   Nicole Vochelle

## Introduction

Among the methods proposed to prevent deep vein thrombosis (DVT) after total hip replacement (THR), we evaluated aspirin (ASP), dextran (DEX), fixed doses of unfractionated heparin (FDUH), fixed doses of unfractionated heparin plus dihydroergotamine (FDUH+DHE), antivitamin K (AVK), adjusted doses of unfractionated heparin (ADUH), intermittent pneumatic compression (IPC), and low molecular weight heparin. The interesting new method of FDUH associated with antithrombin III (Francis, 1989) was not supported by a sufficient number of patients to be realistically appraised.

A consensus now exists on the necessity of a bilateral venographic assessment performed between day 10 to 14, to define the rate of postoperative DVT after THR (Sandler, 1984; Winter-Christensen, 1987; Hoek, 1988, Cruickshank, 1989). Thus, we performed a computer-assisted search (Medline) of the literature as well as manual search on all the papers reporting the venographic incidence of DVT in prospective trials. We rejected trials where DVT was detected by the fibrinogen uptake test (FUT) and dose ranging studies of the same drug.

To evaluate the possibilities of each method, we performed an informal meta-analysis with the results obtained. We pooled the data, compared the means by using the $Chi^2$ test and calculated the relative risk reduction. We used the method of Simonneau and Leizorovicz (1991).

We successively defined the natural history of the disease, the relative risk reduction observed in trials performed against placebo, trials comparing two methods, and lastly we determined the observed rates of DVT with each of these method of prevention.

**Table 25.1**
Methods of prophylaxis against placebo (PLA)

| Method | Authors | Control group n | Control group DVT (%) | Treatment group n | Treatment group DVT (%) | ×2 | % relative risk reduction |
|---|---|---|---|---|---|---|---|
| ASP | Soreff et al, 1975<br>Shondorf et al, 1976<br>Harris et al, 1977 | 80 | 46% | 95 | 39% | 0.67<br>p=0.33 | 16% |
| IPC | Gallus et al, 1983<br>Hull et al, 1990 | 205 | 50% | 195 | 26% | 22.6<br>p<0.0001 | 47% |
| LDUH+DHE | Beisaw et al, 1988<br>Lassen et al, 1988 | 162 | 54% | 175 | 29% | 20.9<br>p<0.00001 | 47% |
| DEX | Evarts et al, 1971<br>Welin-Berger, 1982 | 74 | 47% | 66 | 17% | 13.5<br>p<0.0001 | 65% |
| LMWH | Turpie et al, 1986<br>Hoek et al, 1989 | 149 | 52% | 147 | 14% | 46.9<br>p<0.0001 | 73% |

ASP = Aspirin   IPC = Intermittent pneumatic compression
LDUH+DHE = Low dose unfractionated heparin plus dihydroergotamine
DEX = Dextran   LMWH = Low molecular weight heparin

## Natural history of DVT after THR

We retrieved 11 trials where the control group did not receive a form of protection (Evarts and Feil, 1971; Harris et al, 1977; Moskowitz et al, 1978; Ishak and Morley, 1981; Sikorski et al, 1981; Gallus et al, 1983; Turpie et al, 1986; Beisaw et al, 1988; Lassen et al, 1988; Hoek et al, 1989; Hull et al, 1990). In a total of 908 patients, 459 developed DVT (50.5%) (95% CI: 47.2%-53.7%). Of these DVT, 222 were proximal to the calf (24.4%) (95% CI: 22.7%-28.4%). The incidence was the same in trials reported from Europe as in those from North America.

The natural history of pulmonary embolism (PE) after elective hip surgery is still unknown. No large study has screened the patients by mandatory scintigraphic ventilation and perfusion scans and by a pulmonary angiographic assessment. The observed rates of fatal PE varied between 1.4% (Johnson et al, 1977) and 3.4% (Coventry et al, 1973). It is probable that the natural rate of PE is high. In patients protected by aspirin, Guyer et al (1982) found a PE incidence of 19% and McCardel et al (1990) of 12.6%. Harris et al (1984) found an incidence of 23% of PE in patients receiving various methods of prophylaxis, 83% of them being silent. With prophylaxis with AVK, Guyer et al (1982) in the same study found a reduction of PE to 6%. Recently, Eriksson et al (1991), in patients protected by standard heparin, found an incidence of PE of 30.6% and of 12.3% in patients receiving a LMWH. Thus, as now acknowledged, a reduction in DVT is followed by a reduction in PE. But the relationship is not necessarily a linear one.

Moreover, Johnson et al (1977) observed an incidence of 83 fatal PE, 1.04% (confirmed by autopsy in 88% of cases) in 7959 THR performed between 1962 and 1973. Of these fatal

**Table 25.2**
Comparison of method of prophylaxis

| Authors | Control group | | Treatment group | | ×2 | % relative risk reduction |
|---|---|---|---|---|---|---|
| | n | DVT (%) | n | DVT (%) | | |
| Harris et al, 1974; 1985 | *Aspirin* 141 | 28% | *Dextran* 100 | 19% | 1.95 p=0.11 NS | 31% |
| Harris et al, 1974 | *Aspirin* 50 | 36% | *Antivitamin K* 51 | 20% | 2.61 p=0.064 NS | 45% |
| Harris et al, 1974 Francis et al, 1983 | *Antivitamin K* 104 | 20% | *Dextran* 93 | 35% | 5.02 p=0.016 | 43% |
| Paiement et al, 1987 | *Antivitamin K* 72 | 17% | *IPC* 66 | 17% | NS | 0% |
| Leyvraz et al, 1983 Taberner et al, 1989 | *FDUH* 73 | 33% | *ADUH* 78 | 7.7% | 13.5 p<0.0001 | 76% |
| Barre et al, 1987 Leyvraz et al, 1988 Dechavanne et al, 1989 | *LMWH* 279 | 11% | *ADUH* 279 | 12% | 0.5 NS | 0% |
| Ericksson et al, 1988 Lassen et al, 1990 Mätzsch et al, 1990; 1991 | *LMWH* 275 | 14% | *Dextran* 283 | 28% | 15.1 p<0.00005 | 50% |

FDUH = Fixed doses of unfractionated heparin
ADUH = Adjusted doses of unfractionated heparin

PE, 9.7% were observed in the first week, 54.2% in the second week, 22.9% in the third week, 8.4% in the fourth week, and 4.8% subsequently. This study suggests the need for prolonged protection of the patient after discharge from hospital.

# Summary of results presented in Tables 25.1-25.3

### Aspirin (ASP)
Protection given by aspirin is poor. A recent unpublished meta-analysis (Antiplatelet Triallist Collaboration Group) is in favour of aspirin protection against PE. But the study

**Table 25.3**
Observed rates of DVT with different methods

| Methods and authors | Number of DVT (%) | | 95% Confidence interval |
|---|---|---|---|
| **ASP** Harris et al, 1974; 1977 Harris et al, 1982; 1985 Soreff et al, 1975 | 388 | 42.7% | 37.7%-47.6% |
| **DEX** Evarts et al, 1971 Harris et al, 1974 Nillius and Nylander, 1979 Welin-Berger et al, 1982 Francis et al, 1983 Fredin et al, 1984 Lassen et al, 1990 | 456 | 38.4% | 33.9%-42.9% |
| **FDUH** Collins et al, 1988 After 1988: Planes et al, 1988 Levine et al, 1991 Ericksson et al, 1991 | 371 465 | 21.0% 26.0% | 16.8%-25.1% 22.0%-30.0% |
| Proximal DVT | 387 | 18.3% | 14.4%-22.1% |
| **FDUH + DHE** Fredin et al, 1984 Kakkar et al, 1985 Beisaw et al, 1988 Lassen et al, 1988 Leyvraz et al, 1988 Estoppey et al, 1989 | 925 | 17.3% | 14.8%-19.7% |
| Proximal DVT | 104 | 11.2% | 9.2%-13.2% |
| **IPC** Gallus et al, 1983 Harris et al, 1985 Paiement et al, 1987 Hull et al, 1990 Woolson et al, 1991 | 305 | 23.3% | 18.5%-28.0% |
| Proximal DVT | 337 | 14.8% | 11.0%-18.6% |
| **AVK** Harris et al, 1974 Francis et al, 1983 Paiement et al, 1987 | 176 | 18.7% | 12.9%-23.5% |
| Proximal DVT | 123 | 4.8% | 1.0%- 8.5% |
| **ADUH** Leyvraz et al, 1983 Leyvraz et al, 1989 Barre et al, 1987 Dechavanne et al, 1989 | 370 | 17.0% | 13.1%-20.8% |
| Proximal DVT | 370 | 13.2% | 9.7%-16.6% |

| **ENOXAPARIN** | | | |
|---|---|---|---|
| Turpie et al, 1986 | 536 | 14.5% | 11.5%-17.5% |
| Planes et al, 1988 | | | |
| Lassen et al, 1990 | | | |
| Levine et al, 1991 | | | |
| Proximal DVT | 536 | 5.0% | 3.1%- 6.8% |

Enoxaparin was included in this table due to the large number of published papers with venographically assessed patients

previously reported (Guyer et al, 1982) does not support this concept. So aspirin may be considered in the current state of the art, as a weak antithrombotic protector.

### Unfractionated heparin in standard doses (LDUH)
It has been demonstrated by Collins et al (1988) that LDUH is effective in preventing DVT and PE. Analysis of venographically controlled trials performed after 1988 confirm this assertion. However, the protection remains inferior in comparison to other methods. The increased risk of bleeding, according to Collins, is about one half to two thirds, with the absolute excess being small (about 2%) (Collins et al, 1988).

### Dihydroergotamine plus fixed doses of unfractionated heparin (FDUH+DHE)
This does possibly afford a better protection against proximal DVT, but rare problems of ergotism have been reported (Van den Berg et al, 1982) which have led to this drug being rejected in some countries, such as France and USA.

### Dextran (DEX)
The relative risk reduction by dextran is 65%, but the rate of total DVT remains high. Its effectiveness against PE is the result of preventing growth and extension of the thrombus, probably because of its interference with fibrin polymerisation. It is less effective than the AVK and even less so than LMWHs. The risks consist of overloading the circulation and allergic reactions. In conclusion, it is now a secondary antithrombotic drug. Its synergistic effect in association with other more effective methods has to be defined.

### Antivitamin K (AVK)
Oral anticoagulants have been demonstrated to be more effective than aspirin or dextran, and as effective as IPC. The low dose regimen popularised by the MacMaster University is certainly an attractive method for reducing the bleeding risk. The International Sensitivity Index (ISI) of the reagent must be clearly defined, and the results expressed with the International Normalised Ratio (INR) to obtain and maintain the range of INR between 2 and 3 (Hirsh et al, 1989). Also, the AVK drugs have been demonstrated to be effective in reducing the incidence of fatal PE (Coventry et al, 1973; Amstutz et al, 1989). A comparison with LMWHs is necessary.

### Intermittent Pneumatic Compression (IPC)
IPC reduces the relative risk by 47% without any risk of bleeding or associated complications. The reduction is comparable to that obtained with AVK. But the rate of proximal DVT remains high (14%). The combination with other methods should be explored.

An improved efficacy was not observed when combined with Dextran (Harris et al, 1985).

### Adjusted doses of unfractionated heparin (ADUH)
ADUH have been demonstrated to be more effective in reducing the rates of total and proximal DVT than FDUH. ADUH was as effective as Kabi 3165 (Fragmin[R] LMWH) and CY216 (Fraxiparin[R] LMWH) (which showed a significant superiority in preventing proximal DVT). However, it is difficult to obtain and maintain the adjustment on a day to day basis (Leyvraz et al, 1988).

### Low molecular weight heparin (LMWH)
LMWH reduces the risk by 73% with the advantages of simplicity of administration and elimination of the need for laboratory monitoring. In comparative trials, LMWH was found superior to unfractionated heparin, to dextran and to FDUH+DHE. These trials were conducted with Enoxaparin (Turpie et al, 1986; Planes et al, 1988; Lassen et al, 1990; Levine et al, 1991); Kabi 2165 (Fragmin[R]) (Barre et al, 1987; Dechavanne et al, 1989; Mätzsch et al, 1990; 1991); CY216 (Fraxiparin[R])(Leyvraz et al, 1989); an association of LMWH and DHE[R] (Haas et al, 1987; Lassen et al, 1988); and Organon 10172 (Lomoparan[R]) (Hoek et al, 1989). In Europe, they are given before operation but they may be used after operation (Turpie et al, 1986; Levine et al, 1991). The question of the superiority of a preoperative administration is still debatable. Tolerance has been demonstrated to be better than that to FDUH (Planes et al, 1988; Levine et al, 1991) but is still disputed (ten Cate et al, 1991). LMWH is now the prophylactic treatment of choice.

### Type of anaesthesia
The type of anaesthesia is not a method of prophylaxis by itself, but is of interest. Prins and Hirsh (1990) in a recent meta-analysis found a relative risk reduction of 50% when a lumbar regional anaesthetic was administered instead of general anaesthesia. However, this advantage is lost when an effective method of prophylaxis is given to the patient (Fredin et al, 1984; 1986; Planes et al, 1991).

# Conclusions

- Aspirin is slightly better than nothing.
- FDUH are insufficiently protective.
- DHE possibly adds a protection against proximal DVT yet with some inherent risks.
- Dextran has its own limitations and is inferior to LMWHs.
- IPC is very attractive, without risk and the combined effect with LMWHs should be investigated.
- ADUH is very attractive, but difficult to manage and for that reason inferior to LMWH.
- LMWH is the treatment of choice. Presently, since each LMWH preparation is considered as a different entity, each drug must be assessed separately in independent trials. The administration must conform to the recommendations of the manufacturers and to legal accreditations.

# References

Amstutz HC, Friscia DA, Dorey F, Carney BT. Warfarin prophylaxis to prevent mortality from pulmonary embolism after total hip replacement. J Bone J Surg 71A:321, 1989

Barre J, Pfister G, Potron G et al. Efficacité et tolérance comparée du Kabi 2165 et l'héparine standard dans la prévention des thromboses veineuses profondes au cours des prothèses totales de hanche. J Mal Vascul 2:90, 1987

Beisaw NE, Comerota A, Groth HE et al. Dihydroergotamine/heparin in the prevention of deep vein thrombosis after total hip replacement. J Bone J Surg 70A:2, 1988

Collins R, Scrimgeour A, Yusuf S, Peto R. Reduction in fatal pulmonary embolism and venous thrombosis by perioperative administration of subcutaneous heparin. N Engl J Med 318:1162, 1988

Coventry MB, Nolan DR, Beckenbaugh RD. Delayed prophylactic anticoagulation. A study of results and complications in 2,012 total hip arthroplasties. J Bone J Surg 55A:1487, 1973

Cruickshank MK, Levine MN, Hirsh J et al. An evaluation of impedance plethysmography and $^{125}$I-fibrinogen leg scanning in patients following hip surgery. Thromb Haemostas 62:830, 1989

Dechavanne M, Ville D, Berruyer M, Trepo F, Dalery F, Clermont N, Lerat JL, Moyen B, Fischer LP, Kher A, Barbier P. Randomised trial of a low-molecular weight heparin (Kabi 2165) versus adjusted dose subcutaneous standard heparin in the prophylaxis of deep vein thrombosis after elective hip surgery. Haemostasis 19:5, 1989

Eriksson BI, Zachrisson BE, Teger-Nilsson et al. Thrombosis prophylaxis with low molecular weight heparin in total hip replacement. Br J Surg 75:1053, 1988

Eriksson BI, Kalebo P, Anthmyr B et al. Prevention of deep vein thrombosis and pulmonary embolism after total hip replacement. J Bone J Surg 73A:484, 1991

Estoppey D, Hochreiter J, Breyer GH et al. Org 10172 (Lomoparan) versus heparin-DHE in prevention of thromboembolism in total hip replacement — a multicentre trial. Thromb Haemost 62:356, abstract, 1989

Evarts CM and Feil E. Prevention of thromboembolic disease after elective surgery of the hip. J Bone J Surg 53a:1271, 1971

Francis CW, Marder VJ, Evarts CM et al. Two-step warfarin therapy. JAMA 249:374, 1983

Francis CW, Pellegrini VD, Marder VJ et al. Prevention of venous thrombosis after total hip replacement. J Bone J Surg 71A:327, 1989

Fredin HO, Rosberg B, Arborelius M et al. On thromboembolism after total hip replacement in epidural analgesia: a controlled study of dextran 70 and low dose heparin combined with dihydroergotamine. Br J Surg 71:58, 1984

Fredin HO and Rosberg B. Anaesthetic techniques and thromboembolism in total hip arthroplasty. Eur J Anaesthes 3:273, 1986

Gallus A, Raman K, Darby T. Venous thrombosis after elective hip replacement. The influence of preventive intermittent calf compression and surgical technique. Br J Surg 70:17, 1983

Guyer RD, Booth RE, Rothman RH. The detection and prevention of pulmonary embolism in total hip replacement. J Bone J Surg 64A:1040, 1982

Haas S, Stemberger A, Fritsche HM et al. Prophylaxis of deep vein thrombosis in high risk patients undergoing total hip replacement with low molecular weight heparin plus dihydroergotamine. Arznei Forsch Drug Res 37(II):839, 1987

Harris WH, Salzman EW, Athanasoulis C. Comparison of warfarin, low molecular weight heparin, dextran, aspirin and subcutaneous heparin in prevention of venous thromboembolism following total hip replacement. J Bone Joint Surg 56:1552, 1974

Harris WH, Salzman EW, Athanasoulis C et al. Aspirin prophylaxis of venous thromboembolisn after total hip replacement. N Engl J Med 297:1246, 1977

Harris WH, Athanasoulis C, Waltman AC et al. High and low dose aspirin prophylaxis against venous thromboembolic disease in total hip replacement. J Bone J Surg 64A:63, 1982

Harris WH, McKusick K, Athanasoulis C et al. Detection of pulmonary emboli after total hip replacement using serial $C^{15}O_2$ pulmonary scans. J Bone J Surg 66a; 1388, 1984

Harris WH, Athanasoulis CA, Waltman AC, Salzman EW. Prophylaxis of deep-vein thrombosis after total hip replacement. J Bone Joint Surg Am 67A:57, 1985

Hirsh J, Poller L, Deykin D et al. Optimal therapeutic range for oral anticoagulants. Chest 95:55, 1989

Hoek JA, Lensing AWA, ten Cate JW et al. The clinical utility of objective diagnostic tests for diagnosing deep vein thrombosis of the legs. Br J Clin Pract 43:26, 1989

Hoek JA, Nurmohamed MT, ten Cate JW et al. Prevention of deep vein thrombosis following total hip replacement by a low molecular weight heparinoid (Org10172). Thromb Haemost 62:Abstract 1637, 1989a

Hull RD, Raskob GE, Gent M et al. Effectiveness of intermittent pneumatic leg compression for preventing deep vein thrombosis after total hip replacement. JAMA 263:2313, 1990

Ishak MA and Morley KD. Deep venous thrombosis after total hip arthroplasty: a prospective controlled study to determine the prophylactic effect of graded pressure stocking. Br J Surg 68:429, 1981

Johnson R, Green JR, Charnley J. Pulmonary embolism and its prophylaxis following the Charnley total hip replacement. Clin Orthop 127:123, 1977

Kakkar VV, Fox PJ, Murray WJG et al. Heparin and dihydroergotamine prophylaxis against thromboembolism after hip arthroplasty. J Bone J Surg 67B:538, 1985

Lassen MR, Borris LC, Christensen HM, et al. Heparin/dihydroergotamine for venous thrombosis prophylaxis: comparison of low dose heparin and low molecular weight heparin in hip surgery. Br J Surg 75:686, 1988

Lassen MR, Borris LC, Hauch O et al. Enoxaparin versus dextran 70 in the prevention of postoperative deep vein thrombosis after total hip replacement. A Danish multicentre study. Proceedings of the Danish Enoxaparin Symposium, February 3, 1990

Levine M, Hirsh J, Gent M et al. Prevention of deep vein thrombosis after elective hip surgery. Ann Int Med 114:545, 1991

Leyvraz PF, Richard J, Bachmann F et al. Adjusted versus fixed dose subcutaneous heparin in the prevention of deep vein thrombosis after total hip replacement. N Engl J Med 309:954, 1983

Leyvraz PF, Bachmann F, Vuilleumier B et al. Adjusted subcutaneous heparin versus heparin plus dihydroergotamine in prevention of deep vein thrombosis after total hip arthroplasty. J Arthroplasty 3:81, 1988

Leyvraz PF et al. Prevention of postoperative deep vein thrombosis in elective total hip replacement by low molecular weight heparin (CY216). Satellite symposium (Fraxiparine, Tokyo), 1989

McCardel BR, Lachiewicz PF, Jones K. Aspirin prophylaxis and surveillance of pulmonary embolism and deep vein thrombosis in total hip arthroplasty. J Arthroplasty 5:181, 1990

Mätzsch T, Bergqvist D, Fredin H, Hedner U. Low molecular weight heparin compared with Dextran as prophylaxis against thrombosis after total hip replacement. Acta Chir Scand, 156:445, 1990

Mätzsch T, Bergqvist D, Fredin H, Hedner U, Lindhagen A, Nistor L. Comparison of the thromboprophylactic effect of a low molecular weight heparin versus dextran in total hip replacement. Thromb Haemorrh Disorders 3:25, 1991

Moskowitz PA, Ellenberg SS, Feffer HL et al. Low dose heparin for prevention of venous thromboembolism in total hip arthroplasty and surgical repair of hip fractures. J Bone J Surg 60A:1065, 1978

Nillius A, Nylander G. Deep vein thrombosis after total hip replacement: a clinical and phlebographic study. Br J Surg 66:324, 1979

Paiement G, Weissinger SJ, Waltman AC et al. Low dose warfarin versus external pneumatic compression for prophylaxis against venous thromboembolism following total hip replacement. J Arthoplasty 2:23, 1987

Planes A, Vochelle N, Mazas F, Mansat C, Zucman J, Landais A, Pascariello JC, Weill D, Butel J. Prevention of postoperative venous thrombosis: a randomised trial comparing unfractionated heparin with low molecular weight heparin in patients undergoing total hip replacement. Thromb Haemost 60(3):407, 1988

Planes A, Vochelle N, Fagola M et al. Prevention of deep vein thrombosis after total hip replacement. The effect of low molecular weight heparin with spinal and general anaesthesia. J Bone J Surg 73B:418, 1991

Prins MH, Hirsh J. A comparison of general anaesthesia and regional anaesthesia as a risk factor for deep vein thrombosis following hip surgery: a critical review. Thromb Haemost 64:497, 1990

Sandler DA, Duncan JS, Ward P et al. Diagnosis of deep vein thrombosis: comparison of clinical evaluation, ultrasound, plethysmography, and venoscan with x-ray venogram. Lancet ii:716, 1984

Schondorf TH, Hey D. Combined administration of low dose heparin and aspirin as prophylaxis of deep vein thrombosis after hip joint surgery. Haemostasis 5:250, 1976

Sikorski JM, Hampson WG, Staddon GE. The natural history and aetiology of deep vein thrombosis after total hip replacement. J Bone J Surg 63B:171, 1981

Simonneau G, Leizorovicz A. Conférence de consensus. Document de travail. Faculté de Médecine Xavier Bichat. 8 Mars1991

Soreff J, Johnsson H, Diener L et al. Acetylsalicylic acid in a trial to diminish thromboembolic complications after elective hip surgery. Acta Orthop Scand 46:246, 1975

Taberner DA, Poller L, Thomson JM et al. Randomised study of adjusted versus fixed low dose heparin prophylaxis of deep vein thrombosis in hip surgery. Br J Surg 736:933, 1989

ten Cate JW. Low molecular weight heparins in the prophylaxis of venous thrombosis. A meta-analysis. International symposium of low molecular weight heparins and related polysaccharides. Munich, June 27-28, 1991

Turpie AGG, Levine MN, Hirsh J et al. A randomised controlled trial of a low molecular weight heparin (Enoxaparin) to prevent deep vein thrombosis in patients undergoing elective hip surgery. N Engl J Med 315:925, 1986

Van den Berg E, Rumpf KD, Frohlich H et al. Vascular spasm during thromboembolism prophylaxis with heparin-dihydroergotamine. Lancet ii:268, 1982

Welin-Berger T, Bygdeman S, Mebius C. Deep vein thrombosis following hip surgery. Relation to activated factor X inhibitor activity: effect of heparin and dextran. Acta Orthop Scand 53:937, 1982

Winter-Christensen S, Wille-Jorgensen P, Kjaer L et al. Contact thermography, $^{99m}$Tc-plasmin scintimetry and $^{99m}$Tc-plasmin scintigraphy as screening methods for deep venous thrombosis following major hip surgery. Thromb Haemost 58:831, 1987

Woolson ST, Watt M. Intermittent pneumatic compression to prevent proximal deep venous thrombosis during and after total hip replacement. J Bone J Surg 73A:507, 1991

CHAPTER 26

# Thromboprophylaxis in hip fracture patients

Michael R Lassen    Lars C Borris

## Introduction

Hip fracture, femoral neck fracture, intertrochanteric and subtrochanteric femoral fracture, are conditions with an increasing incidence in most western countries, probably due to improved general health conditions which give a longer life expectancy. The number of fractures, however, is too great to be explained by the increase in mean age of the population alone. The presence of more women than men with hip fractures has resulted in the suggestion that there might be a relation to an increase in the incidence of metabolic bone disease (osteoporosis) in women but, most certainly, other contributing factors are involved also. Not surprisingly, the treatment of these patients places an enormous burden on the hospital resources and occupies a significant part of the work in the orthopaedic wards. Apart from the surgical management of the fractures, many resources are spent on the treatment of postoperative complications which are very common.

Hip fracture is an important cause of mortality with rates up to about 30% within one year after the injury in some series (Colbert and O'Muircheartaigh, 1976). In previous reports on large series of patients from Scandinavian countries, not only was the mortality found to be especially increased within the first months after the fracture (Jensen and Tøndevold, 1979; Dahl, 1980), but also the long-term survival was influenced and in one of these reports survival did not parallel that expected until after 1.6 years (Jensen and Tøndevold, 1979). In a recent retrospective study including 405 patients, who had surgical treatment for hip fractures, risk factors associated with death within 1 year included increasing age, male sex and the presence of dementia or congestive cardiac failure (Clayer and Bauze, 1989).

Postoperative complications other than death are common in hip fracture patients and apart from surgical and medical complications including wound infection, non-union, avascular necrosis of the femoral head, urinary tract infections, lung infections, cardiac failure, cardiac arrythmias, electrolyte and fluid imbalance, and pressure sores, thromboembolic complications are very common. Since the classic study by Sevitt and Gallagher (1959), venous thromboembolism has been recognised as a common cause of mortality and morbidity after hip fracture. In a retrospective study by Riska (1970) comprising 470 patients treated for hip fractures, without the use of pharmacologic thromboprophylaxis, the overall mortality rate within 1 month of the injury was 18.5%. Of the 87 patients who died, autopsy was performed in all but 5 and in 17 patients (19.5%), death was found to be due to pulmonary embolism (PE) which was almost as many deaths from lung infections. In other retrospective studies, the incidence of thromboembolism has been rather low after hip fractures (Clayer and Bauze, 1989), mostly because the clinical diagnosis of deep vein thrombosis (DVT) and PE is very unreliable causing some thromboembolic events to be erroneously registered as primary pulmonary or cardiac complications. An autopsy study showed PE in 46% and DVT in 83% of patients who died after femoral neck fracture (Freeark et al, 1967). The prevalence of DVT after hip fractures varies in different reports depending on the time of diagnosis, the diagnostic method used, and the use of thromboprophylaxis. In studies on patients without prophylaxis the preoperative prevalence of venographic DVT was about 12-15%, depending on the time that elapsed since the injury, and the postoperative prevalance was about 45% (Freeark et al, 1967; Stevens et al, 1968). Most of the thrombi were proximal, clinically silent, involved the injured as well as the uninjured extremity, and were frequently bilateral. In a more recent study, the preoperative frequency of venographic DVT was 9% and the additional postoperative frequency 11% in patients having perioperative prophylaxis with dextran (Roberts et al, 1990).

The aim of this chapter is to review the value of prophylactic modalities in hip fracture patients.

## Oral anticoagulants

In 1941 Butt et al reported that coumarin anticoagulants isolated from spoiled sweet clover (Melitolus alba) were able to prolong the coagulation and prothrombin time of the blood. The first modern clinical study in hip fracture patients using an oral anticoagulant (phenindione) in the prevention of thromboembolic complications was the classic study by Sevitt and Gallagher published in 1959. Although the methodology used has been criticised, the results inaugurated a new era in the prevention of these often fatal complications. The study comprised 300 elderly patients, 150 of whom were allocated to prophylaxis with phenindione and the rest acting as controls. The end points of the study were clinical symptoms of DVT, PE, and autopsy findings of thromboembolic complications. The number of patients who died of fatal PE was lower in the phenindione group than in the control group and there was a reduction in clinically diagnosed DVT from 28.7% to 2.7% (Table 26.1) Subsequently, Borgström et al (1965) confirmed the findings of Sevitt and Gallagher, by prophylactic treatment with dicoumarol in hip fracture patients, but in this study venography for the diangosis of DVT was mandatory in all patients. Table 26.1 shows published prophylaxis studies in hip fracture patients comparing oral anticoagulation with no prophylaxis. Although the methodology varies between the studies, the overall trend is a better efficacy of oral anticoagulation compared with the control, and by compilation of data on mortality from all studies, it appears that oral anticoagulation can reduce the total mortality within the first month of fracture from 22.5% to 16.5%. To investigate whether oral

**Table 26.1**
Oral anticoagulation versus no prophylaxis in hip fracture patients

| Reference | Patients n | Oral anticoagulation | | | | No prophylaxis | | | |
|---|---|---|---|---|---|---|---|---|---|
| | | DVT | PE fatal | Deaths | Bleeding | DVT | PE fatal | Deaths | Bleeding |
| Sevitt & Gallagher, 1959 | 300 | 4/150 | 2 | 25 | 35 | 43/150 | 11 | 42 | 14 |
| Borgström et al, 1965 | 48 | 2/ 23 | 0 | 2 | 1 | 14/ 25 | 2 | 3 | 0 |
| Eskeland et al, 1966 | 200 | 10/100 | 1 | 19 | 6 | 22/100 | 7 | 24 | 3 |
| Salzman et al, 1966 | 166 | 6/ 83 | 1 | 20 | 29 | 18/ 83 | 4 | 22 | 20 |
| Hamilton et al, 1970 | 76 | 10/ 38 | 0 | 4 | 18 | 18/ 38 | 1 | 5 | 6 |
| Morris et al, 1976 | 149 | 23/ 75 | 0 | 16 | 17 | 50/ 74 | 6 | 23 | 7 |
| Powers et al, 1989 | 128 | 13/ 65 | 0 | 2 | 6 | 29/ 63 | 0 | 1 | 6 |

DVT = Deep vein thrombosis  PE = Pulmonary embolism

anticoagulation should start before or after operation, Myhre et al (1973) reported a tendency in favour of the preoperative administration although the difference was not statistically significant. A drawback of oral anticoagulation is an increased risk of operative and postoperative bleeding and the need for laboratory monitoring, and today these compounds are not much used for routine prophylaxis outside North America.

# Dextran

Dextran, a polysaccharide, was originally introduced in the 1940s for use as a plasma expander. One side effect of dextran infusion was a bleeding tendency and this led to intensive research on the mode of action of dextran on haemostasis (Koekenberg, 1961). In the first placebo controlled study with dextran prophylaxis in hip fracture patients by Ahlberg et al (1968), it was found that patients prophylactically treated with Dextran 70 had a significantly lower incidence of venographic DVT than patients in the placebo group. Six of 39 patients in the dextran group died during the study compared with 14 of 45 in the control group (n.s.) Autopsy was performed in all cases, and 2 deaths, both in the control group, were due to pulmonary embolism (Table 26.2). Four similar studies confirmed the superiority of dextran to placebo but in 2 other placebo controlled studies, dextran was not effective (Darke, 1972; Daniel et al, 1972) (Table 26.2). However, direct comparison between studies is not possible due to differences in the dextran regimens used and in most of the studies there is not enough information to make a reasonable comparison on bleeding complications. In a number of studies the thromboprophylactic efficacy and safety of dextran was compared with oral anticoagulation in hip fracture patients and in all studies the regimens were comparable in terms of efficacy. In one study it was emphasised that the bleeding tendency seemed to be less pronounced with dextran than with warfarin (Bergqvist et al, 1972) (Table 26.3). A combined regimen of dextran and oral anticoagulation was compared with dextran alone by Korvald et al (1973). Even though there was a significant

**Table 26.2**
Dextran 70 versus placebo in hip fracture patients

| Reference | Patients n | Dextran 70 DVT | PE fatal | Deaths | Bleeding | Placebo DVT | PE fatal | Deaths | Bleeding |
|---|---|---|---|---|---|---|---|---|---|
| Ahlberg et al, 1968 | 94 | 5/39 | 0 | 6 | — | 16/45 | 2 | 14 | — |
| Johnsson et al, 1968 | 34 | 1/17 | 0 | 0 | 0 | 9/17 | 0 | 0 | 0 |
| Myhre and Holen, 1969 | 110 | 11/55 | 0 | 3 | 1 | 122/55 | 2 | 6 | 0 |
| Stadil, 1970 | 64 | 6/34 | — | — | — | 11/32 | — | — | — |
| Daniel et al, 1972 | 66 | 21/35 | — | — | — | 19/31 | — | — | — |
| Darke et al, 1972 | 24 | 1/12 | — | — | — | 1/12 | — | — | — |
| Bergqvist et al, 1979a | 141 | 33/70 | 0 | 2 | 0 | 64/71 | 0 | 3 | 0 |

For abbreviation see table 26.1

difference in favour of the combination, the authors themselves recommended using dextran alone because the vast majority of the thrombi diagnosed in both groups were limited to the calf veins. Their conclusion, however, may not be valid because the study used screening with the fibrinogen uptake test (FUT), a technique recently shown to be inadequate in hip fracture patients because many thrombi in the proximal veins are overlooked (Faunø et al, 1990). In another study, dextran 70 combined with dihydroergotamine (DHE) was compared with dextran 70 alone and a tenfold decrease in FUT detected DVT was observed in the combination group compared with dextran alone (Bergqvist et al, 1984). However, two later studies failed to confirm this observation (Fredin et al, 1985; Rørbæk-Madsen et al,

**Table 26.3**
Dextran 70 versus oral anticoagulation in hip fracture patients

| Reference | Patients n | Dextran 70 DVT | PE fatal | Deaths | Bleeding | Oral anticoagulation DVT | PE fatal | Deaths | Bleeding |
|---|---|---|---|---|---|---|---|---|---|
| Myhre and Holen, 1969 | 105 | 11/55 | 0 | 3 | 1 | 9/50 | 1 | 4 | 3 |
| Bronge et al, 1971 | 135 | 27/74 | — | — | 0 | 21/61 | 0 | 0 | 1 |
| Bergqvist et al, 1972 | 159 | 24/75 | — | 9 | 0 | 17/63 | — | 12 | 5 |
| Burcharth et al, 1973 | 99 | 0/53 | 1 | 5 | 3 | 1/46 | 0 | 5 | 6 |
| Bergqvist and Dahlgren, 1973 | 87 | 19/43 | 0 | 1 | 0 | 16/32 | 1 | 2 | 1 |

For abbreviations see table 26.1

**Table 26.4**
Dextran 70 versus Dextran 70 + Dihydroergotamine in hip fracture patients

| Reference | Patients n | Dextran 70 DVT | PE fatal | Deaths | Bleeding | Dextran 70 + Dihydroergotamine DVT | PE fatal | Deaths | Bleeding |
|---|---|---|---|---|---|---|---|---|---|
| Bergqvist et al, 1984 | 68 | 11/36 | 0 | 1 | — | 1/32 | 0 | 1 | — |
| Fredin et al, 1985 | 55 | 5/27 | 0 | 2 | 110/28 | 1 | 1 | 1 | |
| Rørbaek-Madsen et al, 1988 | 45 | 4/21 | — | — | — | 6/24 | — | — | — |

For abbreviations see table 26.1

1988) (Table 26.4). Although different regimens of dextran have been introduced, the standard regimen mostly used today is infusion of the first dose (500 ml) during the operation, the second dose 4-6 hours later, and one dose on days 1 and 3 after the operation. To protect against allergic reactions it is recommended to give an infusion of hapten (Dextran 1) just before the first administration. Due to an increased risk of overloading the circulation which may result in cardiac complications, dextran may not seem to be the ideal prophylaxis for use in elderly patients with a fractured hip.

# Low dose heparin

The most intensively investigated prophylactic regimen in hip fracture patients is low dose heparin (LDH) (5000 IU) injected subcutaneously twice or thrice daily. In a study in major surgery by Kakkar et al (1972), low dose heparin was investigated in 50 patients with fracture of the hip and an incidence of 40% of FUT detected DVT was reported. This result was presented as unsatisfactory by the authors although no control group was included in the study. Several comparative studies in hip fracture patients have reported a significantly better efficacy of LDH compared with no prophylaxis, but three studies showed no effect. However, the latter were small and the design not optimal (Moskowitz et al, 1978; Svend-Hansen et al, 1981; Montrey et al, 1985) (Table 26.5). A meta-analysis by Collins et al (1988) on a number of studies concluded that LDH was significantly more efficacious than no prophylaxis, but so far no significant influence on the total mortality or on the incidence of fatal PE after hip fracture has been demonstrated by LDH in any study. In a three parallel group, placebo controlled study by Bergqvist et al (1979a) comparing LDH with a standard regimen of dextran 70, dextran was superior to heparin but the difference was not statistically significant. In a study by Alho et al (1984) comprising 734 patients with hip fractures, aspirin and warfarin were evaluated against LDH. Warfarin was the most effective in decreasing the number of postoperative thromboembolic complications. However, the methodology in this study was not optimal because it was unblinded and clinical diagnosis was used to select patients for venography (Table 26.6). Adjusted dose heparin prophylaxis that has been effective in patients undergoing total hip replacement (Leyvraz et al, 1983) was not effective in hip fracture patients in a very small study by Taberner et

**Table 26.5**
Low dose heparin versus placebo in hip fracture patients

| Reference | Patients n | Low dose heparin DVT | PE fatal | Deaths | Bleeding | Placebo DVT | PE fatal | Deaths | Bleeding |
|---|---|---|---|---|---|---|---|---|---|
| Kakkar et al, 1972 | 50 | 20/ 50 | 0 | 4 | — | | | | |
| Gallus et al, 1973 | 46 | 3/ 23 | 0 | 0 | 0 | 11/23 | 0 | 0 | 0 |
| Checketts and Bradley, 1974 | 51 | 17/ 25 | — | — | — | 13/26 | — | — | — |
| Galasko et al, 1976 | 100 | 8/ 50 | 1 | 15 | 9 | 23/50 | 3 | 11 | 9 |
| Morris and Mitchell, 1977 | 48 | 12/ 24 | — | — | 0 | 16/24 | — | — | 0 |
| Xabregas et al, 1978 | 50 | 0/ 25 | — | — | 3 | 12/25 | — | — | 3 |
| Rogers et al, 1978 | 30 | 5/ 14 | 0 | 1 | 1 | 12/16 | 0 | 1 | 0 |
| Moskowitz et al, 1978 | 52 | 12/ 29 | 0 | 0 | 11 | 9/23 | 1 | 3 | 8 |
| Bergqvist et al, 1979a | 143 | 45/ 72 | 1 | 3 | 0 | 64/71 | 0 | 3 | 0 |
| Lahnborg et al, 1980 | 139 | 15/ 70 | 0 | 0 | — | 28/69 | 0 | 0 | — |
| Svend-Hansen, 1981 | 130 | 15/ 65 | 1 | 1 | — | 28/65 | 1 | 1 | — |
| Montrey et al, 1985 | 184 | 25/103 | — | — | 6 | 22/81 | — | — | 2 |

For abbreviations see table 26.1

**Table 26.6**
Hydroxychloroquine, aspirin and other regimens versus various controls in hip fracture patients

| Reference | Patients n | Treatment DVT | PE fatal | Deaths | Bleeding | Control DVT | PE fatal | Deaths | Bleeding |
|---|---|---|---|---|---|---|---|---|---|
| | | Hydroxychloroquine | | | | Placebo | | | |
| Chrisman et al, 1976 | 100 | 1/ 49 | 0 | 0 | 7 | 8/ 49 | 2 | 2 | 7 |
| | | Hydroxychloroquine + aspirin | | | | Placebo | | | |
| Snook et al, 1981 | 31 | 7/ 26 | 0 | 0 | 7 | 15/ 25 | 0 | 0 | 3 |
| | | Aspirin | | | | Placebo | | | |
| Snook et al, 1981 | 49 | 6/ 24 | 1 | — | 1 | 15/ 25 | 0 | 0 | 3 |
| | | | | | | Low dose heparin | | | |
| Alho et al, 1984 | 434 | 6/197 | 1 | — | — | 10/237 | 4 | — | — |
| | | | | | | Warfarin | | | |
| Alho et al, 1984 | 398 | 6/197 | 11 | — | — | 5/205 | 1 | — | — |

For abbreviations see table 26.1

**Table 26.7**
Low dose heparin + dihydroergotamine versus various controls in hip fracture patients

| Reference | Patients n | Low dose heparin + dihydroergotamine |  |  |  | Control |  |  |  |
|---|---|---|---|---|---|---|---|---|---|
|  |  | DVT | PE fatal | Deaths | Bleeding | DVT | PE fatal | Deaths | Bleeding |
|  |  |  |  |  |  | Low dose heparin |  |  |  |
| Lahnborg, 1980 | 141 | 15/ 70 | 0 | 0 | — | 12/ 71 | 0 | 2 | — |
| Bergqvist et al, 1980 | 54 | 20/ 25 | 1 | 3 | 0 | Dextran 21/ 29 | 0 | 1 | 0 |
|  |  |  |  |  |  | PZ68B |  |  |  |
| Bergqvist et al, 1980 | 54 | 20/ 25 | 1 | 3 | 0 | 21/ 29 | 1 | 4 | 3 |
|  |  |  |  |  |  | Low dose heparin + Acenocumarol |  |  |  |
| Gruber, 1985 | 372 | — | 6 | 19 | 6 | — | 4 | 21 | 7 |
|  |  |  |  |  |  | Dextran + Aspirin |  |  |  |
| Pini et al, 1985 | 83 | 12/ 41 | 0 | 0 | 2 | 14/ 42 | 0 | 2 | 3 |
| Schlag et al, 1986 | 159 | 30/ 75 | 1 | 5 | 2 | 46/ 75 | 0 | 4 | 1 |
|  |  |  |  |  |  | Placebo |  |  |  |
| Lassen et al, 1989 | 108 | 23/ 54 | 0 | 2 | 0 | 23/ 54 | 2 | 3 | 0 |
|  |  |  |  |  |  | Aspirin + dihydroergotamine |  |  |  |
| Orthner et al, 1990 | 404 | 7/211 | 3 | 19 | 21 | 18/193 | 3 | 20 | 17 |

For abbreviations see table 26.1

al (1989). In a placebo controlled study by Montrey et al (1985), LDH was compared with a mechanical prophylactic regimen (cyclic sequential compression) but both regimens failed to decrease the incidence of venographic DVT (Table 26.5). Today, LDH is probably still the most preferred regimen in hip fracture patients although it has not yet been demonstrated in a controlled clinical study whether LDH should be administered twice or thrice daily. In a review of several studies both in general and orthopaedic surgery, it was concluded that there was no indication that a thrice daily regimen was superior to a twice daily regimen in terms of efficacy, but the latter regimen caused less haemorrhage and accordingly the twice daily regimen was recommended (Bergqvist et al, 1979b).

# Low dose heparin and dihydroergotamine

In elective hip surgery a combination of LDH and DHE was more effective than LDH alone (Sagar et al, 1976). A similar comparison was made in hip fracture patients but without a confirmatory result (Lahnborg, 1980) and in a three-parallel group, placebo controlled, randomised study the combination was not significantly more effective than a placebo (Lassen et al, 1989) (Table 26.7).

**Table 26.8**
Ancrod versus placebo in hip fracture patients

| Reference | Patients n | Ancrod | | | | Placebo | | | |
|---|---|---|---|---|---|---|---|---|---|
| | | DVT | PE fatal | Deaths | Bleeding | DVT | PE fatal | Deaths | Bleeding |
| Barrie et al, 1974 | 49 | 3/10 | 0 | 1 | 1 | 5/12 | 3 | 5 | 1 |
| Lowe et al, 1978 | 105 | 24/53 | 0 | 0 | 0 | 38/52 | 0 | 1 | 5 |

For abbreviations see table 26.1

Table 26.7 lists the studies comparing LDH/DHE with different control regimens in hip fracture patients. LDH/DHE was compared with dextran 70 and a sulfated polysaccharide (PZ68B) in a study by Bergqvist et al (1980). There was no difference in the incidence of DVT in the groups, but more bleeding complications were found in the PZ68B group. These findings were confirmed in a study by Fredin et al (1982). Subsequently, Schlag et al (1986) reported a very high incidence of venographic DVT in a study comprising 159 patients, all women, with intertrochanteric fractures operatively treated with Ender nails. The study compared LDH/DHE with a combination of heparin and acenocoumarin. The incidence of DVT was 40% in the LDH/DHE group compared with 61% in the control group. The difference was statistically significant. Prophylaxis in the heparin/acenocoumarin group was adjusted on the basis of an INR between 1.6-2.8 and no differences in bleeding complications were observed between the groups. Another study compared LDH/DHE with the combination of aspirin and DHE in 404 hip fracture patients with clinically diagnosed DVT as an end point (Orthner et al, 1990). The incidence of DVT was low in both groups, but there was a significantly lower incidence of DVT in the LDH/DHE group. However, the incidence of fatal PE and total mortality did not differ between the groups. A study by Gruber et al (1985) compared LDH/DHE with a regimen of dextran 70. The results showed an equal efficacy in terms of number of deaths due to fatal PE and total mortality. The authors concluded that the regimens were comparable in efficacy with oral anticoagulants and more effective than placebo by the use of historic controls. Circulatory disturbances (ergotism) have been reported by many authors to be related to treatment with DHE and, although rather rare, they are serious and most often irreversible (Mattson et al, 1991). These complications are mostly observed in multitrauma patients, but also in patients with hip fractures (Borris et al, 1988). DHE is not recommended in traumatised patients and in patients with arteriosclerosis. Consequently, DHE does not seem to be the ideal prophylaxis to use in elderly patients with hip fractures.

# Other regimens

Ancrod has been investigated in two studies in hip fracture patients (Barrie et al, 1974; Lowe et al, 1978) but further development of this compound has been stopped (Table 26.8). In a study by Chrisman et al (1976), hydroxychloroquine was reported to be superior to placebo (Table 26.6). In combination with aspirin, hydroxychloroquine did not improve the

**Table 26.9**
General versus regional anaesthesia in hip fracture patients

| Reference | Patients n | General anaesthesia |  |  |  | Regional analgesia |  |  |  |
|---|---|---|---|---|---|---|---|---|---|
|  |  | DVT | PE fatal | Deaths | Bleeding | DVT | PE fatal | Deaths | Bleeding |
| Davis et al, 1980 | 74 | 28/37 | 2 | 7 | — | 17/37 | 0 | 3 | — |
| McKenzie et al, 1985 | 40 | 16/20 | — | 2 | — | 8/20 | — | 0 | — |
| Davis et al, 1987 | 538 | — | — | 16/279 | — | — | — | 15/259 | — |

For abbreviations see table 26.1

efficacy of aspirin but both regimens were superior to placebo (Snook et al, 1981) (Table 26.6).

## Regional anaesthesia

The technique of anaesthesia has been reported to be important with respect to postoperative thromboembolism and in a randomised study in elective hip surgery, significantly fewer of the patients operated under regional anaesthesia experienced a postoperative thromboembolic complication compared with patients operated under general anaesthesia (Modig et al, 1985). This has been confirmed in hip fracture patients in two studies (Davis et al, 1980; McKenzie et al, 1985) (Table 26.9). However, in the long term it was not demonstrated that regional anaesthesia had any better effect on mortality (survival) after hip fracture compared with general anaesthesia (Davis et al, 1987).

## Low molecular weight heparin and heparinoids

Two Danish studies in hip fracture patients compared a low molecular weight heparin (LMWH) with placebo (Lassen et al, 1989; Jorgensen et al, 1992). In both studies, FUT was used for screening and venography for confirmation of positive tests. The results were in favour of LMWH in terms of efficacy and no clinically relevant differences in blood loss or bleeding events were reported. In a number of studies, prophylaxis with LMWH has also been compared with LDH in hip fracture patients (Table 26.10). Lassen et al (1989) found a strong trend in favour of LMWH (possibly a high Beta-error) whereas other studies were inconclusive due to very low incidences (Breyer et al, 1986; Korninger et al, 1989; Pini et al, 1989). In a dose finding study with a LMWH (Enoxaparin), using bilateral venography in all patients, Barsotti et al (1990) reported a very low incidence of DVT. However, no control group was included. Wattrise et al (1990) also observed a low incidence of thromboembolism in hip fracture patients prophylactically treated with LMWH. However, the methodology used in the study was not optimal, because clinical diagnosis of DVT was used for selection of patients for venography. In a large well-designed multicentre study from Scandinavia comprising 308 hip fracture patients who were randomly allocated to

**Table 26.10**
Low molecular weight heparin versus various controls in hip fracture patients

| Reference | Patients n | Low molecular weight heparin DVT | PE fatal | Deaths | Bleeding | Control DVT | PE fatal | Deaths | Bleeding |
|---|---|---|---|---|---|---|---|---|---|
| | | | | | | Placebo | | | |
| Lassen et al, 1989 | 107 | 14/ 53 | 0 | 4 | 1 | 23/ 54 | 2 | 3 | 1 |
| Jørgensen et al, 1989 | 68 | 9/ 30 | 0 | 0 | 0 | 22/ 38 | 1 | 1 | 0 |
| | | | | | | Low dose heparin | | | |
| Breyer et al, 1986 | 140 | 5/ 70 | 0 | 0 | 0 | 7/ 70(A) | 0 | 0 | 0 |
| Lassen et al, 1989 | 107 | 14/ 53 | 0 | 4 | 1 | 23/ 54(A) | 0 | 2 | 0 |
| Korninger et al, 1989 | 68 | 3/ 35 | | | | 7/ 33 | | | |
| Monreal et al, 1989 | 90 | 14/ 32 | 0 | 2 | 2 | 6/ 30 | 0 | 3 | 3 |
| Pini et al, 1989 | 49 | 5/ 25 | 0 | 0 | 2 | 7/ 24 | 0 | 2 | 1 |
| Barsotti et al, 1990 | 103 | 14/ 97 | 0 | 0 | 0 | | | | |
| Wattrisse et al, 1990 | 189 | 16/182 | 1 | 21 | 11 | | | | |
| | | | | | | Dextran 70 | | | |
| Bergqvist (B) et al, 1991 | 308 | 14/143 | 0 | 9 | 6 | 43/146 | 3 | 8 | 3 |

For abbreviations see table 26.1
(A) = + Dihydroergotamine    (B) = Heparinoid (Org 10172)

prophylaxis with a heparinoid (Org10172), or a standard regimen of dextran 70 the result showed a highly significant difference in favour of the heparinoid but no differences were observed between the groups regarding bleeding complications or deaths (Table 26.10). In general, many recent prophylaxis studies conducted in hip fracture patients with LMWH show rather low incidences of thromboembolic complications compared with older studies. However, it must be remembered that a variety of other factors contribute to the results of clinical studies, and these factors may well differ between studies and between time periods. Some important factors are the surgical and anaesthetic techniques used, preference of early versus delayed operation, and early versus delayed mobilisation after the operation, the importance of which we have previously reported in elective hip surgery (Lassen and Borris, 1991). In combination with an effective prophylaxis, these factors contribute to the final result of a clinical prophylaxis study.

# Conclusion

Whereas most prophylaxis studies in hip fracture patients have demonstrated a reduction in the number of postoperative thromboembolic complications (DVT and/or PE) with various prophylactic regimens, the classic study by Sevitt and Gallagher from 1959 is still the only study that was able to demonstrate a significant reduction in total mortality by giving prophylaxis with an oral anticoagulant in this high risk group of patients. The newer compounds, LMWHs and heparinoids, have so far given promising results, but further studies are needed before decisions can be made concerning prevention of thromboembolism after hip fracture in the future. Our main recommendation is to implement an efficacious and simple regimen which has a high probability of acceptance by the patients and the nursing staff. Prophylaxis must be started as soon as possible, i.e., just after diagnosis of the fracture, and unnecessary delay of the surgical treatment and postoperative mobilisation should be avoided.

# References

Ahlberg Å, Nylander G, Robertson B, Cronberg S, Nilsson IM. Dextran in prophylaxis of thrombosis in fractures of the hip. Acta Chir Scand Suppl. 387:83, 1968

Alho A, Stangeland L, Røttingen J, Wing JN. Prophylaxis of venous thromboembolism by aspirin, warfarin and heparin with hip fractures — a prospective clinical study with cost-benefit analysis. Ann Chir Gyn 73:225, 1984

Barrie WW, Wood EH, Crumlish P, Forbes CD, Prentice CRM. Low- dosage ancrod for prevention of thrombotic complications after surgery for fractured neck of femur. Br Med J 4:130, 1974

Bergquist E, Bergqvist D, Bronge A, Dahlgren S, Lindquist B. An evaluation of early thrombosis prophylaxis following fracture of the femoral neck. A comparison between dextran and dicoumarol. Acta Chir Scand 138:689, 1972

Bergqvist D, Dahlgren S. Leg vein thrombosis diagnosed by $^{125}$I-Fibrinogen test in patients with fracture of the hip: a study of the effect of early prophylaxis with dicoumarol or dextran 70. VASA 2:121, 1973

Bergqvist D, Efsing HO, Hallböök T, Hedlund T. Thromboembolism after elective and post-traumatic hip surgery — a controlled prophylactic trial with dextran and low dose heparin. Acta Chir Scand 145, 213, 1979a

Bergqvist D. Prophylaxis of postoperative thromboembolic complications with low dose heparin. An analysis of different administration intervals. Acta Chir Scand 145:7, 1979b

Bergqvist D, Efsing HO, Hallböök T, Lindblad B. Prevention of postoperative thromboembolic complications. A prospective comparison between dextran 70, dihydroergotamine heparin and a sulfated polysaccharide. Acta Chir Scand 146:559, 1980

Bergqvist D, Lindblad B, Ljungström K-G, Persson NG, Hallböök T. Does dihydroergotamine potentiate the thromboprophylactic effect of dextran 70? A controlled prospective study in general and hip surgery. Br J Surg 71:516, 1984

Bergqvist D, Kettunen K, Fredin H, Faunø P, Suomalainen O, Soimakallio S, Karjalainen P, Cederholm C, Jensen LJ, Justesen T, Stiekema JCJ. Thromboprophylaxis in hip fracture patients — a prospective randomised comparative study between Org 10172 and dextran 70. Surgery 109:617, 1991

Borgström S, Greitz T, van der Linden W, Molin J, Rudics I. Anticoagulant prophylaxis of venous thrombosis in patients with fractured neck of the femur — a controlled clinical trial using venous phlebography. Acta Chir Scand 129:500, 1965

Breyer HG, Al-Therib J, Bacher P, Werner B. Thrombosis prophylaxis with low molecular weight heparin in trauma surgery. Thromb Res Suppl VI:84, 1986 (abstract)

Borris LC, Lassen MR, Christiansen HM, Møller-Larsen F, Knudsen VE, Nielsen BW. Circulatory insufficiency during thrombosis prophylaxis with heparin/dihydroergotamine. Effect or side-effect? Ugeskr Laeger 150:1682, 1988

Bronge A, Dahlgren S, Lindquist B. Prophylaxis against thrombosis in femoral neck fractures — a comparison between dextran 70 and dicumarol. Acta Chir Scand 137:29, 1971

Burcharth F, Hansen OH, Wolf H, Østegaard AH. Prevention of pulmonary embolism in patients with fractures of the femoral neck. Acta Chir Scand 433:178, 1973

Butt HR, Allen EW, Bollman J. A preparation from spoiled sweet clover (3,3'-methylene-bis-(4-hydroxycoumarin)) which prolongs coagulation and prothrombin time of the blood. Preliminary report of experimental and clinical studies. Proc Staff Mayo Clin 16:388, 1941

Checketts RG, Bradley JG. Low dose heparin in femoral neck fractures. Injury 6:42, 1974

Chrisman OD, Snook GA, Wilson TC, Short JY. Prevention of venous thromboembolism by administration of hydroxychloroquine. J Bone J Surg 58A:918, 1976

Clayer MT, Bauze RJ. Morbidity and mortality following fractures of the femoral neck and trochanteric region: analysis of risk factors. J Trauma 29:1673, 1989

Colbert DS, O'Muircheartaigh I. Mortality after hip fracture and assessment of some contributory factors. Irish J Med Sci 145:44, 1976

Collins R, Scrimgeour A, Yusuf S, Peto R. Reduction in fatal pulmonary embolism and venous thrombosis by perioperative administration of subcutaneous heparin. N Engl J Med 318:1162, 1988

Dahl E. Mortality and life expectancy after hip fractures. Acta Orthop Scand 51:163, 1980

Daniel WJ, Moore AR, Flanc C. Prophylaxis of deep vein thrombosis (DVT) with dextran 70 in patients with a fractured neck of the femur. Aust NZ J Surg 41:289, 1972

Darke SG. Ilio-femoral venous thrombosis after operations on the hip — a prospective controlled trial using dextran 70. J Bone J Surg 54B:615, 1972

Davis FM, Quince M, Laurenson VG. Deep vein thrombosis and anaesthetic technique in emergency hip surgery. Br Med J 281:528, 1980

Davis FM, Woolner DF, Frampton C et al. Prospective, multi-centre trial of mortality following general or spinal anaesthesia for hip fracture surgery in the elderly. Br J Anaesth 59:1080, 1987

Eskeland G, Solheim K, Skjörten F. Anticoagulant prophylaxis, thromboembolism and mortality in elderly patients with hip fractures. A controlled clinical trial. Acta Chir Scand 131:16, 1966

Faunø P, Suomalainen O, Bergqvist D et al. The use of the fibrinogen uptake test in screening for deep vein thrombosis in patients with hip fracture. Thromb Res 60:185, 1990

Fredin HO, Nillius SA, Bergqvist D. Prophylaxis of deep vein thrombosis in patients with fracture of the femoral neck. Acta Orthop Scand 53:413, 1982

Fredin H, Lindblad B, Jaroszewski H, Bergqvist D. Prevention of thrombosis after hip fracture surgery. Acta Chir Scand 151:681, 1985

Freeark RJ, Boswick J, Fardin R. Posttraumatic venous thrombosis. Arch Surg 95:567, 1967

Galasko CSB, Edwards DH, Fearn CBD'A, Barber HM. The value of low dosage heparin for the prophylaxis of thromboembolism in patients with transcervical and intertrochanteric femoral fractures. Acta Orthop Scand 47:276, 1976

Gallus AS, Hirsh J, Tuttle RJ et al. Small subcutaneous doses of heparin in prevention of venous thrombosis. N Engl J Med 288:545, 1973

Gent M, Roberts RS. A meta-analysis of the studies of dihydroergotamine plus heparin in the prophylaxis of deep vein thrombosis. Chest 89:396S, 1986

Gruber UF. Prevention of fatal pulmonary embolism in patients with fractures of the neck of the femur. Surg Gyn Obst 161:37, 1985

Hamilton HW, Crawford JS, Gardiner JH, Wiley AM. Venous thrombosis in patients with fracture of the upper end of the femur — a phlebographic study of the effect of prophylactic anticoagulation. J Bone J Surg 52B:268, 1970

Jensen JS, Tøndevold E. Mortality after hip fractures. Acta Orthop Scand 50:161, 1979

Johnsson SR, Bygdeman S, Eliasson R. Effect of dextran on postoperative thrombosis. Acta Chir Scand, Suppl 387:80, 1968

Jørgensen PS, Knudsen JB, Broeng L et al. The thromboprophylactic effect of a low molecular weight heparin (Fragmin$^R$) in hip fracture surgery. A placebo controlled study. Clin Orthop 278:95, 1992

Kakkar VV, Spindler J, Flute PT et al. Efficacy of low dose heparin in prevention of deep vein thrombosis after major surgery — a double-blind randomised trial. Lancet ii:101, 1972

Koekenberg LJL. Experimental use of macrodex as a prophylaxis against postoperative thromboembolism. Exp Med Amst 40:123, 1961

Korninger C, Schlag G, Poigenfürst et al. Randomised trial of low molecular weight heparin (LMWH) versus low dose heparin/acenocoumarin (H/AC) in patients with hip fracture — thromboprophylactic effect and bleeding complications. Thromb Haemost 62:187, 1989 (abstract)

Korvald E, Stren E, Ongre A. Simultaneous use of warfarin-sodium and dextran 70 to prevent post-operative venous thrombosis in patients with hip fractures. J Oslo City Hosp 23:25, 1973

Lahnborg G. Effect of low dose heparin and dihydrogergotamine on frequency of postoperative deep vein thrombosis in patients undergoing post-traumatic hip surgery. Acta Chir Scand 146:319, 1980

Lassen MR, Borris LC, Christensen HM, et al. Prevention of thromboembolism in hip fracture surgery. Comparison of low dose heparin and low molecular weight heparin combined with dihydroergotamine. Arch Orthop Traum Surg 108:10, 1989

Lassen MR, Borris LC. Mobilisation after hip surgery and efficacy of thromboprophylaxis Lancet i:618, 1991

Leyvraz PF, Richard J, Bachmann F et al. Adjusted versus fixed dose subcutaneous heparin in the prevention of deep vein thrombosis after total hip replacement. N Engl J Med 309:945, 1983

Lowe GD, Campbell AF, Meek DR, Forbes CD, Prentice CR. Subcutaneous ancrod in prevention of deep vein thrombosis after operation for fractured neck of femur. Lancet ii:698, 1978

McKenzie PJ, Wishart HY, Gray I, Smith G. Effects of anaesthetic technique on deep vein thrombosis — a comparison of subarachnoid and general anaesthesia. Br J Anaesth 57:853, 1985

Modig J, Hjelmstedt A, Sahlstedt B, Maripuu E. Comparative influences of epidural and general anaesthesia on deep venous thrombosis and pulmonary embolism after total hip replacement. Acta Chir Scand 147:125, 1981

Monreal M, Lafoz E, Navarro A et al. A prospective double-blind trial of a low molecular weight heparin once daily compared with conventional low dose heparin three times daily to prevent pulmonary embolism and venous thrombosis in patients with hip fracture. J Trauma 29:873, 1989

Montrey JS, Kistner RL, Kong AYT, Lindberg RF, Mayfield GW, Jones DA, Mitsunaga MM. Thromboembolism following hip fracture. J Trauma 25:534, 1985

Morris GK, Mitchell JRA. Warfarin sodium in prevention of deep venous thrombosis and pulmonary embolism in patients with fractured neck of the femur. Lancet ii:869, 1976

Morris GK, Mitchell JRA. Preventing venous thromboembolism in elderly patients with hip fractures: studies of low dose heparin, dipyridamole, aspirin and flurbiprofen. Br Med J 1:535, 1977

Morris GK, Mitchell JRA. Can death from venous thromboembolism be prevented in elderly patients with hip fractures? Am Heart J 95; 139, 1978

Moskowitz PA, Ellenberg SS, Feffer HL, Kenmore PI, Neviaser RJ, Rubin BE, Marma VM. Low dose heparin for prevention of venous thromboembolism in total hip arthroplasty and surgical repair of hip fractures. J Bone J Surg 60A:1065, 1978

Myhre H, Holen A. Thrombosis prophylaxis. Dextran or sodium warfarin? A controlled clinical study (In Norwegian). Nord Med 82:1534, 1969

Myhre HO, Storen EJ, Auensen CA. Pre- or post-operative start of anticoagulation prophylaxis in patients with fractured hips? J Oslo City Hosp 23:15, 1973

Orthner E, Hertz H, Kwasny O et al. Thromboembolieprophylaxe bei hüftgelenknahen Oberschenkelfrakturen-Ergebnisse einer prospektiven randomisierten studie twischen Heparin-DHE und ASS-DHE. Unfallchirurgie 16; 128, 1990

Pini M, Spadini E, Carluccio L, Giovanardi C, Magnani E, Ugolotti U, Uggeri E. Dextran/aspirin versus heparin/dihydroergotamine in preventing thrombosis after hip fractures. J Bone Joint Surg Br 67B:305, 1985

Pini M, Tagliaferri A, Manotti C, Lasagni F, Rinaldi E, Dettori AG. Low molecular weight heparin (Alfa LMWH) compared with unfractionated heparin in prevention of deep vein thrombosis after hip fractures. Int Angiol 8P; 134, 1989

Pinto J. Controlled trial of an anticoagulant (Warfarin sodium) in the prevention of venous thrombosis following hip surgery. Br J Surg 57:349, 1970

Powers PJ, Gent M, Jay RM, Julian DH, Turpie AGG, Levine M, Hirsh J. A randomised trial of less intensive postoperative warfarin or aspirin therapy in the prevention of venous thromboembolism after surgery for fractured hip. Arch Intern Med 149:771, 1989

Riska EB. Factors influencing the primary mortality in the treatment of hip fractures. Injury 2:107, 1970

Roberts TS, Nelson CL, Barnes CL, Ferris EJ, Holder JC, Boone DW. The preoperative prevalence and postoperative incidence of thromboembolism in patients with hip fractures treated with dextran prophylaxis. Clin Orthop 255:198, 1990

Rogers PH, Walsh PN, Marder VJ et al. Controlled trial of low dose heparin and sulfinpyrazone to prevent venous thromboembolism after operation on the hip. J Bone J Surg 60A:758, 1978

Rørbæk-Madsen M, Jakobsen BW, Pedersen J, Sørensen B. Dihydroergotamine and the thromboprophylactic effect of dextran 70 in emergency hip surgery. Br J Surg 75:364, 1988

Sagar S, Stamatakis JD, Higgins AF, Nairn D, Maffei FH, Thomas DO, Kakkar VV. Efficacy of low dose heparin in prevention of extensive deep vein thrombosis in patients undergoing total hip replacement. Lancet i:1151, 1976

Salzman EW, Harris WH, DeSanctis RW. Anticoagulation for prevention of thromboembolism following fractures of the hip. N Engl J Med 275:122, 1966

Schlag G, Gaudernak T, Pelinka H, Kederna H, Welzel D. Thromboembolic prophylaxis in hip fracture. Acta Orthop Scand 57:340, 1986

Sevitt S, Gallagher NG. Prevention of venous thrombosis and pulmonary embolism in injured patients. Lancet ii:981, 1959

Sharnoff JG, Rosen RL, Palazzo PJ, Fethiere DA, Sotudeh S, Alvarez EV, Rosen C. Prevention of fatal pulmonary thromboembolism by small dose heparin prophylaxis in acute hip fracture surgery. Br J Clin Pract 35:390, 1981

Snook GA, Chrisman OD, Wilson TC. Thromboembolism after surgical treatment of hip fractures. Clin Orthop 155:21, 1981

Stadil F. Prophylaxis of postoperative venous thrombosis with dextran-70$^R$. Ugeskr Laeger 132:1817, 1970

Stevens J, Fardin R, Freeark RJ. Lower extremity thrombophlebitis in patients with femoral neck fractures. J Trauma 8:527, 1968

Svend-Hansen H, Bremerskov V, Gøtrik J, Ostri P. Low dose heparin in proximal femoral fractures — failure to prevent deep vein thrombosis. Acta Orthop Scand 52:77, 1981

Taberner DA, Poller L, Thomson JM et al. Randomised study of adjusted versus fixed low dose heparin prophylaxis of deep vein thrombosis in hip surgery. Br J Surg 736:933, 1989

Wattrisse G, Lecoutre D, Groux-Pante C, Mottet D. Prophylaxie thrombo-embolique par héparine de pas poids moléculaire et hémodilution en chirurgie traumatologique gériatrique du col du fémur. Cahiers d'Anesthésiologie 38:319, 1990

Williams JW, Eikman EA, Greenberg SH, Hewitt JC, Lopez-Cuenca E, Jones P, Madden JA. Failure of low dose heparin to prevent pulmonary embolism after hip surgery or above the knee amputation. Ann Surg 188:468, 1978

Xabregas A, Gray L, Ham JM. Heparin prophylaxis of deep vein thrombosis in patients with a fractured neck of the femur. Med J Austr 1:620, 1978

CHAPTER 27

# Combined modalities for hip surgery

Juan I Arcelus  Joseph A Caprini
Clara I Traverso

## Introduction

During the past two decades, a number of prophylactic methods against postoperative venous thromboembolism (VTE) have been evaluated clinically in patients undergoing total hip replacement (THR). These include oral anticoagulants, aspirin, heparin at fixed or adjusted doses, dextran, heparin-dihydroergotamine (H-DHE), graduated elastic stockings (GES), intermittent pneumatic compression (IPC) and, more recently, low molecular weight heparins (LMWH) and heparinoids.

In general surgery, low dose heparin has become the worldwide standard of prophylaxis because of its simplicity and the favourable results reported in several meta-analyses of the literature (Colditz et al, 1986; Collins et al, 1988; Clagett and Reisch, 1988). In contrast, there is not yet a generally accepted standard of prophylaxis for patients undergoing hip surgery. Collins et al (1988) analysed the rates of deep vein thrombosis (DVT) reported in the literature in different surgical specialities and found a significant reduction (68%) in the incidence of this complication when low dose heparin was utilised for orthopaedic patients. However, the frequency of DVT in this population remained unacceptably high (20-30%) despite low dose heparin prophylaxis. A reduction in the incidence of VTE has been reported with other modalities such as oral anticoagulants, dextran, heparin at adjusted doses, and low molecular weight heparins. Yet, the incidence of DVT remains elevated, between 10% and 30% when these modalities are implemented.

What are the reasons for this apparent resistance to achieving a more effective prophylaxis in THR patients? First, most of the aforementioned pharmacological modalities are directed to neutralise hypercoagulability, one of the components of Virchow's triad. However, they do not influence venous stasis, another key factor in the pathogenesis of venous thrombosis. In addition, patients undergoing hip surgery are usually over 60 years of age and present a number of associated risk factors that make them more prone to develop VTE (cardiopulmonary disease, obesity, varicose veins, etc.). Therefore, the protection given by a single prophylactic modality is often inappropriate to the degree of risk. Second, an increasing number of orthopaedic patients are currently being discharged from hospital around the seventh postoperative day; many of these patients remain at home with minimal mobilisation and, in many cases, with less surveillance and protection than in hospital (Scurr et al, 1988).

In order to further reduce the rates of VTE amongst orthopaedic patients, the "ideal" prophylactic regimen should cover most of the factors involved in the pathogenesis of venous thrombosis: stasis, hypercoagulability, and endothelial dysfunction. Moreover, that regimen should be implemented during the whole period that the patient remains at risk; after total hip replacement, this period can extend several weeks beyond the time of operation or discharge from hospital.

A combined approach, using mechanical plus pharmacological modalities or two or more pharmacologic agents, seems to be a reasonable way of addressing the problem of prevention of VTE after hip surgery. After hospital discharge, single or combined modalities can be utilised, according to the patient's characteristics and compliance (Caprini et al, 1988).

In this chapter, we will review the experience gathered by several investigators with combined modalities in elective total hip replacement and the role of post-discharge prophylaxis in this surgical population. Our current protocol and results will also be discussed.

## Combined modalities of prophylaxis

There are three basic types of combined prophylactic approaches: 1. Physical and pharmacological methods; 2. Association of two or more pharmacological agents (antiplatelet, anticoagulant, or vasoconstrictor agents; 3. A combination of physical methods (stockings, intermittent compression).

Again, the rationale of a combined regimen is to achieve a better coverage of the multifactorial pathogenesis of venous thrombosis during and after hip surgery. Another possible theoretical advantage of some combined modalities could be the possibility of reducing doses of anticoagulant agents necessary to overcome postoperative hypercoagulability. This is very important among hip patients because of the bleeding potential inherent in the technical aspects of the operation. Furthermore, bleeding at the operative site can compromise the results of the joint replacement (Hirsh, 1990) and increase the risk of infection.

### Physical-pharmacological combinations

Several authors have reported that the combination of graduated elastic stockings (GES) and low dose heparin (LDH) is effective in general surgery (Torngren, 1980; Borow and Goldson, 1983; Wille-Jorgensen et al, 1985; Chapter 21). The combined use of stockings and anticoagulant or antiplatelet agents is less reported in elective hip surgery. Table 27.1 shows the results of several studies assessing the combined regimen using conventional ascending venography as the routine diagnostic endpoint or as a confirmatory test for DVT detected by noninvasive methods. Although the reported results varied markedly among the different studies, most investigators found a trend towards a reduction in the rate of DVT when the GES were added to the pharmacological agent. Fredin et al (1989) have found a statistically significant reduction in the total rate of postoperative DVT by adding the GES

**Table 27.1**
Results of combined physical and pharmacological prophylaxis for total hip replacement

| Author | Modality | Patients n | % DVT | % Prox DVT | Diagnosis |
|---|---|---|---|---|---|
| Sautter et al, 1983 | GES+ASA+Sulfinpyrazone | 31 | 22.6 | — | Ven |
| | ASA+Sulfinpyrazone | 23 | 13* | — | |
| Nilsen et al, 1984 | GES+intraoperative dextran | 22 | 59 | 31.8 | FUT/Ven |
| Harris et al, 1985 | ASA (0.3 g/24 h) | 43 | 60.4 | 11.6 | FUT/IPG/Ven |
| | ASA (1.2 g/24 h) | 48 | 60.4 | 33.3 | |
| | SIPC+dextran (intra/post-op) | 44 | 20.4 | 11.3* | |
| Patel et al, 1988 | Adjusted IV heparin | 78 | 19.2 | — | Ven |
| | GES+adjusted IV heparin | 72 | 9.7 | — | |
| Christensen et al, 1989 | GES+Heparin-dihydroergotamine | 28 | 10.7 | 3.6 | PS/Ven# |
| | GES+Placebo | 27 | 11.1 | 3.7 | |
| Fredin et al, 1989 | Dextran (intra & postop) | 46 | 45.6 | 19.5 | FUT/Ven |
| | GES+Dextran (intra & postop) | 44 | 29.5* | 11.4 | |
| | Dextran (pre, intra & postop) | 46 | 52.2 | 8.6 | |
| Sharrock et al, 1990 | GES+ASA+IV heparin (intraop) | 60 | 8.3* | 1.6 | Ven |
| | GES+ASA | 66 | 24.2 | 9.1 | Duplex or Ven |
| Woolson et al, 1991 | GES+SIPC | 76 | — | 11.8 | |
| | GES+SIPC+ASA | 72 | — | 9.7 | |
| | GES+SIPC+Warfarin | 69 | — | 8.7 | |
| Lassen et al, 1991 | GES+Logiparin | 93 | 31.2 | 25.8 | Ven |
| | GES+Placebo | 97 | 45.3 | 36.1 | |

GES = Graduated elastic stockings   SIPC = Sequential intermittent pneumatic compression
ASA = Aspirin   FUT = Fibrinogen uptake test   PS = Plasmin Scintigraphy
Ven = Venography   IPG = Impedance plethysmography   *Statistically significant difference ($p<0.05$)   # Venography performed if the other tests positive for DVT

to dextran 70. However, this reduction was not significant for proximal DVT. Promising results have been reported by combining GES to intravenous heparin (Patel et al, 1988), intravenous heparin plus ASA (Sharrock et al, 1990) or to heparin-dihydroergotamine (Christensen et al, 1989).

The combination of external pneumatic compression and dextran achieved a better protection than two different dose regimens of aspirin (Harris et al, 1985). The incidence of proximal DVT (11.3%) was similar to the rates found by Fredin et al (1989) using GES instead of pneumatic compression, and by Woolson and Watt (1991), using intraoperative and postoperative GES and IPC. In the later study, lower incidences of proximal DVT were detected by adding aspirin (9.7%) or warfarin (8.7%) to the combination of physical methods. A possible drawback of this study could be that the diagnosis of DVT relied on venography, duplex scanning, or both. However, the authors only considered the proximal venous system for evaluation, whereas their results with duplex scanning have been very good (Woolson et al, 1990).

**Table 27.2**
Results of studies combining dihydroergotamine with other pharmacological agents in patients undergoing total hip replacement

| Author | Modality | Patients n | % DVT | % Prox DVT | Diagnosis |
|---|---|---|---|---|---|
| Kakkar et al, 1979 | LDH (5,000 IU/8h) | 25 | 72 | 44 | Ven |
|  | H-DHE (5,000 IU-0.5 mg/8h) | 25 | 24* | 12* |  |
| Morris and Hardy, 1981 | Placebo | 27 | 63 | — | FUT |
|  | DHE (0.5 mg/8h) | 27 | 44.4 | — |  |
|  | H-DHE (5,000 IU-0.5 mg/8h) | 27 | 7.4* | — |  |
| Fredin et al, 1984 | Dextran 70 (intra & postop) | 50 | 54 | 22* | Ven |
|  | H-DHE (5,000 IU-0.5 mg/12h) | 49 | 59.2 | 42.8 |  |
| Kakkar et al, 1985 | H-DHE (5,000 IU-0.5 mg/8h) | 500 | 26.2 | 13.1 | Ven |
| Lassen et al, 1988 | H-DHE (5,000 IU-0.5 mg/12h) | 112 | 30.3* | 18.7 | FUT/Ven# |
|  | LMWH-DHE (6,000 AntiXa U-0.5mg) | 107 | 32.7* | 12.1 |  |
|  | Placebo | 97 | 54.6 | 28.9 |  |
| Beisaw et al, 1988 | H-DHE (5,000 IU-0.5 mg) | 63 | 25.4* | 4.8* | FUT/Ven |
|  | Placebo | 65 | 52.3 | 18.4 |  |
| Estoppey et al, 1989 | Org 10172 (705 Anti-XA U/12h) | 146 | 17.1* | 4.8 | Ven |
|  | H-DHE (5,000 IU-0.5 mg/12h) | 149 | 32.2 | 8 |  |

H-DHE = Heparin-dihydroergotamine   LMWH = Low molecular weight heparin
LDH = Low dose heparin   FUT = Fibrinogen uptake test   Ven = Venography
* Statistically significant difference (p<0.05)   # Venography performed if the other tests positive for DVT

An additional favourable effect of the stockings did not appear to be present in other studies in which GES were combined with dextran administered only during the operation (Nilsen et al, 1984), aspirin and sulfinpyrazone (Sautter et al, 1983), or Logiparin (Lassen, 1991). Despite the good results reported by Barnes et al (1978) and subsequently by Ishak and Morley (1981), elastic stockings cannot be recommended as the only prophylactic modality for patients undergoing THR.

**Combinations of pharmacological agents**
The combined pharmacological regimen consisting of heparin and dihydroergotamine (H-DHE) has been extensively assessed in total hip replacement surgery. As shown in Table 27.2, most of the studies have reported a reduction in the rates of DVT when dihydroergotamine was combined with heparin, as compared to heparin alone or DHE alone. However, the incidence of DVT detected by venography in these studies remains high, between 24 and 32 percent, with the rates for proximal thrombosis between 5 and 13 percent. The incidence of bleeding complications after using H-DHE has been low, around 5 percent.

No significant complications derived from the vasoconstrictor effect of DHE have been reported in the studies presented in table 27.2. Nevertheless, several cases of important complications secondary to arterial ischaemia have been documented after using DHE (Cunningham et al, 1985; Gatterer, 1986). For this reason, H-DHE ceased to be approved in the United States for VTE prophylaxis in 1989.

Stern and Vasey (1987) conducted one study in which H-DHE was given during the first five postoperative days. From the sixth postoperative and for at least 21 days they compared two oral regimens. The first consisted of a combination of ASA (500 mg/8h) and DHE (3 mg/24h), and the second of acenocoumarol, at doses based on the prothrombin time and starting on the second postoperative day. By a combination of the fibrinogen uptake test (FUT), Doppler, and confirmatory venography, they found a rate of DVT of 18.5 percent in the ASA-DHE group and of 9.1 percent in the oral anticoagulant population (difference not significant).

Using a combination of sulfinpyrazone (200 mg/6h) and ASA (200 mg/6h), Sautter et al (1983) detected a significant reduction in the incidence of proximal DVT from 38.5 percent in the placebo group to 18.5 percent in the treated group ($p<0.05$).

Francis et al (1989) have reported very encouraging results by combining Antithrombin III intravenously administered (1,500 U two hours before surgery and continuing with 1,000/day for five days) and subcutaneous heparin (5,000 IU/12h). They compared this regimen to another consisting of low dose dextran 40, given intraoperatively and continued intravenously for 5 days. A venogram performed on the tenth postoperative day detected thrombosis in 4.9 percent of the heparin-antithrombin III group and 18.5 percent in the dextran group ($p<0.005$).

## Combination of physical methods

The simultaneous use of elastic stockings and sequential intermittent pneumatic compression (SIPC) has been assessed in few studies. In patients undergoing general surgery, Scurr et al (1987) have reported a reduction in the incidence of DVT, detected by Doppler and strain-gauge plethysmography and confirmatory venography, from 9% in the legs with SIPC to 1% in the legs with GEC and SIPC ($p<0.005$). A possible theoretical explanation for this dramatic reduction in the incidence of DVT when stockings are added is that they improve the venous flow and prevent venous dilatation during the period between the compression cycles. The role of venous dilatation in the pathogenesis of thrombosis has been stressed by Comerota et al (1985; 1989; Chapter 3).

There is not much experience with this type of combination in hip surgery. We conducted a prospective study in which 106 consecutive patients undergoing THR received thigh length GES before and after surgery, with the additional application of SIPC and the continuous passive motion machine (CPM) until the patients were fully ambulatory. We found an incidence of 4% of DVT detected by FUT, Doppler and SPG and confirmed by venography (Caprini et al, 1987). As described above, Woolson and Watt (1991) have reported very good results using a similar approach for patients undergoing THR, with the difference that they applied both stockings and SIPC to both legs during and after the operative procedure.

**Table 27.3**
Effect of prophylaxis on the development of late postoperative DVT in patients undergoing total hip replacement

| Author | Prophylactic modality | Total number of thrombosis[*] | Number after 7th PO day | Proportion |
|---|---|---|---|---|
| Hampson et al, 1974 | Placebo | 28 | 3 | 11% |
|  | Low Dose Heparin | 22 | 13 | 59% |
| Mannucci et al, 1976 | Placebo | 14 | 4 | 28% |
|  | Low Dose Heparin | 5 | 2 | 40% |
| Sagar et al, 1976 | Placebo | 22 | 1 | 5% |
|  | Low Dose Heparin | 17 | 5 | 29% |
| Johnson et al, 1978 | Dextran | 16 | 16 | 100% |
| Sikorski et al, 1981 | None | 107 | 25 | 23% |
|  | Low Dose Heparin | 28 | 15 | 53% |
|  | IPC[**] | 25 | 13 | 52% |
| Erikkson et al, 1988 | Dextran | 22 | 4 | 18% |
|  | LMWH (Kabi 2165) | 10 | 3 | 30% |

[*] Diagnosis of DVT based on $^{125}$I-fibrinogen uptake test, ultrasound or thermography, and confirmed by venography
[**] Intermittent pneumatic compression

## Prophylaxis after hospital discharge in THR patients

The risk of developing VTE extends several weeks after total hip replacement. However, most patients undergoing this procedure receive prophylaxis for a limited period of 7 to 14 days. In the survey conducted by Paiement et al (1987), 30 percent of the US orthopaedic surgeons discontinued prophylaxis when the patient was ambulatory and an additional 65 percent of the surgeons stopped prophylaxis at the time of discharge from hospital. Improved anaesthetic techniques and postoperative rehabilitation in recent years have allowed discharge of many of these patients one week after surgery. Table 27.3 displays the results of several trials in which prophylaxis was given between one and two weeks after surgery. The effect of prophylaxis on the natural history of DVT after THR, delaying its onset, is clearly illustrated. Most prophylactic modalities were associated with an increase in the proportion of thrombi detected after the seventh postoperative day.

During a trial comparing a low molecular weight heparinoid (Org 10172) with a placebo in which bilateral venography was routinely performed on the tenth postoperative day, Hoek et al (1991) detected 15 thrombi in the 97 patients receiving the heparinoid. During an additional follow-up period of eight weeks, there were three additional patients of this grup with symptomatic DVT confirmed by objective testing, representing almost 17 percent of all the thrombi detected in the treated group. Similar results have been reported by Mätzsch et al (1991) using a low molecular weight heparin (13.6 percent of the thrombi were detected after the 14th postoperative day). Likewise, in the experience of Kakkar et al (1985), 23 percent of the thrombi detected in patients receiving heparin-dihydroergotamine developed between the 15th and 24th postoperative days.

We have found similar results in a study currently in progress. Bilateral duplex scanning is performed before operation and seven and 28 days after surgery in all patients undergoing

THR. After 42 patients completed the prophylactic protocol, consisting of pre-, intra- and post-operative GES and sequential intermittent pneumatic compression (SIPC) plus postoperative subcutaneous heparin for four weeks, we found three asymptomatic thrombi, all detected on the 28th postoperative day scan. There were three additional patients who, after receiving GSE-SIPC and heparin during the first postoperative week, were sent home on aspirin (500 mg/24h) because they refused the heparin after discharge. Two of them subsequently developed asymptomatic proximal DVT detected on the 28th day scan and confirmed by venography. These results demonstrate that objective diagnostic endpoints are also needed for the detection of postdischarge DVT. Yet, several authors do not support the use of prophylaxis after discharge in patients undergoing THR (Sharrock et al, 1990; Woolson et al, 1990; Agnelli et al, 1991). These authors base their attitude on the apparently good clinical outcome of their patients after they left the hospital. If we had not performed routine serial duplex scans on our patients, we would probably share that approach after missing most thrombi. But, based on our results, we are more in agreement with other authors who stress the importance of extending prophylaxis for several weeks beyond discharge after hip surgery (Swiestra et al, 1988; Amstutz et al, 1989; Paiement et al, 1991).

Further studies are required to establish whether prolonging prophylaxis after discharge can reduce the incidence of late VTE complications and which are the best modalities. Meanwhile, it is our current standard of practice to utilise low dose heparin and GES or warfarin and GES for at least three weeks after discharge in all our high risk orthopaedic patients (Arcelus and Caprini, 1991). In countries where low molecular weight heparins are clinically available, the use of these agents in combination with stockings would be better accepted by patients as they would require a single daily injection only.

## Our protocol for VTE prevention and results after THR

Our current protocol for VTE prevention in THR consists of a combination of physical methods and adjusted subcutaneous heparin. Two to twelve hours before operation, depending on the time of admission to hospital, our patients are fitted with bilateral thigh-length graduated elastic stockings and SIPC. During the operative procedure, one sterile SIPC sleeve is applied on the operative leg and a standard sleeve on the contralateral limb. Thigh-length GES are used underneath the compression sleeves. This combined physical modality is maintained until the patient is fully ambulating without assistance and spending most of the day out of bed or chair. The patient continues wearing the stockings for at least one month after surgery. Some orthopaedic surgeons in our hospital also use the continuous passive motion machine (CPM), from the first postoperative day.

In addition to the physical methods, we use subcutaneous heparin, starting with 5,000 IU on the night of the day of surgery and then twice a day, adjusting the doses to keep the partial thromboplastin time (PTT) between 1.3 and 1.5 times the control value, performed every other day four hours after the heparin injection. After discharge, we combine the GES with subcutaneous heparin, twice a day. The doses of heparin are dependent on the patient's response to heparin shown in the last PTT prior to hospital discharge. These doses are then readjusted based on the results of another PTT performed 1 and 3 weeks after discharge.

Our preliminary results using this protocol are summarised in table 27.4. So far, our main problem has been the poor compliance of some patients to the subcutaneously injected heparin after they leave the hospital. For that reason, we have recently included another group in which patients receive the same physical regimen. Instead of heparin, warfarin is

**Table 27.4**
Our experience with a combined prophylactic regimen in patients undergoing total hip replacement (see text)

---

Diagnostic Protocol
    Venous duplex scanning of both lower limbs performed preoperatively 1 and 4 weeks after surgery. If the results are equivocal or positive for DVT, ascending venography is ordered

Results
    Number of patients studied: 52
    Three patients refused heparin after discharge and aspirin was prescribed. Seven patients failed to complete the diagnostic protocol
    42 patients completed the prophylactic and diagnostic protocol. There were three asymptomatic proximal DVT, all diagnosed on the 28th postoperative day (7.1%)
    Two of the three patients sent home on aspirin developed asymptomatic proximal thrombosis detected on the 28th postoperative day
    There have not been significant bleeding complications (only one wound haematoma)
    Amount of blood transfused (mostly autologous) 495±275 ml
    Estimated intraoperative blood losses: 765±325 ml
    Postoperative blood losses: 317±290 ml

---

used, starting with 10 mg the night before surgery, followed by 5 mg the night of surgery and continuing by daily dose adjustments to maintain the prothrombin time at 1.2-1.3 times the control value.

# Final considerations

It is clear that the combination of different prophylactic modalities can play an important role in the prevention of VTE after total hip replacement. Yet, the experience with some combined regimens is still limited and further well designed prospective trials are needed. It could be argued that the results of combined physical-pharmacological modalities (Patel et al, 1988; Sharrock et al, 1990; Woolson and Watt, 1991) are similar to the results recently obtained with some low molecular weight heparins (Hoek et al, 1991; Leyvraz, 1991, Mätzsch et al, 1991; Planes et al, 1991). Nevertheless, there are two important considerations regarding this issue. First, the optimal dosage regimen for many of the LMWH preparations is still under investigation (Levine et al, 1989). There is a potential risk of bleeding complications, especially if a preoperative dose is given shortly before the operation. Second, these heparin fractions are not available in all countries. Thus, where they have not yet been approved, other alternatives have to be considered for hip surgery. The administration of heparin at adjusted doses has significantly lowered the incidence of postoperative DVT after THR (Leyvraz et al, 1983; Leyvraz, 1991). In our experience, the combination of physical methods and adjusted heparin will reduce the dose of this drug necessary to modify postoperative hypercoagulability and, hopefully, decrease the incidence of haemorrhage. Possibly, the reduction in venous stasis achieved by the compression modalities decreases the activation of the haemostatic system. In additon, several investigators have shown that intermittent pneumatic compression induces activation of the fibrinolytic system (Tarnay et al, 1980; Summaria et al, 1988; Inada et al, 1988). The importance of this for thrombosis prevention remains to be elucidated.

A significant advantage of physical methods is that they can be combined with pharmacological agents, enhancing their prophylactic effect, without increasing the risk of complications (Caprini et al, 1991). After all, as remarked by Goldhaber (1988), the two modalities should be contemplated as complementary instead of competitive.

With respect to prophylaxis after hospital discharge, it is clear that there is a need to protect THR patients while they remain at risk. There are two alternatives: heparin or oral anticoagulants, either of which can be associated with elastic stockings. More studies are necessary to determine which is the best regimen (Scurr, 1990) and how long prophylaxis should be continued after hospital discharge.

# References

Agnelli G, Ranucci V, Cosmi B, Rinonapoli E, Lupatelli L, Nenci GG. Outcome of hip surgery in patients with lower limb negative venography at discharge. Thromb Haemost 65:1175, 1991

Amstutz HC, Friscia DA, Dorey F, Carney BT. Warfarin prophylaxis to prevent mortality from pulmonary embolism after total hip replacement. J Bone J Surg 71A:321, 1989

Arcelus JI, Caprini JA. Prevention after hospital discharge. In: Goldhaber SZ (ed), Prevention of Venous Thromboembolism, Marcel Dekker Inc., New York 1992

Barnes RW, Brand RA, Clarke W, Hartley N, Hoak JC. Efficacy of graded compression antiembolism stockings in patients undergoing total hip arthroplasty. Clin Orthop Rel Dis 132:61, 1978

Beisaw NE, Comerota A, Groth HE et al. Dihydroergotamine/heparin in the prevention of deep vein thrombosis after total hip replacement. J Bone J Surg 70A:2, 1988

Borow M, Goldson HJ. Prevention of postoperative deep vein thrombosis and pulmonary emboli with combined modalities. The American Surgeon 49:599, 1983

Caprini JA, Scurr JH, Hasty JH. Role of compression modalities in a prophylaxis program for deep vein thrombosis. Sem Thromb Hemostas 14:77, 1988

Caprini JA, Kudrna JC, Mitchell AS. Thrombosis prophylaxis in total hip arthroplasty patients using a combination of physical methods (Abs). Thromb Haemost 58:385, 1987

Caprini JA, Arcelus JI, Traverso CI, Hasty JH. Low molecular weight heparins and external pneumatic compression as options for venous thromboembolism prophylaxis. A surgeon's perspective. Semin Thromb Hemost 17:356, 1991

Christensen sw, Wille-Jorgensen P, Bjerg-Nielsen A, Kjaer L. Prevention of deep venous thrombosis following total hip replacement using epidural anesthesia. Acta Orthop Bel 55:58, 1989

Clagett GP, Reisch JS. Prevention of venous thromboembolism in general surgical patients — results of meta-analysis. Ann Surg 208:227, 1988

Colditz GA, Tuden RL, Oster G. Rates of venous thrombosis after general surgery — combined results of randomised clinical trials. Lancet 2:143, 1986

Collins R, Scrimgeour A, Yusuf S, Peto R. Reduction in fatal pulmonary embolism and venous thrombosis by perioperative administration of subcutaneous heparin. N Engl J Med 318:1162, 1988

Comerota AJ, Stewart GJ, Alburger PD, Smalley K, White JV. Operative venodilation: a previously unsuspected factor in the cause of postoperative deep vein thrombosis. Surgery 106:301, 1989

Comerota AJ, Stewart GJ, White JV. Combined dihydroergotamine and heparin prophylaxis of postoperative deep vein thrombosis: Proposed mechanism of action. Am J Surg 150:39, 1985

Cunningham M, de Torrente A, Ekoe JM, Ackerman JP, Humair L. Vascular spasm and gangrene during heparin-dihydroergotamine prophylaxis. Br J Surg 71:829, 1984

Eriksson BI, Zachrisson BE, Teger-Nilsson et al. Thrombosis prophylaxis with low molecular weight heparin in total hip replacement. Br J Surg 75:1053, 1988

Estoppey D, Hochreiter J, Breyer GH et al. Org 10172 (Lomoparan) versus heparin-DHE in prevention of thromboembolism in total hip replacement — a multicentre trial. Thromb Haemost 62:356, abstract, 1989

Francis CW, Pellegrini VD, Marder VJ et al. Prevention of venous thrombosis after total hip replacement. J Bone J Surg 71A:327, 1989

Fredin HO, Rosberg B, Arborelius M et al. On thromboembolism after total hip replacement in epidural analgesia: a controlled study of dextran 70 and low dose heparin combined with dihydroergotamine. Br J Surg 71:58, 1984

Fredin H, Bergqvist D, Cederholm C, Linblad B, Nyman U. Thromboprophylaxis in hip arthroplasty. Dextran with graded compression or perioperative dextran compared in 150 patients. Acta Orthop Scand 60:678, 1989

Gatterer R. Ergotism as complication of thromboembolic prophylaxis with heparin and dihydroergotamine (letter). Lancet 2:638, 1986

Goldhaber SZ. Venous thromboembolism: How to prevent a tragedy. Hosp Pract 23:164, 1988

Hampson WGJ, Harris BC, Lucas K et al. Failure of low dose heparin to prevent deep vein thrombosis after hip replacement arthroplasty. Lancet 2:795, 1974

Harris WH, Athanasoulis CA, Waltman AC, Salzman EW. Prophylaxis of deep-vein thrombosis after total hip replacement. J Bone Joint Surg Am 67A:57, 1985

Hirsh J. Prevention of venous thrombosis in patients undergoing major orthopedic surgical procedures. Acta Chir Scand 556:30, 1990

Hoek JA, Nurmohamed MT, ten Cate JW et al. Prevention of deep vein thrombosis following total hip replacement by a Lomoparan, Organon Satellite Symposium, Amsterdam, June 30, 1991

Inada K, Koike S, Shirai N, Matsumoto K, Hirose M. Effects of intermittent pneumatic leg compression for prevention of postoperative deep venous thrombosis with special reference to fibrinolytic activity. Am J Surg 155:602, 1988

Ishak MA and Morley KD. Deep venous thrombosis after total hip arthroplasty: a prospective controlled study to determine the prophylactic effect of graded pressure stockings. Br J Surg 68:429, 1981

Johnson R, Carmichael JHE, Almond HGA, Loynes RP. Deep venous thrombosis following Charnley arthroplasty. Clin Orthop 132:24, 1978

Kakkar VV, Fox PJ, Murray WJG et al. Heparin and dihydroergotamine prophylaxis against thromboembolism after hip arthroplasty. J Bone J Surg 67B:538, 1985

Lassen MR, Borris LC, Christiansen HM et al. Prevention of thromboembolism in 190 hip arthroplasties. Comparison of LMW heparin and placebo. Acta Orthop Scand 62:33, 1991

Levine MN, Planes A, Hirsh J, Goodyear M, Vochelle N, Gent M. The relationship between anti-factor Xa level and clinical outcome in patients receiving enoxaparine low molecular weight heparin to prevent deep vein thrombosis after hip replacement. Thromb Hemost 62:940, 1989

Leyvraz PF, Richard J, Bachmann F et al. Adjusted versus fixed dose subcutaneous heparin in the prevention of deep vein thrombosis after total hip replacement. N Engl J Med 309:945, 1983

Leyvraz PF. Prevention of deep vein thrombosis after total hip replacement: comparison between adjusted heparin and a low molecular weight heparin, International Symposium on low molecular weight heparins and related polysaccharides; Munich, Germany, June 27-28, 1991

Mannucci PM, Citterio LE, Panajotopulos N. Low dose heparin and deep vein thrombosis after total hip replacement. Thromb Haemost 36:157, 1976

Mätzsch T, Bergqvist D, Fredin H, Hedner U, Lindhagen A, Nistor L. Comparison of the thromboprophylactic effect of a low molecular weight heparin versus dextran in total hip replacement. Thromb Haemorrh Disorders 3:25, 1991

Nilsen DWT, Naess-Andersen KF, Kierulf P, Heldaas J, Storen G, Godal HC. Graded pressure stockings in prevention of deep vein thrombosis following total hip replacement. Acta Chir Scand 150:531, 1984

Paiement GD, Desautels C. Deep vein thrombosis: prophylaxis, diagnosis, and treatment. Lessons from orthopedic studies. Clin Cardiol 13 (Suppl 6):19, 1990

Paiement GD, Wessinger SJ, Harris WH. Cost effectiveness of prophylaxis in total hip replacement. Am J Surg 161:519, 1991

Paiement G, Weissinger SJ, Waltman AC et al. Low dose warfarin versus external pneumatic compression for prophylaxis against venous thromboembolism following total hip replacement. J Arthoplasty 2:23, 1987

Patel A, Couband D, Feron JM, Signoret F. Prevention of deep venous thrombosis in arthroplastic surgery of the hip by the combination of heparin therapy and the antithrombosis stocking. Presse Medicale 17:1201, 1988

Planes A, Vochelle N, Fagola M et al. Prevention of deep vein thrombosis after total hip replacement. The effect of low molecular weight heparin with spinal and general anaesthesia. J Bone J Surg 73B:418, 1991

Sagar S, Stamatakis JD, Higgins AF, Nairn D, Maffei FH, Thomas DO, Kakkar VV. Efficacy of low dose heparin in prevention of extensive deep vein thrombosis in patients undergoing total hip replacement. Lancet i:1151, 1976

Sautter RD, Koch EL, Myers WO et al. Aspirin-sulfinpyrazone in prophylaxis of deep venous thrombosis in total hip replacement. JAMA 250:2649, 1983

Scurr JH. How long after surgery does the risk of thromboembolism persist? Acta Chir Scand 156; Suppl 556:22, 1990

Scurr JH, Coleridge-Smith PD, Hasty JH. Regimen for improved effectiveness of intermittent pneumatic compression in deep venous thrombosis prophylaxis. Surgery 102:816, 1987

Scurr JH, Coleridge-Smith PD, Hasty JH. Deep venous thrombosis: a continuing problem. Br Med J 297:28, 1988

Sharrock NE, Brien WW, Salvati EA, Mineo R, Garvin K, Sculco TP. The effect of intravenous fixed-dose heparin during total hip arthroplasty on the incidence of deep vein thrombosis. J Bone J Surg 72A:1456, 1990

Sikorski JM, Hampson WG, Staddon GE. The natural history and aetiology of deep vein thrombosis after total hip replacement. J Bone J Surg 63B:171, 1981

Stern D, Vasey H. A combination of dihydroergotamine and acetylsalicyclic acid — prevention of postoperative thromboembolic complications. Clinical study in orthopaedics. Schweiz Med Wochen 117:2084, 1987

Summaria L, Caprini JA, McMillan R et al. Relationship between postsurgical fibrinolytic parameters and deep vein thrombosis in surgical patients treated with compression devices. Am Surg 54:156, 1988

Swiestra BA, Stibbe J, Schouten HJ. Prevention of thrombosis after hip arthroplasty. A prospective study of preoperative oral anticoagulants. Acta Orthop Scand 59:139, 1988

Tarnay TJ, Rohr PR, Davidson MM, Stevenson MM, Byars EF, Hopkims GR. Pneumatic calf compression, fibrinolysis and the prevention of deep venous thrombosis. Surgery 88:489, 1980

Torngren S. Low dose heparin and compression stockings in the prevention of postoperative deep venous thrombosis. Br J Surg 67:482, 1980

Wille Jorgensen P, Thorup J, Fischer A, Holst-Chrisatensen J, Flamshot R. Heparin with and without graded compression stockings in the prevention of thromboembolic complications of major abdominal surgery: a randomised trial. Br J Surg 72:579, 1985

Woolson ST, McRory D, Walter JF, Maloney WJ, Watt JM, Cahill PD. B-mode ultrasound scanning in the detection of proximal venous thrombosis after total hip replacement. J Bone J Surg 72A:983, 1990

Woolson ST, Watt M. Intermittent pneumatic compression to prevent proximal deep venous thrombosis during and after total hip replacement. J Bone J Surg 73A:507, 1991

CHAPTER 28

# Knee surgery

Clara I Traverso   Juan I Arcelus
Joseph A Caprini

## Incidence of venous thromboembolism

The number of surgical procedures of the knee is increasing, and it is estimated that around 15,000 patients in the United Kingdom and 150,000 in the United States undergo total knee replacement (TKR) every year (Editorial, 1991).

Knee surgery is associated with a high risk of developing postoperative venous thromboembolic disease. The reported rate of venographically documented deep vein thrombosis (DVT) after total knee replacement in patients who did not receive prophylaxis is about 50-70% (Table 28.1) The incidence of proximal DVT as a thrombus extension from the calf veins to the popliteal or femoral veins in this surgical population is also significant (10-20%); in contrast, isolated proximal thrombosis is found very uncommonly (Stulberg et al, 1984; Lynch et al, 1988; Stringer et al, 1989; Francis et al, 1990). That represents an important difference with the findings reported after hip surgery, where isolated femoral thrombosis is more prevalent (Hirsh, 1990).

Few studies have investigated by objective outcome endpoints the incidence of pulmonary embolism (PE) after knee surgery in patients who did not receive prophylaxis. McKenna et al (1980) found positive lung perfusion scans in 4 of 12 untreated patients (33.3%) following TKR. Similarly, in a review of their experience with thrombosis prevention, also on TKR, Lynch et al (1990) found an incidence of 22% of postoperative PE in a group of 186 patients, who acted as controls in previous studies (Table 28.2). In some patients with documented segmental defects by the perfusion lung scan, only calf thrombi were identified in the venograms (McKenna et al, 1976; Lotke et al, 1984; Stringer et al, 1989). McKenna et al (1980) reported that six of ten patients with the most proximal portion of the thrombus located at the calf had documented evidence of PE. This could be secondary to the dislodgement and embolisation of part of a thrombus located in the popliteal or femoral vein. Furthermore, it could indicate that fragments of thrombi originating from the calf veins could be big enough to occlude segmental pulmonary arteries and,

**Table 28.1**
Incidence of deep vein thrombosis in knee surgery in patients without prophylaxis

| Author | Procedure | Anaesthesia | Tourniquet | n | % DVT | % Prox DVT | Day of venogram |
|---|---|---|---|---|---|---|---|
| Hull et al, 1979 | TKR | G | Y | 14 | 71.4 | — | 14-17 |
| Stulberg et al, 1984 | TKR# | G | Y | 62 | 67.7 | 11.2 | 4- 5 |
| Stringer et al, 1989 | TKR | G/E | Y | 55 | 56.4 | 9.1 | 7-10 |
|  | Arthroscopy | G/E | Y | 48 | 4.2 | 0 |  |
|  | Meniscectomy | G/E | Y | 151 | 24.5 | 2 |  |
|  | Miscellaneous | G/E | Y | 58 | 31.0 | 5.2 |  |
| Kim, 1990 | Cementless TKR | — | Y | 124 | 23.8 | 1.6 | 10-11 |
|  | Cementless TKR | — | Y | 160 | 25.0 | 1.2 |  |
| Wilson et al, 1991 | TKR | — | Y | 32 | 68.7 | 18.7 | 10 |

TKR = Total Knee Replacement   G = General Anaesthesia   E = Epidural Anaesthesia
# = No separation was made between bilateral and unilateral replacement

in cases of multiple or repeating embolisation, be of clinical significance. The reported incidence of symptomatic PE after TKR when prophylaxis was not used is low — one to three percent (Morrey et al, 1987; Stringer et al, 1989). Likewise, the risk of fatal embolism after TKR appears to be less than one percent (Morrey et al, 1987).

Apart from TKR, other knee operations are associated with a significant thromboembolic risk when prophylaxis is not implemented. Sixty percent of 15 patients undergoing different non-replacement knee procedures developed DVT in the trial conducted by Hull et al (1979). More recently, Stringer et al (1989) found that, of 209 patients who underwent knee surgery other than replacement or arthroscopy, 55 (26.3%) developed DVT. In this study, only four percent of 48 arthroscopies were followed by venous thrombosis (Table 28.1).

**Table 28.2**
Incidence of documented pulmonary embolism (PE) after TKR

| Author | Prophylaxis | Patients n | % PE | Diagnostic method |
|---|---|---|---|---|
| McKenna et al, 1980 | No | 12 | 33.3 | Perfusion scan |
| Lotke et al, 1984 | ASA (1.3g/24h) | 74 | 10.8 | Vent/perfusion scan |
| Stulberg et al, 1984 | ASA (1.3g/24h) | 475 | 8.2 | Perfusion scan |
| Haas et al, 1990 | ASA (1.3g/24h) | 58 | 1.7 | Perfusion scan |
|  | T-SIPC | 61 | 4.9 | Perfusion scan |
| Lynch et al, 1990 | No | 186 | 22.0 | Perfusion scan |
| Sharrock et al, 1991 | ASA (1.3g/24h) | 541 | 7.4 | Perfusion scan |

ASA = Aspirin
T-SIPC = Thigh-length sequential intermittent pneumatic compression

As shown in table 28.1, there are notable differences in the rates of postoperative DVT amongst the different studies. Irrespective of the use of prophylaxis, these differences could be explained by several influencing factors: type of anaesthesia (Jorgensen et al, 1991); use of cemented versus uncemented prostheses (Lynch et al, 1988; Stringer et al, 1989); unilateral versus bilateral replacement (Stulberg et al, 1984; Haas et al, 1990) and both timing and type of diagnostic endpoints (Lotke et al, 1984). The importance of some of these factors will be discussed later. Some authors have reported an association between some of the generally accepted risk factors, such as obesity (Stulberg et al, 1984; Kim, 1990), hypertension (Stulberg et al, 1984), and duration of the anaesthesia (Lotke et al, 1984; Stringer et al, 1989), and an increased risk of developing VTE after TKR. However, other authors did not find such correlations (Kim, 1990; Francis et al, 1990). The weight of advanced age is not yet well-established (McKenna et al, 1980; Stulberg et al, 1984; Stringer et al, 1989; Francis et al, 1990).

## Prophylaxis

There are not many prospective, randomised trials involving large series of patients that analyse the efficacy of different prophylactic modalities to prevent DVT following elective knee surgery. Accordingly, current published information appears to be insufficient to reach a consensus on the effectiveness of any prophylactic modality.

As discussed above, several factors may influence the pathogenesis of thromboembolism after knee surgery. In relation to the procedure, both the employment of a tourniquet during the operation and the anaesthetic regimen appear to be the two more controversial issues (McKenna et al, 1980; Fahmy and Patel, 1981; Francis et al, 1990; Sharrock et al, 1991). This presents additional difficulty when evaluating the reported outcomes.

The paucity of data in elective knee surgery is illustrated in a review of the reported bibliography carried out by Hull and Raskob in 1986. These authors concluded that the prophylactic role of both oral anticoagulants and dextran had not been adequately evaluated. Subcutaneous low dose heparin (LDH) was not even mentioned by them at that time. The results regarding acetylsalicylic acid (ASA) were found inconclusive; thus, they stated that further studies would be needed to establish its role. After having some personal experience with below-knee intermittent pneumatic compression (Hull et al, 1979), these authors concluded in this review that such a modality is both effective and safe.

More recently, the review by Lynch et al (1990) established that mechanical modalities were equal to or more effective than pharmacologic methods, and free of side-effects. The pharmacologic agents studied in this review were considered effective, yet associated with increased risk of bleeding. Another similar review did not reach any conclusion regarding the effectiveness of prophylaxis; however, the authors stressed the urgent need of further investigations on this issue (Lotke and Elia, 1990).

In a large retrospective evaluation involving 638 total knee arthroplasties performed during a five-year period, Stulberg et al (1984) analysed several aspects regarding thromboembolism after that procedure. From a prophylactic viewpoint, the study provides us little information because, as mentioned by these authors, their review was based on data from both non-randomised and non-double-blind prophylactic protocols. It should also be considered that despite prophylaxis instituted before surgery, only the postoperative regimens were evaluated; obviously, the results were biased because the pre- and postoperative regimens administered to some patients were different. Therefore, conclusions regard-

**Table 28.3**
Prospective studies in which venography was used as end-point for the diagnosis of DVT

| Author | Surgical procedure | Prophylaxis | Patients n | % Total DVT | | % Proximal DVT | |
|---|---|---|---|---|---|---|---|
| Hull et al, 1979 | Unilateral | Untreated | 32 | 65.5 | | 24.1 | |
| | | B-IPC | 29 | 6.2 | * | 0 | * |
| McKenna et al, 1980 | Unilateral | Untreated | 12 | 75 | | 41.7 | |
| | GA | LDASA (0.975) | 9 | 78 | | 33.3 | |
| | | HDASA (3.9) | 12 | 8 | * | 0 | * |
| | | T-IPC | 10 | 10 | * | 0 | * |
| Fahmy and Patel, 1981 | Unilateral | ASA (1.2) | 20 | 10 | | — | |
| | GA | ASA (1.2)+ | 20 | 35 | ns | 4 | ns |
| Lynch et al, 1988 | Unilateral | ASA (1.3) | 75 | 37.3 | | 6.7 | |
| | GA++ | ASA (1.3)+CPM | 75 | 54.3 | ns | 4 | ns |
| Francis et al, 1990 | Unilateral (87%) | ATIII-H+CPM | 39 | 36 | | — | |
| | GA++ | LDDextran+CPM | 38 | 81.5 | * | — | |
| Haas et al, 1990 | Unilateral | ASA(1.3)+CPM | 36 | 47 | | 0 | |
| | | T-IPC+CPM | 36 | 22 | * | 0 | |
| | Bilateral | ASA(1.3)+CPM | 32 | 68 | | 3.1 | |
| | GA++ | T-IPC+CPM | 35 | 48 | ns | 5.7 | ns |
| Wilson et al, 1991 | Unilateral | Untreated | 32 | 68.7 | | 18.7 | |
| | | IFP | 28 | 50 | ns | 0 | * |
| Jorgensen et al, 1991 | Unilateral | GEC GA | 22 | 59.1 | | 13.6 | |
| | | GEC RA | 17 | 17.6 | * | 5.9 | ns |

+ = Only in this study a tourniquet was not used
++ = In most patients the above specified anaesthetic regimen was used (RA: Regional; GA: General)
ASA = Acetylsalicylic acid (g/day)   IPC = Intermittent pneumatic compression
CPM = Continuous passive motion   ATIII-H = Antithrombin III plus low dose heparin
IFP = Impulse foot pump   GEC = Graduated elastic compression
* = Significant ($p<0.05$)   ns = Not significant
Note: for information on prophylactic protocols, see the text

ing the efficacy of one method when compared with another could not be reached. In their study, pharmacologic modalities were used in all cases. The incidence of DVT was similar (around 50%) when using ASA, warfarin, and both subcutaneous and intravenous heparin, as assessed by venography. No isolated proximal DVT was diagnosed. Likewise, no complications were recorded. The most frequently used method was ASA, which was administered to 69.5 percent of patients. An unexpected finding for these authors was that

9.5 percent of the patients did not receive any prophylactic drug. Regardless of their results, the authors advocated anti-platelet agents, among which ASA was the one preferred.

## Studies including treated versus untreated groups

Two studies have analysed a certain prophylactic modality exclusively compared with a non-treated group. In both cases, a mechanical method was evaluated. The first study was carried out by Hull et al, in 1979. The authors found statistically significant differences in the incidence of DVT between an untreated group and another group treated with below-knee intermittent pneumatic compression (B-IPC) on various knee procedures, as assessed by venography (Table 28.3). On total knee replacement, the incidence of DVT was reduced from 71.4 percent (10/14) in the control group to 7.7 percent (1/13) in the studied group. On a miscellaneous group, involving several knee operations, only one of nineteen patients (5.3%) in whom a B-IPC device was fitted developed DVT. In contrast, DVT was diagnosed in nine out of fifteen patients (60%) who belonged to the control group. The preoperative intake of ASA only showed a significant benefit in the control group. The second study (Wilson et al, 1991) consisted of a larger number of patients (60 TKR procedures), in which the authors studied a new mechanical device called the arterial-venous impulse foot pump. The rationale for introducing this new device was that the available conventional mechanical methods are not functional in this type of surgery because of the nature of the procedure. The "foot pump" rhythmically compresses and empties the plantar veins of the foot. The authors found a statistically significant reduction of proximal DVT from 18.7 percent in the control group to zero in the treated group ($p<0.05$), as screened by venography. However, there was no difference regarding the total incidence of DVT (68.7% and 50%, respectively). We recently had the opportunity of testing one of these devices in our vascular laboratory. By using a colour-coded duplex unit, we were able to document a clear acceleration of blood flow in the popliteal and common femoral veins during the compression cycles. Therefore, despite the small volume of blood that is ejected from the plantar veins, there are some haemodynamic effects in proximal sectors of the leg veins.

## Studies comparing treated groups

Table 28.3 compiles results from prospective studies involving knee surgery. In most of them, TKR was performed. Exceptions to that are the studies by both Hull et al (1979), as explained above, and Fahmy and Patel (1981), in which knee arthrotomies were analysed. In all of them, venography was used as an end-point for the diagnosis of DVT. The factors that are currently considered the more controversial because of their influence on the results are also specified there.

Regarding *mechanical methods*, the continuous passive motion device (CPM) has been evaluated by Lynch et al (1988) in unilateral TKR. CPM was started at the conclusion of the procedure on the operated leg, and maintained for a period depending on the gained degree of flexion but the minimum prophylactic period was seven days. It is important to realise that all patients in this group received simultaneously 1.3g of ASA per day, beginning on admission to the hospital, and continued for six weeks. The same regimen was instituted in the group used as control for the analysis. As shown in table 28.3, neither modality was effective in preventing DVT. With respect to proximal DVT, ASA administered alone was somewhat more effective than ASA plus CPM, although the results were very close. Obviously, no conclusions on the role of CPM can be reached. Its low acceptance by patients was a major drawback. The advantage of this method was that patients were able to walk at the time of discharge. Other reported advantages of CPM in knee surgery are a faster recuperation of motion (Vince et al, 1987), and its effectiveness and safety in arthroplasties with potential risk of bleeding (Limbird and Dennis, 1987).

CPM is included by some orthopaedic surgeons as part of the postoperative rehabilitation programme, but its effects in preventing DVT have not been evaluated. Thus, Francis et al (1990) mention that such a modality was "frequently" employed, but no additional comments were made. Likewise, Haas et al (1990) fitted CPM in the recovery room, without any further comment on the prophylactic role of this device.

Thigh-length intermittent pneumatic compression (T-IPC) has been analysed in two studies where this mechanical modality was compared with ASA (Table 28.3). In both, ASA was started the day before surgery and maintained until discharge. In the two studies, T-IPC was fitted on the non-operated leg before the procedure and immediately after surgery on the operated leg, and continued for a minimum period of five days. Analysing the total incidence of DVT on the unilateral procedure, T-IPC was effective in both studies, and there were statistically significant differences when compared with both a dosage of ASA equal to 0.975g per day (McKenna et al, 1980) and to 1.3 g per day (Haas et al, 1990). On the non-operated leg, T-IPC abolished DVT (Haas et al, 1990). Dosages of ASA as high as 3.9 g daily were slightly more effective than T-IPC. These methods were significantly more effective than both the untreated and the low-dose of ASA groups (McKenna et al, 1980). In contrast, neither of them reduced the incidence of DVT following the bilateral procedure (Haas et al, 1990). No patients belonging to the high dose ASA group developed proximal DVT after the unilateral TKR, and proximal DVT was also not found in any of the two studies where the T-IPC was used. Regarding the bilateral procedure, ASA was more effective than T-IPC (Table 28.3), although there was not a statistically significant difference (Haas et al, 1990).

A dosage of ASA equal to 1.2 g a day was not effective following knee arthrotomies when the procedures were performed without a tourniquet, compared with a group in which the tourniquet was fitted (Fahmy and Patel, 1981). As shown in table 28.3, the difference was not significant. It could be argued that the lower incidence in the second group could be attributed to the use of the tourniquet. Nonetheless, similar dosages of ASA were not effective in other studies in which all procedures were performed with a tourniquet (McKenna et al, 1980; Lotke et al, 1984; Lynch et al, 1988). The role of the tourniquet on the development of DVT will be analysed later.

Regarding *pharmacological methods*, a few studies are also available. Francis et al (1990) compared an association of Antithrombin III and heparin (ATIII-H) with dextran 40. The optimal doses of ATIII-H had been established prior to this study by these authors (Stulberg et al, 1989). Such dosages consisted of 3,000 IU of intravenous ATIII and 5,000 IU of subcutaneous heparin two hours before the procedure, postoperatively maintaining 2,000 IU for ATIII and the same dosage for heparin every twelve hours per day, during a five-day period. Dextran 40 was also started two hours before surgery at doses of 10 ml/Kg/day, and the maintenance dosage, administered as a constant infusion, was equal to 7 ml/Kg/day, and it was continued for 5.5 days. As mentioned above, CPM was used frequently. ATIII-H significantly reduced the incidence of total DVT (Table 28.3), but it was not more effective than dextran in reducing the incidence of proximal DVT. In addition, no isolated proximal DVT was diagnosed in any of the two treated groups (Francis et al, 1991).

In a previous study, those authors (Francis et al, 1983) analysed a short series comparing eight patients to whom the same regimen of dextran specified above was administered, but maintained 4.5 days, with 14 patients who received a two-step regimen of warfarin. The first step consisted of administering preoperatively (seven to ten days before the operation), doses of warfarin to prolong the prothrombin time (PT) to 1.5 to 3 seconds longer than the control value. The average dose for that was 3 mg, ranging from 0.5 to 100 mg. The second step consisted of administering postoperatively (starting the evening of surgery) dosages of warfarin to prolong the PT 1.5 times the control value. As assessed by venography, all eight patients in the dextran group developed DVT versus three (21%) in the warfarin group. The difference is statistically significant. They also documented a significant reduction in the rate of proximal DVT. In a recent preliminary report involving ten patients, who were not compared with another group, Dale et al (1991) found that 1 mg per day of warfarin, starting on an average of twenty days prior to the procedure and maintained for ten postoperative days, was not appropriate prophylaxis following TKR. On the other hand, the number of bleeding complications reported by Francis et al (1983) was low, and similar in both warfarin and dextran groups. More recently, Sutherland and Schurman (1987) reported that eight of 46 TKR patients (17%) receiving warfarin developed local or systemic bleeding complications. The fear of bleeding complications associated with this pharmacologic agent among US orthopaedic surgeons was well illustrated by the survey conducted by Paiement et al in 1987. In this study, one half of the surveyed surgeons responded that they had used warfarin for prophylaxis in total hip replacement, but they had stopped using it, mainly because of bleeding complications or because they found warfarin to be difficult to monitor.

Apart from the aforementioned ATIII and heparin association, a combined prophylaxis has not yet been studied prospectively. Clayton and Thompson (1987) reported good results combining ASA and mechanical methods. However, it was a review of their experience, and no objective diagnostic test was used. In a review of their experience, Lynch et al (1990) did not document improved results with a combination of CPM and sequential intermittent pneumatic compression after adding warfarin to the prophlactic regimen. Yet, the association of warfarin increased the incidence of haemarthrosis and wound haematomas. Based on these results, the authors concluded that CPM plus sequential IPC appeared to be equal or more effective than some pharmacological modalities, with the additional advantage of being free of complications.

Our current protocol of prophylaxis for TKR consists of a combination of GEC, T-IPC, and warfarin, starting preoperatively and continuing during and after the surgical procedure. Despite the discouraging results reported by Lynch et al (1990) with a similar approach, we feel that, since compression cannot be applied to the operated leg during the operation, warfarin started on the evening before surgery could provide a certain degree of protection at that time. In our experience, this combination has proved to be safe and effective in preventing clinically significant thromboses.

There is not sufficient information regarding prophylaxis and pulmonary embolism following knee surgery. Table 28.2 displays the incidence of PE after TKR, documented by lung scanning, in several studies involving patients untreated or receiving different prophylactic modalities. Although the results are not conclusive, there is a trend towards a reduction in the incidence of postoperative PE when prophylaxis is used.

**Influence of the anaesthetic regimen and the use of a tourniquet**
Nielsen et al (1990) studied the influence of general versus regional anaesthesia on the incidence of DVT in patients undergoing unilateral TKR. DVT was diagnosed by venography in 15.4 percent of the epidural group and in 62.5 percent of the general anaesthesia group (p<0.05). However, the incidence of proximal DVT was slightly higher in the general anaesthesia group (18.7%) than in the regional anaesthesia group (7.7%), without a

statistically significant difference. Recently, these authors have confirmed these outcomes in a similar study (Jorgensen et al, 1991). In a retrospective analysis of 705 knee replacements, Sharrock et al (1991) reported a significant reduction in the incidence of venographically documented DVT in patients operated under epidural anaesthesia, as compared with patients who received general anaesthesia. All patients received ASA. The aforementioned reduction was statistically significant for both total and proximal DVT. Moreover, the reduction derived from the use of epidural anaesthesia was also evident when patients were separated into unilateral or bilateral procedures. However, Haas et al (1990) found prophylaxis to fail on bilateral TKR even when using regional anaesthesia in 97 percent of the procedures. Outcomes are dissimilar. In any case, it appears that effectiveness is more related to the adequate prophylactic method than to the anaesthetic regimen as shown in table 28.3.

As mentioned above, another controversial factor that appears to notably influence the results regarding DVT after knee surgery is the employment of a tourniquet. It has been suggested that the local vein damage caused by the tourniquet could, in part, be responsible for developing DVT after knee surgery (McKenna et al, 1976), as could distal hypoxia induced by the tourniquet (Francis et al, 1991). In both cases, the genesis of a thrombus would be mediated by platelets and endothelial cells (Mustard and Packham, 1970; Hamer et al, 1981; Madden et al, 1986). In contrast, other authors have reported that the tourniquet increases the fibrinolytic response, as assessed by the euglobulin lysis time and the fibrin-plate method (Fahmy and Patel, 1981). In this study, enhanced fibrinolysis was followed by a lower incidence of DVT after total knee arthroplasty, presumably related to the hypoxia. Accordingly, the use of a tourniquet would have a protective effect. Conversely, it has been demonstrated in dogs that, in addition to the effect on fibrinolysis, the tourniquet may contribute to the production of a hypercoagulable state, because platelet count, fibrinogen levels and haematocrit all increased when a tourniquet was fitted (Nakahara and Sakahashi, 1967).

Despite these findings, there is no consensus regarding the influence of the tourniquet on thromboembolism after knee surgery, either as a causal or a protective factor. The tourniquet is employed by most surgeons. Most authors have not found an association between the duration of tourniquet ischaemia and DVT (McKenna et al, 1980; Lotke et al, 1984; Stulberg et al, 1984; Stringer et al, 1989; Kim, 1990). A protective effect was reported by Fahmy and Patel (1981) following the only study which specifically compared a group with tourniquet and the other without it. In the prospective studies conducted by Francis et al (1983; 1990), the use of tourniquet was always considered a disadvantage, although its negative influence was only apparent on groups in which the prophylactic modality was not appropriate. However, in a review of their experience, these authors did not find any relation between DVT and the time of tourniquet ischaemia, when analysing several pharmacological methods (Stulberg et al, 1984). On the other hand, it is not clear if the low incidence of isolated proximal DVT following knee surgery could be partly due to a local effect of the tourniquet. Stringer et al (1989) suggested that, but in other studies where isolated DVT was not diagnosed, the tourniquet effect was shown to be either harmless (Francis et al, 1990) or without influence (Stulberg et al, 1984). However, doses of ASA equal to or greater than 1.2 g per day were effective in decreasing the incidence of proximal DVT in the unilateral TKR when using a tourniquet (Fahmy and Patel, 1981; Lynch et al, 1988; Haas et al, 1990). Obviously, further studies to clarify the influence of the tourniquet are necessary.

The role of other prophylactic modalities, such as heparin at adjusted doses and low molecular weight heparins, remains to be established. More studies are required to determine which is the safest and most effective prophylactic approach for patients undergoing knee surgery. These studies should include detailed information regarding all factors influencing the development of venous thrombosis in this high-risk surgical population.

# References

Clayton ML, Thompson TR. Activity, air boots and aspirin as thromboembolism prophylaxis in knee arthroplasty. A multiple regimen approach. Orthopedics 10:1525, 1987

Dale C, Gallus A, Wycherley A, Langlois S, Howie D. Prevention of venous thrombosis with minidose warfarin after joint replacement. Br Med J 303:224, 1991

Editorial. How good are knee replacements? Lancet 338:447, 1991

Fahmy NR, Patel DG. Hemostatic changes and postoperative deep vein thrombosis associated with use of a pneumatic tourniquet. J Bone J Surg 63-A:461, 1981

Francis CW, Marder VJ, McCollister E, Yaukoolbodi S. Two step warfarin therapy. Prevention of postoperative venous thrombosis without excessive bleeding. JAMA 249:374, 1983.

Francis CW, Pellegrini VD, Harris CM, Stulberg BN, Gabriel R, Marder VJ. Prophylaxis of venous thrombosis following total hip and knee replacement using antithrombin III and heparin. Sem Hematol 28:39, 1991

Francis CW, Pellegrini VD, Stulberg BN, Miller ML, Totterman S, Marder VJ. Prevention of venous thromboembolism after total knee arthroplasty. Comparison of antithrombin III and low-dose heparin and dextran. J Bone J Surg 72A:976, 1990

Haas SB, Insall JN, Scuderi GR, Windsor RE, Ghelman B. Pneumatic sequential compression boots compared with aspirin prophylaxis of deep vein thrombosis after total knee arthroplasty. J Bone J Surg 72-A:27, 1990

Hamer JD, Malone PC, Silver IA. The PO2 in venous valve pockets: Its possible bearing on thrombogenesis. Br J Surg 68:166, 1981

Hirsh J. Prevention of venous thrombosis in patients undergoing major orthopedic surgical procedures. Acta Chir Scand 556:30, 1990

Hull R, Delmore TJ, Hirsh J et al. Effectiveness of intermittent pulsatile elastic stockings for the prevention of calf and thigh vein thrombosis in patients undergoing elective knee surgery. Thromb Res 16:37, 1979

Hull RD, Raskob GE. Prophylaxis of venous thromboembolic disease following hip and knee surgery. J Bone J Surg 68-A:146, 1986

Jorgensen LN, Rasmussen LS, Nielsen PT, Leffers A, Albrecht-Beste E. Antithrombotic efficacy of continuous extradural analgesia after knee replacement. Br J Anaesthesiol 66:8, 1991

Kim YH. The incidence of deep vein thrombosis after cementless and cemented knee replacement. J Bone J Surg 72B:779, 1990

Limbird TJ, Dennis SC. Synovectomy and continuous passive motion (CPM) in hemophiliac patients. Arthroscopy 3:74, 1987

Lotke PA, Elia EA. Thromboembolic disease after total knee surgery: a critical review. Instructional Course Lectures 39:409, 1990

Lotke PA, Ecker ML, Alavi A, Berkowitz H. Indications for the treatment of deep venous thrombosis following total knee replacement. J Bone J Surg 66A:202, 1984

Lynch AF, Bourne RB, Rorabeck CH, Rankin RN, Donald A. Deep vein thrombosis and continuous passive motion after total knee arthroplasty. J Bone J Surg 70A:11, 1988

Lynch JA, Baker PL, Polly RE et al. Mechanical measures in the prophylaxis of postoperative thromboembolism in total knee arthroplasty. Clin Orthop 260:24, 1990

Madden MC, Vender RL, Friedman M. Effect of hypoxia on prostacyclin production in cultured pulmonary artery endothelium. Prostaglandins 31:1049, 1986

McKenna R, Bachmann F, Kaushal SP, Galante JO. Thromboembolic disease in patients undergoing total knee replacement. J Bone J Surg 58A:928, 1976

McKenna R, Galante J, Bachmann F, Wallace DL, Kaushal S, Meredith P. Prevention of venous thromboembolism after total knee replacement by high-dose aspirin and intermittent calf and thigh compression. Br Med J 280:514, 1980

Morrey BF, Adams RA, Ilstrup DM, Bryan RS. Complications and mortality associated with bilateral or unilateral total knee arthroplasty. J Bone J Surg 69A:484, 1987

Mustard JF, Packham MA. Factors influencing platelet function: adhesion, release, and aggregation. Pharmacol Rev 22:97, 1970

Nakahara M, Sakahashi H. Effect of application of a tourniquet on bleeding factors in dogs. J Bone J Surg 49A:1345, 1967

Nielsen PT, Jorgensen LN, Albrecht-Beste E, Leffers M, Rasmussen LS. Lower thrombosis risk with epidural blockade in knee arthroplasty. Acta Orthop Scand 61:29, 1990

Oster G, Tuden RL, Colditz GA. A cost-effectiveness analysis of prophylaxis against deep vein thrombosis in major orthopedic surgery. JAMA 257:203, 1987

Paiement GD, Wessinger SJ, Harris WH. Survey of prophylaxis against venous thromboembolism in adults undergoing hip surgery. Clin Orthop 223:188, 1987

Sharrock NE, Haas SB, Hargett MJ, Urquhart B, Insall JN, Scuderi G. Effects of epidural anaesthesia on the incidence of deep vein thrombosis after total knee arthroplasty. J Bone J Surg 73A:502, 1991

Stringer MD, Steadman CA, Hedges AR, Thomas EM, Morley TR, Kakkar VV. Deep vein thrombosis after elective knee surgery: an incidence study in 312 patients. J Bone J Surg 71B:492, 1989

Stulberg GN, Francis CW, Pellegrinin VD et al. Antithrombin III/low dose heparin in the prevention of deep vein thrombosis after total knee arthroplasty. Clin Orthop 248:152, 1989

Stulberg GN, Insall JN, Williams GW, Ghelman B. Deep vein thrombosis following total knee replacement. An analysis of six hundred and thirty-eight arthroplasties. J Bone J Surg 66A:194, 1984

Sutherland CJ and Schurman JR. Complications associated with warfarin prophylaxis in total knee arthroplasty. Clin Orthop 219:158, 1987

Vince KG, Kelly MA, Beck J, Insall JN. Continuous passive motion after total knee arthroplasty. J Arthroplasty 2:281, 1987

Wilson NV, Das SK, Maurice H, Smibert G, Thomas EM, Kakkar VV. Thrombosis prophylaxis in total knee replacement. A new mechanical device. Thromb Haemost 65:1131, 1991

CHAPTER 29

# Medical patients

Denis I Clement   P Gheeraert
M De Buyzere   D Duprez

## Introduction

Anticoagulant regimens for preventing venous thromboembolism (VTE) in high risk patients have been with us for 50 years and the use of small doses of subcutaneous heparin for this purpose has become standard practice, sanctioned by the 1986 Consensus Development Conference of the US National Institute of Health (1986). Recently published meta-analyses of data from numerous clinical trials (Colditz et al, 1986; Clagett and Reisch, 1988; Collins et al, 1988) supported this point of view. Nevertheless, some important practical questions remain: which are the clinically apparent risk factors for VTE in medical patients? Should all patients "at risk" receive preventive therapy? What are the risks and benefits of preventive measures in medical patients? Should prophylaxis be tailored to individual circumstances or is there a "best" all purpose regimen?

The subject of this review will be restricted to the prevention of deep vein thrombosis (DVT) in the lower extremity veins for the following reasons:
1. Pulmonary thromboembolism (PE) is a leading cause of morbidity and mortality and is responsible for more than 50,000 deaths in the United States annually.
2. Available data indicate that more than 95% of pulmonary emboli arise from thrombi in the deep venous system of the lower extremities. Prevention of DVT in the lower extremity veins is thus the most effective approach to prevention of, and death due to, venous thromboembolism.

The groups of medical conditions in which the evidence of thromboembolism is greatly increased are summarised in table 29.1. There is a growing list of conditions in which the thrombotic risk is increased in the group of medical patients. However, the inherited risk factors are very uncommon in the non-surgical population which develops DVT and are usually discovered after the event.

Fortunately, there are clinically apparent risk factors for DVT and PE which can be used to select medical patients for prophylaxis (Stolley et al, 1975; Havic, 1977; Treffers

**Table 29.1**
Risk factors predisposing to thromboembolism

*Inherited risk factors*
    Antithrombin III deficiency
    Protein C deficiency
    Protein S deficiency
    Dysfibrinogenaemia
    Disorders of plasminogen and plasminogen activation

*Acquired risk factors*
    Lupus anticoagulant
    Nephrotic syndrome
    Paroxysmal nocturnal haemoglobinuria
    Cancer
    Stasis — congestive heart failure, myocardial infarction, cardiomyopathy, constrictive pericarditis, anasarca
    Advancing age
    Oestrogen therapy
    Sepsis
    Immobilisation
    Stroke
    Polycythaemia rubra vera
    Inflammatory bowel disease
    Obesity
    Prior thromboembolism

**Table 29.2**
Clinically apparent risk factors

    Increasing age
    Bed rest for longer than 4 days
    Recent myocardial infarction
    Recent stroke
    Transvenous pacing
    Intensive care
    Obesity
    Cancer
    Oral contraceptive use
    Preeclampsia or eclampsia
    Central venous lines
    Left and right ventricular failure
    Chronic deep venous insufficiency of the legs
    Prior thromboembolism
    Sepsis
    Nephrotic syndrome
    Inflammatory bowel disease
    Pneumonia

et al, 1983; Goldhaber, 1985; Goldhaber et al, 1987; Kierkegaard et al, 1987; Gallus, 1990). Autopsy and screening studies extended by the routine use of the fibrinogen uptake test (FUT) and venography have shown strong associations between VTE and the conditions given in table 29.2.

## Prevention trials in medical patients

There has been a flood of information about a wide selection of prophylactic methods in surgical patients. In the medical population, most evidence derives from small trials in patients with medical catastrophes like myocardial infarction or hemiplegia where the high risk period for VTE is triggered by an acute event so that preventive measures begun at or soon after its onset should succeed. Information is sparse about the success of preventive measures applied during transient severe exacerbations of chronic illness (Gallus, 1990).

### Diagnostic end-points used in studies of DVT prevention
The clinical diagnosis of DVT or PE is sufficiently unreliable to be almost useless for clinical trial purposes (Gallus et al, 1976). Measuring the incidence of DVT or PE postmortem requires a much higher autopsy rate than is presently performed. Total or cause-specific mortality reduction could be measured only through exceedingly large studies including at least 5,000 patients. Providing convenient high frequency "substitute" end-points for clinical trials, most prevention studies since 1970 have used the FUT or routine venography (VG) to screen for DVT. The major limitations of FUT are a relative insensitivity to femoral DVT and complete inability to detect pelvic vein thrombosis (Gallus and Hirsh, 1976). This problem is probably not critical in medical patients where thrombosis usually arises in the calf and extends proximally (Havic, 1977) so that a negative scan indicates a very low risk of proximal DVT (above knee) or PE. A positive scan carries a 20% chance of asymptomatic progression complicated in turn by symptomatic embolism in perhaps 40% of patients if left untreated (Gallus, 1990). Noninvasive approaches include mainly impedance plethysmography (IPG). The use of a DVT screening test as a marker for PE is justified both by the known pathophysiology of PE and the association of a reduction in DVT with a reduction in PE.

### Clinical trials
In patients with myocardial infarction, the incidence of DVT ranges between 17% and 38% (Table 29.3). Positive FUT was the diagnostic end point most used. In those studies full and low dose heparin showed significant reduction in the incidence of DVT. No other preventive measures had been studied. When using PE as an end point, only a few large randomised control trials were performed. Only full dose heparin and warfarin were used in these trials which showed a significant reduction of PE. Most of the studies were too small for safety analyses.

In non-haemorrhagic stroke patients the incidence of DVT ranges between 30% and 75% (Table 29.4). FUT, impedance plethysmography, venography and their combinations were used as diagnostic end points. The lowest incidence was found when venography was included in the end points. The highest incidence was found in the elderly patients where FUT was the end point. A significant reduction in incidence was found in low dose heparin and low molecular weight heparin (LMW-heparin) trials. One study with dextran could not

**Table 29.3**
Clinical trials in patients with myocardial infarction

| Reference | Patients n | Incidence of DVT in: Control group | Incidence of DVT in: Treatment group | p | Endpoint | Method |
|---|---|---|---|---|---|---|
| Med. Res. Council Trial, 1969 | 1,427 | 5.6% | 2.2% | <0.01 | PE | Heparin Phenindione |
| BMH, 1972 | 1,136 | 6.1% | 3.8% | ns | PE | Heparin Phenindione |
| VACT, 1973 | 999 | 2.6% | 0.2% | <0.005 | PE | Heparin Warfarin |
| Nicolaides et al, 1971 | 31 | 38% | 5.5% | 0.03 | LS | Warfarin |
| Wray et al, 1973 | 922 | 1.7% | 6.5% | <0.05 | LS | Warfarin |
| Handley, 1972 | 50 | 29% | 25% | ns | LS | Low dose heparin |
| Warlow et al, 1973 | 127 | 17% | 3.2% | <0.025 | LS | Low dose heparin |
| Emmerson and Marks, 1977 | 78 | 34% | 5% | <0.005 | LS | Low dose heparin |
| SCATI, 1989 | 711 | 9.9% | 5.8% | <0.03 | Mortality | Calcium Heparin |

LS = Fibrinogen leg scan

reduce the incidence in a group of fifty patients. No other preventive measures were studied in control trials for stroke patients.

Few control studies have defined the efficacy of preventive measures for DVT among medical patients admitted to hospital for reasons other than myocardial infarction or stroke

**Table 29.4**
Clinical trials in patients with stroke

| Reference | Number of patients | Incidence of DVT in: Control group | Incidence of DVT in: Treatment group | p | Endpoint | Method |
|---|---|---|---|---|---|---|
| McCarthy et al, 1977 | 32[*] | 75% | 12.5% | <0.01 | LS | Calcium heparin |
| Czechanowski and Heinrich, 1981 | 81 | 48% | 24% | 2p<0.02 | LS | Low dose heparin |
| Turpie et al, 1987 | 67 | 30.4% | 2.3% | 0.002 | IPG+LS+VG | LMWH |
| Mellbring et al, 1976 | 50 | 54% | 50% | ns | LS | Dextran |
| Prins et al, 1986 | 60 | 40% | 20% | 0.05 | LS+VG | LMWH |

[*] mean age 78.2±7.4

**Table 29.5**
Clinical trials in general medical patients

| Reference | Number of patients | Incidence of DVT in: Control group | Incidence of DVT in: Treatment group | p | Endpoint | Method |
|---|---|---|---|---|---|---|
| Belch et al, 1981 | 100 | 26% | 4% | — | LS | LDH |
| Cade, 1982 | 119* | 29% | 13% | — | LS | LDH |
| Halkin et al, 1982 | 1,358 | 10.9% | 7.8% | 0.05 | Mortality | LDH |
| Dogan et al, 1986 | 270(>65y) | 9.1% | 3% | 0.03 | LS | LMWH |
| Harenberg et al, 1987 | 200 | 2% LDH | 1.5% LMWH | ns | IPG | LDH, LMWH |
| Pouievierski et al, 1987 | 192 | 0% LDH | 0% LMWH | — | VG | LDH, LMWH |

LDH = low dose heparin   LMWH = low molecular weight heparin
*Critical care patients

(Table 29.5). FUT, IPG and VG were used as diagnostic end points in these studies. The incidence ranged from 9.1% to 26%. Low dose heparin was found to be effective in general medical patients and critical care patients. However, the studied groups were too small to confirm safety. Low molecular weight heparin (LMWH) was effective in an elderly medical patient group. LMWH and low dose heparin were compared in two double blind randomised control trials and were found to be equally effective. No differences in complication rates were noted. Low dose heparin reduced the mortality rate in one large trial (Halkin et al, 1982). However, the incidence of DVT was not specified.

# Conclusion

Low dose heparin has been shown to be effective in the prevention of DVT in patients with myocardial infarction and non-haemorrhagic stroke in a few clinical trials each covering a small group of patients. There are trials which found low dose heparin to be effective in general medical patients, although its value in this clinical setting is much less well documented. LMWH has proven to be effective in patients with non-haemorrhagic stroke and general medical patients older than sixty years in three small studies. Two studies suggest equal efficacy of low dose heparin and LMWH in general medical patients. Although several approaches other than heparin or dextran such as elastic stockings, physiotherapy, "ultra low dose heparin" and "minidose" warfarin are available, their value in medical patients is not documented by clinical trials.

To prevent DVT and PE in medical patients, it should be instructive to know more about the value of the clinically and biochemically apparent risk factors that can identify the majority of patients who develop DVT. Assuming that DVT prevention is a substitute for PE prevention, more large scale trials on preventive measures for DVT are needed in medical patients. The credibility of DVT prevention trials depends heavily on their choice of diagnostic end points. However, those end points that are clinically the most important and relevant (symptomatic DVT and PE, fatal PE, and total mortality) present practical difficulties. The clinical diagnosis of DVT or PE is unreliable for trial purposes. A reduction in either total or cause specific mortality by prophylaxis can be measured only through extremely large studies. Because of this, more convenient high frequency "substitute" end points for large scale clinical trials are needed.

# References

Belch JJ, Lowe GDO, Ward AG. Prevention of deep vein thrombosis in medical patients by low dose heparin. Scottish Med J 26:115, 1981

Cade JH. High risk of the critically ill for venous thromboembolism. Critical Care Med 10:448, 1982

Clagett GP, Reisch JS. Prevention of venous thromboembolism in general surgical patients. Ann Surg 208:227, 1988

Colditz GA, Tuden RL, Oster G. Rates of venous thrombosis after general surgery: combined results of randomised clinical trials. Lancet ii:143, 1986

Collins R, Scrimgeour A, Yusuf S, Peto R. Reduction in fatal pulmonary embolism and venous thrombosis by perioperative administration of subcutaneous heparin. N Engl J Med 318:1162, 1988

Conference report (1986): Prevention of deep venous thrombosis and pulmonary embolism. Lancet i:1202, 1986

Czechanowski B, Heinrich F. Prophylaxe venöser Trhombosen bei frischem ischaemischem zerebrovaskulariën Insult. Dtsch Med Wschr 106:1254, 1981

Dogan R, Houlbert D, Caulin C et al. Prevention of deep vein thrombosis in elderly medical inpatients by a low molecular weight heparin: a randomised double blind trial. Haemostasis 16:159, 1986

Drapkin A, Mersky C. Anticoagulant therapy after acute myocardial infarction: relation of therapeutic benefit to patient's age, sex and severity of infarction. JAMA 222:541, 1972

Emmerson PA, Marks P. Preventing thromboembolism after myocardial infarction: effect of low dose heparin or smoking. Brit Med J 1:18, 1977

Gallus AS. Anticoagulants in the prevention of venous thromboembolism. Ballières Clin Hematol 3:651, 1990

Gallus AS, Hirsh J. Prevention of Venous Thromboembolism. Semin Thromb Hemost 2:232, 1976

Gallus AS, Hirsh J, Hull R et al. Diagnosis of venous thromboembolism. Semin Thromb Hemost 2:203, 1976

Goldhaber SZ. Pulmonary embolism and deep venous thrombosis. Philadelphia, WB Saunders Co., 1985

Goldhaber SZ, Buring JE, Hennekens CH et al. Cancer and venous thromboembolism. Arch Intern Med 147:216, 1987

Halkin H, Goldberg J, Nodan M et al. Reduction of mortality in general medical inpatients by low dose heparin prophylaxis. Ann Int Med 96:561, 1982

Handley AJ. Low dose heparin after myocardial infarction. Lancet 2:623, 1972

Harenberg J, Kallenbach B, Martin U, Zimmermann R. Randomised double blinded study of normal and a low molecular weight heparin in general medical patients. Thromb Haemost 58:Abstr. 1392, 1987

Havic O. Deep vein thrombosis and pulmonary embolism. Acta Chir Scand 478 (Suppl.):1, 1977

Kierkegaard A, Norgren L, Olsson CG et al. Incidence of deep vein thrombosis in bedridden nonsurgical patients. Acta Med Scand 111:409, 1987

McCarthy ST, Robertson D, Turner JJ et al. Low dose heparin as a prophylaxis against deep vein thrombosis after stroke. Lancet 2:800, 1977

Mellbring G, Strand T, Eriksson S. Venous thromboembolism after cerebral infarction and the prophylactic effect of dextran 40. Acta Med Scand 220:425, 1986

Nicolaides AN, Kakkar VV, Renney TJG et al. Myocardial infarction and deep vein thrombosis. Brit Med J 1:432, 1971

Pouievierski I, Barthels M, Poliwoda H. The safety and efficacy of a low molecular weight heparin (Fragmin) in the prevention of deep vein thrombosis in medical patients: a randomised double blind trial. Thromb Haemost 58:Abstr. 425, 1987

Prins MH, Gelsema R, Sing AK et al. Prophylaxis of deep venous thrombosis with a low molecular weight heparin (Kabi 2165/Fragmin) in stroke patients. Haemostasis 19:245, 1989

Report of the working party on anticoagulation therapy in coronary thrombosis to the Medical Research Council. Assessment of short term anticoagulant administration after cardiac infarction. Br Med J 1:335, 1969

SCATI Group (1989). Randomised controlled trial of subcutaneous calcium heparin in acute myocardial infarction. Lancet 2:182, 1989

Stolley PD, Tonascia JA, Tockman MS et al. Thrombosis with low estrogen oral contraceptives. Am J Epidemiol 102:197, 1975

Treffers PE, Huidekoper BL, Weenink GH, Kloosterman GI. Epidemiological observations of thromboembolic disease during pregnancy and in the perperium in 56,022 women. Int J Gynaecol Obstet 21:327, 1983

Turpie AGG, Hirsh J, Jay R et al. Double blind randomised trial of ORG 10172 low molecular weight heparinoid in prevention of deep vein thrombosis in thrombotic stroke. Lancet 1:523, 1976

VAHI. Veterans Administration Hospital Investigators. Anticoagulants in acute myocardial infarction: results of a cooperative clinical trial. JAMA 225:724, 1973

Warlow C, Terry G, Kenmere AC et al. A double blind trial of low dose of subcutaneous heparin in the prevention of deep vein thrombosis after myocardial infarction. Lancet 2:934, 1973

Wray R, Maurer B, Shillingford J. Prophylactic anticoagulant therapy in the prevention of calf vein thrombosis after myocardial infarction. N Engl J Med 288:815, 1973

Chapter 30

# Stroke and neurosurgical patients

Alexander G G Turpie

## Neurosurgery

Deep vein thrombosis (DVT) and pulmonary embolism (PE) are common causes of morbidity and mortality in neurosurgical patients. The incidence of DVT detected by $^{125}$I-labelled fibrinogen leg scanning and impedance plethysmography (IPG) in neurosurgical populations has been reported to be 20% to 30% (Turpie et al, 1977; Skillman et al, 1978; Turpie et al, 1979; 1985). Fatal PE occurs in approximately 1% of neurosurgical patients (Sigel et al, 1974; Watson, 1974).

Several methods for preventing DVT following neurosurgery are available, but the most attractive are the physical methods which include graduated compression stockings or intermittent pneumatic compression (IPC) devices (Turpie and Hirsh, 1984). Anticoagulant prophylaxis with low-dose heparin is effective in general surgical patients, but the use of anticoagulants in neurosurgical patients is problematic because of the potential for serious bleeding. Intermittent pneumatic compression is an effective method of prophylaxis in both general surgical patients and neurosurgical patients (Turpie et al, 1977; Skillman et al, 1978; Turpie et al, 1979; Turpie and Hirsh, 1984). Despite its demonstrated efficacy, IPC is not widely used for the prevention of DVT in neurosurgical patients, possibly because of the perception that it is inconvenient to both patients and nursing staff. Graduated compression stockings which are much easier to use, are also effective in the prevention of DVT in general surgical patients (Holford, 1976; Scurr et al, 1977; Allan et al, 1983; Bergqvist et al, 1984; Colditz et al, 1986). In a study in neurosurgical patients, graduated compression stockings alone were as effective as graduated compression stockings plus IPC for the prevention of venous thrombosis in neurosurgical patients (Turpie et al, 1979).

There have been few reports on the use of low-dose heparin prophylaxis in neurosurgical patients. Powers and Edwards (1982) in a review of the low-dose heparin studies, concluded that low-dose heparin was indicated in all patients undergoing elective neurosurgical procedures and that the regimen was efficacious and safe. However, the studies were too small to exclude clinically important bleeding, including intracranial bleeding, in the heparin group. Therefore, low-dose heparin is not widely used in these patients. The main attraction of physical methods of prophylaxis in neurosurgical patients is that they are free of the potential for haemorrhagic side-effects.

## Spinal Cord Trauma

In patients with spinal cord injuries, venous thrombosis has been reported to occur in 15% to 60% of patients depending upon the severity of the injury, the presence of lower limb paralysis, and the presence of other associated risk factors (Cook and Lyons, 1949; Brach et al, 1977; Rossi et al, 1980; Frisbie and Sasahara, 1981). The reported incidence of fatal pulmonary embolism ranged from 2% to 16% of patients within two to three months of spinal cord injury (Schull and Rose, 1966; Naso, 1974; diRicco et al, 1984).

Because of the evidence for the efficacy of low-dose heparin prophylaxis in general surgical and medical patients without an increased risk of significant haemorrhage, low-dose heparin has been proposed as the method of preventing deep vein thrombosis in spinal cord injured patients. There have been several reports on the use of low-dose heparin in spinal cord injury patients, but these studies have been non-randomised and involved only small numbers of patients (Silver, 1974; Rocha Casas et al, 1976; 1977). In one study using retrospective controls, there was a highly significant reduction in the frequency of deep vein thrombosis in spinal cord injured patients using objective tests. In none of the studies was there a significant increase in bleeding reported. In one randomised controlled trial involving 32 patients with spinal cord injury, the frequency of venous thrombosis was unexpectedly low in both the control and in the heparinised groups, but in this study, only impedance plethysmography was used, which would be insensitive to calf vein and non-occluding thrombi. The majority of the reports indicate that venous thrombosis is most common during the period of flaccidity, and most authors recommend the use of low-dose heparin or other prophylaxis for the first three months following injury (Silver, 1974; Rocha Casas et al, 1976; 1977; Colditz et al, 1986).

In a recent study (Green et al, 1990), a low molecular weight heparin (Logiparin) was compared with standard low-dose heparin for the prevention of DVT in spinal cord injured patients. Twenty-one patients were randomised to standard heparin and 20 to Logiparin. Five patients in the standard heparin group had thrombotic events, including two patients with fatal pulmonary embolism; two other patients had bleeding severe enough to necessitate withdrawing the heparin. The cumulative event rate in the heparin group was 34.7 percent (95% CI, 13.7% to 55.2%). None of the patients treated with low-molecular weight heparin had thrombosis or bleeding (95% CI, 0% to 14%). The difference between the two groups was significant (p=0.006). The results of this study indicate that Logiparin is safe and effective in the prevention of thromboembolism in patients with spinal cord injury and is superior to standard heparin given in a dose of 5,000 units three times per day.

## Stroke

Venous thromboembolism is a common complication in patients with acute ischaemic stroke. Without prophylaxis, deep vein thrombosis (DVT) occurs, usually in the paralysed limb, in 60-75% of patients with dense hemiplegia (Warlow et al, 1972; McCarthy et al, 1977), and 1-2% suffer fatal pulmonary embolism (Brown and Glassenberg, 1973). Several methods of preventing DVT have been shown to be safe and effective in other high-risk medical patients. Of these, low-dose subcutaneous heparin has been the most extensively evaluated (Turpie and Leclerc, 1990). Three randomised trials using low-dose heparin prophylaxis in patients with acute stroke have been reported. In two studies (McCarthy et al, 1977; McCarthy and Turner, 1986), low-dose heparin given subcutaneously in doses of 5,000 units every eight hours reduced the frequency of DVT from 75% of 16 patients to 13% of 16 patients and from 73% of 161 patients to 22% of 144 patients in the placebo and heparin-treated groups, respectively. In the third study (Czechanowski and Heinrich, 1981), a combination of low-dose heparin 5,000 units with dihydroergotamine (DHE) subcutaneously every 12 hours reduced the frequency of DVT from 56% of 41 patients in the placebo-treated group to 28% of 40 patients in the combined heparin/DHE group. Despite the demonstration in all three studies of a significant benefit of treatment, low-dose heparin is not widely used in stroke patients because of concern about a possible increased risk of intracranial haemorrhage. In addition, the rates of venous thrombosis in patients with paralytic stroke remain high even with low dose heparin prophylaxis.

There have been two studies using low molecular weight heparin for the prevention of deep vein thrombosis in patients with ischaemic stroke (Prins et al, 1989; Sandset et al, 1990). The results of these studies are conflicting. The first study (Prins et al, 1989) compared Fragmin in a dose of 2,500 units twice a day with placebo and demonstrated a reduction in the rate of venous thrombosis from 50% to 22%. In the second study (Sandset et al, 1990), Fragmin was given in a dose of 50-65 units/km/body weight once daily (equivalent to 3500-4550 anti-Factor Xa units daily) but in contrast to the first study, there was no difference in the frequency of deep vein thrombosis in the Fragmin-treated patients (36%) compared with the placebo-treated patients (34%).

Orgaran, a low-molecular weight heparinoid which has been shown to be effective in preventing venous thrombosis in high-risk surgical patients without significant bleeding risk has been evaluated for the prevention of deep vein thrombosis in patients with acute ischaemic stroke in two studies. In a double-blind, placebo-controlled study (Turpie et al, 1987), 75 patients were randomised to receive Orgaran (50 patients) in a loading dose of 1,000 anti-Xa units intravenously followed by 750 anti-Xa units subcutaneously 12-hourly or placebo (25 patients). Prophylaxis was commenced within seven days of stroke onset, continued for 14 days or until discharge from hospital, if earlier. Venous thrombosis was diagnosed by $^{125}$-Iodine labelled fibrinogen leg scanning and impedance plethysmography. Deep vein thrombosis was confirmed by venography which occurred in 2 of 50 (4%) in the Orgaran group and 7 of 25 (28%) in the placebo group (p=0.005). The corresponding rates for proximal deep vein thrombosis were 0% and 16% respectively (p=0.01). There was one major haemorrhage in the Orgaran-treated group and one minor haemorrhage in the placebo group. Plasma heparin levels (anti-factor Xa units/ml: mean ± SED) gradually rose from 0.18 to ± 0.001 and 0.06 ± 0.001, six and 12 hours after injection on the first day to 0.24 ± 0.02 and 0.12 ± 0.01 after 11 days of treatment. The results of the placebo-controlled trial demonstrate that Orgaran is highly effective in the prevention of deep vein thrombosis in stroke patients without causing bleeding. In the second study (Turpie et al, 1992), the safety and efficacy of Orgaran was compared with unfractionated heparin in the prevention of deep vein thrombosis in a double-blind randomised trial in patients with acute ischaemic stroke. Eighty-seven patients with marked lower limb paralysis secondary to stroke were randomised to receive Orgaran (45 patients) in a dose of 750 anti-factor Xa units subcutaneously 12-hourly or unfractionated heparin (42 patients) in a dose of 5,000 units subcutaneously 12-hourly. Prophylaxis was commenced within five days of the onset of stroke on average and continued for 14 days. Venous thrombosis surveillance was carried out with

**Table 30.1**
DVT prevention in stroke

|  | Placebo | LDH | LMWH | Orgaran |
|---|---|---|---|---|
| Warlow et al, 1972 | 60% | — | — | — |
| McCarthy et al, 1977 | 75% | 12% | — | — |
| Czechanowski & Heinrich, 1981 | 56% | 28%* | — | — |
| McCarthy & Turner, 1986 | 73% | 22% | — | — |
| Turpie et al, 1987 | 28% | — | — | 4% |
| Prins et al, 1989 | 50% | — | 22% | — |
| Sandset et al, 1990 | 34% | — | 36% | — |
| Turpie et al, 1992 | — | 31% | — | 9% |

*Plus DHE
LDH = Low dose heparin   LMWH = Low molecular weight heparin

$^{125}$Iodine-labelled fibrinogen leg scanning and impedance plethysmography confirmed by ascending venography. Venous thrombosis occurred in 4 of 45 (8.9%) of the Orgaran group and 13 of 42 (31%) in the unfractionated heparin group (2p=0.02). The corresponding rates for proximal vein thrombosis were 2.2% and 11.9% respectively (2p=0.17). There were no clinically significant haemorrhagic complications in either group and the frequency of haemorrhagic conversion of the infarct was 6.9% overall with no difference in the incidence between the two treatment groups (p>0.1). The results of this study indicate that Orgaran is more effective prophylaxis against deep vein thrombosis than conventional low-dose subcutaneous heparin in patients with acute stroke. The results of these two studies demonstrate that deep vein thrombosis prophylaxis with Orgaran is more effective than standard low-dose subcutaneous heparin without causing bleeding complications in patients with acute ischaemic stroke.

The incidence of DVT in the control and treatment groups in randomised trials of venous thrombosis prophylaxis in stroke are shown in the table.

# References

Allan A, Williams JT, Bolton JP et al. The use of graduated compression stockings in the prevention of postoperative deep vein thrombosis. Br J Surg 70:172, 1983

Bergqvist D, Lindblad B. The thromboprophylactic effect of graded elastic compression stockings in combination with dextran 70. Arch Surg 119:1329, 1984

Brach BB, Moser KM Cedar L et al. Venous thrombosis in acute spinal cord paralysis. J Trauma 17:189, 1977

Brown M, Glassenberg M. Mortality factors in patients with acute stroke. JAMA 224:1493, 1973

Colditz GA, Tuden RL, Oster G. Rates of venous thrombosis after general surgery: Combined results of randomized clinical trials. Lancet 2:143, 1986

Cook AW, Lyons HA. Venous thromboembolic phenomena: their absence in paraplegic or tetraplegic patients. Am J Med Sci 218:155, 1949

Czechanowski B, Heinrich F. Prophylaxe venoser Thrombosen bei frischem ischamischem zerebrovaskularem Indult — Doppelblind studie mit Heparin-Dihydrogot. Dtsch Med Wochenschr 106:1254, 1981

diRicco G, Marini G, Rindi M et al. Pulmonary embolism in neurosurgical patients; diagnosis and treatment. J Neurosurg 60:972, 1984

Frisbie JH, Sasahara AA. Low dose heparin prophylaxis for deep venous thrombosis in acute spinal cord injury patients: A controlled study. Paraplegia 19:141, 1981

Green D, Lee MY, Lim AC et al. Prevention of thromboembolism after spinal cord injury using low-molecular-weight heparin. Ann Intern Med 113:571, 1990

Holford CP. Graded compression for preventing deep venous thrombosis. Br Med J 2:969, 1976

McCarthy ST, Robertson D, Turner JJ, Hawkey CJ. Low-dose heparin as a prophylaxis against deep vein thrombosis after acute stroke. Lancet 2:800, 1977

McCarthy ST, Turner J. Low-dose subcutaneous heparin in the prevention of deep vein thrombosis and pulmonary emboli following acute stroke. Age and Ageing 15:84, 1986

Naso F. Pulmonary embolism in acute spinal cord injury. Arch Phys Med Rehabil 55:275, 1974

Powers SK, Edwards MSB. Prophylaxis of thromboembolism in the neurological patient: A review. Neurosurgery 10:509, 1982

Prins MH, Gelsema R, Sing AK et al. Prophylaxis of deep venous thrombosis with a low-molecular weight heparin (Kabi 2165/Fragmin) in stroke patients. Haemostas 19:245, 1989

Rocha Casas E, Sanchez MP, Arias CR et al. Prophylaxis of venous thrombosis and pulmonary embolism in patients with acute traumatic spinal cord lesions. Paraplegia 14:178, 1976

Rocha Casas E, Sanchez MP, Arias CR et al. Prophylaxis of venous thrombosis and pulmonary embolism in patients with acute traumatic spinal cord lesions. Paraplegia 15:209, 1977

Rossi EC, Green D, Rosen JS et al. Sequential changes in factor VIII and platelets preceding deep vein thrombosis in patients with spinal cord injury. Br J Haematol 45:143, 1980

Sandset PM, Dahl T, Stiris M et al. A double-blind and randomized placebo-controlled trial of low molecular weight heparin once daily to prevent deep vein thrombosis in acute ischemic stroke. Semin Thromb and Hemost 16:25, 1990

Schull JR, Rose DL. Pulmonary embolism in patients with spinal cord injuries. Arch Phys Med Rehabil 47:444, 1966

Scurr JH, Ibrahim SZ, Faber RG et al. The efficacy of graduated compression stockings in the prevention of deep vein thrombosis. Br J Surg 64:371, 1977

Sigel B, Ipsen J, Felix WR. The epidemiology of lower extremity deep venous thrombosis in surgical patients. Ann Surg 179:278, 1974

Silver JR. The prophylactic use of anticoagulant therapy in the prevention of pulmonary emboli in one hundred consecutive spinal injury patients. Paraplegia 12:188, 1974

Skillman JJ, Collins EC, Coe NP et al. Prevention of deep vein thrombosis in neurosurgical patients: A controlled randomized trial of external pneumatic compression boots. Surgery 83:354, 1978

Turpie AGG, Gallus AS, Beattie WS et al. Prevention of venous thrombosis in patients with intracranial disease by intermittent pneumatic compression of the calf. Neurology 27:435, 1977

Turpie AGG, Delmore T, Hirsh J et al. Prevention of venous thrombosis by intermittent sequential calf compression in patients with intracranial disease. Thromb Res 15:611, 1979

Turpie AGG, Hirsh J, Gent M, Julian D, Johnson J. Prevention of deep vein thrombosis in potential neurosurgical patients: A randomized trial comparing graduated compression stockings alone or graduated compression stockings plus intermittent pneumatic compression with control. Arch Intern Med 149:679, 1979a

Turpie AGG, Hirsh J. Venous thromboembolism: II. Current concepts. Hosp Med November pp 13-14, 1984

Turpie AGG, Gent M, Doyle DJ et al. An evaluation of suloctidil in the prevention of deep vein thrombosis in neurosurgical patients. Thromb Res 39:173, 1985

Turpie AGG, Hirsh J, Jay RM et al. Double-blind randomized trial of ORG 10172 low-molecular weight heparinoid in prevention of deep vein thrombosis in thrombotic stroke. Lancet 1:523, 1987

Turpie AGG, Leclerc J. Prophylaxis of venous thromboembolism. In: Venous Thromboembolic Disorders, J. Leclerc (ed) 303, 1991, Lea and Sebiger, Philadelphia

Turpie AGG, Gent M, Cote R, Levine MN, Ginsberg JS, Powers P, et al. A low-molecular-weight heparinoid compared with unfractionated heparin in the prevention of deep vein thrombosis in patients with acute ischaemic stroke. Ann Intern Med 117: 353, 1992

Warlow C, Ogston D, Douglas AS. Venous thrombosis following strokes. Lancet 1:1305, 1972

Watson N. Anticoagulant therapy in the treatment of venous thrombosis and pulmonary embolism in acute spinal injury. Paraplegia 12:197, 1974

CHAPTER 31

# Urologic surgery

Gianni Belcaro    Andrew Nicolaides

## Incidence of deep vein thrombosis (DVT) and pulmonary embolism (PE) in patients having urological operations

In 1945 Colby reported a 2.54% overall incidence of fatal pulmonary embolism in patients undergoing prostatic surgery (2.13% with transurethral (TUR) operations, 2.17% with perineal procedures and 8.69% with suprapubic prostatectomy (SPP)). In his report pulmonary embolism was the most common single cause of postoperative mortality (30% of total mortality) in patients undergoing urological surgery.

Similar results were reported two decades later by Antila and his colleagues (1966) who found a 2.6% incidence of fatal pulmonary embolism after surgery for benign hyperplasia which accounted for more than 50% of the total mortality. In subsequent reports, mortality due to pulmonary embolism (mainly prostatectomy) varied from 1.2% to 5.5% (Storm et al, 1967; Allgood et al, 1970; Becker et al, 1970; International Multicenter Trial, 1975; Holbraad et al, 1976). It should be noted that the incidence reported in these studies had been mostly obtained from clinical data. When perfusion lung scans were used before and after operation, a 22% incidence of pulmonary embolism was found (Allgood et al, 1970).

It has been calculated by Moser (1983) that at least 10 nonfatal emboli occur for each fatal one. Therefore an incidence of death from pulmonary embolism from 1% to 2% suggests a total incidence of perioperative embolism of at least 10% to 20%.

The incidence of postoperative DVT in urological patients determined by the fibrinogen uptake test (FUT) or venography is shown in table 31.1. The total number of patients reported in the 15 studies listed is 598 with an overall incidence of DVT of 168 (28%). In two studies in which patients having both transurethral (TUP) and retropubic prostatectomy (RPP) the results indicated that the incidence was five to seven times higher in the latter (Mayo et al, 1971; Nicolaides et al, 1972b).

**Table 31.1**
Incidence of deep vein thrombosis (DVT) in urology patients

| Reference | Diagnostic method | Type of operation | Number of patients | Incidence of DVT(%) |
|---|---|---|---|---|
| Becker and Borgstrom, 1968 | Venography | RPP | 43 | 7 (16%) |
| Becker et al, 1970 | Venography | RPP | 187 | 39 (21%) |
| Williams, 1971 | FUT | RPP | 5 | 4 |
| Mayo et al, 1971 | " | RPP | 41 | 21 (51%) |
|  |  | TUP | 20 | 2 (10%) |
| Gordon-Smith et al, 1972 | " | RPP | 32 | 9 (28%) |
| Nicolaides et al, 1972a | " | RPP | 23 | 8 (28%) |
| Nicolaides et al, 1972b | " | RPP | 21 | 10 (48%) |
|  |  | TUP | 29 | 2 (7%) |
| Rosenberg et al, 1975 | " | RPP | 33 | 11 (33%) |
| Sebeseri et al, 1975 | " | Kidney, Ureter, Bladder | 31 | 18 (58%) |
| Hedlund, 1975 | " | TUP | 40 | 18 (43%) |
| Kutnowski et al, 1977 | " | RPP, Renal, Ureteric | 25 | 12 (48%) |
| Coe et al, 1978 | " | RPP, Renal, Bladder | 24 | 6 (25%) |
| Bergqvist and Hallbook, 1980 | ", | Miscellaneous | 19 | 6 (31%) |
| Vandendris et al, 1980 | ", | RPP | 33 | 13 (39%) |

RPP = Retropubic prostatectomy   TUP = Transurethral prostatectom
FUT = Fibrinogen uptake test

## Incidence of DVT and PE after renal transplantation

The European Dialysis and Transplant Association Report of 1983 showed a mortality rate attributable to PE of 4.4% after renal transplantation (1983).

The incidence of thromboembolic complications in patients having renal transplantation has been reported to vary from 8.8% to 14.9% in several retrospective studies (Nestrom et al, 1973; Rao et al, 1976; Arnadottir et al, 1983; Allen et al, 1987). It was higher in a prospective series using noninvasive techniques: 14% which increased to 24.1% if diabetic patients were included (Bergqvist et al, 1985). In a review of 480 consecutive patients having renal transplants over a period of 10 years, an 8.3% incidence of thromboembolic events were found, comprising 25 lower limb DVT alone, 11 DVT with PE and four with PE alone. Four deaths were directly attributable to PE which was the fourth major cause of death in this 10-year period. The incidence was low in the first month after transplantation (1.7%), but it increased subsequently reaching a peak in the fourth month. Age (>40), prolonged bedrest (>4 days) because of infection or further surgical procedures, pelvic pathology and the administration of steroids were factors associated with an increased incidence of DVT (Allen et al, 1987).

Table 31.2
Randomised controlled studies of DVT prevention in patients having urological operations using the fibrinogen uptake test (FUT)

| Reference | Type of operation | Control group n | DVT | Low Dose Heparin Group n | DVT | Intermittent pneumatic compression n | DVT | Electrical stimulation n | DVT | Dextran-70 n | DVT |
|---|---|---|---|---|---|---|---|---|---|---|---|
| Williams, 1971 | RPP | 7 | 4 | 5 | 4* | | | | | | |
| Nicolaides et al, 1972b | RPP | 25 | 7 (28%) | 22 | 0 | | | | | | |
| Sebeseri et al, 1975 | Renal, Ureteric, Bladder | 31 | 18 (58%) | 34 | 4 (12%) | | | | | | |
| Rosenberg et al, 1975 | Bladder, RPP | 32 | 11 (34%) | 23 | 8 (34%)* | | | 24 | 8 (33%) | | |
| Hedlund et al, 1975 | Transvesical, Prostatect'y | 40 | 18 (45%) | 38 | 13 (34%)* | | | | | 37 | 10 (27%) |
| Kutnowski et al, 1977 | Renal, Ureteric, RPP | 25 | 12 (48%) | 22 | 3 (14%) | | | | | | |
| Coe et al, 1978 | Renal, Bladder, RPP | 24 | 6 (25%) | 28 | 6 (21%) | 29 | 2 (7%) | | | | |
| Vandendris et al, 1980 | RPP | 33 | 13 (35%) | 31 | 3 (6%) | | | | | | |
| Saltzman et al, 1980 | Renal, Ureteric Misc. | | | | | 50 50 | 3 (6%) 5 (10%) | | | | |
| Bergqvist & Hallböök, 1980 | Misc. | 19 | 6 (32%) | 18 | 3 (17%) | | | | | 22 | 8 (36%) |

*not statistically significant

# Prophylaxis

Two randomised controlled studies of approximately 200 patients in each using dicoumarol (Storm, 1967) and marcoumar (Holbraad, 1976), but relying on clinical diagnostic methods have produced conflicting results. Anticoagulation was commenced before operation in both; EACA was also administered in the first (Storm, 1967). A significant decrease in the incidence of both DVT and PE was reported in the first, but not in the second study. Anderson et al (1966) had already reported that a group of 368 consecutive patients having prostatectomy had a clinical incidence of venous thromboembolism of 0.8%. Studies using objective diagnostic criteria to study the efficacy of oral anticoagulants are not available.

Ten randomised controlled studies using objective diagnostic criteria (FUT and/or venography) are listed in table 31.2. Low dose heparin was used in 9, electrical calf stimulation in one, dextran in two and intermittent pneumatic compression in two.

A significant reduction was produced by low dose heparin in five out of the nine studies. In all nine studies there were 236 patients in the control groups, with an incidence of DVT of 40%; there were 221 patients in the heparin groups with a 20% incidence of DVT. These results indicate a 50% reduction in DVT.

Electrical stimulation did not have any significant effect on the incidence of DVT (Hedlund et al, 1975). Dextran reduced DVT in the first of the two studies (Hedlund et al, 1976) but not in the second (Bergqvist and Hallböök, 1980). The overall effect of Dextran when the results of both studies are combined is a 25% reduction in the incidence of DVT (from 40% to 30%).

Intermittent pneumatic compression in one study (Coe et al, 1978) reduced the incidence of DVT from 25% in the control group to 7% in the treatment group. The incidence of DVT in 100 patients treated with intermittent pneumatic compression (in 50 during the operation and in the recovery room, and in 50 for an additional 3 days until fully ambulant) was also 8%.

The results of these studies indicate that low dose heparin is effective in patients having urological surgery, producing a 50% overall reduction in the incidence of DVT, without increase in haemorrhagic complications. A greater reduction (70%) in the incidence of DVT by intermittent pneumatic compression is suggested by two studies (Coe et al, 1978; Saltzman et al, 1980). Intermittent pneumatic compression may well prove to be a better alternative method if the results were to be reinforced by further studies.

We are not aware of any studies on the prevention of DVT in patients with renal transplants. The high risk subgroup identified merits prophylaxis.

# References

Allen RDM, Murie JA, Morris PJ. Deep venous thrombosis after renal transplantation. Surg Gynaecol Obst, 164:137, 1987.

Allgood RJ, Cook JH, Weedn RJ et al: Prospective analysis of pulmonary embolism in the postoperative patient. Surgery 68:116, 1970

Arnadottir M, Bergentz SE, Bergqvist D et al. Thromboembolic complications after renal transplantation. World J Surg 7:757, 1983

Anderson R, Jensen P. Prophylactic anticoagulant therapy in prostatic surgery. Acta Chir Scand 132:144, 1966

Antila LE, Markulla H and Iisaly E. Ten years experience of geriatric aspects of surgery of patients with benign prostatic hypertrophy. Acta Chir Scand (Suppl) 357:95, 1966

Becker J, Borgstrom S. Incidence of thrombosis associated with epsilon aminocaproic acid administration and with combined epsilon-aminocaproic acid and subcutaneous heparin therapy. Acta Chir Scand 134:343, 1968

Becker J, Borgstrom S and Saltzman GF. Occurrence and course of thrombosis following prostatectomy. Acta Radiol (Diagn) 10:513, 1970

Bergqvist D, Bergentz SE, Bornmyr S et al. Deep vein thrombosis after renal transplantation. Eur J Surg Res, 17:69, 1985

Bergqvist D, Hallböök T. Prophylaxis of postoperative venous thrombosis in a controlled trial comparing Dextran 70 and low dose heparin. World J Surg 4, 239, 1980

Coe ND, Collins REC, Klein LA et al. Prevention of deep venous thrombosis in urological patients: A controlled randomised trial of low-dose heparin and external pneumatic compression boots. Surgery 83:230, 1978

Combined report on Regular Dialysis and Transplantation in Europe. European Dialysis and Transplant Association, London: Pitman, 1983

Gordon-Smith IC, Hickman JA, Elmastei SH. The effect of the fibrinolytic inhibitor epsilon aminocaproic acid on the incidence of deep vein thrombosis after prostatectomy. Br J Surg 59:222, 1972

Hedlund PO. Postoperative venous thrombosis in benign prostatic disease. Scand J Urol Nephrol (Suppl 27):1, 1975

Holbraad L, Thybo E and VeNnits H. A controlled investigation of the value of anticoagulant therapy in cases of prostatectomy. Scand J Urol Nephrol 10:39, 1976

Kakkar VV. International multicentre trial prevention of fatal post-operative embolism by low doses of heparin. Lancet 2:45, 1975

Kutnowski M, Vandendris M, Steinberger R, Kraytman M. Prevention of Deep Vein Thrombosis by low-dose heparin in urological surgery. Urological Research 5:123, 1977

Mayo ME, Halil T and Browse NL. The incidence of deep vein thrombosis after prostatectomy. Br J Urol 43:738, 1971

Moser KM. Thromboembolic disease in the patients undergoing urologic surgery. Urol Cl N Amer 10 1:101-107, 1983

Nestrom B, Ladefoged J, Lund FL. Vascular complications in 155 consecutive kidney transplantations. Scand J Urol Nephrol Suppl 15, 6:65, 1973

Nicolaides AN, Dupont PA, Desai S, Lewis JD, Douglas JN, Dodsworth H, Fourides G, Luck RJ. Small doses of subcutaneous sodium heparin in preventing deep venous thrombosis after major surgery. Lancet 2:890, 1972a

Nicolaides AN, Field ES and Kakkar VV. Prostatectomy and deep vein thrombosis. Br J Surg 50:487, 1972b

Rao KV, Smith EJ, Alexander JW et al. Thromboembolic disease in renal allograft recipients. Arch Surg 111:1086, 1976

Rosenberg IL, Evans M and Pollock AV. Prophylaxis of post-operative leg vein thrombosis by low dose subcutaneous heparin or pre-operative calf muscle stimulation. Br Med J 1:649, 1975

Salzman EW, Ploetz J, Bettman M, Skillman J, Klein L. Intraoperative external pneumatic calf compression to afford long-term prophylaxis against deep vein thrombosis in urological patients. Surgery 87:239, 1980

Sebeseri O, Kummer H, Zingg E. Controlled prevention of post- operative thrombosis in urological diseases with depot heparin. Eur Urol J 1:229, 1975

Storm O. Suprapubic prostatectomy with pre-operative dicumarol and epsilon-aminocaproic acid prophylaxis. Scand J Urol Nephrol 1:1, 1967

Vandendris M, Kutnowski M, Futeral B, Giannakopoulos X, Krayman M and Gregoir W. Prevention of postoperative deep vein thrombosis by low dose heparin in open prostatectomy. Urological Research 8:219, 1980

Williams HT. Prevention of post-operative deep vein thrombosis with peri-operative subcutaneous heparin. Lancet 2:950, 1971

CHAPTER 32

# A protocol plan for preventing deep vein thrombosis

Philip D Coleridge-Smith

## Introduction

Deep vein thrombosis is a common event in patients receiving medical and surgical treatment in hospital. This problem increases with age, obesity, a previous history of deep vein thrombosis, varicose veins and in the presence of malignant disease. It is frequently not diagnosed correctly, and its more serious sequel, pulmonary embolism still causes the death of 10-17% of surgical patients dying in hospital (Sandler and Martin, 1989; Lindblad et al, 1991).

## Patients at risk

### Surgical patients
The factors which predispose to deep vein thrombosis are well established (Nicolaides and Irving, 1975). Patients less than 40 years of age undergoing short surgical procedures (less than 30 minutes duration) are at low risk (less than 6%). Above the age of 40 years with procedures lasting more than 30 minutes the risk rises towards 40%. Particular groups of patients are at very high risk of suffering a deep vein thrombosis. These include the elderly, those with a previous history of deep vein thrombosis, and those suffering major trauma. Certain types of surgical procedure are associated with frequent deep vein thrombosis; these include hip, knee and pelvic surgery and patients undergoing such procedures must be considered in the high risk category. The risk of developing a DVT in this group is 60-100% (Table 32.1).

**Table 32.1**
Categories of risk in surgical patients

**Low risk — Less than 6%**
  Age under 40 years
  Minor surgery

**Moderate risk — 6-40%**
  Age 40-60 years
  Abdominal, pelvic or thoracic surgery
  Duration of procedure >30 minutes

**High risk**
  Age >60 years
  Complex, protracted surgery
  Malignancy
  Hip or knee replacement
  Previous history of DVT

## Medical Patients

Patients being treated in medical wards are as likely to suffer deep vein thrombosis as general surgical patients although this group has never been studied in as much detail. Certain groups of medical patients are at particularly high risk of suffering a DVT and these include those with strokes and myocardial infarction (Table 32.2) (Nicolaides et al, 1971).

# DVT prophylaxis

Several means are available to reduce the risk of deep vein thrombosis in hospital patients. These have been widely studied in many trials published during the last twenty years which have mainly relied on the use of the fibrinogen uptake test (Flanc et al, 1968) as the diagnostic determinant of thrombosis.

**Table 32.2**
Categories of risk in medical patients

**Low risk**
  Age under 40 years
  Uncomplicated patient confined to bed

**Moderate risk**
  Age 40-60 years
  Uncomplicated myocardial infarction

**High risk**
  Age >60 years
  Previous DVT
  Coagulation defect — deficiency of proteins C or S, AT III deficiency
  Stroke or neurological problem resulting in paralysis

### Efficacy of heparin in surgical patients

Collins has undertaken a meta-analysis of data addressing the efficacy of aspirin in surgical patients. This shows that the incidence of DVT was 23% of 3,396 general surgical patients without prophylaxis and 47% in 619 orthopaedic patients. Using low dose subcutaneous heparin (unfractionated) the incidence was reduced to 9% in 3,966 general surgical patients and 24% in 635 orthopaedic patients (Collins et al, 1988).

More recently, new preparations of heparin have become available. In these new products low molecular weight fractions of the original heparin have been separated which retain anti-thrombotic activity but have reduced potential to cause haemorrhage and may be administered once daily by the subcutaneous route (Hirsh, 1990) (see also chapters 12-15).

### Efficacy of mechanical methods of prophylaxis

Fewer patients have been investigated in studies where the efficacy of mechanical methods of prophylaxis have been investigated. Colditz reported that in a meta-analysis of seven studies, full-length graduated compression stockings reduced the incidence of DVT to 11% in 598 general surgical patients (Colditz et al, 1986). Intermittent pneumatic compression devices reduce the incidence of DVT to 17% (see also chapters 19 and 20).

### Combined modalities of prophylaxis

Combinations of methods of prophylaxis which achieve their effect by different mechanisms have an additive effect in preventing deep vein thrombosis. The efficacy of subcutaneous heparin may also be improved by combination with graduated compression stockings (DVT incidence of 6% in 142 patients in two trials). Intermittent pneumatic compression probably has an additive effect when combined with graduated compression stockings (Scurr et al, 1988) (see also chapters 21 and 27).

### Less frequently used methods

Intravenous infusion with dextran (Borow and Goldson, 1983; Chapter 17) and treatment with warfarin (Goldhaber, 1985; Chapter 18) have also been shown to reduce the incidence of deep vein thrombosis to a useful degree. Aspirin has been investigated as a prophylactic agent, but although a detectable reduction in the incidence of postoperative deep vein thrombosis has been found, this is probably not clinically useful (Harris et al, 1982; Chapter 18).

## Protocols for prophylaxis

Despite the large number of patients studied in trials and the proven efficacy of prophylactic measures, it is estimated that only 50% of general surgeons, 20% of orthopaedic surgeons and fewer physicians employ any of the methods described above in the United Kingdom (Chapter 11). Arguably the most significant factor reducing the efficacy of currently available prophylactic measures is the failure to employ them on a regular basis in patients at risk of venous thromboembolism.

### Surgical patients

It has been recommended that the methods of prophylaxis employed should be related to the likely risk of a DVT (Dalen et al, 1986). Classification of surgical patients according to

**Table 32.3**
Prophylactic regimens for general surgical patients

**Low risk**
  Graduated compression stockings
**Moderate risk**
  Low dose heparin or intermittent pneumatic compression
  or
  Graduated compression stockings combined with either modality
**High risk**
  Combined methods: Intermittent pneumatic compression
  and
  graduated compression stockings
  and
  low dose heparin

table 32.1 will assist in determining the correct prophylactic measures. The methods suggested in table 32.3 are based on large series of patients, and the efficacy of these measures is well established. In general, urological and orthopaedic surgical patients the risk of deep vein thrombosis is reduced by approximately 70% by the use of low dose heparin, at the price of a small increase in the risk of bleeding which amounts to a 2% excess incidence (Collins et al, 1988). Graduated compression stockings are as effective as heparin in preventing deep vein thrombosis, according to data presently available and stockings do not carry the risk of increased haemorrhage. The principal contraindication to the use of stockings is the presence of significant peripheral vascular arterial disease, so these may be used in virtually all patients deemed to be at appreciable risk of DVT. In very high risk patients it is probably worth using all available modalities of prophylaxis, since combinations of different methods increase the overall protection.

Orthopaedic patients are at substantial risk of deep vein thrombosis, especially those undergoing joint replacement of the lower limb (Table 32.1). There is some reluctance to use low dose heparin in the prevention of thromboembolism in these patients because of the belief that it is ineffective and may lead to haemorrhage. Both of these assumptions are incorrect, as demonstrated in many clinical trials presented in earlier chapters, although a small increase in the incidence of haemorrhage is reported. Recently the protection afforded by anticoagulants has been improved by the introduction of low molecular weight heparins, of which two are presently marketed in the United Kingdom. In comparative trials with unfractionated heparin, the incidence of proximal deep vein thrombosis has been halved by the new agents in patients undergoing hip surgery (Planes et al, 1988; Chapter 25). The frequency of distal thrombosis has been unaltered by these drugs. The recommendations made in table 32.4 are based on these data, as well as the advantage that once daily dosage of low molecular weight heparin affords. These advantages are gained at the price of increased cost, which is some 3-5 times that of unfractionated heparin. These drugs are not included in table 32.3 since no increase in efficacy over unfractionated heparin alone has been shown in general surgical patients (Chapter 15). In addition, the theoretical advantage of reduced incidence of haemorrhage with low molecular weight heparin has not been confirmed in clinical trials.

**Table 32.4**
Prophylactic regimens for orthopaedic surgical patients

**Low risk**
 Graduated compression stockings

**Moderate risk**
 Low dose low molecular weight heparin or intermittent pneumatic compression
 or
 Graduated compression stockings combined with either modality

**High risk**
 Combined methods: Intermittent pneumatic compression
 and
 graduated compression stockings
 and
 low dose low molecular weight heparin

Mechanical methods are also effective in patients undergoing orthopaedic surgery. Intermittent pneumatic compression may be applied by sterile sleeves included in the drapes during surgery, arguably the period of greatest risk for the patient, and continued in the ward until ambulation. Graduated compression stockings may be used in a wide range of orthopaedic procedures, although lower limb operations precludes their use during surgery.

**Medical patients (Table 32.5)**
Far less has been studied of the efficacy of prophylaxis in medical patients. However, the incidence of deep vein thrombosis and frequency of death of these patients from throm-

**Table 32.5**
Prophylactic regimens for medical patients

*Low risk*
 Graduated compression stockings

*Moderate risk*
 *Suggested as suitable for patients with myocardial infarction*
 Low dose heparin or intermittent pneumatic compression
 or
 Graduated compression stockings combined with either modality

*High risk*
 Combined methods: Intermittent pneumatic compression
 and
 graduated compression stockings
 and
 low dose heparin

NB: *In patients with a haemorrhagic diathesis, or with a stroke of uncertain origin, the use of heparin is contraindicated in view of the potential for further haemorrhage*

boembolism, indicates that the use of prophylactic measures is highly desirable (Lindblad et al, 1991; Chapter 29).

Certain groups of patients deserve particular consideration. These include those with stroke as the presenting condition. Here it would be inadvisable to administer heparin unless objective evidence had been obtained that haemorrhage is not the cause of the stroke (Chapter 30). Mechanical methods may provide an effective alternative, although the restrictions of movement imposed by intermittent pneumatic compression devices may retard mobilisation. Elderly, poorly nourished patients may not tolerate regular injections, making graduated compression stockings more attractive.

## Obstetric patients

Pregnancy increases the risk of developing a deep vein thrombosis and this is increased further still in those patients having an operative delivery. Pulmonary embolism is the most common cause of maternal death (Bonnar, 1975). Many post thrombotic limbs are the results of an undiagnosed deep vein thrombosis during pregnancy. Heparin can be administered subcutaneously to pregnant women without risk to the fetus since it does not cross the placental barrier but in the long term administration may cause thrombocytopenia and osteoporosis (Jaffe and Willis, 1965; Towne et al, 1979). Warfarin is contraindicated during pregnancy due to its teratogenic potential in the first trimester, and the risk of fetal haemorrhage in the third trimester. Graduated compression stockings may assist in preventing deep vein thrombosis as well as protecting from lower limb oedema. The use of heparin at full term may be considered inadvisable by some anaesthetic services since this provides a relative contraindication to the administration of epidural analgesia. The complication of a peridural haematoma is feared, but appears to be more of a theoretical than actual hazard (Chapter 24).

## Thrombophilic disorders

All young patients presenting with a deep vein thrombosis for which no good aetiological factor can be identified should be investigated for a thrombophilic disorder such as antithrombin III deficiency, protein C deficiency, protein S deficiency and lupus anticoagulant (Chapter 4). No specific treatment yet exists for these conditions, but adequate prophylaxis should be offered to such patients when they undergo surgery, suffer medical illnesses or become pregnant. This may be one or more of the measures described above, although heparin is ineffective in patients with antithrombin III deficiency. Full anticoagulation may be appropriate for cover during surgical procedures in those patients with a history of frequent deep vein thrombosis. Alternatively, missing plasma proteins may be replaced by transfusion with fresh frozen plasma. Long term prophylaxis (outside hospital) may be necessary in patients who suffer recurrent thrombotic episodes.

## Prophylaxis after discharge from hospital

Patients are now discharged from hospital at ever earlier phases of their recovery from surgery. There can be little doubt that the risk of a deep vein thrombosis or fatal pulmonary embolism does not subside as soon as the patient leaves the doors of the hospital, but persists for several weeks (Bergqvist and Lindblad, 1985; Scurr et al, 1988). No study has so far been completed to indicate the most appropriate measures which might be taken to prevent these complications developing at home. It seems reasonable to recommend that patients who were supplied with stockings should continue to wear these after discharge from hospital. Studies are currently in progress to evaluate low dose heparin as a prophylactic measure in this setting.

# References

Berqvist D, Lindblad B. A 30 year survey of pulmonary embolism verified at autopsy: an analysis of 1,274 surgical patients. Br J Surg 72:108, 1985

Bonnar J. Thromboembolism in obstetric and gynaecology patients. In Nicolaides AN (ed) Thromboembolism. MTP Publishing Co, Lancaster, p 311, 1975

Borow M, Goldson HJ. Prevention of postoperative deep vein thrombosis and pulmonary emboli with combined modalities. American Surgery 49:599, 1983

Colditz GA, Tuden RL, Oster G. Rate of venous thrombosis after venous surgery: combined results of randomised clinical trials. Lancet ii:143, 1986

Collins R, Scrimgeour A, Yusuf S, Peto R. Reduction in fatal pulmonary embolism and venous thrombosis by perioperative administration of subcutaneous heparin. New Engl J Med 318:1162, 1988

Dalen J, Hull RD, Nicolaides AN. Deep vein thrombosis and pulmonary embolism: developing a protocol for effective prophylaxis. Phlebology 1:75, 1986

Flanc C, Kakkar VV, Clarke MB. The detection of venous thrombosis of the legs using $^{125}$-I labelled fibrinogen. Br J Surg 1968, 55:742

Goldhaber SZ. In: Goldhaber SZ (ed). Pulmonary embolism and deep venous thrombosis. W.B. Saunders Co, Philaphia, p 148, 1985

Harris WH, Athanasoulins CA, Waltman AC et al. High and low dose aspirin prophylaxis against venous thromboembolic disease in total hip replacement. J Bone Joint Surg 64A:63, 1982

Hirsh J. From unfractionated heparins to low molecular weight heparins. Acta Chir Scand (Suppl.) 556:42, 1990

Jaffe MD, Willis PW III. Multiple fractures associated with long term heparin therapy. JAMA 193:158, 1965

Lindblad B, Sternby NH, Bergqvist D. Incidence of venous thromboembolism verified by necroscopy over 30 years. Br Med J 302:709, 1991

Nicolaides AN, Irvine D. Clinical factors and the risk of deep vein thrombosis. In: Nicolaides AN (ed.) Thromboembolism: aetiology, advances in prevention and management, MTP Co. Ltd, Lancaster, p. 193, 1975

Nicolaides AN, Kakkar VV, Renney JTG, Kidner PH, Hutchison DCS, Clarke MB. Myocardial infarction and deep vein thrombosis. Br Med J 1:432, 1971

Planes A, Rochelle N, Mazas F. Prevention of postoperative venous thrombosis: a randomised trial comparing unfractionated heparin with low molecular weight heparin in patients undergoing total hip replacement. Thromb Haemostasis 60:407, 1988

Sandler DA, Martin JF. Autopsy proven pulmonary embolism in hospital patients: are we detecting enough deep vein thrombosis? J Roy Soc Med 82:203, 1989

Scurr JH, Coleridge-Smith PD, Hasty JH. Deep venous thrombosis: a continuing problem. Br Med J 297:28, 1988

Scurr JH, Coleridge-Smith PD, Hasty JH. An improved DVT prophylactic regimen: the combined utilisation of elastic compression stockings with intermittent sequential pneumatic compression. Swiss Med 10:77, 1988

Towne JB, Bernhard VM, Hussey C, Garancis JC. White clot syndrome. Peripheral vascular complications of heparin therapy. Arch Surg 114:372, 1979

PART IV

# Secondary Prevention

Chapter 33

# The combination of liquid crystal thermography and duplex scanning in DVT diagnosis

**Evi Kalodiki**
**Charles M Fisher**
**Andrew N Nicolaides**

## Introduction

Several studies have demonstrated that acute deep vein thrombosis (DVT) can be detected by ultrasonic duplex scanning with a sensitivity of 96% and specificity of 95% (Elias et al, 1987; Cranley et al, 1989; Comerota et al, 1990; Nicolaides and Renton, 1990) so that in centres where this technique is available, venography is now rarely performed. Because of the accuracy and cost-effectiveness of duplex scanning compared to venography the demand for this method has increased to such an extent that the availability of scanning time has become a limiting factor. It is now apparent that a simple screening method that could identify legs without DVT and avoid the need for duplex scanning would be highly desirable.

Thermography is a noninvasive method used in the past to detect DVT (Cooke and Pilcher, 1973). The principle of the test was based on the observation that the skin temperature of the limb with DVT was increased and could be detected with an infra-red telecamera. However, the cost and bulkiness of the equipment which had to be placed in a constant temperature room limited its widespread use. In recent years liquid crystal thermography (LCT) has overcome these limitations and has provided a method that can detect DVT with a sensitivity of 97% and a specificity of 62% (Pochaczevsky et al, 1982; Sandler and Martin, 1985), providing a screening test for determining absence of DVT. In addition, LCT can be performed at the bedside with minimal training (Sandler and Martin, 1985).

The aim of our study was to demonstrate that by combining LCT with duplex scanning one could avoid not only venography, but also duplex scanning in a large proportion of patients with clinically suspected acute DVT, saving time not only in the angiography room but also in the ultrasonic service. Therefore, it was necessary as a first step to determine the accuracy of both LCT and duplex scanning against venography in the same group of patients. The results could subsequently be used to formulate the most appropriate and cost effective application.

## Material and methods

### Patients
100 patients with clinically suspected acute DVT have been included in the study. They were all tested with LCT and duplex scanning. Ascending venography was performed within the subsequent 12-48 hours. Reporting on the noninvasive and venographic results was done blind.

### Liquid Crystal Thermography (LCT)
The equipment consists of latex sheets impregnated with cholesteric crystals (Novamedix Ltd, Andover, UK) which change in colour with variations in temperature from brown (cool) to yellow, green and finally blue (warm). The latex sheets are 34 by 43 cm and are enclosed in special boxes with a perspex viewing face. Six different detectors are available which are calibrated to cover temperature ranges of 2 °C above and below a mean temperature of 22 °C, 24 °C, 26 °C, 28 °C, 30 °C, 32 °C, 34 °C, and 36 °C. A frame holds the latex sheets to a Polaroid camera and a flash unit, so that a colour photograph of each thermographic image can be taken. The detector is placed over the calves, with the patient prone on a bed or couch having first elevated and exposed the legs to room temperature for ten minutes. After 20-30 seconds, an image is formed, showing the temperature patterns of both legs. The image can be assessed immediately and photographed if necessary. The procedure is repeated with the patient supine and the legs elevated 30° with the thermographic detectors placed on the shins and thighs.

    The presence of an homogeneous area with a temperature difference of 0.8 °C or more in the symptomatic limb, compared with the same area of the asymptomatic limb, is considered to be a positive thermographic diagnostic criterion. The thermograph is considered to be negative when the temperature distribution is similar in both limbs (temperature difference less than 0.8 °C).

### Duplex Scanning
Duplex scanning was performed using the ATL Ultramark 9 instrument (Advanced Technology Laboratories, Seattle, USA) using the 5 MHz linear array probe. Whenever possible, examination of the external iliac and femoral veins was performed with the patient standing. The patient was asked to place the weight of the body on the opposite leg and externally rotate the examined limb with slight knee flexion. In order to be steady in this position and avoid involuntary muscle contractions, the patient was holding onto an orthopaedic frame, or the duplex scanner. A few patients who were too ill and unable to stand were examined supine in the reversed Trendelenburg position with the trunk at 45 °C to the horizontal. These positions ensured that the veins were full. For the examination of the popliteal and calf veins the patient was seated on the edge of the couch with the heel of the tested leg resting on the examiner's stool or chair so that the calf muscles were relaxed.

    The criteria for thrombosis are summarised in table 33.1. Scanning was performed with the probe held both longitudinally and transversely. Initially the common femoral vein was

**Table 33.1**
Duplex Scanning: Diagnostic Criteria for DVT

| B-Mode Image | Colour flow/Doppler signal |
| --- | --- |
| Intraluminal echogenic material<br>Noncompressibility of vein<br>Blood flow (red cell aggregates) around a lucent filling defect | Absent intraluminal signal<br>Continuous signal, not phasic with respiration (iliac veins)<br>Reduced or absent flow with augmentation manoeuvres<br><br>Colour flow imaging: blue or red colour, indicating flow around a lucent filling defect |

scanned longitudinally as proximally as possible and the patient was asked to take deep breaths and perform a Valsalva manoeuvre. Absence of flow which was phasic with respiration and a continuous Doppler signal were the criteria for iliac vein thrombosis (Comerota et al, 1990). The femoral vein was then scanned longitudinally and transversely moving the probe distally as far as the adductor canal. Throughout the scanning, one looked for intraluminar echogenicity or blood flow around a lucent filling defect, whether the walls of the vein could be made to approximate on external compression, and for the presence of augmentation of blood flow on manual compression of the thigh or calf using the colour flow facility.

The popliteal, gastrocnemius, soleal and axial veins of the leg were also examined systematically using the same manoeuvres. Colour flow imaging was first used to localise the artery (anterior tibial, peroneal, posterior tibial) shown red and the veins were subsequently localised on either side of the artery by calf compression producing a blue colour flow image indicating flow in the opposite direction. The probe was then rotated 90° (transverse image) and was used to compress the veins demonstrating approximation of the venous walls. Failure to elicit a venous augmentation signal with failure to approximate the venous walls on compression of the skin with the probe indicated DVT.

**Ascending Venography**

A screening table with the facility to tilt erect was used. With the patient supine an 18G butterfly needle was introduced into a superficial vein on the dorsum of each foot. A two cm wide pneumatic cuff was then applied just above the ankle and another to the lower thigh of the limb being studied. The two cuffs were connected via a T piece allowing independent inflation. The lower cuff was inflated so as to prevent filling of the superficial veins and direct the injected contrast into the deep venous system. The upper cuff was inflated to a lesser degree to contain the contrast in the leg during the initial part of the study.

A non ionic low osmolar contrast medium of 300 mg I/ml concentration (Omnipaque) was used and it was injected until the popliteal vein was opacified. Using a $35 \times 35$ cm film, a posterior-anterior and two oblique views of the calf veins are obtained. The upper cuff was then released, further contrast injected and films of the upper thigh were obtained. Centering over the iliac veins and lower inferior vena cava with the patient in the oblique position to project the iliac vein off the hip joint, the lower cuff was also released and as the final bolus of contrast reached the iliac vein a $24 \times 30$ cm film was exposed. The table was then tilted with the patient using hand grips for support and further exposures of the thigh and popliteal veins were obtained if necessary, Finally the leg was elevated and the veins were flushed with saline.

**Table 33.2**
LCT findings compared with venography

|  |  | Liquid Crystal Thermography Positive | Negative | Total |
|---|---|---|---|---|
| Venography | DVT | 42 (93%) | 3[*] | 45 |
|  | No DVT | 15 | 38 (72%) | 53 |
|  | Total | 57 | 41 | 98 |

Sensitivity 93%   Specificity 72%
Positive predictive value 74% (42/57)   Negative predictive value 93% (38/41)
Overall accuracy 83%

[*] 2 patients had symptoms suggestive of DVT for more than one week (venography demonstrated calf DVT in one and proximal DVT in the other); the third patient had peroneal DVT found on venography only

The venographic criteria used for the diagnosis of DVT were those established by DeWeese and Rogoff (1963): the presence of well defined filling defects present on at least two radiographs. Non-visualisation of one or more calf veins was not considered diagnostic of thrombosis since, in normal extremities, these veins are frequently not all visualised. Non-visualisation of the femoral vein with good opacification of the proximal and distal veins in the presence of collaterals was considered evidence of thrombotic obstruction.

# Results

Of the 100 patients admitted to the study, 55 were male and 45 female. Mean age was 53.3 years (range 20-90). DVT was demonstrated by venography in 46 patients. Thirty (64%) of the 46 thromboses were in the left leg and 17 (36%) in the right leg. Twelve (26%) of the thrombi were confined to the calf and 34 (74%) were extending to or arising from the popliteal or more proximal veins.

The comparison of LCT with venography is shown in table 33.2. One patient had one leg amputated previously and another had a plaster of Paris cast so that LCT could be performed in 98 patients only. There was an overall accuracy of 83% and a negative predictive value of 93%. Out of 41 patients with negative LCT 38 patients had a normal venogram. The remaining 3 patients had false negative thermograms. One patient had a small thrombus in the left peroneal vein. In the remaining 2 patients the history of DVT was 10 and 21 days old, and venography demonstrated soleal vein thrombosis in one, and calf/popliteal/femoral vein thrombi respectively in the other. The history of symptoms and signs suggestive of DVT was less than one week in 39 of the 41 patients with negative LCT. There were 15 positive thermograms without DVT (Table 33.2). Of these, 4 patients had arthritis, 2 had had a recent operation, 2 gave a history of muscular strain, 1 had short saphenous vein thrombosis and 1 patient had a haematoma. In 5 of the patients there was no apparent reason for the increase in temperature.

The comparison of the duplex scan with venography is shown in table 33.3. There was an overall accuracy of 92% with a sensitivity of 93% and a specificity of 91%. There were 3 false negative duplex scans. Two of them were in patients who had extremely tense and tender oedematous legs that made the examination difficult. Both had femoral thrombi. The

**Table 33.3**
Duplex scanning findings compared with venography

|  |  | Duplex Scanning DVT | No DVT | Total |
|---|---|---|---|---|
| Venography | DVT | 43 (93%) | 3[*] | 46 |
|  | No DVT | 5[**] | 49 (91%) | 54 |
|  | Total | 48 | 52 | 100 |

Sensitivity 93%   Specificity 91%
Positive predictive value 89% (43/48)   Negative predictive value 94% (49/52)
Overall accuracy 92%
[*] 2 patients with femoral DVT (tense and tender oedematous thighs); 1 patient with peroneal (<2 cm long) DVT
[**] 2 falsely diagnosed as femoral DVT (groin and thigh wounds) 3 falsely diagnosed as calf DVT

third patient had a small (<2cm long) peroneal DVT. The latter was the one missed also on LCT. There were 5 false positive results on duplex scanning. Two patients had a recent operation (iliofemoral and femoropopliteal bypass) and in both the leg was very oedematous making compression of the femoral veins very difficult. In the remaining three patients calf vein thrombosis was falsely diagnosed on duplex.

# Discussion

It has been demonstrated that the symptoms and signs of DVT are unreliable and as many as 46% of patients who present with clinical DVT have normal veins on venography (McLachin et al, 1962; Soulen et al, 1972). Because of this, venography became the standard method of investigation in the 1970s before deciding to treat patients with anticoagulants which are expensive and not without risk.

The results of the LCT in our hands are similar to those of others (Pochaczevsky et al, 1982; Sandler and Martin, 1985). The negative predictive value of 93% means that in the presence of a negative thermogram, the likelihood of DVT being present is small. Previous studies have indicated that many pathological conditions other than DVT will produce an increased skin temperature. They include ruptured Baker's cysts, cellulitis, muscular or joint trauma and superficial thrombophlebitis, and are responsible for the relatively poor specificity of thermography. However, few conditions produce false negative thermograms. The latter may occur when the history of thrombosis is older than one week, when the thrombi are small (less than 2cm in length) and are limited to a compartment not closely related to the skin surface or when there is peripheral neuropathy (Aronen et al, 1981; Pochaczevsky et al, 1982). The results of our study suggest that if the two patients with a history of DVT longer than one week were excluded because thermography would have been an inappropriate test (Table 33.2), and we adopted the practice of neither proceeding to other tests nor treating any of the remaining 39 patients in whom thermography was negative then we would have missed one calf DVT (negative predictive value: 97%).

The results of duplex scanning in our hands are also similar to those of others (Elias et al, 1987; Cranley et al, 1989; Comerota et al, 1990). The sensitivity of 93% indicates that this method will detect most thrombi. Previous studies have indicated that the thrombi missed are usually in the calf (Elias et al, 1987; Cranley et al, 1989; Comerota et al, 1990). In the presence of severe oedema, tenderness or surgical wounds compression of the veins cannot be adequately achieved and this test is inappropriate. If the duplex examination is inadequate or inapplicable because of such conditions, then venography may be the only available method for making the diagnosis. In our series of 100 patients, six limbs fell into this category.

If we were to adopt the practice of excluding such limbs from the duplex study (using venography only), then the sensitivity and specificity of the duplex scanning would have risen to 97%. (43/44 × 100) and 94% (47/50 × 100). One small (less than 2 cm in length) peroneal DVT would have been missed (also missed by LCT) and three calf DVTs would have been falsely diagnosed. The safety of withholding treatment in patients suspected of DVT confined to the calf, has been demonstrated already by several studies (Stallworth et al, 1981; Hull et al, 1985; Huisman et al, 1986).

On the basis of the above, a policy for the investigation of patients with clinically suspected DVT has been formulated (Figure 33.1). According to this policy, LCT is the first diagnostic test to be applied unless inappropriate (symptoms suggestive of DVT longer than one week) or technically impossible. If LCT is negative then no further investigation or treatment is necessary. If LCT is inappropriate, technically not possible or if positive, duplex scanning should be performed unless a surgical wound or severe tenderness and oedema make such a test impossible to perform, when a venogram would be requested instead. Had this policy been adopted for the 100 patients in our study, a decision of no DVT and therefore no treatment would have been made in 49 patients: in 39 because of a negative thermogram, and in 10 because of a negative duplex scan. As a result of this, DVT in the calf would have been missed in one patient. A decision to admit to hospital and treat would have been made in 34 patients with thrombosis in veins proximal to the calf: 31 on the basis of a positive duplex scan and 3 on the basis of a positive venogram. Fourteen patients would have been diagnosed by the duplex scan as having DVT confined to the calf (11 true positive; 3 false positive) (see Figure 33.1). These patients, if ambulant, would have been rescanned every two days until free of symptoms in order to ensure that there is no proximal extension into the popliteal. On the basis of the proposed policy (Figure 33.1) only six venograms would have been performed. Although this policy is rational, it should be validated prospectively with follow-up of all the patients for at least 1 year in order to ensure that none of the untreated patients developed further deep vein thrombosis or pulmonary embolism.

The cost of LCT is £10, that of duplex scanning £70 and of venography £140. It can be calculated that to do venography as a routine test in all patients (Policy A) would cost £14,000, duplex scanning in all patients (Policy B) would cost £7,000 and to follow the plan suggested figure 33.1 (Policy C), would cost £5,640. Thus, policy C would result in a 60% reduction in cost when compared to policy A and 20% when compared to policy B. In addition, policy C would save 39% of the scanning sessions which could be used for other useful tests such as the detection and grading of carotid stenosis and mesenteric or renal artery stenosis offered by the noninvasive service using the same duplex scanner. Also, the identification of 49% of patients (39 with LCT and 10 with duplex: Figure 33.1) as not having DVT without a venogram means that they would not be admitted to hospital, saving beds for those who really need them. It is not uncommon for patients to be admitted with the clinical diagnosis of DVT and to have heparin therapy until the following day (or the Monday morning if admitted during the weekend: Friday to Sunday) when venography is performed, only to be discovered that there is no evidence of DVT. The results of our study support the hypothesis that the combination of LCT with duplex scanning can contribute

Figure 33.1
Suggested policy for investigating patients with clinically suspected DVT (n=100)

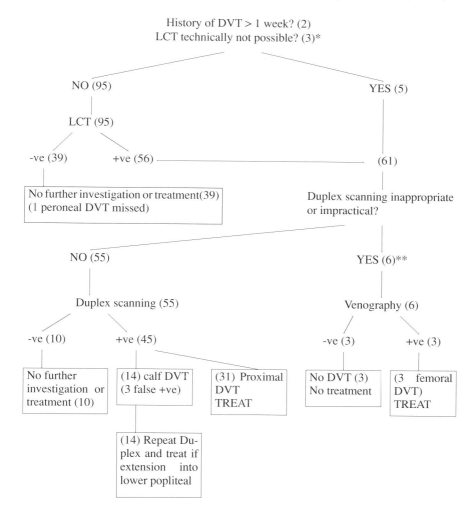

NOTE: Numbers in brackets indicate the number of patients from our study that would have passed through various points of the algorithm
* One amputee, one in plaster of Paris and one with leprosy
**Very oedematous, tense tender legs with a surgical wound in four

not only towards an accurate, but also a more cost effective diagnosis of DVT (Nicolaides and Sumner, 1991).

Whether a district general hospital can afford to be without duplex scanning has already been questioned (Nicolaides and Renton, 1990). Departments and noninvasive vascular laboratories now providing a duplex scanning service and facing the problem of being unable to deal with the large number of referrals due to time available on the ultrasonic scanner should consider adding liquid crystal thermography to their practice.

## References

Aronen HJ, Suorant HT, Taaritsainen MJ. Thermography in deep venous thrombosis of the leg. Am J Radiol 137:1179, 1981

Comerota AJ, Katz ML, Greenwald LL et al. Venous duplex imaging: Should it replace hemodynamic tests for deep venous thrombosis? J Vasc Surg 11:53-60, 1990

Cooke ED, Pilcher MF. Thermography in diagnosis of deep venous thrombosis. Br Med J 2:523, 1973

Cranley JJ, Canos AJ, Sull WJ. The diagnosis of deep venous thrombosis. Fallibility of clinical symptoms and signs. Arch Surg 111:34, 1976

Cranley JJ, Higgins RF, Berry RE et al. Near parity in the final diagnosis of deep venous thrombosis by duplex scan and phlebography. Phlebology 4:71, 1989

DeWeese JA, Rogoff SM. Phlebographic patterns in acute deep venous thrombosis of the leg. Surgery 53:99, 1963

Elias E, Le Gorff G, Bouvier JL, Benichou M, Serrandimigni A. Value of real-time B-mode ultrasound imaging in the diagnosis of deep vein thrombosis of the lower limbs. Int Angiol 6:175, 1987

Huisman M, Buller HR, ten Cate JW, Vreeken J. Serial impedance plethysmography for suspected deep venous thrombosis in outpatients. The Amsterdam general practitioners' study. N Engl J Med 314:823, 1986

Hull RD, Hirsh J, Carton CJ, Jay RM, Ockelford PA, Buller HR, Turpie AG, Powers P, Kinch D, Dood PE, Gill GS, Leclerc JR, Gent M. Diagnostic efficacy of impedance plethysmography for clinically suspected deep vein thrombosis. Ann Int Med 102:21, 1985

McLachin J, Richards T, Paterson JC. An evaluation of clinical signs in the diagnosis of venous thrombosis. Arch Surg 85:738, 1962

Nicolaides AN, Renton SC, Duplex scanning: The second sight of the vascular surgeon. Eur J Vasc Surg 4:445, 1990

Nicolaides AN, Sumner DS. Investigation of patients with deep vein thrombosis and chronic venous insufficiency. London, Med-Orion Publishing Company, 1991, p21.

Pochaczevsky R, Pillari G, Feldman F. Liquid crystal contact thermography of deep venous thrombosis. Amer Roentg 138:717, 1982

Sandler DA and Martin JF. Liquid crystal thermography as a screening test for deep vein thrombosis. Lancet 1:665, 1985

Soulen RL, Lapayowker MS, Tyson RR et al. Angiography, Ultrasound and Thermography in the study of peripheral vascular disease. Radiol 105:115, 1972

Stallworth J, Plong CW Jr, Horne JB. Negative phleborheography. Clinical followup in 593 patients. Arch Surg 116:795, 1981

CHAPTER 34

# The value of thrombectomy

Bo Eklof

## Introduction

Modern venous reconstructive surgery using valvuloplasty can show good longterm results in primary venous insufficiency while the results of vein segment transfer and autologous vein transplantation in the post-thrombotic syndrome are much less promising (Kistner, 1991). It is therefore important to treat thrombosis of the leg early and successfully to preserve valvular function and avoid obstruction of the venous outflow tract to prevent the development of a severe post-thrombotic syndrome. There are three modalities of treatment: anticoagulation, thrombolysis and thrombectomy.

Conservative treatment with heparin started in the 1930s and in the beginning of the 1940s dicoumarol was introduced. In the early 1960s thrombolytic therapy was introduced and clinically evaluated. The objectives of therapy for iliofemoral venous thrombosis are to prevent fatal pulmonary embolism and proximal extension of the thrombus; progressive swelling of the leg resulting in increased compartmental pressure which can lead to phlegmasia cerulea dolens, venous gangrene and limb loss; and later, development of a severe postthrombotic (PT) syndrome.

The risk of developing pulmonary embolism (PE) and the subsequent mortality appear to increase with the proximity of the thrombus in the venous system (Mavor and Galloway, 1967). At admission, patients with iliofemoral venous thrombosis have been found to have scan/angiography verified *symptomatic* PE in 9-18% (Norris et al, 1985, Plate et al, 1985; Neglen et al, 1992) with an additional 25-36% of cases having *asymptomatic* but scan-positive emboli (Plate et al, 1985; Neglen et al, 1992). When the IVC is involved symptomatic PE rate increases to 30-34% (Farber et al, 1984; Girard et al, 1987, Radomski et al, 1987). Despite the anticoagulant treatment, 4% of cases with iliofemoral deep vein thrombosis (DVT) had recurrence of PE within one month (Plate et al, 1985; Girard et al, 1987) being higher (18%) following IVC thrombus (Radomski et al, 1987). However, others have shown no further scan-positive PE in patients with IVC thrombosis nor with iliofemoral DVT 10 days after initiating anticoagulant treatment (Farber et al, 1984). There is no doubt that patients with IVC thrombosis have a higher frequency of PE at the onset of the disease compared to those with more distal DVT. Anticoagulant treatment appears to control recurrence of PE at least in the iliofemoral DVT. It is still debatable if this is so when the IVC is involved.

Killewich et al (1985) described the "natural course" of DVT treated with anticoagulation and found 14% early extension (7 days) and 19% late extension (30-160 days). Heparin infusion usually gives immediate symptomatic relief of swelling and pain, possibly due to its antiinflamatory effect. The main disadvantage is that lysis of the thrombus depends on the endogenous fibrinolytic mechanisms and requires weeks to months. It often leads to incomplete recanalisation and invariably results in destruction of the venous valves involved in the thrombotic process (Porter and Taylor, 1985). Thus anticoagulant treatment is of less value in prevention of the post-thrombotic syndrome.

Thrombolytic therapy seems then to be the rational way to attempt to solve the problem as it may allow early lysis with preservation of normal venous valve function. Several prospective randomised studies have been published comparing the efficacy of heparin with streptokinase (SK) treatment (Porter and Taylor, 1985). It is obvious that the dissolution of deep vein thrombi is more rapid and more complete with streptokinase (SK) therapy. Half of the patients receiving thrombolytic therapy within three days of onset of symptoms have total clot resolution with preservation of functional valves. It is likely that the delicate valve leaves are destroyed within 3-5 days so the lysis has to be quick and complete. Our own experience with standard dosage SK therapy in 47 patients revealed only 2/35 (6%) patients having normal venous function after 29 months (Albrechtsson et al, 1981). In addition, severe complications were encountered during the SK treatment including spontaneous rupture of intraabdominal organs with life threatening bleeding (Eklof et al, 1977). There are only a few reports with longterm follow up comparing the development of post-thrombotic (PT) sequelae. Two studies find better results with SK treatment (Elliot et al, 1979; Arnesen et al, 1982) while one does not show any difference between the two treatment groups (Kakkar et al, 1986). Severe PT syndrome occurred in around 30% during a follow up of 5.7 years. A disadvantage for the SK treatment is the numerous contraindications, which reduce the availability of the latter as a treatment alternative. Porter found that only 15% of DVT patients in his clinical practice presented within 3 days of onset of symptoms and had no contraindications (Porter and Taylor, 1985). Others have reported frequencies of contraindications between 24-80% (Kadji, 1984; Einarsson et al, 1986; Juhan et al, 1987). It seems as though thrombolysis cannot be used in half of cases with iliofemoral venous thrombosis. Although the induced thrombolysis appears the most logical treatment for extensive DVT, the many contraindications, the potential risks and the doubtful long-term results have made us turn to the surgical alternative in acute iliofemoral venous thrombosis.

In our present management to preserve the outflow tract and valvular function we also advocate a surgical approach in acute IVC thrombosis, in acute iliac vein obstruction and in acute superficial thrombophlebitis with extension of the thrombus in the long saphenous vein above the knee. The first thrombectomy (TE) of a leg vein was ascribed to Läwen (1938). This was the same year that Dos Santos (1938) described venography. Gregoire (1938) showed that DVT of the lower limb may lead to phlegmasia cerulea dolens and Haimovici (Audier and Haimovici, 1938) described its further progress to venous gangrene. During the 1950s and early 1960s several enthusiastic reports on the clinical success of venous thrombectomy were published in the USA (Mahorner et al, 1957, De Weese et al, 1960; Haller and Abrams, 1963). The invention of the Fogarty catheter substantially facilitated removal of the thrombus (Fogarty et al, 1966). Mavor showed an improvement of patency of the thrombectomised iliac vein from 61 to 79% (Mavor and Galloway, 1969). His conclusion in 1969 was that "(therefore) it is all the more unfortunate that thrombectomy is not yet generally accepted as the most rational, most effective and safest way of dealing with iliofemoral thrombosis". Lansing and Davis' report (1968) with a five year follow-up of Haller and Abrams (1963) material, unfounded as it may seem, stopped the enthusiastic wave of thrombectomy, and the procedure was abandoned by most surgeons in the USA as well as Europe. However, during the 1970s, TE revived in continental Europe (Gillot and Imbert, 1980). Inspired by a report from Jean Kunlin (1953) on the use of a temporary arteriovenous fistula (AVF) to improve the outcome of venous reconstructive surgery and Joerg Vollmar's clinical application thereof we performed our first iliofemoral TE with a temporary AVF in Lund, Sweden, in 1974. Our personal experience of this surgical procedure now comprises 203 patients: in Lund, Sweden (1974-78) 70 patients, in Helsingborg, Sweden (1978-1981) 31 patients and in Kuwait (1981-1990) 102 patients. Based on this and the results of others, we will argue that TE with temporary AVF is the method of choice for the treatment of acute iliofemoral venous thrombosis.

## Surgical management

The immediate work-up has to detect the extension of the thrombosis proximally. This will affect the surgical management, especially if the inferior vena cava (IVC) is involved. Duplex scanning will verify the thrombus with high accuracy, but can rarely determine its proximal end. A femoral venogram from the contralateral side is usually required to achieve this. When the diagnosis is established, heparin infusion is started. Prophylactic antibiotics are given to reduce the rate of wound infection (Christenson et al, 1977). Surgery is performed under intubation anaesthesia. Ten centimetres water PEEP is added during manipulation of the thrombus to prevent perioperative embolisation. The involved leg and abdomen are prepared. A longitudinal incision is made in the groin to expose the long saphenous vein (LSV), which is followed to its confluence with the common femoral vein (CFV). The anterior wall of the CFV is exposed, avoiding detachment of the lateral and posterior walls. The vein is not encircled and proximal and distal control is maintained by external pressure using a sponge on a stick. The superficial femoral artery 3-4 cm below the femoral bifurcation is dissected free in preparation for the construction of the AVF. When the dissection is completed, 5,000 IU of heparin is given intravenously. A transverse venotomy is made in the CFV just above the confluence. A venous Fogarty thrombectomy catheter 8/10 is passed through the thrombus into the IVC. The balloon is inflated and repeated exercises with the Fogarty catheter are performed until no more thrombotic material is extracted. With the balloon inflated in the common iliac vein, a suction catheter is introduced to the level of the internal iliac vein to evacuate thrombi from this vein. Backflow is not a reliable sign of clearance since a proximal valve in the external iliac vein may be present (25% of cases) (Basmajean, 1952) preventing retrograde flow in a cleared vein. On the other hand, backflow can be excellent from the internal iliac vein and its tributaries despite a remaining occlusion of the common iliac vein. Therefore, an intraoperative completion venogram is mandatory. An alternative is the use of an angioscope which enables removal of residual thrombus material under direct vision (Winter et al, 1989). The distal thrombus in the leg is removed by manual massage of the leg starting at the foot. The Fogarty catheter can sometimes be gently advanced in retrograde fashion. The aim is to remove all fresh thrombi from the leg. If the thrombus is old and adherent to the venous wall, we have already lost the battle to preserve the valves. The venotomy is closed with continuous prolene suture and an AVF is created using the LSV, anastomosing it end-to-side to the superficial femoral artery. The use of a cell-saving device minimises the use of bank blood. An intraoperative venogram is performed through a catheter inserted in a branch in the AVF. After a satisfactory completion venogram, a suction drain is applied for 24 hours and the wound closed in layers.

If phlegmasia cerulea dolens or venous gangrene is present, we start the operation with fasciotomy of the calf compartments in order to release the pressure and reestablish the circulation. If there is an extension of the thrombus into the IVC, the cava is approached transperitoneally through a subcostal incision. The IVC is exposed by deflecting the duodenum and ascending colon medially. An Adams-DeWeese interruption clip is applied just below the renal veins. The cava is opened and the thrombus is removed by massage, especially of the iliac venous system. If the iliofemoral segment is involved, the operation is continued in the groin as described above. When total clearance is achieved, the caval clip can be removed before closure of the abdomen. When laparotomy is contraindicated in patients in poor condition a caval filter of the Greenfield or Gunther type can be introduced before the TE to protect against fatal pulmonary embolism.

Heparin is continued for at least 5 days after operation and warfarin is started the first postoperative day and continued routinely for 6 months. The patient is ambulant the day after the operation wearing a compression stocking. If there is an immediate reocclusion of the iliac vein, resulting in a severely compromised outflow from the leg, previously uninvolved or cleared distal veins and a picture of phlegmasia cerulea dolens, an immediate reconstruction with a synthetic femorofemoral crossover bypass graft is considered to prevent retrograde formation of thrombus and subsequent valve insufficiency (Eklof, 1989). The patient is usually discharged on the 10th to 12th postoperative day to return after 6 weeks for closure of the fistula.

## Complications of surgical management

### Mortality
One of the reasons that induced surgeons to abandon TE in the 1960s was a high perioperative mortality due to pulmonary embolism. Surgery still bears a risk but with the present pre- and postoperative precautions, the results have improved. In our series, two patients died (1% mortality). One patient succumbed to an acute respiratory failure due to chronic pulmonary fibrosis. Autopsy did not reveal any fresh pulmonary emboli. The other patient had a preoperatively undetected cirrhosis of the liver. He also had an IVC extension of the thrombus. The patient died from multiorgan failure on the 32nd postoperative day following intraabdominal haemorrhage and severe shock due to postoperative over-anti-coagulation.

### Pulmonary embolism
In our series we have had no case of fatal pulmonary embolism in the perioperative period. To avoid this problem it is of the utmost importance to perform a preoperative venogram that can exclude an extension of the thrombus into the IVC, which can be fractured during manipulation with the Fogarty catheter. We do not use a separate balloon catheter to occlude

**Table 34.1**
Early patency of the iliac vein following thrombectomy with temporary AVF

| Author | Number of patients | Patent iliac vein (%) |
|---|---|---|
| Delin et al, 1982 | 13 | 85 |
| Plate et el, 1984 | 31 | 87 |
| Piquet et al, 1985 | 92 | 80 |
| Einarsson et al, 1986 | 51 | 88 |
| Kniemeyer, 1987 | 157 | 90 |
| Juhan et al, 1987 | 42 | 93 |
| Vollmar et al, 1989 | 93 | 82 |
| Neglen et al, 1990 | 48 | 89 |
| TOTAL | 527 | 87 |

the IVC but routinely ask the anaesthetist to apply a PEEP during the operative manipulation of the thrombotic vein. In a randomised study (Plate et al, 1985) we found positive perfusion scans at admission in 45% of all patients with additional defects seen after 1 and 4 weeks in the conservatively treated group in 11% and 12% respectively and in the thrombectomised group in 20% and 0% respectively. Mavor and Gallaway (1969) demonstrated that an incomplete clearance of the thrombus in the iliac vein increased the incidence of rethrombosis and pulmonary embolism. In our series no additional perfusion defects developed after the first postoperative week following thrombectomy with AVF. Since the AVF effectively prevented rethrombosis it can be assumed that the fistula was one reason for the low incidence of postoperative pulmonary embolism.

The reasons for the decreased risk of developing significant symptomatic and fatal pulmonary embolism with the present technique are listed below:
- Careful selection of patients.
- Preoperative demonstration by venography of the extension and level of the top of the thrombus, requiring an extended surgical approach if the IVC is involved.
- Use of PEEP during surgery to decrease the risk for perioperative pulmonary embolism.
- Atraumatic surgery.
- Utilisation of an AVF to decrease the risk of immediate rethrombosis with subsequent pulmonary embolism.

### Early morbidity
Thrombectomy combined with temporary AVF compared with conservative treatment has shown no difference in leg swelling and hospital stay (Plate et al, 1985). Complications were infrequent in both groups. The rate of early rethrombosis of the iliac vein is only 13% (Table 34.1). The important factors are listed below:
- Rarely operating if the symptoms of iliofemoral obstruction are more than 7 days old.
- Use of the Fogarty catheter with special consideration to the internal iliac vein
- Direct caval approach when the IVC is involved.
- Intraoperative venography or venoscopy to demonstrate clearance of the iliac vein.
- Liberal and early indication for decompressive leg fasciotomy in patients with phlegmasia cerulea dolens.

- Use of a temporary AVF.
- Early ambulation wearing compression stockings.
- Carefully monitored postoperative anticoagulant administration.

## Role and closure of AVF

The objectives of a temporary AVF are to increase blood flow in the thrombectomised segment to prevent immediate rethrombosis, to allow time for healing of the endothelium and to promote the development of collaterals in case of incomplete clearance or immediate rethrombosis of the iliac segment. Closure of the fistula is performed after 6-10 weeks. An experimental study in dogs was performed to assess the time for full endothelialisation (Einarsson et al, 1984). Following the near complete loss of endothelial cells lining the vein after thrombectomy, new endothelium grew out from small branch openings and valve pockets within 4 weeks, except in the proximity of the AVF where endothelial regrowth was still incomplete after 4 months. This study supports our routine tpractice of keeping the temporary fistula for at least 4 weeks. During the first few years of our experience, the fistula was closed under local anaesthesia by ligation and division. Early in our experience we had more problems with the closure of the AVF than with the original operation (Einarsson et al, 1986). With the new percutaneous technique developed by Endrys in Kuwait (Endrys et al, 1989), these problems have almost vanished. Through a puncture of the femoral artery on the contralateral surgically untouched side, a catheter is inserted and positioned at the fistula level. Prior to inflation and release of the balloon, an arterio-venogram can be performed to evaluate the patency of the iliac and caval veins, which is of prognostic value. More than 10% of patients have been shown to have remaining significant stenosis despite initially successful surgery. A transvenous percutaneous angioplasty can immediately be performed under the protection of the AVF, which is closed 4 weeks later after repeat arterio-venogram.

## Results of thrombectomy with arteriovenous fistula

### Early results
In the 1960s the early clinical results after thrombectomy were reported as successful on clinical grounds alone since venography was rarely performed. Table 34.1 shows published reports regarding patency of the iliac vein less than three months after removal of the thrombus. Totally there are 527 patients collected with an average patency rate of 87 percent. Einarsson et al (1986) reported that arteriovenography performed on 60 legs of originally 70 patients visualised a patent AVF in 85 percent. In Piquet's material, all patients had an extension of the thrombus into the IVC and an Adams-DeWeese clip was applied in addition to the thrombectomy (Piquet et al, 1985). A temporary AVF was utilised in 59% of the cases. In the group of 27 patients with excellent patency of the iliocaval vein, 21 had a fistula to prevent reocclusion. Vollmar et al (1989) confirmed the advantage of the AVF showing 82% patency in 93 patients with AVF versus 54% in 26 patients without an AVF.

**Table 34.2**
The frequency of clinical success (i.e., asymptomatic patients with no signs of PT syndrome) at 6-60 months follow-up after thrombectomy with temporary AVF

| Author | Number of patients | Follow-up (months) | Clinical success (%) |
| --- | --- | --- | --- |
| Poilleux et al, 1975 | 27 | — | 78 |
| Plate et al, 1984 | 31 | 6 | 42 |
| Piquet et al, 1985 | 82 | 51 | 51 |
| Einarsson et al, 1986 | 55 | 10 | 75 |
| Kniemeyer, 1987 | 37 | 36 | 62 |
| Juhan et al, 1987 | 36 | 12-48 | 93 |
| Winter et al, 1989 | 100 | 12 | 64 |
| Plate et al, 1990 | 19 | 60 | 37 |
| Neglen et al, 1990 | 37 | 24 | 83 |
| TOTAL | 424 | | 65 |

## Late results

There are few studies on longterm results after TE and AVF. Table 34.2 shows the clinical results of those that have been done. To develop a post-thrombotic syndrome takes many years so the final clinical outcome of success is too early to assess in most of the presented material. In Plate's randomised study a highly significant difference in asymptomatic patients was found (42% in the operated group vs 7% in the conservative group) (Plate et al, 1984). Moderate leg swelling, secondary varicose veins and venous claudication were more frequently observed in the conservative treatment group. In Plate's report of 5 years' follow-up, 37% of the operated patients were free of symptoms compared to 18% in the conservative treatment group (Plate et al, 1990).

Table 34.3 shows the "long-term" results of iliac patency, which seems to be maintained in several series. The average patency of 289 patients was 76 percent. In Plate's randomised study after 6 months there was a patency of 76% in the operated group compared to 35% in the conservative group (Plate et al, 1984). After 5 years radionuclide venography showed

**Table 34.3**
The patency rate of the iliac vein at 6-60 months follow-up after thrombectomy with temporary AVF

| Author | Number of patients | Follow-up (months) | Patent iliac vein (%) |
| --- | --- | --- | --- |
| Plate et al, 1984 | 31 | 6 | 76 |
| Piquet et al, 1985 | 57 | 39 | 80 |
| Einarsson et al, 1986 | 58 | 10 | 61 |
| Juhan et al, 1987 | 36 | 12-48 | 93 |
| Törngren et al, 1988 | 54 | 19 | 54 |
| Plate et al, 1990 | 19 | 60 | 77 |
| Neglen et al, 1990 | 34 | 24 | 88 |
| TOTAL | 289 | | 76 |

**Table 34.4**
The frequency of patent and competent femoropopliteal vein segments at 6-60 months follow-up after thrombectomy with temporary AVF

| Author | Number of patients | Follow-up (months) | Competence (%) |
| --- | --- | --- | --- |
| Plate et al, 1984 | 31 | 6 | 52 |
| Einarsson et al, 1986 | 53 | 10 | 42 |
| Kniemeyer, 1987 | 157 | 42 | 45 |
| Plate et al, 1990 | 14 | 60 | 36 |
| Neglen et al, 1990 | 34 | 24 | 46 |
| TOTAL | 289 |  | 44 |

a patency of 77% in the surgical group. The iliac vein was normal in 71% of cases in the surgical group compared to 30% in the conservative group (Plate et al, 1990).

Table 34.4 shows the "long-term" valvular competence and reflux of the femoropopliteal segment following thrombectomy combined with AVF. Very few reports contain information on valvular competence after surgery. Among the collected 289 patients an average of 44% had patent and competent valves in the femoropopliteal segment. It is vital to preserve these valves and retain a normal calf pump function in order to prevent the development of the post-thrombotic syndrome. Plate et al (1984) found after 6 months, patent and competent valves in the femoropopliteal segment in 52% in the surgical group compared with 26% in the conservatively treated group. Browse predicted that the incidence of the post-thrombotic syndrome would not differ between the groups after 5 years (Browse et al, 1988). However, after 5 years, Plate et al (1990) found a decreased risk of developing the severe post-thrombotic syndrome after surgery and more pronounced venous hypertension amongst patients treated with anticoagulants only. The thrombectomised patients had a significant reduction in ambulatory venous pressure (AVP), and improved venous emptying as shown by plethysmography and a better calf pump function with less reflux measured by foot volumetry. Taking the results of all functional tests into account at the 5-year follow up, 36% of the operated patients had a normal venous function, compared to 11% of those conservatively treated. Kniemeyer (1987) and Einarsson et al (1986) have reported a similar rate of preservation of valvular function. An interesting difference in Kniemeyer's technique is the more distal placement of the temporary AVF, in 72% of cases at the adductor canal or lower in the popliteal vein (Kniemeyer et al, 1985). Using Doppler ultrasound and photoplethysmography, Neglen et al (1992) reported slightly better results.

## Results of thrombectomy without AVF

Table 34.5 lists the clinical results after TE *without* AVF. Different adjunctive measures, such as perioperative local infusion of thrombolytic agents, ligation of the superficial femoral vein and postoperative local heparin infusion have been added to TE. In 2,437 thrombectomies, the average clinical success was 76% with a range from 6% (Lansing and Davis, 1968) to 100% (Goto et al, 1980). In many papers it is difficult to find out the time for follow-up and definition of clinical success. Very few authors have followed their patients with venography or studies of venous function. In Mavor's study (Mavor and

**Table 34.5**
The frequency of clinical success at follow-up after thrombectomy with temporary AVF

| Author | Number of thrombectomies | Follow-up (months) | Clinical success (%) |
| --- | --- | --- | --- |
| Mahorner et al, 1957 | 11 | 15 | 64 |
| Haller et al, 1963 | 34 | 18 | 76 |
| Bradham et al, 1964 | 13 | early | 100 |
| DeWeese, 1964 | 31 | 24 | 68 |
| Fontaine et al, 1965 | 72 | >12 | 83 |
| Hafner et al, 1965 | 41 | 42 | 98 |
| Kaiser et al, 1965 | 49 | 36 | 65 |
| Smith, 1965 | 18 | 17 | 78 |
| Britt, 1966 | 19 | early | 42 |
| Fogarty et al, 1966 | 21 | 22 | 86 |
| Little et al, 1966 | 19 | early | 95 |
| Wilson and Britt, 1967 | 39 | early | 39 |
| Lansing and Davis, 1968 | 17 | 60 | 6 |
| Bertelsen, 1969 | 15 | early | 87 |
| Mavor and Galloway, 1969 | 110 | 96 | 89 |
| Mavor and Galloway, 1969 | 54 | 36 | 95 |
| Edwards et al, 1970 | 61 | 54 | 80 |
| Johansson et al, 1976 | 21 | 24 | 19 |
| Senn et al, 1973 | 130 | early | 75 |
| Baumann, 1976 | 44 | early | 80 |
| Matsubara et al, 1976 | 17 | 6 | 67 |
| Stephens, 1976 | 16 | late | 75 |
| Denck, 1977 | 123 | late | 85 |
| Lindhagen et al, 1978 | 21 | 6 | 77 |
| Lindhagen et al, 1978 | 12 | 12 | 100 |
| Hortsch et al, 1979 | 21 | early | 86 |
| Kistner and Sparkuhl, 1979 | 58 | 12-60 | 84 |
| Kistner and Sparkuhl, 1979 | 19 | 60-96 | 83 |
| Kistner and Sparkuhl, 1979 | 19 | 96-132 | 89 |
| Nadjabat et al, 1979 | 63 | 12 | 94 |
| Provan et al, 1979 | 12 | <96 | 67 |
| Goto et al, 1980 | 43 | 46 | 100 |
| Metz et al, 1980 | 52 | 36 | 80 |
| Andriopoulos et al, 1982 | 134 | 28 | 80 |
| Røder et al, 1984 | 45 | 5 | 77 |
| Røder et al, 1984 | 30 | 120 | 67 |
| Shionoya et al, 1989 | 43 | late | 85 |
| Vollmar et al, 1989 | 26 | 52 | 54 |
| Husfeldt et al, 1991 | 900 | — | 80 |
| Paquet et al, 1991 | 44 | 60 | 76 |
| TOTAL | 2,437 | | 76 |

Gallaway, 1969) of 23 legs 3 years after TE, venography showed normal venous morphology in 79%. Kistner published the results of TE combined with ligation of the superficial femoral vein in 1979 (Kistner et al, 1979). Follow-up of 57 patients after 49 months with venography confirmed patency of the iliac vein in 75%. The philosophy behind ligation of the superficial femoral vein was to avoid early pulmonary embolism and the severe postthrombotic syndrome due to reflux in the deep venous system. In a recent follow-up after more than 15 years the approach seems to be valid (Personal communication).

An interesting finding in some reports on TE without AVF is the early rethrombosis of the iliac vein in 21-37% (Mavor and Galloway, 1969; Lindhagen et al, 1978; Røder et al, 1984) which should be compared with 13% in TE with AVF (Table 34.1).

## The postthrombotic syndrome

One of the main objectives in the treatment of DVT is to preserve venous patency and normal valves, thereby avoiding the development of the postthrombotic syndrome. Anticoagulant treatment has been shown to give immediate symptomatic relief and to efficiently prevent fatal pulmonary embolism, at least when the IVC is not involved. The following unavoidable recanalisation is often incomplete and results in destruction of valves. Only 30% of iliac vein segments remain open and almost invariably a severe reflux will occur five years later (Akesson et al, 1990). Venous hypertension leads to postthrombotic sequelae in 66-82% of patients (Bradham and Buxton, 1964; Arnesen et al, 1982). Its severe form with venous claudication or venous ulcers will develop in 1/3 of cases with time (O'Donnell et al, 1977; Raju and Fredericks, 1986; Akesson et al, 1990). Thus, conservative treatment of iliofemoral venous thrombosis with anticoagulation alone is not an optimal method.

In the series that are cited here regarding results following thrombectomy, the observation time is short but clinical success with no symptoms and signs of the PT syndrome is found in 65% after TE and AVF (Table 34.2). The early patency of the iliac vein (87%) seems to hold up in some material, but there is a decrease on average to 76% (Table 34.3) with observation times ranging from 6-60 months. Preservation of patency and valvular competence in the femoropopliteal segment is reported in 44 percent (Table 34.4). There is only one prospective randomised study performed by Plate et al (1984; 1990). Unfortunately, almost 1/3 of the patients had died between the 6-month and 5-year follow up, since the mean age in the material was high with frequent concomitant malignant disease. This makes proper statistical analysis inconclusive, but the study certainly indicates strong trends. Six months after treatment 42% of patients after thrombectomy were asymptomatic compared with 7% following medical treatment. At 5-year follow-up, this difference was maintained, but was not as obvious, 37% vs 18%. Iliac vein patency after 6 months was 76% in the operated group compared to 35% in the conservative group. After five years radionuclide venography showed a patency of 77% in the surgical group with a normal iliac vein in 71% vs 30% in the conservative group. In the early follow-up period, twice as many TE cases had preserved valves (52 vs 26%) and valve reflux was four times more common in cases conservatively treated (9 vs 37%). Observations after 5 years indicate that there is a higher risk of developing venous hypertension after conservative treatment and if all tests for reflux, obstruction and calf pump function are taken together, 36% of the operated patients had a normal venous function compared to 11% of the conservatively treated patients.

## Follow up

As mentioned above, all patients are anticoagulated for at least 6 months, and are carefully monitored to keep them in the therapeutic range. After six months, a coagulation survey is performed including fibrinolytic activity, AT III, protein C and protein S. The result will determine the indication to prolong anticoagulation treatment.

In patients with a functioning AVF an arteriovenogram is performed after 6 weeks. If the venous outflow is satisfactory, the AVF is closed as described. If there is a significant stenosis of the iliac vein, an attempt is made to dilate the stenosis, keeping the AVF for another 4-6 weeks before closure.

The longterm follow-up should include a study of morphology and function with duplex colour flow imaging (Bemmelen et al, 1989; Vasdekis et al, 1989) and air plethysmography (APG) (Nicolaides et al, 1990) which seem to be the best tools at present. As we have a preoperative colour flow imaging study we repeat this before discharge after surgery. We recommend repeat studies after closure of the AVF, six months after surgery and then annually. In the later follow-up APG will be added as a noninvasive modality to study function. This will give us an indication whether the patient resumes normal venous function or develops a postthrombotic syndrome. Necessary measures can be instituted and in the severe cases venous reconstruction could be considered.

## Indications for surgery

The rational way to treat thromboembolic venous disease is by induced thrombolysis. Unfortunately, about 50% of patients presenting with acute iliofemoral venous thrombosis will have contraindications for this treatment. Thrombectomy combined with a temporary AVF appears to give superior results compared with conservative anticoagulant treatment. The results of surgery have improved because of better preoperative management and surgical technique with special precautions in patients with extension of the thrombus into the IVC. The use of perioperative venography or venoscopy to demonstrate clearance of the iliac vein as well as the temporary AVF will decrease the risk of early rethrombosis. With the new technique of percutaneous closure of the AVF with a detachable balloon the closing procedure has been simplified. Until results of a prospective study comparing surgery with thrombolysis is at hand, thrombectomy with a temporary AVF is our method of choice to treat all patients with acute iliofemoral venous thrombosis if the thrombus is less than seven days old, and the patient is less than 70 years old.

In patients with phlegmasia cerulea dolens or venous gangrene, there is an absolute indication for surgery to try to save limb and life. We do not advise surgery in patients with metastatic malignant disease, severe arteriosclerotic disease, limited life expectancy due to concurrent disease, and those who are immobilised.

We agree with Rutherford (1986) that "... thrombectomy now is a better operation which can achieve specific goals in carefully selected patients".

## References

Akesson H, Brudin L, Dahlstrom JA, Eklof B, Ohlin P, Plate G. Venous function assessed during a 5-year period after acute iliofemoral venous thrombosis treated with anticoagulation. Eur J Vasc Surg 4:43, 1990

Albrechtsson U, Andersson J, Einarsson E, Eklof B, Norgren L. Streptokinase treatment of deep venous thrombosis and the post-thrombotic syndrome. Follow-up evaluation of venous function. Arch Surg 116:33, 1981

Andriopoulos A, Wirsing P, Botticher R. Results of iliofemoral venous thrombectomy after acute thrombosis. Report on 165 cases. J Cardiovasc Surg 23:123, 1982

Arnesen H, Hoiseth A, Ly B. Streptokinase or heparin in the treatment of deep vein thrombosis. Acta Med Scand 211:65, 1982

Audier M, Haimovici H. Les gangrènes des membres d'origine veineuse. Press Med 46:1403, 1938

Basmajean JV. The distribution of the valves in the femoral, external iliac and common iliac veins and their relation to varicose veins. Surg Obstet Gynecol 95:537, 1952

Baumann G. Indikation, Teknik und Ergebnisse der Thrombektomie. Chirurg 47:108, 1976

Bemmelen PS, Bedford G, Beach K, Strandness DE Jr. Quantitative segmental evaluation of venous valvular reflux with duplex ultrasound scanning. J Vasc Surg 10:425, 1989

Bertelsen S. Surgical management of iliofemoral thrombophlebitis. Acta Chir Scand 135:149, 1969

Bradham RR, Buxton JT. Thrombectomy for acute iliofemoral venous thrombosis. Surg Gynecol Obstet 119:1271, 1964

Britt LG. Iliofemoral veno-occlusive disease. Results with thrombectomy in 16 cases. Am Surg 32:103, 1966

Browse NL, Burnand KG, Thomas ML. Deep vein thrombosis: treatment. In: Browse NL, Burnand KG, Thomas ML (Eds): Diseases of the veins. Edward Arnold, London, Baltimore, Melbourne, Auckland, p, 501, 1988

Christenson J, Einarsson E, Eklof B. Infection complications after thrombectomy in deep venous thrombosis. Acta Chir Scand 144:431, 1977

Delin A, Swedenborg J, Hellgren M, Jacobson H, Nilsson E. Thrombectomy and arteriovenous fistula for iliofemoral venous thrombosis in fertile women. Surg Gyne Obstet 154:169, 1982

Denck H. Operative Therapie. (Thrombektomie, Schirmfilter, Cavaligatur). Langenbecks Arch Chir 345:381, 1977

DeWeese JA. Thrombectomy for acute iliofemoral venous thrombosis. J Cardiovasc Surg 5:703, 1964

DeWeese JA, Jones TI, Lyon J, Dale WR. Evaluation of thrombectomy in the management of iliofemoral venous thrombosis. Surgery 47:140, 1960

Dos Santos JC. La phlebographie directe. Conception, technique, premier resultats. J Int Chir 3:625, 1938

Edwards WH, Sawyers JL, Foster JH. Iliofemoral venous thrombosis: reappraisal of thrombectomy. Ann Surg 171:961, 1970

Einarsson E, Eklof B, Kuenzig M, von Mecklenburg C, Schwartz SI. Scanning electron microscopy and Evans blue staining for assessing endothelial trauma and reconstitution after venous thrombectomy. Scan Electron Microsc 1:273, 1984

Einarsson E, Albrechtsson U, Eklof B, Norgren L. Follow up evaluation of venous morphologic factors and function after thrombectomy and temporary arteriovenous fistula in thrombosis of iliofemoral vein. Surg Obstet Gynecol 163:111, 1986

Einarsson E, Albrechtsson U, Eklof B. Thrombectomy and temporary AV-fistula in iliofemoral vein thrombosis. Technical considerations and early results. Int Angio 5:65, 1986

Eklof B. Temporary arteriovenous fistula in reconstruction of iliac vein obstruction using PTFE grafts. In: Eklof B, Gjores JE, Thulesius O, Bergqvist D (Eds): Controversies in management of venous disorders. Butterworths, London, Boston, Sydney, Singapore, Toronto, Wellington, P. 280, 1989

Eklof B, Gjores JE, Lohi A, Staszkiewicz W, Norgren L. Spontaneous rupture of liver and spleen with severe intra-abdominal bleeding during streptokinase treatment of deep venous thrombosis. VASA 6:369, 1977

Elliott MS, Immelmman EJ, Jeffery P, Benatar SR, Funston MR, Smith JR et al. A comparative randomised trial of heparin versus streptokinase in the treatment of acute proximal venous thrombosis: an interim report of a prospective trial. Br J Surg 66:838, 1979

Endrys J, Eklof B, Neglen P, Zyka I, Peregrin J. Percutaneous closure of femoral arteriovenous fistula after venous thrombectomy. J Cardiovasc Intervent Radiol 12:226, 1989

Farber SP, O'Donnell TJ Jr, Deterling RA, Millan VF, Callow AD. The clinical implications of acute venous thrombosis of the inferior vena cava. Surg Gynecol Obstet 158:141, 1984

Fogarty TJ, Dennis D, Kripaehne WW. Surgical management of iliofemoral venous thrombosis. Am J Surg 112:211, 1966

Fontaine R, Tuchmann L, Suhler A. Surgical treatment of deep and recent venous thrombosis. Its role, methods and results. J Cardiovasc Surg Suppl, 174, 1965

Gillot C, Imbert P. Les thromboses iliocaves. Rapport au 82e Congrès Francais de Chirurgie. Masson, Paris, 1980

Girard P, Mathieu M, Simonneau G, Petitpretz P, Cerrina J, Hervé P et al. Recurrence of pulmonary embolism during anticoagulant treatment: a prospective study. Thorax 42:481, 1987

Girard P, Hauuy MP, Musset D, Simonneau G, Petitpretz P. Acute inferior vena cava thrombosis. Early results of heparin therapy. Chest 95:284, 1989

Goto H, Wata T, Matsumoto A, MatsumuraH, Soma T. Iliofemoral venous thrombectomy. Follow-up studies of 88 patients. J Cardiovasc Surg 21:341, 1980

Gregoire R. La phlebite blue (Phlegmasia coerulea dolens). Press Med 46:1403, 1938

Hafner CD, Cranley JJ, Krause RJ, Strasser ES. Venous thrombectomy. Current status. Am Surg 161:411, 1965

Haller JA, Abrams BL. Use of thrombectomy in the treatment of acute iliofemoral venous thrombosis in forty-five patients. Ann Surg 158:561, 1963

Horsch S, Zehle A, Eisenhardt JH, Landes T, Pichlmaier H. Chirurgische Behandlung der akuten Bein- und Beckenvenenthrombose. Med Klin 74:101, 1979

Husfeldt KJ, Raschke R, Wesch G. Reoperations after reconstructive surgery of the veins. XII International Vascular Workshop. April 6-13, 1991, Obergurgl, Austria

Johansson E, Nordlander S, Zetterquist S. Venous thrombectomy in the lower extremity — clinical, phlebographic and plethysmographic evaluation of early and late results. Acta Chir Scand 139:511, 1973

Juhan C, Cornillon B, Tobiana F, Schlama S, Barthelemy P, Denjean-Massia JP. Patency after iliofemoral and iliocaval venous thrombectomy. Ann Vasc Surg 1:529, 1987

Kadji H. Traitment chirurgical des thromboses veineuse hautes des membres inferierus. A propos de 186 cas. Theses Université de Marseille, 1980

Kaiser GC, Murray RC, Willman VL, Hanlon CR. Iliofemoral thrombectomy for venous occlusion. Arch Surg 90:574, 1965

Kakkar VV, Paes TRF, Murray WJG. Does thrombolytic therapy prevent the postphlebitic syndrome. In: Negus D, Jantet G (Eds): Phlebology 85, John Libbey, London, Paris, p. 481, 1986

Killewich LA, Bedford GR, Beach KW, Strandness DE Jr. Spontaneous lysis of deep venous thrombi: rate and outcome. J Vasc Surg 9:89, 1989

Kistner RL, Sparkuhl MD. Surgery in acute and chronic venous disease. Surg 85:31, 1979

Kistner RL. Valve repair and segment transposition in primary valvular insufficiency. In: Bergan JJ, Yao JST (Eds): Venous disorders. WB Saunders, Philadelphia, London, Toronto, Montreal, Sydney, Tokyo, p. 261, 1991

Kniemeyer HW, Sandmann W, Waller S. Die embolisierende Venenthrombose. Therapiekoncept, Ergebnisse. Akt Chir 20:204, 1985

Kniemeyer HW. Personal communication, 1987

Kunlin J. Les greffes veineuses. 15 Congress of International Surgical Society, Lisbon 15:875, 1953

Lansing AM, Davis WM. Five-year follow-up study of iliofemoral venous thrombectomy. Ann Surg 168:620, 1968

Lawen A. Weitere Ehrfahrung uber operative Thrombenentfernung bei Venenthrombose. Zentralbl Chir 64:961, 1938

Lindhagen J, Haglund M, Haglund U, Holm J, Schersten T. Iliofemoral venous thrombectomy. J Cardiovasc Surg 19:319, 1978

Little JM, Loewenthal J, Mills FH. Venous thromboembolic disease. Br J Surg 53:657, 1966

Mahorner H, Castleberry JW, Coleman WO. Attempts to restore function in major veins which are the site of massive thrombosis. Ann Surg 146:510, 1957

Matsubara J, Ban J, Nakata Y, Shinjo K, Hirai M et al. Longterm follow-up results of iliofemoral venous thrombosis. J Cardiovasc Surg 17:234, 1976

Mavor GE, Galloway JMD. The iliofemoral venous segment as a source of pulmonary emboli. Lancet 22:871, 1967

Mavor GE, Galloway JMD. Iliofemoral venous thrombosis. Pathological considerations and surgical management. Br J Surg 56:45, 1969

Metz L, Weber H. Die chirurgische Behandlung der akuten Becken-Beinvenenthrombose. Zentralbl Chir 105:1211, 1980

Nadjabat T, Birtel FJ, Neuhas G, Thelen M, Schmidt J. Atiologie, Diagnostik und operative Behandlung der akuten Bein, Becken- und unteren Hohlvenenthrombose. Zentralbl Chir 104:529, 1979

Neglen P, Al-Hassan H, Endrys J, Nazzal M, Christenson J, Eklof B. Iliofemoral venous thrombectomy followed by percutaneous closure of the temporary arterio-venous fistula. Surgery, 1992

Nicolaides AN, Christopoulos DC. Optimal methods to assess the deep venous system in the lower limb. Acta Chir Scand 555 (Suppl.):175, 1990

Norris CE, Greenfield LJ, Herrman JB. Free-floating iliofemoral thrombus. A risk of pulmonary embolism. Arch Surg 120:806, 1985

O'Donnell TF Jr, Browse NL, Burnand KG, Thomas ML. The socioeconomic effects of an iliofemoral thrombosis. J Surg Res 22:483, 1977

Paquet KJ, Koussouris P, Siemens F. Late results after thrombectomy in deep vein thrombosis of the leg and pelvis. XII International Vascular Workshop. Obergurgl, Austria, April 6-13, 1991

Piquet P, Tournigand P, Joss B, Mercier C. Traitement chirurgical des thromboses ilio-caves: exigences et resultats. In: Kieffer E (ed.): Chirurgie de la vein cave inferierur et de ses branches, Expansion Scientifique Francaise, Paris, p. 210, 1985

Plate G, Einarsson E, Ohlin P, Jensen R, Qvarfordt P, Eklof B. Thrombectomy with temporary arteriovenous fistula in acute iliofemoral venous thrombosis. J Vasc Surg 1:867, 1984

Plate G, Ohlin P, Eklof B. Pulmonary embolism in acute iliofemoral venous thrombosis. Br J Surg 72:912, 1985

Plate G, Akesson H, Einarsson E, Ohlin P, Eklof B. Long-term results of venous thrombectomy combined with a temporary arteriovenous fistula. E J Vasc Surg 4:483, 1990

Poilleux J, Chennet J, Bigot JM, Deliere T. Recent iliofemoral venous thrombosis. With a report of 27 cases treated by surgery. Ann Chir 29:713, 1975

Porter JM, Taylor LM. Current status of thrombolytic therapy. J Vasc Surg 2:239, 1985

Provan JL, Rumble EJ. Re-evaluation of thrombectomy in the management of iliofemoral venous thrombosis. Can J Surg 22:378, 1979

Radomski JS, Jarrell BE, Carabasi RA, Yang SL, Koolpe H. Risk of pulmonary embolus with inferior vena cava thrombosis. Am Surg 53:97, 1987

Raju S, Fredericks R. Late hemodynamic sequelae of deep venous thrombosis. J Vasc Surg 4:73, 1986

Røder OC, Lorentzen JE, Buchardt-Hansen HJ. Venous thrombectomy for iliofemoral thrombosis. Early and long-term results of 46 consecutive cases. Acta Chir Scand 150:31, 1984

Rutherford RB. Role of surgery in iliofemoral venous thrombosis. Chest 89 (Suppl.):434S, 1986

Senn A, Althaus V. Die chirurgische Behandlung der Phlebothrombose. Chirurg 44:193, 1973

Shionoya S, Yamada J, Sakurai T, Ohta T, Matsubara J. Thrombectomy for deep vein thrombosis: prevention of post-thrombotic syndrome. J Cardiovasc Surg 30:484, 1989

Smith GW. Therapy of iliofemoral venous thrombosis. Surg Gynecol Obstet 121:1298, 1965

Stephens GL. Current opinion on iliofemoral venous thrombectomy. Am Surg 42:108, 1976

Torngren S, Swedenborg J. Thrombectomy and temporary arteriovenous fistula for iliofemoral venous thrombosis. Int Angiol 7:14, 1988

Vasdekis SN, Clarke GH, Nicolaides AN. Quantification of venous reflux by means of duplex scanning. J Vasc Surg 10:670, 1989

Vollmar JF, Hutschenreiter S. Surgical treatment of acute thromboembolic disease: the role of vascular endoscopy. In: Veith F (Ed.) Current critical problems in vascular surgery. QMP, St Louis, p. 154, 1989

Wilson H, Britt LG. Surgical treatment of iliofemoral thrombosis. Am Surg 165:855, 1967

Winter G, Weber H. Loeprecht H. Surgical treatment of iliofemoral vein thrombosis: technical aspects. Possible secondary interventions. Int Angiol 8:188, 1989

CHAPTER 35

# The value of fibrinolysis in secondary prevention

Arthur A Sasahara   Cecilia C St Martin

## Introduction

Venous thromboembolism, including both venous thrombosis and its potentially fatal complication of pulmonary embolism (PE) continues to be a major health problem that arises mainly as a complication in the immobilised hospital patient, but also occurs in ambulant, otherwise healthy individuals. The incidence of deep vein thrombosis (DVT) and PE has been estimated in a number of epidemiologic studies dealing with a variety of data sources (Chapter 1), all of which are probably gross underestimates of the true occurrence rates. However, in order to put into perspective the scope of the problem in the United States, several series can be cited. Hume and colleagues (1970) estimated on the basis of hospital statistics in the US in 1966, that the total number of diagnosed cases of PE was about 106,000 and the total number of diagnosed cases of DVT was about 182,000, bringing the number with diagnosed venous thromboembolism to over a quarter of a million patients. Coon and Willis (1973), in a longitudinal study on the prevalence and incidence of venous thromboembolism in a Michigan community, extrapolated their data to the US census (1970) and estimated the annual incidence of DVT in the US to be over 250,000 cases. Additionally, data from this study was used to estimate the prevalence of the post-thrombotic syndrome in the US. The approximate frequency of stasis changes in the skin of the legs was 6-7 million persons and about 500,000 have or have had leg ulcers. These figures for the prevalence of the post-thrombotic changes would represent a frequency of about 5% of the US adult population in 1970, indicating that both the acute effects and longterm sequelae of venous thromboembolism represent a very significant public health problem.

# Secondary prevention

### Treatment objectives
In selecting therapy for patients with acute venous thromboembolism, several objectives should be borne in mind: (1) stop clot propagation and prevent acute PE in those with DVT; (2) stop clot propagation and prevent recurrent PE in those with PE. Additionally, longterm objectives should also be considered: (1) prevent recurrent DVT and the post-thrombotic syndrome; (2) prevent recurrent PE and chronic pulmonary hypertension. In both DVT and PE, an additional goal should be to remove, as completely as possible, the obstructing thromboemboli.

### Heparin
Although heparin anticoagulation has been the cornerstone of therapy for many years (Salzman et al, 1975), its function is principally one of prevention: it prevents propagation of the clot and it generally prevents pulmonary embolism. However, it does not prevent chronic venous insufficiency and the post-thrombotic syndrome, nor does it prevent chronic pulmonary hypertension in patients with previous PE, nor is it an effective clot remover.

### Thrombolysis
Thrombolytic therapy can also achieve the same objectives as heparin in preventing both clot propagation and PE. Additionally and uniquely, it appears to prevent or minimise the development of chronic venous insufficiency and it now seems to prevent or minimise chronic pulmonary hypertension. In contrast to heparin, it is much more efficient in removing clot mass.

Comerota (1988) cites 13 studies in which anticoagulant therapy has been compared with thromblytic therapy in patients with acute DVT. Contrast venography was used to evaluate efficacy, with post-therapy venography being performed on an average of 7 days following initiation of therapy. In the 227 patients treated with heparin, only 6% showed complete or significant clot lysis and an additional 12% showed partial lysis. The remaining 82% showed no change or had some enlargement of the clot mass.

In the 227 patients treated with thrombolytic therapy, 48% showed complete or near-complete lysis and an additional 20% showed partial lysis. The remaining 32% showed no change or had some enlargement of the clot mass.

In a meta-analysis of a number of randomised, comparative trials of streptokinase and heparin therapy of DVT, Goldhaber et al (1984) showed that improvement by clot mass reduction was achieved 3.7 times more often by thrombolytic therapy than by heparin anticoagulation. However, this benefit of lytic therapy was achieved with a bleeding complication that was 2.9 times higher than in the anticoagulant group.

# Factors influencing thrombolytic efficacy

Responsiveness of DVT to thrombolytic treatment is influenced by several factors: (1) age of clot; (2) mass of clot; (3) degree of cross-sectional venous obstruction, and (4) local concentration of the thrombolytic agent.

### Age of clot
Clots that are most susceptible to lysis are fresh ones that are friable because of loose cross-linking of fibrin, with high water content and little or no cellular infiltration. There is also minimal adherence to the vein wall. Clinically, this translates to a period of about 5-7 days from the onset of symptoms to the time of thrombolytic therapy for both DVT and PE. Fewer patients with symptoms up to 10-14 days will respond satisfactorily to lytic therapy. Theiss et al (1983) found the best response to streptokinase occurred in those patients who had symptoms of DVT for 3 days or less; Seaman et al (1976) noted a poor result in those with symptoms of DVT over 5 days, while Marder's (1977) results extended the window of therapy to 7 days. Our own experience parallels that of Marder's and also the National Institutes of Health sponsored Urokinase Pulmonary Embolism Trial (Sasahara et al, 1973) that showed the window of therapy for PE to be most effective up to 7 days. However, recent studies have demonstrated the efficacy of thrombolysis up to 14 days (Goldhaber et al, 1988). Nonetheless, it is clear that maximal lysis of clots can be achieved only in those that are particularly fresh.

### Mass of clot
The mass or quantity of the clot is also important as it primarily influences the duration of thrombolytic therapy. Whereas small thrombi causing acute myocardial infarction can be lysed within 1-2 hours, large thrombi in DVT or emboli in PE require hours to days to lyse completely.

### Degree of venous obstruction
Closely related to quantity of clot are its surface area and the degree of cross-sectional vessel obstruction. Clots that are completely occlusive are generally more difficult to lyse because only the small surface area of the clot end is exposed to the thrombolytic agent, whereas clots that are only partially occlusive tend to lyse readily because of the greater surface area that is exposed to the thrombolytic agent. Arnesen and his colleagues (1978) however, found no difference in complete or partially obstructive thrombi. Similarly, Kakkar and his co-workers (1969) frequently obtained complete lysis of thrombi that were completely occlusive. Nevertheless, partially obstructive clots usually require less time to lyse and if other factors are favourable, they lyse completely.

### Concentration of drug
Local concentration of the thrombolytic agent should be "enough" to overcome circulating inhibitors and to work effectively on and around the clot surface. It should be high enough to equilibrate rapidly in columns of static blood produced by complete occlusions.

## Venous insufficiency
The post-thrombotic syndrome, characterised by leg pain, oedema, hyperpigmentation and skin ulceration, occurs as a result of the venous insufficiency and venous hypertension that follow previous DVT in the majority of patients treated with anticoagulants. As many as 48% of patients treated with heparin may develop stasis ulcers two years after treatment. Thrombolytic therapy, in contrast, can lyse clots relatively rapidly, preserving the integrity of the fragile venous valve cusps. The presence of normal functioning venous valves may well prevent the cascade of events and anatomic changes leading to the post-thrombotic

syndrome. Rogers and Lutcher (1990) in a meta-analysis of all studies directly comparing streptokinase and heparin in patients with DVT showed that 49% (28/57) of the patients treated with streptokinase had normal venograms many months later while only 4% of those treated previously with heparin had normal venograms. Functional testing for venous valve function showed that it was normal in 41% of those treated with streptokinase, while it was normal in only 15% of those previously treated with heparin. Normal venograms correlated well with valve function studies and a reduction in post-thrombotic symptoms. Rogers and Lutcher (1990) concluded that complete lysis of DVT with thrombolytic therapy was associated with normal follow-up venograms, normal valve functions and absence of post-thrombotic symptoms. They also noted that duration of symptoms less than three days before treatment with thrombolytic agents was associated with normal follow-up venograms and normal valve functions. And, patients with femoral or iliac vein thrombosis developed a severe post-thrombotic syndrome five times more often than patients with thrombosis of the popliteal or calf veins.

## Restoration of pulmonary vasculature

As in the treatment of DVT, heparin has been the cornerstone of therapy for acute PE. Although it has been shown by serial perfusion lung scans that incomplete reperfusion generally follows anticoagulant therapy of the acute episode (Tow and Wagner, 1967), the long-term impact of this deficit was not thought to be clinically important. This served to hinder the more widespread application of thrombolytic therapy in patients with PE which would have been expected, following the demonstration of faster and more complete clot removal from the pulmonary vasculature. In the large, multicentre, Urokinase Pulmonary Embolism Trial (1974), it was shown that when clinical benefits are assessed by serial pulmonary angiography, perfusion lung scans and serial measurements of pulmonary arterial and right heart pressures, patients treated with urokinase and streptokinase showed significantly greater resolution of the abnormalities caused by the pulmonary embolic event (Figs 35.1-35.3). Aside from the perfusion lung scans which were performed one year later at follow-up, no other studies were obtained to detect any differences in treatment results (Figs 35.4 and 35.5). The lung scans showed no significant differences in the degree of reperfusion in either the heparin or thrombolysis group. In fact, there was no significant difference in the lung scan findings after 5-7 days following initial therapy.

### Assessment for Residual Pulmonary Emboli
To determine the effects of residual pulmonary emboli, Sharma et al (1980) studied 40 patients with PE who had no other underlying cardiopulmonary disease, and measured pulmonary capillary blood volume and pulmonary diffusing capacity. These parameters of pulmonary vascular function were measured at two weeks and one year following initial therapy with either heparin or with the thrombolytic agents. These results showed that at two weeks and one year later, the pulmonary capillary blood volume and the lung diffusing capacity were abnormally low in the patients treated with heparin, contrasted with the normal values in those treated with either Urokinase or streptokinase. These observations strongly suggested that thrombolytic therapy of patients with PE resulted in more complete resolution of pulmonary thromboemboli than that which occurred with heparin therapy, and that it may reduce associated longterm morbidity.

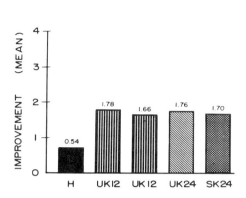

Fig. 35.1 Phase I and II results: Angiographic change. The degree of thromboembolic obstruction was assessed in pulmonary angiograms before treatment and 24 hours after initiation of therapy with heparin or a thrombolytic agent. Clot resolution, rated on a 4-point scale, was equivalent in the lytic groups and minimal with heparin

Fig. 35.2 Scan defect changes. Comparison of lung scans made before treatment and 24 hours after its initiation showed that improvements in perfusion were essentially similar with the lytic agents and significantly greater than with heparin

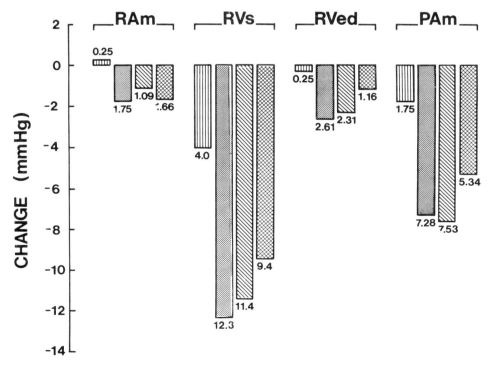

Fig. 35.3 Phase II: Haemodynamic changes. Improvements over baseline in 4 important pressure measurements 24 hours after initiation of therapy were significantly greater with the 3 lytic therapy regimens than with heparin

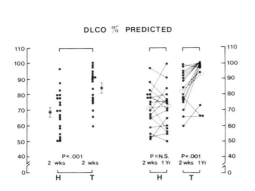
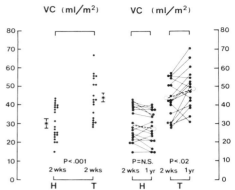

Fig. 35.4 To compare the integrity of the pulmonary microcirculation after therapy with heparin or a thrombolytic agent, the lung diffusing capacity was measured at two weeks and one year after treatment. The mean diffusing capacity was abnormally low in the heparin group and did not improve with time. By contrast, the mean diffusing capacity of the lytic group was in the low normal range at two weeks and showed a significant improvement at one year

Fig. 35.5 The pulmonary capillary blood volume is a major determinant of the lung diffusing capacity. The abnormally low diffusing capacity show in in figure 35.4 is a function of the abnormally low capillary blood volume as shown in this figure. Similarly, the normal diffusing capacity of the lytic treated group is a function of the normal capillary blood volume

## Longterm follow-up for residual damage

Further observations were reported by Sharma et al (1990) in a 7-10 year follow-up study. Twenty-three of these original 40 patients were restudied by right heart cardiac catheterisation during which supine exercise was carried out to measure pulmonary vascular responses to an exercise load. Additionally, exercise studies were carried out to determine functional capacity and classification according to the New York Heart Association criteria for functional disability. The patients with PE treated with anticoagulant therapy showed higher and abnormal pulmonary arterial pressures and pulmonary vascular resistances at rest and during supine exercise, than those patients initially treated with thrombolytic agents. This separation of abnormal pulmonary pressures and vascular resistances in the heparin group from the normal values in the thrombolytic group was highly significant. Additionally, there were more functionally impaired patients in the anticoagulant group (Class II-III) than there were in the thrombolytic group. Hence, these data support the hypothesis that more complete removal of the clot load in acute pulmonary embolism is a desirable therapeutic objective that is likely to lead to less functional impairment of the patient.

# Drug administration

### Urokinase
The recommended and approved dose regimen for urokinase was established by the two large NIH-sponsored trials of pulmonary embolism. This regimen is based upon weight and is administered as a loading dose, followed by an infusion for 12-24 hours:
*Loading dose:* 4,400 IU/kg body weight, administered over several minutes, followed immediately by a
*Maintenance dose:* 4,400 IU/kg body weight/hour × 12 hrs.
Following completion of the infusion, standard anticoagulant practices with heparin and subsequently with warfarin should be implemented.

### Streptokinase
The recommended and approved regimen for streptokinase was also established by the two large NIH sponsored trials of pulmonary embolism. This regimen is not based upon weight and is administered as a fixed loading dose, followed by an infusion for at least 24 hours: loading dose: 250,000 IU administered over 30 minutes, followed by a maintenance dose: 100,000 IU/hour for at least 24 hours. Following completion of the infusion, standard anticoagulation practices with heparin and subsequently with warfarin should be implemented.

### r-Tissue Plasminogen Activator
Recombinant tissue plasminogen activator (r-tPA) is the first of the newer, relatively fibrin-specific thrombolytic agents to be approved for use in PE. Investigations in Europe and the United States have shown it to be an effective agent when 100 mg is administered over a period of 2-7 hours. Goldhaber et al (1986) administered 100 mg over 2 hours and obtained good results, while Verstraete and his colleagues (1988) found that a prolonged infusion of 7 hours (100 mg) was superior to an infusion of 50 mg over 2 hours.

Additionally, Verstraete et al (1988) also compared the relative efficacy of administering r-tPA intravenously and by catheter delivery into the pulmonary artery. The results were similar with either route of administration.

### New treatment strategies
Several recent investigations of urokinase therapy of PE have been concerned with shortening the duration of drug administration, without sacrificing efficacy. Petitpretz et al (1984) began this trend by administering urokinase only as a bolus injection (15,000 IU/kg body weight). Though it was not a randomised, controlled study, objective assessments by pulmonary angiography showed excellent results.

More recently, Goldhaber et al (1991) initiated a multicentre study of PE in which a 2-hour bolus/infusion of 3 million units of urokinase was compared with a 2-hour bolus/infusion of 100 mg of r-tPA. Preliminary analysis has shown no difference in the extent of clot resolution as assessed by pulmonary angiography and by perfusion lung scanning.

These two studies are indeed promising and have demonstrated that urokinase thrombolysis can be accelerated by a high dose, short infusion regimen. Such a regimen should reduce the frequency of bleeding complications without compromising efficacy.

# References

Arnesen H, Heilo A, Jakobsen E, Ly B, Skaga E. A prospective study of streptokinase and heparin in the treatment of deep vein thrombosis. Acta Med Scand 203:457, 1978

Comerota AJ. An overview of thrombolytic therapy for venous thromboembolism. In: Comerota AJ (Ed.): Thrombolytic Therapy, Grune & Stratton, Orlando, p. 65, 1988

Coon WW, Willis PW, Keller JB. Venous thromboembolism and other venous disease in the Tecumseh Community Health Study. Circulation 48:839, 1973

Goldhaber SZ, Buring JE, Lipnick RJ, Hennekins CH. Pooled analysis of randomised trials of streptokinase and heparin in phlebographically documented acute deep venous thrombosis. Am J Med 76:393, 1984

Goldhaber SZ, Vaughan DE, Markis JE et al. Acute pulmonary embolism treated with tissue plasminogen activator. Lancet 2:885, 1986

Goldhaber SZ, Kessler CM, Heit JA et al. TPA vs urokinase in acute pulmonary embolism. Circulation 84:(Suppl. II), 357, 1991

Hume M, Sevitt S, Thomas DP. Venous thrombosis and pulmonary embolism. Harvard University Press, Cambridge MA, USA, p. 4, 1970

Kakkar VV, Flanc C, Howe CT, O'Shea M, Flute PT. Treatment of deep vein thrombosis: a trial of heparin, streptokinase and arvin. Brit Med J 1:806, 1969

Marder VJ, Soulen RL, Atichartakarn V et al. Quantitative venographic assessment of deep vein thrombosis in the evaluation of streptokinase and heparin treatment. J Lab Clin Med 89:1018, 1977

Petitpretz P, Simmoneau G, Cerrina J et al. Effects of a single bolus of urokinase in patients with life-threatening pulmonary emboli: a descriptive trial. Circulation 70:861, 1984

Rogers LQ, Lutcher CL. Streptokinase therapy for deep vein thrombosis: a comprehensive review of the English literature. Am J. Med 88:389, 1990

Salzman EW, Deykin D, Shapiro RM et al. Management of heparin therapy: controlled prospective trial. N Engl J Med 292:1049, 1975

Sasahara AA, Hyers, Cole CM et al. The urokinase pulmonary embolism trial: a national cooperative study. Circulation 47:(Suppl. 2), 1, 1973

Seaman AJ, Common HH, Rosch J et al. Deep vein thrombosis treated with streptokinase or heparin. Angiology 27:549, 1976

Sharma GVRK, Burleson VA, Sasahara AA. Effect of thrombolytic therapy on pulmonary capillary blood volume in patients with pulmonary embolism. N Engl J Med 303:842, 1980

Sharma GVRK, Folland ED, McIntyre KM et al. Longterm benefit of thrombolytic therapy in pulmonary embolic disease. J Am Coll Cardiol 15:65A, 1990

Theiss W, Wirtzfeld A, Fink U, Maubach P. The success of fibrinolytic therapy in fresh and old thrombosis of the iliac and femoral veins 4:61, 1983

Tow DE, Wagner NH Jr. Recovery of pulmonary arterial blood flow in patients with pulmonary embolism. N Engl J Med 276:1053, 1967

Urokinase streptokinase pulmonary embolism trial. Phase 2 results. JAMA 229:1606, 1974

Verstraete M, Miller GAH, Bounameaux H et al. Intravenous and intrapulmonary recombinant tissue plasminogen activator in the treatment of acute massive pulmonary embolism. Circulation 77:353, 1988

CHAPTER 36

# Air plethysmography

**Dimitris Christopoulos   Andrew N Nicolaides**

## Introduction

The physician who is often confronted with painful, swollen or ulcerated legs must first determine the existence of a venous problem and secondly, must decide whether the venous disease involves the superficial or deep veins. His third task is to determine whether the problem is the result of outflow obstruction, reflux, or both. More detailed and quantitative information is required to determine the prognosis and develop a rational plan of management. Air plethysmography has come a long way in providing answers to these questions by supplementing the history and clinical examination.

Chronic swelling, lipodermatosclerosis, pigmentation or ulceration of the lower limb due to chronic venous disease affect a considerable number of patients. In the United Kingdom, half a million people may be affected by this disease with 150,000 suffering from ulceration (Widmer et al, 1978; Fisher et al, 1981). The health service spends an estimated 200 and 400 million pounds per year on treatment. In recent years, this social problem has stimulated the evolution of surgery of superficial as well as deep veins by aiming to correct valvular incompetence and overcome venous obstruction (Palma et al, 1960; Husni, 1971; Gruss, 1983; Taheri et al, 1985; Raju, 1986). However, the absence of a satisfactory objective and quantitative method for the correct selection of patients and the evaluation of the results of these operations are reasons why surgery of the deep veins is still at an experimental stage.

Although venography and ambulatory venous pressure measurements (Nicolaides et al, 1985) are established venous investigations, they are invasive, expensive, and time consuming. Also, information provided is incomplete: venography shows mainly anatomy and ambulatory pressure measurements provide a measure of the overall severity of venous disease but fail to give enough information to determine how much of the problem is the result of venous reflux, venous obstruction or reduction of the ejection capacity of the calf muscle pump. In recent years noninvasive techniques have attempted to replace the above

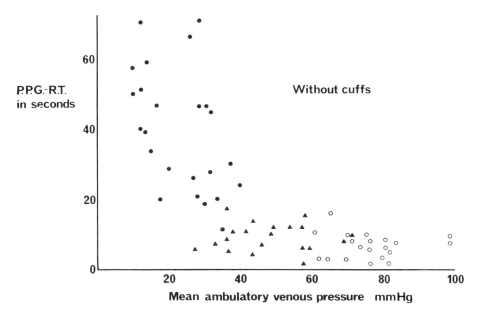

Fig. 36.1 Correlation between ambulatory venous pressure measurement (AVP) and photoplethysmography 90% recovery time (RT90). Note that for AVP ranging between 45 and 80 mmHg, the PPG 90% RT remains in the same abnormal range 1-5 sec

methods. Photoplethysmography (Abramowitz et al, 1979) has provided indirect and qualitative information to distinguish normal limbs from limbs and superficial and/or deep venous disease (Fig 36.1) (Nicolaides and Miles, 1987). Although this could be achieved, venography was still necessary in serious cases because photoplethysmography could not provide a measure of the severity of deep venous disease (Nicolaides and Miles, 1987) (Figure 36.1). Strain gauge plethysmography (Barnes et al, 1973; Fernandes e Fernandes et al, 1979), although quantitative, provided information on a segment not necessarily representative of the whole leg (Ludbrook and Loughlin, 1964). This test was difficult to use during changes in posture and exercise because tissue shifts interfered with the measurements (Strandness and Sumner, 1976).

Doppler ultrasound (Nicolaides et al, 1981) and Duplex scanning (Szendro et al, 1986) proved to be valuable tools in the detection of reflux and obstruction in individual veins. However, the results were operator-dependent and did not provide information on the severity of outflow obstruction or the efficacy of collateral circulation.

To overcome the problems of segmental devices air plethysmography used experimentally in the past (Allan, 1964; Ludbrook, 1966) has been recently developed for clinical use with the aim of replacing venography and ambulatory venous pressure measurements in the assessment of complicated cases (Christopoulos et al, 1987). As a result this noninvasive technique can provide quantitative information on the amount of venous reflux, (Christopoulos et al, 1988) the degree of venous obstruction (Christopoulos et al, 1989) and the ejection capacity of the calf muscle pump (Christopoulos et al, 1989b).

The efficacy of heparin, thrombolysis and oral anticoagulants in the treatment of thromboembolic disease has been assessed in terms of venographic clearance and recurrence. Relatively little work has been done to assess the changes in venous haemodynamics

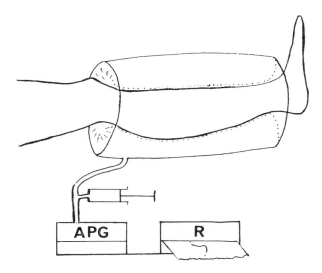

Fig. 36.2 The air-plethysmograph (APG) consists of an air-chamber that surrounds the whole leg, the calibration syringe (c) connected to a pressure transducer, amplifier and recorder. Note the position of the occluding tourniquet for venous occlusion

that lead to the post-thrombotic syndrome, changes that occur as a result of residual obstruction or recanalisation with destruction of valves producing reflux. The purpose of this chapter is to demonstrate the potential of air-plethysmography, a noninvasive technique that can provide objective follow up in short and longterm studies on the natural history of DVT and the efficacy of therapeutic measures in preventing the post-thrombotic haemodynamic changes that so often lead to ulceration.

## The air plethysmograph and its calibration

The air plethysmograph (APG) consists of a 35cm long polyurethane air chamber (5 litres capacity) which surrounds the whole leg connected to a pressure transducer, amplifier and recorder (Figure 36.2). The patient is placed in the supine position with the knee of the examined leg slightly flexed and the heel on a support; the air chamber is inflated to 6 mmHg.

Calibration is performed by depressing the plunger of the syringe (Fig. 36.2), compressing the air included in the air plethysmograph (air chamber and tubing), reducing its volume by 100 ml and observing the corresponding pressure change. After the calibration the plunger is pulled back to its original position when the pressure in the air chamber returns to 6 mmHg. The pressure of 6 mmHg has been selected because it is the lowest pressure that ensures good contact between the air chamber and the limb with minimum compression of the veins. Tissue movements during changes in posture and exercise are unlikely to interfere with the measurements because the air chamber includes almost all the tissues from the knee to the ankle. The air plethysmograph is calibrated in ml, so that consecutive measurements in the same limb are not influenced by changes in tissue volume due to increase or decrease of oedema.

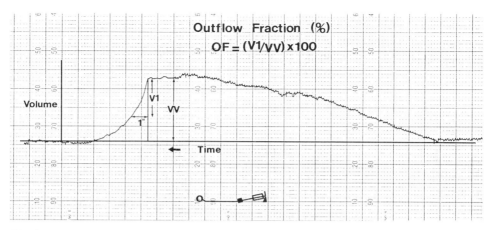

Fig. 36.3 Typical recording of venous occlusion air plethysmography. Low chart paper speed has been used during the filling phase (6 cm/min) and high during the outflow phase (60 cm/min). The outflow fraction (OF) is derived from OF= (V1/V) × 100

## Evaluation of venous outflow

With the patient in the supine position, an 11 cm wide pneumatic tourniquet is placed around the proximal part of the thigh and inflated to 80 mmHg (Figure 36.2). There is an increase in volume (Figure 36.3). When a plateau is reached, the tourniquet is suddenly deflated. The observed rapid decrease in volume is a result of venous outflow. The ratio of the amount of blood that leaves the leg in the first second (V1) over the total venous volume (TVV), times 100, is the outflow fraction (OF) expressed as a percentage. The procedure is repeated

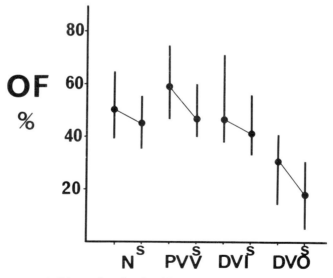

Fig. 36.4 Measurement of the outflow fraction (OF) in five groups of limbs, presented as median and 95% range before and after occlusion of the superficial veins (S). N = normal limbs, PVV = limbs with primary varicose veins, DVI = limbs with deep venous incompetence, without obstruction, DVO = limbs with deep venous obstruction with or without incompetence

with the long saphenous and/or other prominent superficial veins occluded by finger compression.

In limbs with normal deep veins the outflow fraction is higher than 40% (range 40-70%) (Christopoulos et al, 1989b) (Figure 36.4). Limbs with chronic deep venous obstruction on venography have an OF ranging 15-38% which is reduced further after occlusion of the superficial veins. This manoeuvre not only assists in the diagnosis of obstruction in borderline cases but also shows if any dilated superficial veins are important collateral channels bypassing the obstruction, which the surgeon should not ligate.

The OF measurements correlate well with invasive quantification of the severity of venous obstruction, obtained by measuring the arm/foot pressure differential with cannulation of a vein in the arm and a vein in the foot when the patient is in the supine position (Figure 36.5) (Raju, 1986; Christopoulos et al, 1989b). For practical purposes, we have considered that there is no functional venous obstruction for OF greater than 40%, moderate obstruction for OF 30-39% and severe obstruction for OF less than 30%.

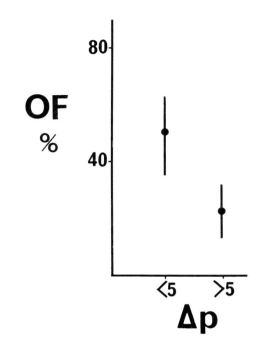

Fig. 36.5 Outflow fraction (OF) (median and 90% range) in 15 limbs with deep venous reflux but no obstruction (arm/foot pressure differential p<5 mmHg) and eight limbs with venographic deep venous obstruction (p>5 mmHg.)

## Evaluation of venous reflux

With the patient in the supine position and the air chamber of the APG inflated to 6 mmHg the examined limb is elevated (45 degrees) to empty the veins. The patient is then asked to stand up with the weight mainly on the opposite limb. The observed increase in volume is a result of venous filling (Figure 36.6). The functional venous volume (VV) ranges from 100-150 ml in normal limbs and up to 350 ml in limbs with venous diseases (Figure 36.6b) (Allan, 1964; Christopoulos et al, 1988). The ratio of 90% of VV divided by the time taken for 90% filling (VFT90) is defined as the venous filling index (VFI=90% VV/VFT90) (Figure 36.6). This is a measure of the average filling rate of the veins expressed in ml/sec. VFI is less than 2 ml/sec in normal limbs which fill slowly from the arterial circulation. It is increased up to 30 ml/sec in limbs with venous reflux (Figure 36.7). In limbs without outflow obstruction on venography, the incidence of ulceration increases with increasing values of VFI. It is zero for VFI less than 5ml/sec, 46% for VFI 5-10 ml/sec and 58% for

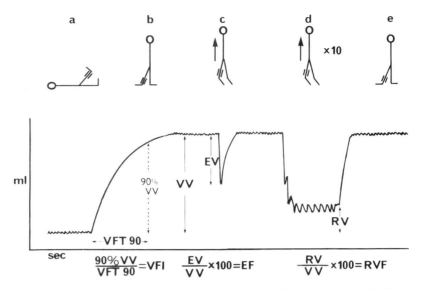

Fig. 36.6 Diagrammatic representation of a typical recording of volume changes during standard sequence of postural changes and exercise: (a) patient in supine position with leg elevated 45 degrees; (b) patient standing with weight on nonexamined leg; (c) single tiptoe movement; (d) ten tiptoe movements; (e) return to resting standing position as in (b). VV = functional venous volume; VFT = venous filling time; VFI = venous filling index; EV = ejected volume; RV = residual volume, EF = ejection fraction; RVF = residual volume fraction

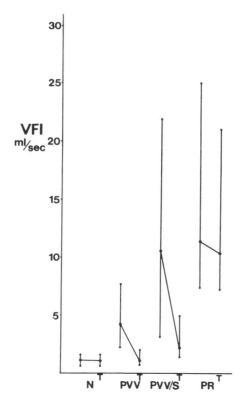

Fig. 36.7 Venous filling index (VFI) (median and 90% range) with and without a tourniquet (T) that occluded the superficial veins at the knee in (N) normal limbs, (PVV) limbs with primary varicose veins and no sequelae of chronic venous disease (liposclerosis and ulceration), (PVVS) primary varicose veins with sequelae of chronic venous disease, and (PR) limbs with popliteal reflux

# AIR PLETHYSMOGRAPHY

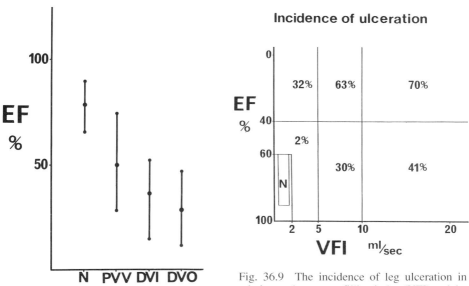

Fig. 36.8 Ejection fraction (EF) (median and 90% range in normal (N) limbs,

Fig. 36.9 The incidence of leg ulceration in relation to the venous filling index (VFI) and the ejection fraction (EF) of the calf muscle pump in 175 limbs with venous problems

VFI greater than 10 ml/sec, irrespective of whether reflux is in superficial or deep veins (Christopoulos et al, 1988).

The measurement of VFI can be repeated after abolition of reflux in the superficial veins at the level of the knee, by using narrow tourniquets or finger compression. VFI is reduced to less than 5 ml/sec in limbs with primary varicose veins and competent deep venous valves but not in limbs with reflux in the popliteal vein (Christopoulos and Nicolaides, 1988b). Abolition of venous reflux has also been demonstrated after conventional surgery for superficial venous incompetence (Christopoulos et al, 1988c).

## Evaluation of the ejection capacity of the calf muscle pump

The amount of blood ejected as a result of a single calf muscle contraction can be quantified, by measuring the decrease in volume produced after a single tiptoe movement (Fig. 36.6c). The ejection volume (EV) is about 100 ml in normal limbs and also in the majority of limbs with primary varicose veins. Limbs with deep venous disease eject less (down to 20ml) because of obstruction of the deep veins or retrograde ejection via incompetent perforating veins (Christopoulos et al, 1987; 1989c).

The ejection fraction (EF) of the calf muscle pump is derived from EF = (EV/VV) × 100 (Fig. 36.6). The EF is more than 60% in normal limbs and down to 10% in limbs with deep venous obstruction (Fig. 36.8). The incidence of venous ulceration is also related to the EF. As shown in figure 36.9, a poor EF was the primary cause of venous ulceration in limbs with minimal reflux. A good ejection fraction, however, significantly reduced the incidence of ulceration in limbs with marked reflux.

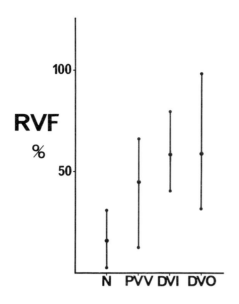

Fig. 36.10 Residual volume fraction (RVF) (mean and 90% range) in normal limbs (N), limbs with primary varicose veins (PVV), deep venous incompetence (DVI) and deep venous obstruction (DVO)

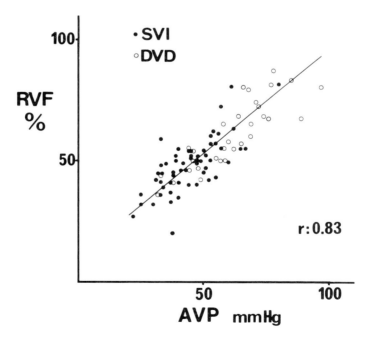

Fig. 36.11 Relationship between residual volume fraction (RVF) and ambulatory venous pressure (AVP) at the end of 10 tiptoe movements. (o = limbs with superficial venous incompetence, • = limbs with deep venous disease)

**Table 36.1**
The incidence of leg ulceration in relation to the residual volume fraction (RVF) in 175 limbs with venous disease

| n | RVF (%) | Incidence of ulceration (%) |
|---|---|---|
| 20 | <30 | 0 |
| 24 | 31-40 | 8 |
| 48 | 41-50 | 18 |
| 43 | 51-60 | 42 |
| 32 | 61-80 | 72 |
| 8 | >80 | 88 |

# Evaluation of the overall performance of the calf muscle pump

The combined effect of venous reflux, obstruction and ejection capacity of the calf muscle pump is evaluated by measuring the residual volume (RV) and residual volume fraction (RVF = RV/VV × 100) after ten tiptoe movements, at the rate of one per second (Fig. 36.6). The measurements of RVF are shown in figure 36.10. RVF correlates well with the measurements of ambulatory venous pressure (r = 0.81), so that the latter can be estimated noninvasively (Fig. 36.11) (Allan, 1964; Christopoulos et al, 1988); also, it correlates well with the incidence of ulceration. The latter is zero for RVF <30% and increases gradually to 88% for RVF >80% (Table 36.1).

# The value and the potential of air plethysmography

The air plethysmographic measurements are easily performed in 10-15 minutes with excellent tolerance from the patient and minor training requirements from the user. Although APG can be used as a simple screening test, it has the potential for and can offer a

**Table 36.2**
Reproducibility of air plethysmographic measurements (one normal limb, three limbs with primary varicose veins and one limb with deep venous disease studied on five different days)

| Measurements | Coefficient of Variation (%) |
|---|---|
| VV (ml) | 10.8 - 12.5 |
| VFT90 (sec) | 8.0 - 11.5 |
| EV (ml) | 6.7 - 9.4 |
| RV (ml) | 6.2 - 12.0 |
| VFI (ml/sec) | 5.3 - 7.9 |
| EF (%) | 2.9 - 9.7 |
| RVF (%) | 4.3 - 8.2 |

complete analysis of venous haemodynamics, useful in the routine clinical management of the patient as well as in research. The reproducibility of the air plethysmographic measurements is shown in table 36.2.

Limbs with oedema or ulceration due to causes other than venous disease (i.e., arterial, lymphatic, cardiac or rheumatoid) can be easily distinguished from those with venous disease (Christopoulos and Nicolaides, 1988). Also, in cases of combined disease (i.e., arterial and venous) the degree of venous involvement can be precisely assessed. Limbs with primary varicose veins can be distinguished from those with deep venous disease, and in patients with combined deep and superficial disease the pathological contribution of each system can be determined. Also, in limbs with prominent varicosities one can determine whether the latter are acting as outflow channels.

Deep venous disease is usually the result of the combined effect of reflux, obstruction, or poor ejection. By using air plethysmography, the contribution of each parameter can be measured, and the appropriate surgical intervention can be considered for each patient. The abolition of venous reflux by conventional surgery on the superficial system has already been shown to normalise the calf muscle pump function (Christopoulos et al, 1989b).

One of the advantages of the APG is that it can be applied over an elastic stocking. Thus, it has been demonstrated that graduated elastic compression reduces the residual volume fraction (and consequently ambulatory venous pressure) by 20-30% and that this is the result of a reduced venous reflux and an increased ejection fraction (Christopoulos et al, 1987). The ability of APG to assess different kinds of compression (graduated or uniform, high or low) has opened a new avenue of investigation in this area.

Table 36.2 shows that the reproducibility of the air plethysmographic measurements would detect any change in venous haemodynamics as a result of therapy provided it is greater than 10%.

Air plethysmography is used in our hospital investigations in all cases where the clinical and pocket Doppler examination fails to produce a clear diagnosis. This is approximately in 10% of all patients seen. In the past, venography was indicated in this group of patients because of a history of deep venous thrombosis, the presence of chronic swelling, liposclerosis and/or ulceration, and recurrent varicose veins. The use of air plethysmography with Doppler ultrasound or duplex scanning (if available) to localise incompetent sites (Nicolaides et al, 1981; Szendro et al, 1986) means that venography in chronic venous disease is now indicated only in patients considered for deep venous surgery.

# References

Abramowitz HB, Querel LA, Flinn WR et al. The use of photoplethysmography in the assessment of venous insufficiency. A comparison to venous pressure measurement. Surgery 86:434, 1979

Allan JC. Volume changes in the lower limb in response to postural alterations and muscular exercise. S Afr J Surg 2:75, 1964

Barnes RW, Collicott PE, Sumner DS, Strandness DE. Noninvasive quantitation of venous hemodynamics in the post-phlebitic syndrome. Arch Surg 107:807, 1973

Christopoulos D, Nicolaides AN, Szendro G, Irvine AT, Bull ML, Eastcott HHG. Air Plethysmography and the effect of elastic compression on the venous haemodynamics of the leg. J Vasc Surg 5:148, 1987

Christopoulos D and Nicolaides AN. Noninvasive diagnosis and quantitation of popliteal reflux in the swollen and ulcerated leg. J Cardiovasc Surg 29:535, 1988

Christopoulos D, Nicolaides AN, Szendro G. Venous reflux quantification and correlation with the clinical severity of chronic venous disease. Br J Surg 75, 1988a

Christopoulos D, Nicolaides AN, Galloway JMD, Wilkinson A. Objective noninvasive evaluation of venous surgical results. J Vasc Surg 8:683, 1988b

Christopoulos D, Nicolaides AN, Duffy P. Functional diagnostic assessment of the swollen and ulcerated leg. In: Strano A, Nono S: Advances in Vascular Pathology p. 185, 1989a

Christopoulos D, Nicolaides AN, Duffy P, Georgiou I. Noninvasive quantification of outflow obstruction. J Cardiovasc Surg 30:72, 1989b

Christopoulos D, Nicolaides AN, Cook A, Irvine A, Galloway GMD, Wilkinson A. Pathogenesis of venous ulceration in relation to the calf muscle pump function. Surgery 106:829, 1989c

Fernandes e Fernandes J, Horner J, Needham T, Nicolaides AN. Ambulatory calf volume plethysmography in the assessment of venous insufficiency. Br J Surg 66:327, 1979

Fisher H, Biland L, Da Silva A, Herwing E, Mehringer G, Mucker A, Widmer MTH, Scheibler P, Widmer LK. Venenleiden. Eine Reprasentative-Untersuchung in der Bevolkerung der Bundesrepublik Deutschland (Tubinger Studie). Munchen-Wien-Baltimore, Urban u Schwarzenberg; 1981

Gruss JD, Der Heutige Stand der Rekonstruktiven Venechirurgie. Schwerpunktmed 6:21, 1983

Husni EA, Venous reconstruction in postphlebitic disease. Circulation 43 (Suppl. 1):147, 1971

Ludbrook J, Loughlin J. Regulation of the lower limb. Am Heart J 67:493, 1964

Ludbrook J. The musculovenous pumps of the lower limb. Am Heart J 71:635, 1966

Nicolaides AN, Fernandes e Fernandes J, Zimmerman H. Doppler ultrasound in the investigation of venous insufficiency. Investigation of Vascular Disorders, Churchill-Livingstone, New York, p. 478, 1981

Nicolaides AN, Zukowski A, Lewis P, Kyprianou P, Malouf M. The value of ambulatory venous pressure measurements. In: Bergan JJ, Yao JST (Eds). Surgery of the veins. Grune and Stratton Inc, Orlando, p. 111, 1985

Nicolaides AN, Miles C. Photoplethysmography in the assessment of venous insufficiency. J Vasc Surg 5:405, 1987

Palma EC, Esperon R. Vein transplants and grafts in the surgical treatment of the postphlebitic syndrome. J Cardiovasc Surg 1:94, 1960

Raju S. New approaches to the diagnosis and treatment of venous obstruction. J Vasc Surg 4:42, 1986

Strandness DE, Sumner DS. Hemodynamics for Surgeons. New York: Grune and Stratton Inc; 1976:404

Szendro G, Nicolaides AN, Zukowski AJ, Christopoulos D, Malouf M, Christodoulou C. Duplex scanning in the assessment of deep venous incompetence. J Vasc Surg 4:237, 1986

Taheri SA, Predergast DR, Lazar E, et al. Vein Valve Transplantation. Am J Surg 150:201, 1985

Widmer LK, Stahelin HB, Nissen C, Da Silva A, Venen-Arterien-Krankheiten, Koronare-Herzkreinheit bei Berufstatigen. Propektiv-Epidimiologische Untersuchung. Basler Studie 1959-1978, Verlag Hans Huber, Bern, p 1-11, 1978

CHAPTER 37

# Indications and efficacy of vena caval filters

Lazar J Greenfield

## Introduction

Mechanical protection against pulmonary thromboembolism began with ligation and plication techniques which required operative access under general anaesthesia. Technical progress over the past 20 years has made it possible to insert vena caval filter devices from peripheral veins, originally by operative access and most recently by percutaneous techniques. The indications for insertion of vena caval filters and the results of published follow-up experience will be reviewed.

## Indications for vena caval filters

The premise for insertion of a vena caval filter is that there has been objective documentation that the patient has developed deep vein thrombosis or has had pulmonary thromboembolism confirmed by pulmonary angiography or a high probability ventilation/perfusion lung scan. The risk of pulmonary embolism from venous thrombosis appears to be proportionally related to the site and size of the involved vein and whether or not there is attachment of the tail of the proximal thrombus. Five currently accepted indications for filter placement are described, along with special situations which may necessitate filter placement with or without concomitant anticoagulation.

### Contraindication to anticoagulation
This is the most common indication in virtually every series reported and has been responsible for 38% of cases in our own experience (Greenfield and Michna, 1988). Heparin is contraindicated in patients with preexisting bleeding disorders, severe hypertension,

active or recent neurologic, pulmonary, gastrointestinal or urologic bleeding, as well as after recent ophthalmic or neurological surgical procedures. Any recent surgical procedure or major trauma is considered to be a relative contraindication. Longterm anticoagulation with warfarin is contraindicated in patients in whom major renal or hepatic dysfunction may exaggerate its effect and in patients unwilling or unable to follow a strict dosing and monitoring protocol. In some series, old age or a generally debilitated medical condition have been considered contraindications to anticoagulation.

**Failure of anticoagulation**
Most failures of anticoagulation are a result of improper dosage, poor patient compliance or inadequate monitoring of coagulation status. In the case of warfarin therapy, other drugs or diet may influence the coagulation status of the patient, resulting in excessive or inadequate anticoagulation. The determination of failure of anticoagulation should be based on objective evidence of progressive thrombosis or recurrent pulmonary embolism. If anticoagulation has been suboptimal due to inadequate dosage, then a second trial may be warranted. If the problem is patient compliance, however, there is less likelihood of improving the situation and the patient becomes a candidate for filter placement. Failure of anticoagulation with recurrent embolism was the second most common indication for filter insertion in our experience, accounting for 27% of cases (Greenfield and Michna, 1988).

Some patients develop asymptomatic progressive thrombosis despite therapeutic anti-coagulation. This occurs without pulmonary embolism and it would be unsuspected without repetitive duplex scans (Krupski et al, 1990). The clinical significance of this finding remains unknown (Strandness, 1990) but in a high-risk patient it could become an indication for filter insertion based on anticoagulant failure.

**Complication of anticoagulation**
The development of a complication of anticoagulation such as thrombocytopenia or bleeding usually requires that the anticoagulant be discontinued. Once the anticoagulant is discontinued, the patient is unprotected against further propagation of thrombus and pulmonary embolism. This situation represents an indication for filter insertion provided that the original thrombus has not reached a stage of healing that has reduced its thrombogenic potential. In our experience, this was responsible for 17% of cases (Greenfield and Michna, 1988).

Although the period during which the patient is at risk of developing further thrombosis has not been determined, there appears to be less concern if the patient has completed at least one month of anticoagulant therapy.

**Prophylaxis**
Since all filters are inserted for prophylaxis against pulmonary embolism, this term has been subject to considerable variation in interpretation. Regardless of their anticoagulation status and prior to sustaining a pulmonary embolism, patients with severe cardiac or pulmonary disease who develop a thrombosis of a major vein were considered to have a prophylactic indication for filter placement. Further research indicated that the geometry of the proximal thrombus was predictive of recurrent embolism (Norris et al, 1985). The relative risk of recurrent embolism was ten times greater for patients who had a free-floating tail of at least 5 cm, despite adequate anticoagulation. Although this concept has been questioned, high risk patients have been successfully identified for maximal protection against recurrent embolism which includes filter placement and anticoagulation. Additional support for this

concept comes from Alexander et al (1986) who found that patients with residual venous thrombi in the lower extremities detected by noninvasive venous tests were at high risk for recurrent embolism despite adequate anticoagulation and from Radomski et al (1987) who found that the risk of embolism despite adequate anticoagulation was 27% in patients with free-floating inferior vena caval thrombosis as contrasted with 17% in the case of adherent thrombi ($p<0.05$). Therefore, although anticoagulation provides 90% protection against recurrent thromboembolism, it is most likely to prove inadequate where there is residual thrombus that is free-floating in a major vein. Given this situation in a high-risk patient who can least tolerate pulmonary embolism, a vena cava filter should be considered.

### Following massive pulmonary embolism
The patient who has sustained massive pulmonary embolism resulting in refractory hypotension despite inotropic support usually requires pulmonary embolectomy to survive. These patients are particularly likely to sustain recurrent embolism with a high fatality rate and are therefore candidates for filter placement at the time of embolectomy, whether performed by open technique on cardiopulmonary bypass or by catheter (Greenfield, 1987).

### Infrequent special circumstances
*Pulmonary hypertension*
Patients with pulmonary hypertension, whether primary or secondary to recurrent thromboembolism, usually die from an embolic event due to the precarious status of their right ventricular function. In the case of primary pulmonary hypertension, the development of right heart failure often is associated with venous thrombosis and the first pulmonary embolism becomes the last (Greenfield et al, 1979). Severe pulmonary hypertension is also found in the morbidly obese who represent another high risk group.

*Mechanical method failure*
No mechanical method or device is perfect and each fails to protect against recurrent embolism for a variety of reasons. First, the source may be outside of the protected drainage area, such as the superior vena caval tributaries or the right heart. Secondly, occlusive techniques such as ligation, occlusion by Hunter balloon, or total occlusion of any filter allow further thrombus to form in the cul-de-sac above the occlusion. Similarly, if a filter is placed on top of a thrombus, it may propagate through the filter, or an occasional trapped embolus in a thrombogenic patient may be associated with proximal propagation. Rarely, the entire device may detach from the vena cava and embolise, as has occurred with the Mobin-Uddin umbrella (Cimochowski et al, 1980) and more recently with the Birds Nest filter (Roehm et al, 1988), usually with a fatal outcome.

When recurrent embolism occurs in a patient after filter placement, it is essential to obtain a venacavogram to look for thrombus proximal to the filter. If only a small amount of thrombus is found, lytic therapy may be employed. If there is a long tail of thrombus, however, it is advisable to place a second filter above it in the suprarenal location (Stewart et al, 1982). This provides excellent protection and in a recent unpublished review of 69 filters placed suprarenally, none was found to be occluded. Suprarenal placement is usually reserved for thrombus that has extended to the level of the renal veins, thrombus propagating from the renal veins or above, and for pregnant patients or young women anticipating pregnancy to avoid compression of the filter by the gravid uterus.

*Septic thromboembolism*
Most episodes of septic thromboembolism can be managed by evacuation of the source of sepsis, antibiotics and anticoagulation. Rarely, septic pulmonary thromboembolism occurs

and becomes an indication for Greenfield filter placement. Since the filter is made of inert stainless steel or a titanium alloy, it does not perpetuate the infection and only the entrapped thrombus becomes infected. We have demonstrated both experimentally and clinically (Payton et al, 1983) that the infected thrombus within the Greenfield filter can be sterilised by a two week course of intravenous antibiotics. This is preferred to the earlier approach of caval ligation which allowed recurrent emboli through collaterals and was associated with the development of caval abscess in the experimental model.

*Subclavian vein thrombosis*
Deep vein thrombosis of the upper extremity is much less common than in the lower extremity, although the incidence is increasing with the use of indwelling catheters and chemotherapy. It was originally believed that the risk of pulmonary embolism was very low in this circumstance but it is now recognised that it can occur in 12-15% of patients and be lethal (Horratas et al, 1988; Monreal et al, 1991). Patients who have a contraindication to pharmacological management should be considered for filter placement, particularly if they are in a high risk category. We have demonstrated that the inverted Greenfield filter is safe and effective in the superior vena cava (Hoffman and Greenfield, 1986).

## Expanded indications for Greenfield filter insertion

The combination of ease of insertion, low morbidity, effectiveness of prevention of recurrent embolism and longterm patency exceeding 95% (Greenfield and Michna, 1988) has led some authors to advocate expanded indications for filter insertion. Vena caval filters have been used as primary therapy instead of anticoagulation for a variety of patients with venous thrombosis: older patients (Gomez et al, 1983), cancer patients (Cohen et al, 1991), those with chronic obstructive pulmonary disease (Pomper and Lutchman, 1991), heart transplant recipients and those over age 65 with venous thromboembolic disease (Fink and Jones, 1991). Other authors have supported liberalisation of the indications for prophylactic filter insertion in the elderly and in other patients at high risk of pulmonary embolism. These include total hip or knee joint replacement patients with a history of venous thrombosis (Golucke et al, 1988), paraplegic patients after spinal cord injury who have a 62% incidence of venous thrombosis and in whom anticoagulation is difficult to regulate (Jarrell et al, 1983), and trauma patients with combined pelvic or extremity fractures and abdominal or neurological injury whose risk of pulmonary embolism ranges from 4% to 22% (Rohrer et al, 1989). Despite the lack of randomised trials to support these recommendations, the safety and efficacy of the Greenfield filter provides support for such more liberalised indications.

## Efficacy of vena caval filters

The current standard for implantable vena caval devices is the stainless steel Greenfield filter based on longterm follow-up information which has accumulated since its introduction in 1972 (Fig. 37.1) (Greenfield and Michna, 1988). In these patients, the recurrent embolism rate is 4% and the longterm patency rate of the filter is 98% (Table 37.1). Similar results have been obtained in other follow-up series with longterm patency rates in excess of 95% (Cimochowski et al, 1980; Gomez et al, 1983). The patency rate of the Greenfield filter does not depend on prolonged anticoagulation and the termination of anticoagulant therapy should be dictated by the patient's underlying thrombotic disorder. Although it was

# INDICATIONS AND EFFICACY OF VENA CAVAL FILTERS

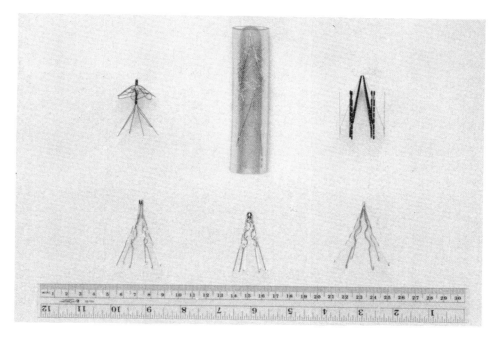

Fig.37.1 Lateral view of the currently available vena caval filters. Beginning in the upper left corner: The Nitinol filter, the Birds Nest filter in a plastic tube, the VenaTech filter and the lower row showing the standard stainless-steel Greenfield filter (centre), the modified hook titanium Greenfield filter (right) and the modified-hook, percutaneous stainless steel Greenfield filter (left) currently under clinical investigation

originally designed for operative insertion via the jugular or femoral vein, percutaneous insertion of the Greenfield filter using a dilator-sheath technique was reported in 1984 (Tadavarthy et al, 1984) from the jugular approach and subsequently from the femoral vein (Denny et al, 1985). However, the necessity for a large sheath (28 French) to accommodate the carrier and consequently for prolonged compression of the vein was associated with a 30-41% incidence of insertion site venous thrombosis (Glanz et al, 1987). In order to minimise this problem yet retain the advantages of the percutaneous technique, a titanium model of the Greenfield filter has been developed which allows the carrier system to be reduced to size 12 Fr (Fig. 37.1) (Greenfield and Savin, 1989). Alternative filter devices have also been developed which utilise smaller carrier systems for percutaneous introduction. The following devices are currently available in the United States for clinical use (Fig. 37.1 and Table 37.1):

## Birds Nest Filter

The birds nest filter was reported initially in 1984 and a larger series of 568 patients was reported in 1988 (Roehm et al, 1988). The device is constructed of 4 stainless steel wires, each of which is 25 cm long and 0.18 mm in diameter (Fig. 37.1). The wires are pre-shaped with nonmatching bends and each end of the wire is attached to a strut which ends in a hook for fixation to the wall of the vena cava. One strut is z-shaped so that a pusher wire can be screwed onto it. The original model was preloaded into an 8 Fr. teflon catheter, but in 1986 the struts were modified with the use of a stiff wire measuring 0.46 mm to improve fixation

**Table 37.1**
Results reported using different vena caval filters

| Filter | Greenfield SS | Greenfield Titanium | Vena Tech | Birds Nest | Simon Nitinol |
|---|---|---|---|---|---|
| *Description* | 6 stainless steel wires attached to a central hub configured as a cone | 6 titanium wires attached to a central hub configured as a cone | 6 side rails attached to 6 radiating diagonal struts with barbs on mural side rails | 2 rigid 0.46 mm struts with "stops" at 2.5 and 5 mm attached to 4 strands of stainless steel forming a maze | 2 sections: upper = dome of 7 wires lower = 6 limbs |
| *Size* | | | | | |
| Device | Length 41 mm Base 30mm | Length 47 mm Base 38 mm | Length 47 mm Base 30 mm | 40 or 75 cm of 0.18 mm wire | Dome diameter 28 mm Length 38 mm |
| Delivery system | Sheath 28 F Carrier 24 F | Sheath 14 F Carrier 12 F | Sheath 12 F Carrier 10 F | Sheath 12 F Carrier 11 F | Sheath 9 F Carrier 7 F |
| Material | 316 stainless steel | Beta-titanium | Stainless steel with cobalt | 304 stainless steel alloy | Nitinol (nickel, titanium alloy) |
| *Maximum Cava* | | | | | |
| Size | 28 mm | 28 mm | 28 mm | 40 mm | 28 mm |
| Insertion | Surgical or percutaneous | Surgical or percutaneous | Percutaneous | Percutaneous only | Percutaneous |
| MR | Yes | Yes | Not reported | Significant local artifact but no displacement | Yes |
| *Evaluation* | Registry (1988) | Clinical Trial (1991) | Clinical Trial (1990) | Clinical Trial (1988) | Clinical Trial (1990) |
| Duration | 12 years | 30 days | 1 year | 6 months | 6 months |
| Number | 469 | 97 (77 at follow-up) | 186 (123 at follow-up) | 568 (440 at 6 months) | 224 (102 at follow-up) |
| Recurrent PE | 4% | 3% | 2% | 2.7% (33-67% in subset with obj. follow-up) | 4% based upon those who had follow-up |
| Caval Patency | 98% | 100% | 92% | 97% | 81% |
| Filter Patency | 98% | Not reported | 63% without thrombus | 81% | Not reported |
| Insertion site DVT | 41% (percutaneous) | 8.7% | 23% | "Few" None obj. | 11% |
| Migration | 35% >3 mm | 11% >10 mm | 14% >1 mm | 9% with original model | 1.2% of those with follow-up |
| Penetration | Not reported | 1% | Not reported | Not reported | 0.6% of those with follow-up |
| Misplacement | 4% | 0% | Not reported | Not reported | Not reported |
| Incomplete opening | Not reported | 2% | 6% | Not reported | Not reported |
| Means of follow-up | PE, IVC Scan, X-ray, non-invasive vascular exam | PE, X-ray, CT (noninvasive vascular exam 2 sites | Objective data are variable by site (cavagram, duplex, CT, X-ray) | Phone interview, objective data random & available for 40/440 | Clinical, X-ray, lab |

| Problems | Misplacement: corrected with use of guide wire | Incomplete opening: corrected with guidewire manipulation  Leg assymetry: under investigation | Incomplete opening: improved with experience  Tilt: ?  Non-radio-opaque sheath: change patency rated based on life-table rates Largest # followed with any modality = 48 | Significant migration: changed hook design  MRI: High degree of artifact due to nature of material  Study design: lack of objective documentation | Failure of legs to release from delivery sheath: change procedure for delivery  Caudal drop of filter after release: related to lg cava  Tilt of filter dome: related to sm. cava  Occlusion rate: decreased during the study |

in an effort to prevent proximal migration which had occurred with the original design. The broader struts required an increase in diameter of the preloaded catheter to size 12 Fr. The insertion procedure consists of pushing the first set of hooks into the wall of the vena cava after which the wire is extruded in an effort to pack the loops of wires closely in the vena cava. Finally, the second pair of hooks is pushed into the vena cava wall. The pusher wire is rotated to free it and allow removal of the catheter. The intention is to pack the wires into approximately a 7 cm length of the vena cava in order to provide multiple barriers to the passage of emboli.

Follow-up information on the birds nest filter is limited, since only 37 of the 481 patients in whom the filter had been in place for six months or more had objective evaluation of their vena cavas by means of cavography or ultrasound (Table 37.1) (Roehm et al, 1988). Seven patients (19%) had caval occlusion. Three symptomatic patients had pulmonary angiograms for recurrent thromboembolism which was confirmed in one. In addition to problems with thrombosis, the birds nest filter has demonstrated migration proximally following what appeared to be secure placement. This has been seen both experimentally and clinically with reports of 5 events and one death. In the latter patient, the birds nest filter was found with a massive embolus in the pulmonary artery 10 days after placement. It was this experience that led to modification of the struts to prevent proximal migration. The University of Arkansas reported their experience with three cases of filter migration out of 32 placements (9%). The two cases identified within 24 hours were successfully retrieved percutaneously and the partially migrated filter was retracted to the infrahepatic segment of the inferior vena cava. The third case of migration was not detected for six months, at which time it was embedded in the right atrium and ventricle and could not be recovered. This experience was prior to the change in hook design. Additional clinical studies of the modified filter are in progress.

## Nitinol Filter
Nitinol is a nickel titanium alloy that can exist as a pliable straight wire when cooled but rapidly transforms into a previously imprinted rigid shape when warmed (Fig. 37.1). Although a filter made of this material was described in 1977, only limited clinical experience has been reported (Simm et al, 1989) with additional data available from a recent clinical trial (Table 37.1) (Dorfman, 1990). The filter design includes a 28 mm dome with 8 overlapping loops and below that the wire is shaped into six diverging legs with terminal

hooks to engage the vena caval wall in the configuration of a cone. The initial report on the clinical experience with this device indicated that it was inserted in 103 patients in 17 participating centres. Detailed information was only available on 44 patients. The insertion procedure utilises iced normal saline infused through a 9 Fr. delivery catheter. The filter wire is advanced rapidly with the feeder pump and then discharged from the storage tube. It is said to expand instantly into the appropriate shape and lock into place. In the multi-centre study, for the brief period of follow-up, there were three cases of recurrent pulmonary embolism and seven cases of confirmed vena caval occlusion with two additional suspected occlusions on the basis of clinical findings. Five of 18 patients studied by ultrasound showed thrombosis at the site of insertion. Of the 44 patients followed, 10 were studied at 3 months but only 4 completed the 6-month follow-up. Within this group, six occlusions of the vena cava were documented and two additional suspected for an occlusion rate of 18%. An additional five patients developed oedema with signs of thrombus within the filter. In one of the two patients with recurrent embolism, a proximal propagating thrombus above the filter was identified by venacavography. Migration of one filter was mentioned in an addendum to the report. The more recent update on the clinical experience shows that 224 patients have receive nitinol filters, 102 are being followed and 65 have completed 6 months follow-up. There were 4 patients who sustained recurrent embolism (4%) with one fatality and 20 documented caval occlusions (19%) to which the author added 3 deaths associated with massive caval thrombosis (Dorfman, 1990). The high rate of vena caval thrombosis in this series with very short follow-up suggests that the filter material and/or design may be thrombogenic.

**Venatech Filter**

In 1986, another cone shaped filter with added stabilising struts on each limb was introduced from France as the "LGM" filter (Fig 37.1) (Ricco et al, 1988). It is currently being marketed in the United States as the Venatech filter, designed for percutaneous introduction. The filter is made of Phynox, which is said to be similar to Elgiloy used in temporary cardiac pacing wires. It is a stamped, six-pronged device on which there are hooked stabilisers with sharp ends intended to centre and fix the device. It is inserted through a 12 Fr. single use catheter system, preferentially via the right internal jugular vein. A guidewire is used and the filter is ejected after it has been passed through the full length of the catheter. The initial reported experience was from France and consisted of 100 attempted insertions resulting in 98 filters discharged, 82 of which were positioned correctly (Table 37.1). Eight filters had a 15$ tilt or more, five opened incompletely and an additional three were both incompletely opened and tilted. All of the filters were implanted via the jugular route. Nine of the filters were observed to migrate distally and four in a cephaled direction for a 13% migration rate. The follow-up experience was limited to one year, at which time there were seven occlusions for a 92% patency rate. Recurrent pulmonary embolism was seen in two patients, both of whom had incompletely opened filters. At the end of one year, 13 filters were observed to have migrated, nine to the iliac vein and four to the renal veins. Twenty-nine patients had lower limb oedema in spite of the use of elastic support hose and seven of them had vena caval thrombosis. A subsequent report had a 13% rate of tilting or partial opening and a caudal migration rate of 13%. Caval occlusion was seen in 8% at follow-up and there was a 2.5% incidence of recurrent embolism (Maquin et al, 1989). The most recent report showed a 2% incidence of recurrent embolism, a 23% rate of insertion site venous thrombosis, a 63% filter patency without thrombus, a 14% migration rate and a 6% rate of incomplete opening (Murphy et al, 1991). There have been isolated reports of breakage of the stabiliser struts and it is surprising that the incidence of tilting has been so high in a device that was designed to prevent a tilt.

## Titanium Greenfield filter

Although it is possible to reduce the size of the carrier system to 19.5 Fr. without deforming the stainless steel filter, the optimal reduction in size occurs when a titanium alloy is used instead of stainless steel. The added flexibility of titanium, however, was presumably responsible for less secure fixation and distal slippage seen in a pilot series when the standard hook model was tested in patients (Greenfield et al, 1989). Several subsequent configurations of limb angulation and hook design were tested before the current recurved hook design with 80° angle was selected (Fig. 37.1), (Greenfield et al, 1990). The recurved portion of the hook should serve as a barrier to penetration beyond the axis of the limb and the 80° hook should limit both upward and downward ventors of force which might induce migration.

In a multicentre study of the modified hook titanium Greenfield filter (TGF-MH), percutaneous filter insertion using the sheath dilator was successful in 97% of cases (Table 37.1)(Greenfield et al, 1992). The primary route of insertion was the right femoral vein (120 cases, 70%). Other insertion sites included the right jugular vein in 35 cases (19%), the left femoral vein in 19 cases (10%), and the left jugular vein in 1 case (5%). Overall there were 148 femoral insertions (80%) and 36 jugular insertions (20%). Insertion site haematoma occurred in one patient. At the time of discharge of the filter, initial incomplete opening was seen in 4 cases (2%) but manipulation with a wire or catheter produced complete deployment of the filter limbs in each case. Leg asymmetry felt to be due to positioning of the carrier catheter against one side of the vena cava at the time of discharge was seen in 10 cases (5.4%). In several cases, the leg spacing corrected itself on follow-up radiograph or was corrected by catheter manipulation. Misplacement of a filter into a lumbar vein occurred in one case and there was penetration of the vena cava during placement in one case when the tip of the filter was pushed outside of the vena cava. No extravasation of contrast medium was noted and there were no long-term sequelae. Because of the misplacements, additional filters were inserted for a total of 184 filters in 181 patients with one patient receiving 3 filters and one patient receiving 2 filters. One filter was inserted in the superior vena cava (1%) and the remainder in the inferior vena cava: 175 infrarenal (95%) and 8 (4%) suprarenal. Angulation of the iliac vein was the most common reason for failure of insertion, but should be amenable to use of a stiffer sheath or an alternative insertion site. The left femoral vein route will always incur a relative disadvantage due to compression by the left common iliac artery. The sheath provides additional security against misplacement due to premature discharge since the filter would remain within the sheath. The apical end of the filter can perforate the wall of the vena cava, however, as demonstrated in one case. There should be particular caution when entering the vena cava from the left femoral approach to avoid this possibility.

Operative insertion of the TGF-MH was used in 2 patients and has previously been used at the time of laparotomy for direct placement of the carrier into the vena cava by palpation. When the carrier system is not centred in the vena cava but against the wall, the filter can be discharged into a narrower folded area of the cava. Because the recurved filter hooks are at a greater angle than the standard hook, there is immediate fixation with less ability to equalise the position of the legs, and some asymmetry of the limbs may result. This raises the possibility of impairment of filtration in the area of wider limb spread. There was no statistically significant association in this series between suspected or documented recurrent embolism and asymmetrical leg spacing. Incomplete opening also was seen in four instances and presumably reflects a transient binding of the limbs, since it was corrected in each case by further manipulation by guidewire or catheter. Aside from one haematoma, the morbidity at the insertion site was minimal. Limited routine follow-up duplex examination for thrombosis showed an incidence of insertion-site venous thrombosis of 8%.

A potentially important technical difference in the insertion technique is the absence of the guide wire which facilitates axial centering of the filter. Although there is some potential for tilting of the filter in its absence, concern that this has an adverse effect on filter effectiveness has not been substantiated. The only obvious deleterious effect of tilting occurs when the apex of the filter is displaced to the wall of the cava where a nidus of thrombus can form.

In a 30 day follow-up experience, the 3% incidence of recurrent pulmonary embolism was within the range observed previously. The fatal pulmonary embolism rate (1.9%) is always a concern, but it is never possible to cover all potential sources of embolism or to be sure of the cause of death without an autopsy. Change in filter position occurred in 11% of placements which was lower than the 27% incidence observed with the earlier titanium model ($p<0.035$). No adverse effects of this movement were noted and there was no significant proximal migration. Suspected caval penetration was observed in only two cases and confirmed by CT in one (0.8%). This is a distinct improvement over the previous model titanium filter where 9/30 (30%) penetrations were suspected and four confirmed (13%). Including all suspected or confirmed penetrations, the difference between filter series is statistically significant ($p<0.005$). There were no adverse effects from the suspected or confirmed penetrations and none would be expected unless the limbs entered the peritoneal cavity or an adjacent structure. There was no evidence of new bilateral oedema in any of the patients at early follow-up but long term assessment of caval patency must await further studies.

We have also developed a percutaneous model of the stainless steel Greenfield filter which can be inserted using a 12 Fr. carrier system (Fig. 37.1). This model is currently undergoing clinical trials and has the advantage of allowing the use of a guide wire at the time of filter positioning and release which should improve axial centering and minimise the remaining concerns about tilting and asymmetry.

As evidence accumulates that the indications for the Greenfield filter should be broadened (Maquin et al, 1989) it is appropriate that efforts continue to minimise cost and patient risk. A recent report has documented that the total cost of percutaneous insertion of the Greenfield filter is 58% of the cost of a surgical approach (Hye et al, 1990). Fortunately, anyone with experience using the stainless steel filter will find the percutaneous approach much easier as well as cost effective.

# References

Alexander JJ, Gewertz, BL, Lu Ct et al. New criteria for placement of a prophylactic vena cava filter. Surg Gynecol Obstet 163:405, 1986

Cimochowski GE, Evans RH, Zarins CK et al. Greenfield filter versus Mobin-Uddin umbrella. The continuing quest for the ideal method of vena caval interruption. J Thorac Cardiovasc Surg 79:358, 1980

Cohen JR, Tenenbaum N, Citron M. Greenfield filter as primary therapy for deep venous thrombosis and/or pulmonary embolism in patients with cancer. Surgery 109:12, 1991

Denny DF, Cronon JJ, Dorfman GS, Esplin C. Percutaneous Kimray-Greenfield filter placement by femoral vein puncture. AJR 145:827, 1985

Dorfman GS. Percutaneous inferior vena caval filters. Radiol 174:987, 1990

Fink JA, Jones BT. The Greenfield filter as the primary means of therapy in venous thromboembolic disease. Surg Gynaecol Obstet 172:253, 1991

Glanz S, Gordon DH, Kantor A. Percutaneous femoral insertion of the Greenfield vena cava filter: incidence of femoral vein thrombosis. AJR 149:1065, 1987

Golucke PJ, Garrett WV, Thompson JE et al. Interruption of the vena cava by means of the Greenfield filter: Expanding the indications. Surgery, 103:111, 1988

Gomez GA, Cutler BS, Wheeler HB. Transvenous interruption of the inferior vena cava. Surgery 93:612, 1983

Greenfield LJ. Intraluminal techniques for vena caval interruption and pulmonary embolectomy. World J Surg 2:45, 1987

Greenfield LJ, MIchna BA. Twelve year clinical experience with the Greenfield vena caval filter. Surgery 104:706, 1988

Greenfield LJ, Savin MA. Comparison of titanium and stainless steel Greenfield vena caval filters. Surgery 106:820, 1989

Greenfield LJ, Scher LA, Elkins RC. KMA-Greenfield[R] filter placement for chronic pulmonary hypertension. Ann Surg 189:560, 1979

Greenfield LJ, Cho KJ, Pais SO, Van Aman M. Preliminary clinical experience with the titanium Greenfield vena caval filter. Arch Surg 124:657, 1989

Greenfield LJ, Cho KJ, Tauscher JR. Evolution of hook design for fixation of the titanium Greenfield filter. J Vasc Surg 9:345, 1990

Greenfield LJ, Cho KJ, Proctor M, et al. Results of a multicenter study of the modified hook titanium Greenfield filter. J Vasc Surg 14:253, 1991

Hoffman MJ, Greenfield LJ. Central venous septic thrombosis managed by superior vena cava Greenfield filter and venous thrombectomy: A case report. J Vasc Surg 4:606, 1986

Horattas MC, Wright DJ, Fenton AH, et al. Changing concepts of deep venous thrombosis of the upper extremity: report of a series and review of the literature. Surg 103:561, 1988

Hye RJ, Mitchell AT, Dory CE, Freischlag J, Roberts AC. Analysis of the transition to percutaneous placement of Greenfield filters. Arch Surg 125:1550, 1990

Jarrell BE, Posuniak E, Roberts J et al. A new method of management using the Kim-Ray Greenfield filter for deep venous thrombosis and pulmonary embolism in spinal cord injury. Surg Gyecol Obstet 157:316, 1983

Krupski WC, Bass A, Dilley RB et al. Propagation of deep venous thrombosis identified by duplex ultrasound. J Vasc Surg 12:467, 1990

Maquin P, Fajadet P, Railhac N, Bloom E, et al. Two complementary vena cava filters. Radiol 173(p):476, 1989

McGowan TC, Ferris EJ, Keifsteck JE et al. Retrieval of dislodged birds nest inferior vena caval filters. J Intervent Radiol 3:179, 1988

Monreal M, LaFoz E, Ruiz J, et al. Upper-extremity deep venous thrombosis and pulmonary embolism. A prospective study. Chest 99:280, 1991

Murphy TP, Dorfman G, Yedlicka JW et al. LGM vena cava filter: objective evaluation of early results. J Vasc Interv Radiol 2:107, 1991

Norris CS, Greenfield LJ, Barnes RW. Free-floating iliofemoral thrombus: a risk of pulmonary embolism. Arch Surg 120:806, 1985

Pomper SR, Lutchman G. The role of intracaval filters in patients with COPD and DVT. Angiology 42:85, 1991

Payton JWR, Hylemon MB, Greenfield LJ et al. Comparison of Greenfield filter and vena caval ligation for experimental septic thromboembolism. Surgery 93:533, 1983

Radomski JS, Jarrell BE, Carabasi RA et al. Risk of pulmonary embolus with inferior vena cava thrombosis. Am Surg 53:97, 1987

Ricco JB, Crochet D, Sebilotte P, et al. Percutaneous transvenous caval interruption with the "LGM" filter: early results of a multicenter trial. Ann Vasc Surg 3:242, 1988

Roehm JOF Jr, Johnsrude IS, Barth MH, Gioanturco C. The birds nest inferior vena cava filter: progress report. Radiol 168:745, 1988

Rohrer MJ, Scheidler MG, Wheeler HB, Cutler BS. Extended indications for placement of an inferior vena caval filter. J Vasc Surg 10:44, 1989

Simm M, Athanasoulis CA, Kim D et al. Simon nitinol inferior vena cava filter: initial clinical experience. Radiol 172:99, 1989

Stewart JR, Payton JWR, Crute SL, Greenfield LJ. Clinical results of suprarenal placement of the Greenfield vena caval filter. Surgery 92:1, 1982

Strandness DE. Thrombus propagation and level of anticoagulation. J Vasc Surg 12:497, 1990

Tadavarthy SM, Castaneda-Zunigba W, Salamonowitz E et al. Kimray-Greenfield filter: percutaneous introduction. Radiol 151:525, 1984

Walker HSJ, Pennington DG. Inferior vena caval filters in heart transplant recipients with perioperative deep vein thrombosis. J Heart Transpl 9:579, 1990

CHAPTER 38

# Cost effectiveness of prevention

Graham A Colditz

## Introduction

Without prophylaxis, approximately one in four patients more than 40 years of age who undergo general surgery lasting more than one hour have a deep vein thrombosis (Multi-unit controlled trial, 1974; Int. Multicentre Trial, 1975; Gruber et al, 1977), and approximately one half of patients undergoing orthopaedic surgery without prophylaxis develop deep vein thrombosis (Oster et al, 1987). Thromboembolic disease has important longterm consequences in addition to acute morbidity and mortality. Persistent pulmonary circulatory abnormalities add to the social and economic costs of venous thromboembolism, as does venous insufficiency in the lower limbs following thrombotic occlusion of the deep venous system of the thigh.

Drummond specifies several advantages of an economic analysis of alternative approaches to health care problems (Drummond, 1980). Such an analysis embodies a systematic approach to a clinical situation allowing the analyst to test the implications of each decision or treatment option, and it recognises the scarcity of resources and the principle that decisions should depend upon benefits foregone as well as benefits obtained. In addition, an economic assessment offers a framework in which assumptions are made explicit and can be tested.

An analysis in which costs are related to a single common effect that differs in magnitude between the alternative treatment approaches is usually referred to as a cost-effectiveness analysis. In the context of thromboembolic disease, the results of such an

---

Acknowledgement: The assistance of Christine L Pappas in preparing this material is gratefully acknowledged

Some material in this chapter is reproduced from detailed reports of our cost-effectiveness studies reported in Oster, Tuden, Colditz, JAMA 257:203-208, 1987; and Oster, Tuden, Colditz, Am J Med 82:889-899, 1987 and from a chapter "Cost-effectiveness of Prophylaxis against Thromboembolism" by Colditz, appearing in Goldhaber SZ, editor, Prevention of Venous Thromboembolism, Marcel Dekker, NY, 1991

analysis may be expressed as costs per unit of outcome (death averted) or in terms of the outcome unit per cost (life-years gained per dollar spent). In economic terms, costs refer to sacrifices made of benefits gained when a resource is consumed in a treatment or a programme. Therefore, it is important to consider all resources, not just those that may be reflected in the market price (or hospital charges). For example, in a fee-for-service health care system, charges for diagnostic procedures may subsidise the operating costs for other areas of a hospital; this point is illustrated by the results of a survey of Boston area hospitals, in which the charges for a bilateral venogram varied by more than three-fold.

In this chapter we review the cost-effectiveness of approaches to prophylaxis against thromboembolism. First we compare primary prevention through heparin with secondary prevention through postoperative surveillance and treatment of detected thromboembolic disease. We then present a detailed analysis of the relative cost-effectiveness of the various approaches to primary prevention.

The following questions are addressed:
- Given the available data and alternative sets of assumptions about parameters for which data are lacking, to what extent is prophylaxis against thromboembolism among patients undergoing surgery a cost-effective use of scarce healthcare resources?
- To what extent does prophylaxis "pay for itself" in that its costs are recovered in expected savings from treatment of thromboembolic complications of surgery?
- To what extent do side effects of prophylaxis mitigate benefits?
- What groupings of patients should be given highest priority for prophylaxis?

## Primary prevention versus secondary prevention

Several investigators have addressed aspects of the cost-effectiveness of prevention of thromboembolic disease. Hull and colleagues (1981) evaluated the cost-effectiveness of primary prevention of fatal pulmonary embolism in patients undergoing abdominothoracic surgery. They compared *primary prevention* (subcutaneous heparin, intravenous dextran; intermittent pneumatic compression of legs) with *secondary prevention* (scanning with the fibrinogen uptake test (FUT) or treatment of clinically apparent thromboembolism). The probabilities of clinical events (i.e., degrees of effectiveness) were obtained from studies performed in Hamilton, Ontario, that included 1,042 patients treated in a six-year period. Over 70% of patients in the studies had operations that involved the gall bladder, stomach or large bowel. Costs for the analysis were based on third-party and operating expenses incurred in a single university teaching hospital in Ontario. Although the costs reported may not reflect the true resource costs incurred when thromboembolism is diagnosed and treated outside that institution, the relative ranking of cost-effectiveness is unlikely to change.

The cost of each prophylactic strategy included the diagnosis and treatment of venous thromboembolism and varied over an eightfold range. Subcutaneous administration of low dose heparin was the least costly strategy. Compared with this form of prophylaxis, intermittent pneumatic compression was 33% more expensive, the traditional approach (treating clinically detected thromboembolism) was 100% more expensive, intravenous dextran was 240% more expensive, and secondary prevention with the FUT was over eight times as expensive.

The efficacy of strategies varied widely. With the traditional approach, there were 80 deaths per 10,000 patients. These data are summarised in table 38.1. Given the equal

### Table 38.1
Cost effectiveness of alternative strategies for prevention of fatal pulmonary embolism in surgical patients, Ontario, Canada, 1982

| Strategy | Result with indicated approach | | Incremental comparison | | |
|---|---|---|---|---|---|
| | Cost*/10,000 patients | Deaths/10,000 patients | Cost | Lives saved | Cost/life saved |
| "No programme"* | 800,000 | 80 | — | — | — |
| Intravenous dextran | 1,350,000 | 10 | 550,000 | 70 | 7,900 |
| Low dose subcutaneous heparin | 400,000 | 10 | -400,000 | 70 | <0 |
| Intermittent pneumatic compression of legs | 530,000 | NS | -270,000 | NS | — |
| Leg scanning with FUT | 3,500,000 | NS | 2,700,000 | NS | — |

Adapted from data in Hull et al, 1981. Costs in 1982 Canadian dollars
*Clinical surveillance only    FUT = Fibrinogen uptake test    NS = not specified

efficacy of the latter two approaches, subcutaneous heparin is preferred over dextran because of its much lower cost. Further, dextran prophylaxis carries a risk of anaphylactic reaction and fluid overload (Gallus et al, 1976; Chapter 17). Because of insufficient data on the prevention of pulmonary embolism by intermittent pneumatic compression of the legs and by leg scanning with the FUT, no conclusions were drawn regarding the efficacy of these modalities.

An incremental analysis of costs and consequences is an important component of a cost-effectiveness analysis (Drummond et al, 1987). The measurement of effectiveness associated with primary and secondary prophylaxis strategies is the number of deaths due to pulmonary embolism that are averted. The incremental data presented in table 38.1 show that compared to "no programme" (clinical surveillance only), intravenous dextran costs $7,900 per life saved (1982 Canadian dollars), while low dose subcutaneous heparin saves both dollars and lives and thus has a negative incremental cost.

On the basis of these analyses, we conclude that, among patients undergoing abdominothoracic surgery, primary prevention with low dose heparin given subcutaneously is more cost-effective than primary prevention with dextran given intravenously. Furthermore, both of the latter approaches are less costly than secondary prevention through the FUT leg scanning. Clinical surveillance alone is ineffective: failure to use more aggressive prophylaxis results in unnecessary loss of life.

In an elegant and simple analysis, Bergqvist and colleagues (1988) compared both low dose heparin prophylaxis (primary prevention) and selective treatment following diagnosis (secondary prevention) with no prophylaxis. The authors base estimates of the frequency of thromboembolism on a literature review and obtain costs for diagnosis and treatment of thromboembolism from records for 28 patients hospitalised with thromboembolism, pulmonary embolism, and/or haemorrhagic complications at Malmo General Hospital, Sweden. Treatment costs (in 1990 US Dollars) are as follows: $1,875 for distal deep vein thrombosis; $3,482 for proximal thrombosis; $3,562 for pulmonary embolism; and $1,063 for haemorrhagic complications. Prophylaxis with low dose heparin costs $53.56. These

**Table 38.2**
Expected clinical and economic outcomes with and without prophylaxis at different initial frequencies of thromboembolism, based on a hypothetical population of 10,000 patients

| Initial frequency of thrombo- embolism | No prophylaxis Clinical outcome (n/10,000) ||||Heparin prophylaxis Clinical outcome (n/10,000) ||||
|---|---|---|---|---|---|---|---|---|
| | Thrombo- embolism | Fatal pulmonary embolism | Haemo- rrhage | Cost/ patient | Thrombo- embolism | Fatal pulmonary embolism | Haemo- rrhage | Cost/ Patient |
| 0.000 | 0 | 0 | 0 | 0 | 0 | 0 | 900 | 149 |
| 0.050 | 500 | 43 | 50 | 133 | 150 | 13 | 900 | 188 |
| 0.115 | 1,150 | 99 | 130 | 303 | 350 | 30 | 910 | 241 |
| 0.150 | 1,500 | 129 | 160 | 395 | 450 | 39 | 910 | 266 |
| 0.250 | 2,500 | 215 | 270 | 658 | 750 | 64 | 920 | 345 |
| 0.500 | 5,000 | 429 | 550 | 1,316 | 1,500 | 129 | 930 | 538 |

Adapted from data reported by Bergqvist et al, 1988. Costs approximate 1990 U.S. Dollars

costs are considerably lower than costs estimated for U.S. hospitals in 1984 (by about one third).

Bergqvist and associates assume that low dose heparin reduces the frequency of thromboembolism to only 30% of that among observed patients who get no prophylaxis. This assumption exceeds the estimates of efficacy obtained in a simple meta-analysis of clinical trials that included patients undergoing general surgery (Colditz et al, 1986). Colditz and colleagues estimated that the rate of thromboembolism is 27.0% among general surgical patients (29 trials) and 9.6% among patients receiving heparin prophylaxis (30 trials). These figures represent a reduction of 35.6% of the rate without prophylaxis or, in absolute terms, a reduction of 17.4 thromboembolic events per 100 patients receiving heparin.

In the case of major orthopaedic surgery, Oster et al (1987) combined data from multiple randomised studies and estimated a rate of thromboembolism of 53.1% for patients receiving no prophylaxis (16 trials) and a rate of 32.5% for patients receiving heparin (12 trials). Thus, heparin was considerably less efficacious among this high-risk group, reducing the rate of thromboembolism to only 62.4% of the rate observed without prophylaxis. Again, in absolute terms, heparin prophylaxis averted 20.6 (53.1 minus 32.5) thromboembolic events per 100 patients — a result very similar to the absolute reduction noted for lower-risk patients.

Thus the assumption of a constant relative reduction in thromboembolic events with prophylaxis across increasing levels of initial thromboembolic risk is not supported. However, since Bergqvist et al (1988) do report a sensitivity analysis in which they vary the efficacy of prophylaxis, we can see how this assumption influences their results. This sensitivity analysis is discussed in detail below.

With their baseline assumptions, Bergqvist and colleagues (1988) show that secondary prevention with routine surveillance fibrinogen scanning is more costly than either no prophylaxis or primary prevention. These authors also note that when the frequency of thromboembolism is high prophylaxis is followed by fewer deaths than no prophylaxis. At lower frequencies of thromboembolism, prophylaxis reduces the number of thromboembolic events, but this reduction is counterbalanced by haemorrhagic complications. In table

**Table 38.3**
Incremental comparison of heparin prophylaxis in place of no prophylaxis at different levels of initial frequency of thromboembolism

| Initial frequency | Additional lives saved/10,000 patients | Incremental cost/10,000 patients | Cost/additional life saved |
| --- | --- | --- | --- |
| 0.000 | 0 | +1,487,000 | — |
| 0.050 | 30 | +543,000 | +18,100 |
| 0.115 | 69 | -625,000 | -9,058 |
| 0.150 | 90 | -1,298,000 | -14,422 |
| 0.250 | 151 | -3,139,000 | -20,788 |
| 0.500 | 300 | -7,788,000 | -25,960 |

Adapted from data reported by Bergqvist et al, 1988. Costs approximate 1990 U.S. Dollars

38.2 the probability of thromboembolism, mortality from pulmonary embolism, and cost per patient are set forth for no prophylaxis and for prophylaxis with low-dose heparin.

Rather than absolute cost per patient, the incremental cost per additional life saved is a better measure of the cost-effectiveness of prophylaxis. In table 38.3 we present data calculated from the model used by Bergqvist and colleagues (1988) to estimate the incremental cost of adding heparin prophylaxis at each initial frequency of thromboembolism.

As seen in table 38.3, when the baseline frequency of thromboembolism is zero, the addition of heparin prophylaxis adds $1.49 million to the cost of care for 10,000 patients, and saves no lives. At an initial frequency of thromboembolism of 0.05, the addition of heparin prophylaxis saves 30 lives/10,000 patients at an incremental cost of $550,000 or $18,333 per death averted. At a frequency of thromboembolism equal to or greater than 0.115, heparin prophylaxis saves lives and saves dollars (hence the minus sign for expenditure per life saved).

As mentioned earlier, the figure for efficacy of prophylaxis used in this model may be an overestimate. The sensitivity analysis reported by Bergqvist and colleagues (1988) allows us to recalculate the data in table 38.2 for the number of fatal pulmonary emboli and then to recalculate the incremental cost-effectiveness of adding heparin prophylaxis. Focussing on initial frequencies of 0.250 and 0.500 and allowing prophylaxis to reduce the number of thromboembolism to 50% of the rate without prophylaxis, the number of fatal pulmonary emboli increases to 107 and 214, respectively, and the cost increases slightly to $464 and $782 per patient, respectively. In this sensitivity analysis, the incremental cost per life saved remains negative, indicating that prophylaxis saves lives and dollars.

In summary, this sensitivity analysis shows that prophylaxis with heparin saves both lives and dollars. This relative saving with prophylaxis is due, in large part, to the higher cost of treating thromboembolic events than of prophylaxis.

The study by Bergqvist and colleagues, like other studies discussed in this chapter, does not include costs of the post-thrombotic syndrome. Clearly, inclusion of these costs would render prophylaxis an even more cost-effective alternative. These authors do, however, include costs for complications of prophylaxis. At extremely low levels of thromboembolism (5/100 patients without prophylaxis), these haemorrhagic complications outweigh the benefits of prophylaxis.

**Table 38.4**
Methods of prophylaxis considered for prevention of thromboembolic disease among patients undergoing general or orthopaedic surgery

| Prophylaxis | Type of surgery | |
| --- | --- | --- |
| | General Surgery | Orthopaedic Surgery |
| Low dose subcutaneous heparin | X | X |
| Intermittent pneumatic compression | X | X |
| Graduated compression stockings | X | X |
| Heparin plus dihydroergotamine | X | X |
| Heparin plus stockings | X | X |
| Intermittent pneumatic compression plus stockings | X | |
| Warfarin | | X |

Among orthopaedic patients undergoing total hip replacement, Paiement and colleagues (1987) have evaluated primary prevention with warfarin as well as two approaches to secondary prevention: clinical surveillance and routine venography on day 10. Using charge data from Massachusetts General Hospital, these authors show that routine venography prevents the majority of fatal pulmonary emboli that occur with clinical surveillance alone, with a cost of approximately $50,000 per death averted (1987 U.S. Dollars). However, like Bergqvist et al (1988), these authors demonstrate that primary prevention (with warfarin or external compression) averts fatal pulmonary emboli and *saves* dollars (approximately $260 per patient) among orthopaedic patients. Paiement and associates (1987) also show that adding venographic surveillance to strategies of primary prevention will save additional lives but at considerable incremental cost.

On the basis of this review of studies comparing primary with secondary prevention, we conclude that primary prevention is more cost-effective for patients undergoing abdominothoracic surgery or major orthopaedic surgery. Further, among high risk patients, primary prevention saves both lives and dollars.

## Comparison of approaches to primary prevention

An early study by Salzman and Davies (1980) examined the cost-effectiveness of prophylaxis against deep vein thrombosis among patients undergoing general or orthopaedic surgery. In some of the trials, these authors used to assess the effectiveness of prophylaxis, patients were not randomly assigned to treatment groups. Moreover, several methods of prophylaxis were not considered, presumably because of insufficient clinical data at the time. Finally, cost estimates were based on charges at a single urban teaching hospital in New England and may not be representative of the actual resource costs of prophylaxis, diagnosis and treatment, either at the institution from which these charges were drawn or at other institutions.

Because a range of prophylactic methods is available to clinicians, we examined the cost-effectiveness of several methods — first, for patients undergoing abdominothoracic surgery (Oster et al, 1987) and second, for those undergoing major orthopaedic surgery (Oster et al, 1987). The methods of prophylaxis that we considered are set out in table 38.4. We did not examine strategies that involve the screening and early treatment of subclinical

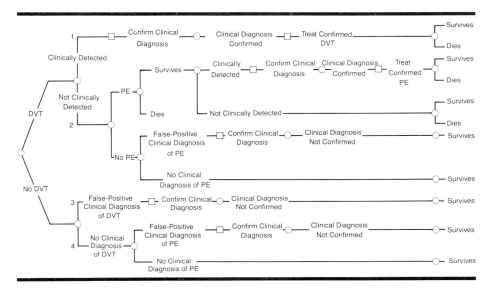

Fig. 38.1 Decision tree for the management of venous thromboembolism. DVT = deep vein thrombosis; PE pulmonary embolism

thrombi because, as has already been discussed, these approaches, while effective, are more costly than primary prophylaxis. Neither did we consider dextran 40 for orthopaedic surgery because it has a significant rate of complications and can induce hypersensitivity reactions that may be life-threatening. Furthermore, as discussed earlier in this chapter, Hull and colleagues (1981) have shown that heparin is more cost-effective than dextran.

We incorporated several important factors into this analysis. First, using meta-analysis we combined results from published reports of randomised trials to obtain our measure of efficacy for each method of prophylaxis. Thus, we used an estimate of efficacy that most closely represents the experience in a wide range of institutions, although efficacy may vary further when applied outside the setting of a clinical trial. Second, we based our cost estimates on measures of actual resource utilisation; other studies have used hospital charge data, which may not be representative of true resource use, either at that institution or elsewhere.

## Methods
### General model
To evaluate the cost effectiveness of prophylaxis against venous thrombosis, we set forth a general model in the form of a decision tree of the possible outcomes of care and the clinical management of venous thromboembolism.

At the beginning of the tree, the choice is that of an approach to prophylaxis. Subsequent clinical events are depicted in figure 38.1. Some patients develop venous thrombosis, which may be either clinically apparent or silent and thus may be either diagnosed or not. Other patients have an incorrect clinical diagnosis of venous thrombosis, and still others neither have venous thrombosis nor receive a clinical diagnosis of venous thrombosis.

**Table 38.5**
Minimal regimens of prophylaxis for inclusion of reports of clinical trials

| Method of prophylaxis | Preoperative administration | Postoperative administration |
|---|---|---|
| Warfarin sodium | Loading dose of 15 mg | Adjusted to maintain prothrombin time at 10-30% of normal |
| Heparin sodium | 2,500 IU | 5,000 IU every 12 hrs for 5 days |
| Intermittent pneumatic compression | Bilaterally applied prior to anaesthesia and continued for 16 hrs | — |
| Graduated compression stockings | Bilateral stockings applied | Stockings worn continuously until ambulation or discharge |
| Heparin and dihydroergotamine mesylate | Heparin sodium 2,500 IU, and dihydroergotamine mesylate 0.5 mg | Heparin sodium 2,500 IU, and dihydroergotamine mesylate 0.5 mg every 12 hrs for 5 days |
| Heparin and stockings | Heparin sodium 2,500 IU, plus bilateral stockings applied | Heparin sodium 5,000 IU every 12 hours for 5 days, plus bilateral stockings worn continuously until ambulation or discharge |

Reprinted with permission: Oster, Tuden, Colditz; JAMA 257: 203-208, 1987. Copyright, 1987, American Medical Association

*Likelihood of deep vein thrombosis*
We determined probabilities for all of the clinical events in our model on the basis of a review of the published literature. For this review we used a computerised literature search (Medline) to identify all English-language reports of trials of thromboembolic prophylaxis published between January 1976 and June 1984; we supplemented our search with a review of citations from the retrieved articles. We then performed a meta-analysis to calculate the expected rate of venous thrombosis for patients receiving each type of prophylaxis as well as for those receiving no prophylaxis.

Of trials identified, we used only those that met the following criteria: (1) either inclusion only of those patients undergoing abdominothoracic, gynaecologic or prostatic surgery, or — for orthopaedic surgery — inclusion only of those patients undergoing routine hip replacement, surgery for neck of femur fractures, or total knee replacement; (2) use of a randomised, controlled design; (3) use of FUT or venography to detect venous thrombosis; (4) adherence to a minimal regimen of prophylaxis.

For general surgery the minimal prophylactic regimens for trial inclusion were as follows: *low dose subcutaneous heparin*, 2,500 IU administered before operation and 5,000 IU administered every 12 hours for five days after operation; *intermittent pneumatic compression*, bilateral, applied prior to induction of anaesthesia and continued for 16 hours; *graduated compression stockings*, bilateral, applied before operation and worn continuously after operation until ambulation or discharge; *heparin plus dihydroergotamine*, 2,500 IU of heparin and 0.5 mg of dihydroergotamine administered every 12 hours for five days after operation; *low dose heparin plus stockings*, heparin and stockings as just described; and *intermittent pneumatic compression plus stockings*, intermittent pneumatic compression as just described, with stockings applied upon removal of intermittent pneumatic compression and worn continuously until ambulation or discharge. For orthopaedic surgery, we also considered *warfarin therapy*. These criteria are summarised in table 38.5.

We also excluded studies comprising only patients undergoing surgery for malignancy. We then determined a mean rate of venous thrombosis for each method of prophylaxis by combining the rates of venous thrombosis from the comparable arms of all eligible trials, weighting the rate from each trial according to its reported precision. Full details of the individual studies used to estimate rates for patients undergoing general surgery and of the methods of analysis employed have been reported by Colditz, Tuden and Oster (1986). The mean age of the patients in these trials was 58 years.

*Costs of prophylaxis, diagnosis and treatment*

To estimate costs for prophylaxis, diagnosis and treatment of venous thromboembolism, we defined protocols for patient care that were established on the basis of a review of recent clinical literature and practices in the Boston area. Using reports from the US Department of Labour, we then determined the cost (in 1984 dollars) of each of these protocols, adjusting price data when necessary for temporal changes in the cost of medical care. In this chapter, these cost estimates are updated through 1990; the medical component of the consumer price index has been used to adjust for increases since 1984 (Hyattsville, 1990). Our cost estimates are intended to reflect full resource utilisation and therefore do not necessarily equal the expenses that would actually be incurred by any particular patient, provider, or third-party payer.

For general surgery, additional days of hospitalisation for the treatment of venous thrombosis (and pulmonary embolism) were estimated according to the average length of stay between patients who had received a secondary diagnosis of venous thrombosis (and pulmonary embolism) after undergoing cholecystectomy and those who had not (Commission of Professional and Hospital Activities, 1983). For orthopaedic surgery, additional days of hospitalisation for treatment of deep vein thrombosis (and pulmonary embolism) were estimated for patients undergoing major joint procedures (diagnosis-related group 209) by the difference in average length of stay between those who receive secondary diagnosis of deep vein thrombosis (pulmonary embolism) and those with no reported diagnosis of deep vein thrombosis (pulmonary embolism). The costs of inpatient laboratory tests and diagnostic procedures, as well as general ward and coronary care unit bed charges, were estimated on the basis of bed-day-weighted average charges from all Maryland hospitals (Maryland Health Services Cost Review Commission, 1984) with more than 250 beds; these charges are established by state rate-setting authorities at a level intended to reflect average cost. Fees for supervision and interpretation of diagnostic procedures were obtained from physicians affiliated with the Maryland hospitals from which charge data were collected. Fees for inpatient and office visits were derived from a national follow-up survey of physicians (Kirchner, 1982). Drug costs for both inpatient and follow-up care were estimated on the basis of average wholesale prices (Annual Pharmacists' Reference, 1984), and were adjusted upward by 60% to reflect resource use associated with ordering, inventorying, and dispensing these agents. The costs of stockings and intermittent pneumatic compression sleeves were estimated on the basis of market-share-weighted average wholesale prices and also were adjusted upward by 60%.

*Costs of prophylaxis*

Cost estimates for each of the prophylactic methods were based on seven-day usage and did not include nursing time. These estimates are summarised in table 38.6. The cost of heparin prophylaxis was based on 5,000 IU administered twice a day; that of heparin plus dihydroergotamine was based on the formulation for combined administration of these

**Table 38.6**
Average per-patient cost of prophylaxis against thromboembolic disease

| Method of prophylaxis | Cost |
| --- | --- |
| Heparin | 138.41 |
| Intermittent pneumatic compression | 110.07 |
| Graduated compression stocking | 31.18 |
| Heparin plus dihydroergotamine | 172.85 |
| Heparin plus stockings | 169.66 |
| Intermittent pneumatic compression plus stockings | 142.25 |
| Warfarin | 88.24 |

Costs per patient are given in 1990 U.S. dollars

agents (5,000 IU and 0.5 mg, respectively), also twice a day. Patients receiving either type of prophylaxis also were assigned the costs of a baseline blood cell count, three platelet counts, urinalysis, and determination of partial thromboplastin time. Costs for stockings were based on the assumed use of two pairs of thigh-length stockings. The costs of intermittent pneumatic compression were based on (1) an average of the price of thigh-length and knee-length sleeves; (2) one hour of technician time; and (3) a pro rata share of annual compressor maintenance and depreciation, assuming 52 uses per year and a useful life of five years. The costs of heparin plus stockings and of intermittent pneumatic compression plus stockings were based on the costs of the individual prophylaxes.

*Costs of confirming a clinical diagnosis of venous thrombosis*
We assumed that bilateral venography, which we estimated to cost $543.40 (test and interpretation), would be used to confirm a clinical diagnosis of venous thrombosis.

*Cost of treating confirmed venous thrombosis*
Venous thrombosis lengthens the stay of patients undergoing general surgery by seven days (Commission of Professional and Hospital Activities). We assumed that these patients would receive intravenous heparin (1,000 IU hourly) (Goldhaber, 1985) and would require one additional physician visit on each of the added days of hospitalisation. To the costs for these services we added the cost of eight determinations of partial thromboplastin time and two complete blood cell and platelet counts. Follow-up care was assumed to consist of 7.5 mg of warfarin daily, monthly office visits, and a total of eight prothrombin time determinations over a four-month period. The total cost of treatment for confirmed venous thrombosis was estimated to be $3255.78 comprised of $2,972.14 for inpatient care and $283.64 for follow-up care.

*Cost of confirming a clinical diagnosis of pulmonary embolism*
We assumed that chest roentgenography and ventilation-perfusion lung scanning would be used to confirm a clinical diagnosis of pulmonary embolism. We also assumed that 10% of these patients would have neither high-probability nor low-probability results and would therefore undergo selective pulmonary angiography. The average cost of confirming a clinical diagnosis of pulmonary embolism was determined to be $605.28.

*Cost of treating confirmed pulmonary embolism*
Pulmonary embolism lengthens the hospital stay of patients undergoing general or orthopaedic surgery by an average of 11 days (Kirchner, 1982). We assumed that the first three of these days would be spent in a coronary care unit, with patients receiving two physician

**Table 38.7**

Outcomes of alternative strategies for preventing venous thromboembolism in general surgery, based on absolute rates of venous thrombosis

| Method of prophylaxis | Outcomes: Number/10,000 patients | | |
|---|---|---|---|
| | Deep vein thrombosis | Pulmonary embolism | Deaths |
| None | 324 | 42 | 48 |
| IPC | 211 | 27 | 32 |
| Stockings | 133 | 17 | 20 |
| Heparin + DHE | 119 | 15 | 18 |
| Heparin | 115 | 15 | 17 |
| Heparin + stockings | 75 | 10 | 11 |
| IPC + stockings | 54 | 7 | 8 |

\* Confirmed and treated only    DHE = Dihydroergotamine
IPC = Intermittent pneumatic compression
Reprinted with permission : Oster, Tuden, Colditz; JAMA 257: 203-208, 1987. Copyright, 1987, American Medical Association

visits daily; cost estimates for the remaining eight days were based on general ward rates, with patients receiving one additional visit daily. Treatment was assumed to consist of seven days of continuous intravenous heparin (1,000 IU hourly). To this cost was added that of eight determinations of partial thromboplastin time, two complete blood cell counts, platelet counts, and prothrombin time determinations. Finally, half of all patients with confirmed pulmonary embolism were assumed to undergo ventilation-perfusion lung scanning prior to discharge. Follow-up care was assumed to consist of 7.5 mg of warfarin daily, monthly office visits, and 12 prothrombin time determinations over a six-month period. The total cost of treatment for confirmed pulmonary embolism was estimated to be $6,410.03 comprised of $5,984.55 for inpatient care and $425.48 for follow-up care.

### Results
*Cost-effectiveness of venous thrombosis prophylaxis among general surgery patients*
For each prophylactic strategy, estimates of the number of cases of venous thrombosis, the number of cases of pulmonary embolism, and the number of thromboembolic deaths per 10,000 general surgery patients are presented in table 38.7.

Our results indicate that among 10,000 general surgery patients receiving no prophylaxis, there will be 324 confirmed cases of deep vein thrombosis, 42 confirmed cases of pulmonary embolism, and 48 deaths. (Only those patients who are actually treated for venous thrombosis or pulmonary embolism are included in these respective counts; deaths as a result of undetected venous thrombosis and pulmonary embolism are not counted as cases of venous thrombosis or pulmonary embolism). The number of thromboembolic deaths is high primarily on account of deaths among patients with undetected pulmonary embolism. Recent advances in patient care may have substantially reduced the likelihood of such deaths over the past decade. With most methods of prophylaxis among general surgery patients, the incidence of thromboembolic events is at least halved, and the most effective strategies may reduce the incidence to about one-quarter of that for patients receiving no prophylaxis.

**Table 38.8**
Costs per patient of alternative strategies for preventing thromboembolism in general surgery

| Method of prophylaxis | Cost per patient ($) | | |
| --- | --- | --- | --- |
| | ophylaxis | Diagnosis and treatment | Total |
| None | — | 166.59 | 166.59 |
| IPC | 111.06 | 117.96 | 229.02 |
| Stockings | 31.14 | 84.06 | 115.20 |
| Heparin + DHE | 172.88 | 77.93 | 250.81 |
| Heparin | 138.52 | 76.39 | 214.91 |
| Heparin + stockings | 169.66 | 59.21 | 228.87 |
| IPC + stockings | 142.20 | 50.32 | 192.52 |

DHE = Dihydroergotamine   IPC = Intermittent pneumatic compression
Costs are given in 1990 US dollars. Adapted from Oster, Tuden, Colditz, 1987a

The costs of prophylaxis and of diagnosis and treatment of clinical venous thrombosis and pulmonary embolism are set forth in table 38.8. The sum of the two columns represents the expected total cost of care per patient. The expected cost of a no-prophylaxis strategy ($155.59 per patient) is lower than that of all other approaches except for stockings ($115.20 per patient). This approach reduces the cost by $43.55. The expected costs of other strategies range from $192.52 to $250.81 per patient.

Although our findings suggest that intermittent pneumatic compression is less effective at preventing thromboembolic events than is the use of stockings, this result is strongly influenced by the report from a single trial (Nicolaides et al, 1980); exclusion of the results of this study from the calculation of a thromboembolic rate for intermittent pneumatic compression results in an estimate of 8.0%. Stockings, heparin, and heparin plus dihydroergotamine are roughly equal in efficacy; there is a range of $135.61, however, in the expected cost per patient of these three methods of prophylaxis. Heparin plus stockings and intermittent pneumatic compression plus stockings are the most effective methods of those considered; their expected costs, however, are comparable to those of the other prophylactic methods (except stockings).

The incremental costs and benefits of these strategies of thromboembolic prophylaxis are presented in table 38.9. Graduated compression stockings are compared with the no-prophylaxis strategy since they represent the least costly method. All other methods substantially increase care costs and hence are compared with stockings. The number of additional lives saved is the difference between the number of deaths with a given strategy and the number that would occur with the comparison strategy. The incremental cost of each strategy is the difference between its expected total cost and the total cost of the comparison strategy. The cost per additional life saved for a given method of prophylaxis, which is a measure of cost-effectiveness is simply the ratio of incremental cost to the number of additional lives saved. Intermittent pneumatic compression is excluded from consideration here because it is costlier yet no more effective than stockings.

When the use of stockings is compared with a no prophylaxis strategy, there are 28 fewer deaths and the expected total costs of care decline by $34 per patient. Thromboembolic risk can be further reduced through the use of more effective prophylaxis; these

### Table 38.9
Incremental costs and additional lives saved with alternative strategies of prophylaxis among general surgery patients

|  | Additional lives saved per 10,000 patients | Incremental cost per 10,000 patients | Cost per additional life saved |
|---|---|---|---|
| **Strategies compared: Stockings to no prophylaxis** | | | |
| None | 0 | 0 | — |
| Stockings | 28 | -513,890 | -18,354 |
| **Strategies compared: All other methods to stockings** | | | |
| Stockings | 0 | 0 | — |
| Heparin and DHE | 2 | 1,356,056 | 678,028 |
| Heparin alone | 3 | 997,100 | 332,367 |
| Heparin and stockings | 9 | 1,136,694 | 126,929 |
| IPC and stockings | 12 | 773,136 | 64,428 |

DHE = Dihydroergotamine
IPC = Intermittent pneumatic compression
NOTE: Results for each method of prophylaxis based on mean rate of venous thrombosis for patients assigned to receive this method across all randomised, controlled trials
Adapted from Oster, Tuden, Colditz (1987b)

methods, however, increase care costs. The cost of additional thromboembolic protection varies widely, ranging from about $75 per patient for intermittent pneumatic compression plus stockings to $135 per patient for heparin plus dihydroergotamine. Variation in cost-effectiveness is even more marked, ranging from $64,428 per additional life saved (for intermittent pneumatic compression plus stockings) to $678,028 (for heparin plus dihydroergotamine).

*Cost-effectiveness of deep vein thrombosis prophylaxis among orthopaedic surgery patients*
The outcomes of alternative strategies of prophylaxis against deep vein thrombosis among patients undergoing orthopaedic surgery are given in table 38.10. Estimates of the numbers of deep vein thromboses, pulmonary embolisms, and deaths per 10,000 patients are presented for each strategy. Strategies are ranked in decreasing order of the expected incidence of thromboembolic events.

Our results indicate that among 10,000 orthopaedic patients, there will be 860 confirmed deep vein thromboses, 132 confirmed pulmonary embolisms, and 153 deaths when no prophylaxis is used. (Only those patients who are actually treated for deep vein thrombosis or pulmonary embolism are included in these respective counts; deaths as a result of undetected deep vein thrombosis and pulmonary embolism are not counted as deep vein thromboses or pulmonary embolisms). Averaged for all patients, the expected cost for the diagnosis and treatment of clinical deep vein thrombosis and pulmonary embolism among patients receiving no prophylaxis is $560.52 per patient.

The cost of prophylaxis, the expected cost per patient for the diagnosis and treatment of clinical deep vein thrombosis and pulmonary embolism, and the sum of these two costs — which is the expected total cost per patient — are set forth in table 38.11. The cost saving per patient represents the difference in expected total cost between patients receiving no prophylaxis and those receiving the prophylaxis indicated.

**Table 38.10**
Outcomes of alternative strategies for preventing venous thromboembolism in orthopaedic surgery, based on absolute rates of venous thrombosis

| Method of prophylaxis | Outcome (n/10,000 patients) | | |
|---|---|---|---|
| | Deep vein thrombosis[*] | Pulmonary embolism[*] | Death |
| None | 860 | 132 | 153 |
| Heparin | 526 | 81 | 93 |
| Heparin and stockings | 5143 | 79 | 91 |
| Stockings | 392 | 60 | 70 |
| Warfarin | 380 | 58 | 67 |
| Heparin and DHE | 201 | 31 | 36 |
| Intermittent pneumatic compression | 183 | 28 | 32 |

[*]Confirmed and treated only
Reprinted with permission: Oster, Tuden, Colditz; JAMA 257: 203-208, 1987a. Copyright, 1987, American Medical Association

With most methods of prophylaxis, the incidence of thromboembolic events is at least halved, and the most effective strategies may reduce this incidence to less than one-fourth of that for orthopaedic patients receiving no prophylaxis. In addition, the expected total cost per patient (including that of prophylaxis) for each of these strategies is substantially lower than for no prophylaxis, ranging from $291.94 to $530.76. Thus, in addition to saving between 60 and 121 lives per 10,000 patients undergoing orthopaedic surgery, prophylaxis reduces the average cost of care by between $29.76 and $278.57 per patient. Sensitivity analyses that varied the costs of prophylaxis and the costs of confirming and treating thromboembolic events did not alter these conclusions.

**Table 38.11**
Costs and estimated cost savings per patient for alternative strategies for preventing thromboembolism in orthopaedic surgery

| Method of prophylaxis | Costs per patient | | | |
|---|---|---|---|---|
| | Prophylaxis | Diagnosis and treatment | Total | Cost saving per patient |
| None | — | 560.52 | 560.52 | — |
| Heparin sodium | 138.48 | 368.35 | 506.82 | 53.69 |
| Heparin and stockings | 169.66 | 361.10 | 530.76 | 29.76 |
| Stockings | 31.18 | 291.27 | 322.45 | 238.08 |
| Warfarin | 88.24 | 284.52 | 372.76 | 187.76 |
| Heparin + DHE | 172.85 | 181.35 | 354.20 | 206.32 |
| IPC | 111.07 | 170.88 | 281.95 | 278.57 |

DHE = Dihydroergotamine   IPC = Intermittent pneumatic compression
Costs are given in 1990 US dollars. Adapted from Oster, Tuden, Colditz, 1987a

Several limitations of this study must be considered. First, we used a decision tree to simplify the complex process of clinical medical practice. In this analysis, we have not accounted for complications of prophylaxis, which would make the cost-effectiveness of pharmacologically based methods decline in comparison with that of physical prophylaxis. Second, we inferred the efficacy of thromboembolic prophylaxis in reducing the incidence of pulmonary embolism and related mortality, because few prophylaxis trials have used either of these rates as endpoints.

## Conclusions

From the available data relating prophylaxis to reduced mortality from pulmonary embolism, it is clear that prophylaxis with low dose heparin is cost-effective and superior to secondary prevention. Although data are lacking on the efficacy of intermittent pneumatic compression, graduated compression stockings, and heparin plus mechanical approaches to prophylaxis against pulmonary embolism and death, a decision tree provides a reassuring model and indicates that these methods are cost-effective. When used for patients who are undergoing orthopaedic surgery and are at high risk of thromboembolism, all forms of primary prophylaxis save dollars and avert deaths.

Among patients at very low risk of thromboembolism, data from the published studies suggest that haemorrhagic side effects may mitigate the benefits of low-dose heparin. However, Bergqvist and colleagues suggest that once the baseline risk among patients without prophylaxis rises above 8.5%, then the benefits outweigh the costs of treating these side effects. The more recent results from trials of low molecular weight heparin suggest that haemorrhagic complications of prophylaxis may be reduced to the rate observed when placebo is used (Turpie et al, 1986). If this level of efficacy and the low rate of side effects persist, then prophylaxis may be even more cost-effective as benefits may outweigh costs of treating side effects at even lower baseline risks of thromboembolism.

With regard to identifying subgroups of patients who will benefit most from prophylaxis, the studies reviewed in this chapter suggest that the benefit will be greatest among orthopaedic patients; in this subgroup prophylaxis both saves dollars and prevents deaths due to pulmonary embolism.

## References

Ann Arbor, Michigan: Commission of Professional and Hospital Activities (1983). Estimated frequency and average length of stay of select diagnoses in US short-term general hospital by DRG and age groups

Bergqvist D, Jendteg S, Lindgren B et al. The economics of general thromboembolic prophylaxis. World J Surg 12:349, 1988

Colditz, GA, Tuden, RL, Oster G. Rates of venous thrombosis after general surgery: combined results of randomised trials. Lancet II:143, 1986

Drummond MF. Principles of economic appraisal in health care. Oxford University Press, New York, 27, 1980

Drummond MF, Stoddart GL, Torrance GW. Methods for the Economic Evaluation of Health Care Programmes. Oxford University Press, New York, 74, 1987

Gallus AS, Hirsh J, O'Brien, SE et al. Prevention of venous thrombosis with small, subcutaneous doses of heparin. JAMA 235:1980, 1976

Goldhaber SZ. Prevention of venous thromboembolism. In: Goldhaber SZ ed. Pulmonary embolism and deep venous thrombosis. WB Saunders, Philadelphia, 135, 1985

Gruber UF, Duckert F, Fridrich R et al. Prevention of postoperative thromboemolism by dextran 40, low-dose heparin or xantinol nicotinate. Lancet I:207, 1877

Hull RD, Hirsh J, Sackett DL et al. Cost-effectiveness of clinical diagnosis, venography, and non-invasive testing in patients with symptomatic deep vein thrombosis. N Engl J Med 304:1561, 1981

International Multicare Trial. Prevention of fatal postoperative pulmonary embolism by low doses of heparin. Lancet II:45, 1975

Kirchner M. Fee increases: restraint takes over. Med Econ 58:218, 1982

Maryland Health Services Cost Review Commission, 1884. Current rate report: 11.30.84, Baltimore, Maryland.

Multi-unit controlled trial. Heparin versus dextran in the prevention of deep vein thrombosis. Lancet II:118, 1974

National Center for Health Statistics. Health, United States 1989. Hyattsville, Maryland,. Public Health Service, 231, 1900

Nicolaides AN, Fernandez JF, Pollock AV. Intermittent sequential pneumatic compression of the legs in the prevention of venous stasis and postoperative deep venous thrombosis. Surgery 87:69, 1980

Oster G, Tuden RL, Colditz GA. A cost-effectiveness analysis of prophylaxis against deep-vein thrombosis in major orthopedic surgery. JAMA 257:203, 1987a

Oster G, Tuden RL, Colditz GA. Prevention of venous thromboembolism after general surgery. Cost effectiveness analysis of alternative approaches to prophylaxis. Am J Med 82:889, 1987b

Paiement GP, Bell D, Wessinger SJ. New advances in the prevention, diagnosis, and cost effectiveness of venous thromboembolic disease in patients with total hip replacement. In: The Hip. Brand RA, ed. The CV Mosby Co.,St. Louis, 94, 1987

Redbook: Annual Pharmacists Reference. Medical Economics, Oradell, New Jersey, 1984

Salzman EW, Davies GC. Prophylaxis of venous thromboembolism: Analysis of cost-effectiveness. Ann Surg 191:207, 1980

Turpie, AG, Levine MN, Hirsh J et al. A randomized controlled trial of a low-molecular-weight heparin (enoxaparin) to prevent deep-vein thrombosis in patients undergoing elective hip surgery. N Eng J Med 315:925, 1986

CHAPTER 39

# Prevention of venous thromboembolism: key questions that need to be answered

Russell D Hull

## SECTION 1 - BACKGROUND

## Introduction
Pulmonary embolism remains a leading cause of death in hospital. In the absence of prophylaxis, the frequency of postoperative fatal embolism ranges from 0.1 to 0.8% in patients undergoing elective general surgery, from 0.3 to 1.7% in patients having elective hip surgery, and from 4 to 7% in patients undergoing emergency hip surgery. Most patients who die from pulmonary embolism succumb abruptly or within two hours of the acute event, before treatment can be initiated or take effect. Therefore, prevention is the key to reducing death and morbidity from venous thromboembolism. Effective and safe prophylaxis is now available for most patient groups.

## Risk factors and classification of risk
Multiple clinical risk factors for venous thromboembolism have been identified, including advanced age, previous venous thromboembolism, recent surgery or trauma, prolonged immobility or paralysis, malignant disease, obesity, varicose veins, oral contraceptive use and congestive heart failure. Certain surgical procedures, such as major orthopaedic surgery to the lower limbs or extensive pelvic or abdominal surgery for advanced malignant disease, are associated with a particularly high risk of postoperative venous thromboembolism.

In general, patients can be classified as being at low, moderate or high risk for developing venous thromboembolism as summarised in table 39.1.

**Table 39.1**
Risk categories in surgical patients

|  | Risk of venous thromboembolism (assessed by objective tests) | | |
|---|---|---|---|
| Risk category | Calf-vein thrombosis | Proximal-vein thrombosis | Fatal pulmonary embolism |
| *High risk*<br>General and urological surgery in patients over 40 years with recent history of DVT or PE<br>Extensive pelvic or abdominal surgery for malignant disease<br>Major orthopaedic surgery of lower limbs | 40-80% | 10-30% | 1-5% |
| *Moderate risk*<br>General surgery in patients over 40 years lasting 30 minutes or more and in patients below 40 years on oral contraceptives | 10-40% | 2-10% | 0.1-0.7% |
| *Low risk*<br>Uncomplicated surgery in patients under 40 years without additional risk factors<br>Minor surgery (i.e. less than 30 minutes) in patients over 40 years without additional risk factors | <10% | <1% | <0.01% |

# Approaches to prophylaxis

Two approaches can be taken to prevent fatal pulmonary embolism. These are: (a) primary prophylaxis, using either drugs or physical methods that are effective for preventing deep vein thrombosis and pulmonary embolism, and (b) secondary prevention by the early detection and treatment of subclinical venous thrombosis (before pulmonary embolism occurs) by screening postoperative patients with objective tests that are sensitive for venous thrombosis. Primary prophylaxis is preferred in most clinical circumstances. Secondary prevention by screening should never replace primary prophylaxis. It is reserved for patients in whom effective primary prophylaxis is either contraindicated or unavailable. Postoperative screening may also be used to supplement primary prophylaxis in very high risk patients, such as those who have suffered a recent episode of venous thrombosis and who require surgery.

The ideal primary prophylactic method should be effective, free of clinically important side effects, and be well accepted by patients, nurses and medical staff. It should also be easily administered, inexpensive, and require minimal monitoring. Multiple primary prophylactic approaches have been evaluated by randomised clinical trials and are effective for preventing venous thrombosis and pulmonary embolism. The recommended primary prophylactic approach depends on the patient's risk category (Table 39.1) and the type of surgery.

In North America low molecular weight heparin is under clinical evaluation and has just become available for clinical use. The potential routine use of low molecular weight heparin is specifically discussed under the heading "Key Questions to be Answered by Future Research". Based on adequate randomised clinical trials evaluating low dose heparin, graded pressure stockings, intermittent pneumatic compression, dextran and oral anticoagulant prophylaxis the following approaches can be recommended for routine use:

**Low Risk Patients:**
These patients should receive graduated compression stockings.

**Moderate Risk Patients:**
*General Abdominal or Thoracic Surgery:*
Low dose heparin (5,000 units every 8 or 12 hours) is effective (Collins et al, 1988; Chapters 12 and 23) and is the approach of choice in most patients. Intermittent pneumatic compression (Sabri et al, 1971; Chapter 20) is indicated in patients with a high risk of bleeding.
*Neurosurgery or Genitourinary Surgery:*
Intermittent pneumatic compression is the approach of choice (Skillmann et al, 1978; Coe et al, 1978; Turpie et al, 1979; Chapters 30 and 31).

**High Risk Patients**
*General Abdominal or Thoracic Surgery:*
Several approaches could be used. The optimal approach remains uncertain because the different approaches have not been directly compared in this high risk patient category. The recommended approaches include oral anticoagulants, low dose heparin using the 8 hourly regimen, intravenous dextran, or adjusted subcutaneous heparin. Any of these approaches could be combined with intermittent pneumatic compression. Primary prophylaxis could also be supplemented by postoperative screening to detect patients who break through prophylaxis.
*Elective Hip Replacement:*
Several approaches have been evaluated and are effective. Prophylaxis with oral anticoagulants adjusted to maintain the prothrombin time between 1.3 and 1.5 times control (using a conventional insensitive rabbit brain thromboplastin), corresponding to an INR of 2.0 to 3.0 is effective and is associated with a low risk of bleeding (Francis et al, 1983; Paiement et al, 1987; Chapters 18 and 25). It is indicated in patients with a high risk of bleeding. Other effective approaches include adjusted dose subcutaneous heparin (Leyvraz et al, 1983; Chapters 11 and 25), intravenous dextran, and intravenous dextran combined with intermittent pneumatic leg compression.
*Fractured Hip:*
Oral anticoagulant prophylaxis is the preferred approach. Intravenous dextran is effective but inconvenient and relatively expensive.
*Major Knee Surgery:*
Intermittent pneumatic compression is the preferred approach.

# SECTION II - KEY QUESTIONS TO BE ANSWERED BY FUTURE RESEARCH

Low molecular weight heparin has the advantage that, because of high bioavailability (90% or more) after subcutaneous injection and a long half life of certain preparations, it can be given subcutaneously once a day, and does not require laboratory monitoring. Thus, low

**Table 39.2**
A firm recommendation is made when the following criteria have been met

1. The clinical trial should be prospective, with a concurrent control group;
2. The patients should be randomly allocated to the alternative prophylactic approaches in order to avoid the potential for conscious or unconscious bias in selection of patients;
3. Ideally, the study should be double blind; if double blinding is not possible, the end-points should be interpreted by an independent observer without knowledge of the patient's treatment category;
4. Comparability of the treatment groups with respect to important prognostic variables should be demonstrated.
5. Properly defined end-points should be used for the evaluation of effectiveness and safety;
6. A sufficient number of patients should be studied to allow valid conclusions;
7. Appropriate statistical methods should be used to analyse the data.

molecular weight heparin has the potential to improve both the effectiveness of prophylaxis against venous thrombosis in surgical patients and to simplify its use.

Low molecular weight heparin is increasingly used in many countries in Europe. There is an extensive European clinical trials data base supporting both the relative efficacy and safety of low molecular weight heparin (Chapters 13-15, 23-31).

A recent meta-analysis of the findings of multiple randomised clinical trials evaluating low molecular weight heparin for prophylaxis against deep vein thrombosis suggests indeed that low molecular weight heparin is more effective than low-dose unfractionated heparin but with an increased risk of bleeding (Rosendaal et al, 1991; Chapter 15). A meta-analysis of 62 comparative studies to assess the efficacy and safety of LMWH. The results, for deep vein thrombosis (DVT), pulmonary embolism and major bleeding are expressed as the risk relative to the control group (RR, Mantel-Haenszal method) with 95% confidence intervals (CI 95%, test-based method). The studies were also scored on predefined methodological quality criteria.

All 62 studies, with a total of over 20,000 patients, were randomised studies, with a control treatment of placebo (n = 12), standard heparin (n = 44) or dextran/warfarin (n = 6). The indications for anticoagulation were general surgery (n = 35) orthopaedic surgery (n = 24) or stroke (n = 3).

As compared to placebo, LMWH proved effective in preventing deep vein thrombosis (RR = 0.4) and pulmonary embolism (RR = 0.3); the relative risk of major bleeding was 2.6.

Compared with standard heparin, prophylaxis with LMWH resulted in less deep vein thrombosis (RR = 0.8), CI 95%: 0.7-0.9), less pulmonary embolism (RR= 0.5, CI 95%: 0.3-0.8), less mortality (RR=0.7, CI 95%: 0.5-1.1). The relative risk for DVT was about equal in general and orthopaedic surgery, which implies a larger absolute reduction in the latter category. Analysis based on the quality criteria yielded a higher bleeding risk and a smaller protective effect in the studies that were of a higher methodological standard.

Based on this large body of data, we concluded that the LMWH have not fulfilled the expectations of a major improvement of the benefit-risk ratio in thrombosis prophylaxis (Rosendaal et al, 1991)

**Table 39.3**
Key parameters

---

1. Effectiveness compared with placebo or active approaches
2. Safety compared with placebo or active approaches
3. Patient, physician and nursing staff compliance
4. Ease of administration
5. Need for laboratory monitoring
6. Cost effectiveness

---

In forming a European consensus statement all data from adequately performed randomised trials should be considered. The criteria of defining an adequate randomised clinical trial are shown in table 39.2. For each prophylactic regimen considered, key parameters should be addressed (Table 39.3) (Hull and Raskob, 1986).

For many of the prophylactic approaches currently used in Europe much of the information necessary to form a consensus is available in the literature. For some, future clinical research will be directed at conducting formal clinical trials to address unanswered questions.

The key questions to be addressed are defined in more detail below. These key questions can be researched from the literature. If for a particular approach the answer to a key question remains unknown this should be addressed by future clinical trials.

### Relative effectiveness

How does the prophylactic approach compare with placebo or other active approaches for preventing venous thrombosis? Is it equivalent to, or more effective than the comparative approach?

Prophylactic approaches which have not yet been evaluated in Phase III studies (i.e., randomised clinical trials evaluating effectiveness and safety) will by necessity be compared with active prophylactic means. This is because it is now clearly unethical to use an inactive placebo which places the patients at an unacceptable risk of post-operative venous thromboembolism. It is important that the trials are large enough to evaluate both promixal deep vein thrombi as well as calf vein thrombi. This is because proximal vein thrombi are associated with a poor prognosis because of their propensity for embolising to the lungs massively or fatally. In contrast it is rare for calf deep vein thrombi to result in clinically evident pulmonary embolism.

### Relative safety

The major endpoint for safety in the evaluation of antithrombotic approaches is of course haemorrhagic complications. Their relative frequencies are best determined by well conducted double blind randomised trials.

Rare side effects may not be readily detected in randomised trials because of the necessity of studying extremely large populations. Thus, formal post-marketing surveys will be important (for example, dihydroergotamine preparations have been withdrawn because of untoward serious vasospastic side-effects).

### Compliance and ease of administration

To ensure widespread use the prophylactic approach should be well accepted by the patient, nursing staff and doctor caring for the patient. This is a function of both knowledge of an approach's effectiveness and safety, but also ease of administration and freedom from patient discomfort. In addition, simplicity of administration encourages both patient and nursing compliance.

### Need for laboratory monitoring

The necessity for laboratory monitoring of an antithrombotic approach is an inherent disadvantage. Laboratory monitoring increases the complexity of the approach. Because of the need to dose determination by laboratory monitoring there is the inherent risk of giving either too little or too much prophylaxis due to errors in processing. This latter problem is important given the universal need for prophylaxis in patients at risk.

### Cost-effectiveness analysis

Many hospitals lack organised strategy for preventing venous thromboembolism. There are several reasons. First, because death from pulmonary embolism is infrequent, a general surgeon may have to operate on a relatively large number of patients before losing one patient to pulmonary embolism and being reminded of this condition's lethality. Second, there have been doubts about the safety of antithrombotic drugs and the effectiveness of all forms of prophylaxis. Finally, at the institutional level there has been reluctance to add interventions whose cost effectiveness has not been adequately evaluated.

The extensive literature on the safety and efficacy of measures to prevent venous thromboembolism contrasts with the virtual absence of studies on the cost-effectiveness of commonly used prophylactic approaches (Bergqvist et al, 1990). Salzman et al (1980) reported a cost-effectiveness analysis of prophylaxis based on a literature review and Hull et al (1982) reported a cost-effectiveness analysis of low molecular weight heparin prophylaxis.

The results of our cost-effectiveness analysis of the traditional methods warrant three conclusions (Hull et al, 1990). First, the traditional approach to preventing fatal pulmonary embolism is ineffective, resulting in unnecessary loss of life, and is costly because of the large numbers of cases of venous thromboembolism, with their attendant diagnostic and treatment costs. Second, primary prevention through routine subcutaneous administration of low doses of heparin to high risk patients is highly effective and relatively inexpensive. Third, primary prevention with low dose heparin given subcutaneously is more cost-effective than primary prevention with dextran given intravenously, and both are less costly than secondary prevention with the fibrinogen uptake test (FUT).

Clinical surveillance is ineffective because half or more of the patients who die from pulmonary embolism do so without warning (the majority of postoperative venous thromboembolic events are silent); furthermore, most of the patients who die do so within two hours, before any treatment could take effect. Primary prophylaxis, however, provides the opportunity for preventing venous thrombosis, the precursor of pulmonary embolism, and secondary prevention with screening for subclinical venous thrombosis with the FUT provides the opportunity for treating silent thromboses early, before they can embolise.

An ideal prophylactic method should be effective, safe and easily administered, require minimal or no monitoring and be well accepted by patients, nurses and physicians. Furthermore, it should be cost-effective. None of the current methods fulfil all of these criteria but low dose subcutaneous heparin prophylaxis fulfils most of them. It is effective in high risk patients undergoing abdominothoracic surgery and does not cause clinically significant bleeding. Subcutaneous administration of heparin is relatively simple, does not require monitoring and is well accepted by patients. In the setting we studied, it is also less expensive than the traditional approach, although sensitivity analysis demonstrated that in certain circumstances the heparin approach may be more costly. The increased cost, however, has to be weighed against the ineffectiveness of the traditional approach.

Intermittent leg compression is a potentially attractive alternative because it is effective in preventing deep vein thrombosis, is free of any risk of bleeding and is relatively inexpensive. Its effectiveness in preventing fatal pulmonary embolism must be inferred, however, and for this reason its use should be confined to patients at high risk of bleeding (e.g., those with a familial bleeding tendency or spinal anaesthesia), in whom subcutaneous heparin prophylaxis is contraindicated.

Although intravenous dextran prophylaxis is effective for preventing fatal pulmonary embolism, it is expensive and carries a risk of anaphylactoid reaction and fluid overload. For these reasons it is not widely accepted in North America for preventing venous thromboembolism in general surgery patients.

FUT is the least effective of the active prophylactic approaches studied here and the most expensive, as it necessitates full dose anticoagulant treatment of large numbers of patients with subclinical venous thrombi. It should therefore be reserved for patients in whom primary prophylaxis is either contraindicated or unavailable.

Future research directed at evaluation of the cost-effectiveness of the newer modalities and in particular the low molecular weight heparins will be necessary before a firm consensus about their role can be reached.

**On the horizon**
Antithrombotic modalities directed against thrombin are currently being evaluated in Phase I and II trials (for example, hirudin, hirulog, monoclonal antibodies). The role of these agents will become clearer once Phase III trials evaluating their effectiveness and safety have been completed. These agents are exciting from the biological point of view because of their specificity and potency.

# References

Bergqvist D, Matzsh T, Jendteg S et al. The cost-effectiveness of prevention of post-operative thromboembolism. Acta Chir Scand Suppl 556:36, 1990

Coe NP, Collins REC, Klein LA et al. Prevention of deep-vein thrombosis in urological patients: a controlled randomized trial of low-dose heparin and external pneumatic compression boots. Surgery 83:230, 1978

Collins R, Scrimgeour A, Yusef S, Peto R. Reduction in fatal pulmonary embolism and venous thrombosis by perioperative administration of subcutaneous heparin. N Engl J Med 318:1162, 1988

Eriksson BI, Kalebo P, Anthymyr BA et al. Prevention of deep vein thrombosis and pulmonary embolism after total hip replacment. Comparison of low-molecular weight heparin and unfractionated heparin. J Bone Joint Surg 73:484, 1991

Francis CW, Marder VJ, Evarts CM. Yaukoubodi S. Two-step warfarin therapy: prevention of post-operative venous thrombosis without excessive bleeding. JAMA 249:374, 1983

Hull RD, Hirsh J, Sackett DL et al. Cost-effectiveness of primary and secondary prevention of fatal pulmonary embolism in high-risk surgical patients. Can Med Assoc J. 127:990, 1982

Hull RD, Raskob GE. Prophylaxis of venous thromboembolic disease following hip and knee surgery. J Bone Joint Surg 68:146, 1986

Hull R, Raskob G, Gent M et al. Effectiveness of intermittent pneumatic leg compression for preventing deep-vein thrombosis after total hip replacement. JAMA 263:2313, 1990

Levine MN, Hirsh J, Gent M et al. Prevention of deep vein thrombosis after elective hip surgery. A randomized trial comparing low molecular weight heparin with standard unfractionated heparin. Ann Intern Med 114:545, 1991

Leyvraz PF, Richard J, Bachmann F et al. Adjusted versus fixed-dose subcutaneous heparin in the prevention of deep-vein thrombosis after total hip replacement. N Eng J Med 309:954, 1983.

Paiement G, Wessinger SJ, Waltman WC, Harris WH. Low-dose warfarin versus external pneumatic compression for prophylaxis against venous thromboembolism following total hip replacement. J Arthroplasty 2:23, 1987

Rosendaal FR, Nurmohamed MI, Büller HR et al. Low molecular weight heparin in the prophylaxis of venous thrombosis: a meta-analysis. Thromb and Hemost 65:927, 1991

Sabri S, Roberts VC, Cotton LT. Prevention of early postoperative deep-vein thrombosis by intermittent compression of the leg during surgery. Br Med J 4:394, 1971

Salzman EW, Davies GC. Prophylaxis of venous thromboembolism. Analysis of cost effectiveness. Ann Surg 191:207, 1980

Skillman JJ, Collins RE, Coe NP et al. Prevention of deep-vein thrombosis in neurosurgical patients: a controlled, randomized trial of external pneumatic compression boots. Surgery 83:354, 1978

Turpie AG. Efficacy of a postoperative regimen of enoxaparin in deep vein thrombosis prophylaxis. Am J Surg 161:532, 1991

Turpie AG, Delmore T, Hirsh J et al. Prevention of venous thrombosis by intermittent sequential calf compression in patients with intracranial disease. Thromb Res 15:611, 1979

Turpie AG, Levine MN, Hirsh J et al. Double-blind randomized trial of Org 10172 low-molecular-weight heparinoid in the prevention of deep vein thrombosis in thrombotic stroke. Lancet 1:523, 1987

Turpie AG, Levine MN, Hirsh J et al. A randomized controlled trial of a low molecular weight heparin (Enoxaparin) to prevent deep vein thrombosis in patients undergoing elective hip surgery. N Engl J Med 315:925, 1987

# CHAPTER 40

# Anticoagulant therapy

Russell D Hull

## Introduction

The classic treatment for acute deep vein thrombosis is initial therapy with continuous intravenous heparin (Salzman et al, 1975; Glazier and Crowell, 1976; Mant et al, 1977; Wilson and Lampman 1979; Hull et al 1986) followed by long-term oral anticoagulant therapy (Coon et al, 1969; Hull et al, 1979; Hull, Delmore et al, 1982; Hull et al, 1982a). Improvements in the methods of clinical trials and the use of accurate objective tests to detect venous thromboembolism (Rabinov and Paulin, 1972; Wheeler et al, 1974; Hull et al, 1977; Hull et al, 1983; Dalen et al, 1971) have made it possible to perform a series of randomised trials (Salzman et al, 1975; Glazier and Crowell, 1976; Mant et al, 1977; Wilson and Lampman 1979; Hull et al, 1986; Hull et al, 1979; Hull et al, 1982; Hull et al, 1982a; Gallus et al 1986; Hull et al, 1990) to evaluate various treatments for venous thrombosis. The results of these trials have resolved many of the uncertainties that a clinician confronts in selecting an appropriate course of anticoagulant therapy. These trials have shown that the intensity of initial heparin treatment must be sufficient to prevent unacceptable rates of recurrent venous thromboembolism (Hull et al, 1986). Patients with proximal deep vein thrombosis who receive inadequate anticoagulant therapy have a risk of recurrent venous thromboembolism that approaches 50% (Hull et al, 1979). Most recently, trials have demonstrated that the duration of initial heparin therapy can be shortened from 10-14 days to approximately five days (Gallus et al, 1986; Hull et al, 1990). In an era of fiscal constraint, short-course heparin allows effective treatment without detracting from patient care (Gallus et al, 1986; Hull et al, 1990) and by shortening the in-hospital stay, offers a substantial financial benefit (Rooke and Osmundson, 1986).

Although continuous intravenous heparin therapy is both highly effective and relatively safe, it requires patient hospitalisation and cannot be given on an outpatient basis (Salzman et al, 1975; Glazier and Crowell, 1976; Mant et al, 1977; Wilson and Lampman 1979; Hull et al, 1986; Coon et al, 1969; Hull et al, 1990; Hirsh, 1990). If an approach for the initial treatment of proximal vein thrombosis is developed which can be given on an outpatient basis and does not require laboratory monitoring, it would markedly simplify treatment and improve cost-effectiveness. A conservative estimate of the number of hospital days that would be saved by an outpatient approach to initial therapy is 5-6 days. It has been estimated that such a decrease in the duration of hospitalisation would result in savings to the health care system in the order of at least $500 million annually in the United States alone (Rooke and Osmundson, 1986).

The optimal management of patients with calf vein thrombosis has not been completely resolved. Venous thrombosis which remains confined to the deep calf veins is associated with a low risk of clinically important pulmonary embolism (Kakkar et al, 1969; Moser and LeMoine et al, 1981; Huisman et al, 1986; Hull et al, 1985; Lagerstedt et al, 1985). Untreated, approximately 20% of calf vein thrombi extend into the proximal venous segment (Kakkar 1969; Lagerstedt, 1985). Recent prospective clinical trials (Huisman et al, 1986; Hull et al, 1985) in patients with suspected venous thrombosis indicate that anticoagulant therapy can be safely withheld if the results of impedance plethysmography (which is insensitive for calf vein thrombosis but highly sensitive for proximal vein thrombosis) remain negative on repeated testing over 10-14 days. Negative findings by serial impedance plethysmography are associated with a low risk of clinically important pulmonary embolism (<1%) or recurrent venous thrombosis (2%) (Huisman et al, 1986; Hull et al, 1985). Thus, surveillance with serial impedance plethysmography can be used to separate the 20% of patients with calf vein thrombosis who develop proximal extension (and require treatment) from the remaining 80% without extension, in whom the risks and costs of anticoagulant therapy may outweigh the benefits. It is likely that B-mode ultrasonography, a noninvasive test with a high sensitivity and specificity for symptomatic proximal DVT will be as effective as impedance plethysmography (White et al, 1989). This approach is particularly useful in patients with isolated calf vein thrombosis who are at high risk for bleeding. If this non-invasive approach is not available to monitor for extension, then patients with calf vein thrombosis should be treated with initial heparin therapy followed by adequate long-term anticoagulant therapy (Lagerstedt et al, 1985).

## Initial intravenous heparin therapy

Heparin is given as an initial intravenous bolus of 5,000 U, followed by a maintenance dose of 30,000 to 40,000 U/24 hours by continuous intravenous infusion. Laboratory monitoring with the APTT is performed four to six hours after the initial bolus injection and then daily (or more frequently if necessary) to ensure that an adequate heparin response is achieved. Randomised clinical trial data in patients with proximal vein thrombosis indicated that failure to achieve an adequate anticoagulant response (APTT >1.5 times control) is associated with a high risk (20%) of recurrent venous thromboembolism. Therefore, sufficient heparin should be administered to maintain the APTT above 1.5 times the control value (Hull et al, 1986; Basu et al, 1972; Hyers et al, 1992; Hull et al, 1992). If the APTT response is below 1.5 times control, the 24 hour heparin dose should be augmented by 3,000 to 6,000 U and the APTT repeated 4 to 6 hours later. If the APTT shows little or no prolongation, then to obtain an adequate anticoagulant response immediately, an intravenous heparin bolus of 5,000 U may be given in addition to the increase in the infusion dose. If the APTT response is excessive, the total daily heparin dose should be reduced by

3,000 to 6,000 U (depending on the degree of prolongation) and the APTT repeated 4 to 6 hours later (Hyers et al, 1992; Hull et al, 1992).

It has been conventional clinical practice to continue intravenous heparin for 7 to 10 days, beginning oral anticoagulant therapy on the 5th to 10th day, overlapping heparin and oral anticoagulant treatment for 4 to 5 days before discontinuing heparin. Randomised clinical trials in patients with proximal vein thrombosis indicate that the length of initial heparin therapy can be shortened to 5 days without loss of effectiveness or safety (Gallus et al, 1986; Hull et al, 1990). Oral anticoagulant therapy is begun on the 1st or 2nd day. In patients at extremely high risk of bleeding (eg. immediately post-operatively or patients in the intensive care unit with multiple invasive lines or patients who have conditions predisposing to major bleeding), it would be prudent to delay oral anticoagulant treatment (Hull et al, 1990) since the effect of heparin can be instantly reversed whereas it may take at least 6 to 8 hours to reverse the oral anticoagulant effect.

Alternate methods of heparin administration include intermittent intravenous injection or subcutaneous injection. Intermittent intravenous heparin is associated with a greater risk of bleeding than continuous intravenous infusion, therefore, it is reserved for situations in which continuous infusion and anticoagulant monitoring are not possible. A practical intermittent intravenous regimen is 5,000 U every 4 hours (30,000 U/24 hours (Hull et al, 1986).

The effectiveness and safety of intermittent subcutaneous heparin for the initial treatment of patients with proximal vein thrombosis has been evaluated in a randomised double blind trial. Subcutaneous heparin started at a dose of 15,000 U every 12 hours and adjusted once daily to maintain the APTT between 1.5 and 2 times control resulted in an inadequate anticoagulant response (APTT <1.5 times control) during the first 24 hours in most patients and a high frequency (20%) of recurrent venous thromboembolism. In contrast, continuous intravenous heparin achieved an adequate anticoagulant response (APTT >1.5 times control) in most patients and a low frequency (5%) of recurrent events. In both treatment groups, the recurrences were limited to patients with an inadequate initial anticoagulant response. The results of this trial definitively establish the efficacy of intravenous heparin in patients with proximal vein thrombosis. The findings also strongly suggest that an adequate initial anticoagulant effect (APTT >1.5 times control) is required to prevent recurrent venous thromboembolism and support the practice of monitoring heparin therapy with the APTT to ensure an adequate anticoagulant response is obtained (Hull et al, 1986). It is possible that a larger starting dose of subcutaneous heparin, more frequent injection (eg. every 8 hours) with more frequent APTT monitoring, or both, will achieve an adequate anticoagulant effect and be effective for preventing recurrent venous thromboembolism.

The best mode of heparin administration in the treatment of venous thromboembolism is still a much debated issue. Hommes et al (1991) therefore quantitatively assessed the efficacy and safety of published randomised trials comparing subcutaneous heparin administration with continuous intravenous heparin for the initial treatment of deep vein thrombosis.

Studies published between 1966 and April 1990 were identified through computer searches using Medline data base and through reviewing Science Citations Index, Current Contents and the references cited in the identified articles. Full manuscripts were obtained from the authors if only abstracts were available. Eight clinical trials comparing subcutaneous with intravenous heparin administration in patients with documented deep vein thrombosis were obtained. Each study was independently analysed for the percentage distribubution of thrombosis, the method of outcome measurement and the heparin dose. Also the methodologic strength of each study was assessed using predefined standards for the proper evaluation of a therapeutic intervention with particular reference to the type of patient allocation and objective measurements. The overall relative risk for efficacy (defined as prevention of extension and recurrence of venous thromboembolism) of subcutaneous versus intravenous heparin treatment was 0.62 (95% confidence interval 0.39-0.98) while for safety (defined as absence of major haemorrhage) it was 0.79 (95% confidence interval 0.42-1.48). The outcome of the meta-analysis suggests that subcutaneously administered heparin twice daily in the initial treatment of deep vein thrombosis is at least as effective and safe as continuous intravenous heparin administration. Administration of heparin subcutaneously may simplify patient treatment and could possibly facilitate "home treatment" (Hommes et al, 1991).

At present, intravenous administration, preferably by continuous intravenous infusion, remains the approach of choice for initial heparin therapy. This is because of concern that in individual patients the subcutaneous route may be less effective because of delays in achieving a therapeutic APTT response.

## Adverse effects of heparin

The side effects of heparin therapy include bleeding, thrombocytopenia, arterial thromboembolism, hypersensitivity to heparin, and osteoporosis.

Bleeding is the most common side effect of heparin, and occurs in 5-10% of patients during initial continuous intravenous heparin therapy (Salzman et al, 1975; Glazier and Crowell, 1976; Wilson and Lampman, 1979; Hull et al, 1986; Basu et al, 1972; Andersson et al, 1982; Doyle et al 1987). Patients at particular risk are those who have been exposed to recent surgery or trauma, and those with an underlying haemostatic defect or predisposing clinical risk factor (for example, an unsuspected duodenal ulcer or occult carcinoma). The risk of bleeding complications is greater with intermittent intravenous heparin than for continuous intravenous heparin (Salzman et al, 1975; Glazier and Crowell, 1976; Wilson and Lampman, 1979). The risk of bleeding may increase with increases in the total 24 hour heparin dose (Glazier and Crowell, 1976; Kernohan and Todd, 1966; Walker and Jick, 1980).

Thrombocytopenia is now a well recognised complication of heparin treatment (Bell and Royall, 1980; Green et al, 1984; Cimo et al, 1979; Babcock et al, 1976; Cines et al, 1980), which usually has its onset 7 to 10 days after the initiation of therapy. Heparin-induced thrombocytopenia occurs more frequently in patients given beef lung heparin (a frequency of about 10%) than in those receiving porcine gut heparin (a frequency of about 5% or less) (Bell and Royall, 1980; Green et al, 1984). Arterial thromboembolism is a rare but potentially devastating complication that occurs together with heparin induced thrombocytopenia (Cimo et al, 1979), and which requires immediate cessation of heparin therapy. The precise mechanism of heparin-induced thrombocytopenia is currently unknown, but probably involves immune mechanisms (Babcock et al, 1976; Cines et al, 1980).

Osteoporosis occurs rarely in patients receiving long-term subcutaneous heparin (Sackler and Liu, 1973; Squires and Pinch, 1979; Wise and Hall, 1980) The earliest clinical manifestation is usually the onset of nonspecific low back pain primarily involving the vertebrae or ribs; patients may also present with spontaneous fracture in these areas. The frequency of osteoporosis appears to be related to the total daily heparin dose, and also to the duration of therapy. Osteoporosis associated with heparin therapy usually occurs in patients receiving 15,000 units or more of heparin daily for longer than three months.

Hypersensitivity to heparin is uncommon and may take the form of a skin rash or less commonly, anaphylaxis. Other rare complications of heparin include alopoecia, and a bluish discolouration of the toes, associated with a burning sensation.

The anticoagulant effect of heparin can be reversed by the intravenous injection of protamine sulphate. Protamine sulphate should be injected slowly over a 10-30 minute period to avoid a hypotensive response.

## Oral anticoagulant therapy

Oral anticoagulants (eg. warfarin sodium) inhibit the effect of vitamin K on the hepatic synthesis of factors II, VII, IX, X, resulting in the synthesis of biologically inactive forms of these coagulation proteins (Bell, 1978). The anticoagulant effect of the vitamin K antagonists is delayed until the normal clotting factors are cleared from the circulation, and the peak effect does not occur until 36 to 72 hours after drug administration. Oral anticoagulants also inhibit the vitamin K-dependent synthesis of protein C, a naturally occurring proenzyme activated by thrombin to form activated protein C. Activated protein C inhibits activated factors V and VIII (Clouse and Comp 1986).

Oral anticoagulant therapy with warfarin sodium is initiated in a dose of 10 mg per day for the first day, and the daily dose is then adjusted according to the results of laboratory monitoring. The laboratory test most commonly used to monitor oral anticoagulant therapy is the one-stage prothrombin time, which is sensitive to reduced activity of factors II, VII and X but is insensitive to reduced activity of factor IX. In North America, the thromboplastin reagents used to measure the prothrombin time are usually obtained from rabbit brain tissue, whereas in the United Kingdom and parts of Europe the thromboplastin was, until recently, obtained from human brain. The rabbit brain thromboplastins that are commercially available in North America (eg. Simplastin, Dade-C) are generally less sensitive to reductions in the vitamin K-dependent coagulation factors than is standardised human brain thromboplastin (Hirsh et al, 1986) A prothrombin time ratio of 1.5 to 2 times control using a rabbit brain thromboplastin is equivalent to a ratio of 4 to 6 times control using standardised human brain thromboplastin. Conversely, a prothrombin time ratio using standardised human brain thromboplastin of 2 to 3 times control is equivalent to a ratio of 1.25 to 1.5 times control using a rabbit brain thromboplastin (Hull et al, 1982; Hirsh et al, 1986). The traditionally recommended therapeutic range in North America (i.e., a prothrombin time ratio at 1.5 to 2 times control using a rabbit brain thromboplastin), although effective, is associated with a high risk (20%) of bleeding (Hull et al, 1979; Hull, Delmore et al, 1982; Hull, Hirsh et al, 1982; Turpie et al, 1988; Saour et al, 1990; Boston Area Anticoagulation Trial for Atrial Fibrillation Investigators, 1990). Randomised clinical trials indicate that the risk of bleeding can be reduced to less than 5%, without loss of effectiveness for preventing recurrent venous thromboembolism, by adjusting the dose of warfarin sodium to achieve a less intense anticoagulant effect (a prothrombin time ratio of 1.25 to 1.5 times control using a rabbit brain thromboplastin (Hull et al, 1982; Turpie et al, 1988; Saour et al, 1990; Boston Area Anticoagulation Trial for Atrial Fibrillation Investigators, 1990).

To promote standardisation of the prothrombin time for monitoring oral anticoagulant therapy, the World Health Organisation (WHO) has developed an international reference thromboplastin from human brain tissue and has recommended that the prothrombin time ratio be expressed according to a uniform system known as the International Normalized Ratio (INR). The INR is the prothrombin time ratio obtained by testing a given sample using the WHO reference thromboplastin. For practical clinical purposes, the INR for a given plasma sample is equivalent to the prothrombin time ratio obtained using a human brain thromboplastin known as the Manchester comparative reagent which is widely used in the United Kingdom. The recommended less intense therapeutic range for warfarin therapy of 1.25 to 1.5 times control using a rabbit brain thromboplastin such as Simplastin or Dade-C corresponds to an INR of 2 to 3 (Hirsh et al, 1986).

A 4- or 5-day overlap with intravenous therapy with heparin during the initiation of warfarin sodium therapy is important (Gallus et al, 1986; Hull et al, 1990). Experimental evidence indicates that the maximal antithrombotic effect of warfarin sodium is delayed for as long as five days, even though the anticoagulant effect, reflected by an increase in the prothrombin time (due mainly to a reduction in factor VII), may be evident within 2 to 3 days. Factor VII and protein C (a naturally occurring anticoagulant) have similar short half-lives (4-5 hours), and during the first 24 to 48 hours of warfarin sodium therapy the levels of functional factor VII and protein C fall while the levels of functional factors II, IX and X remain relatively normal. During the initial 24 to 48 hours of therapy, oral anticoagulants have the potential to be thrombogenic because the anticoagulant effect of low functional VII is counteracted by the potentially thrombogenic effect of low levels of functional protein C, with near-normal levels of functional factors II, IX, and X. After 72-96 hours, the levels of functional factors II, IX, and X fall and the optimal anticoagulant activity of warfarin therapy is expressed (O'Reilly and Aggeler, 1968). For these reasons, it is important to overlap warfarin sodium with heparin for 4 or 5 days even though the prothrombin time may be prolonged into the therapeutic range after 2 or 3 days (Hyers et al, 1992).

Once the anticoagulant effect and the patient's warfarin dose requirements are stabilised, the prothrombin time is monitored weekly throughout the course of long-term therapy. If there are factors that may produce an unpredictable response to warfarin sodium, the prothrombin time should be monitored more frequently to minimise the risk of complications due to poor anticoagulant control. A large number of drugs interact with oral anticoagulants and may produce either a prolongation or a reduction in the anticoagulant effect. A commonly encountered drug interaction with warfarin sodium, resulting in an increased anticoagulant effect, occurs with the concurrent administration of trimethoprim-sulfamethoxazole (eg. in patients with urinary tract infection). Other factors that cause an increased sensitivity to oral anticoagulants are vitamin K deficiency, impaired liver function, and thyrotoxicosis (due to the more rapid metabolism of the vitamin K-dependent clotting factors) (Hyers et al, 1992).

The major side effect of oral anticoagulant therapy is bleeding. Non haemorrhagic side effects of coumarin anticoagulants are uncommon. Coumarin-induced skin necrosis is a rare but serious complication that requires immediate cessation of oral anticoagulant therapy (Hyers et al, 1992).

Vitamin K is the antidote to the oral anticoagulants.

## Adjusted subcutaneous heparin for long-term therapy

Adjusted-dose subcutaneous heparin therapy is the long-term regimen of choice in pregnant patients, in patients who return to geographically remote areas in whom long-term anticoagulant monitoring is unavailable or impractical, and in patients at high risk of bleeding (Hull et al, 1982). The starting dose of long-term subcutaneous heparin is determined from the patient's initial intravenous heparin dose requirements, a starting subcutaneous dose equivalent to one third of the patient's 24 hour intravenous heparin dose is administered every 12 hours. For example, if the patient required 30,000 U per 24 hours of continuous intravenous heparin to maintain the APTT above 1.5 times the control value, the starting dose of long-term subcutaneous heparin would be 10,000 U every 12 hours. The subcutaneous dose is adjusted during the first three days of long-term therapy to maintain the mid interval APTT (determined 6 hours after injection) at 1.5 times the control value. After this initial adjustment, further monitoring is not obligatory and the dose can be fixed (Hull et al, 1982). Randomised clinical trials indicate that this approach is effective for preventing recurrent venous thromboembolism and is associated with a low risk (2%) of bleeding complications (Hull, Delmore et al, 1982). In pregnant patients, continued monitoring is desirable because of changes in heparin requirements throughout the course of pregnancy (Salzman et al, 1975).

Long-term subcutaneous heparin has the potential disadvantage of inducing osteoporosis if administered for longer than three months, and if treatment for longer than three months is necessary, these patients should be evaluated at regular intervals with an objective technique for measuring bone density.

## Contraindications to anticoagulants

Inferior vena caval interruption using a transvenously inserted filter (the Greenfield filter), is the management of choice for preventing pulmonary embolism in patients with proximal vein thrombosis in whom anticoagulant therapy is absolutely contraindicated, and in the very rare patient in whom anticoagulant therapy is ineffective (Hyers et al, 1992).

## Low molecular weight heparin therapy for venous thromboembolism

In recent years, low molecular weight (LMW) derivatives of commercial heparin have been prepared that have a mean molecular weight of 4,000 to 5,000 daltons in contrast to unfractionated heparin, which has a mean molecular weight of 12,000 to 16,000 daltons (Salzman 1986; Verstraete 1990). The excellent bioavailability of LMW-heparin, together with a longer half-life (Aiach et al, 1983; Bara et al, 1985; Bergqvist et al, 1983, Bratt et al, 1986; Frydman et al, 1988; Matzsch et al, 1987; Harenberg et al, 1986; Arneson et al, 1987)(anti F Xa activity) than unfractionated heparin suggests that it may be possible to develop an effective regimen for initial treatment with LMW-heparin using once daily subcutaneous injections. The anticoagulant response (F Xa units/ml) observed with a given dose of LMW-heparin was highly correlated with body weight (Frydman et al, 1988), so it is possible that LMW-heparin may be effective when given in standard doses (F Xa units/kg) without laboratory monitoring.

Studies in experimental animal models of venous thrombosis have shown that some LMW fractions have equal (or greater) antithrombotic efficacy, but less haemorrhagic effects, by comparison to heparin (Salzman, 1986; Verstraete, 1990; Cade et al, 1984; Carter et al, 1981; Carter et al, 1982; Holmer et al, 1982). Whether this latter experimental observation applies clinically is currently uncertain (Hirsh 1990; Salzman 1986; Green et al, 1990; Kakkar and Murray, 1985; Turpie et al, 1986); demonstration of this property in man has remained elusive. A meta-analysis (Rosendaal et al, 1991) of the findings of multiple randomised clinical trials evaluating LMW-heparin for prophylaxis against deep-vein thrombosis (Hirsh, 1990; Salzman, 1986; Kakkar and Murray 1985; Turpie et al, 1986) suggests that LMW-heparin is more effective than low-dose heparin but has an increased risk of bleeding. In contrast, a large randomised trial (Levine et al, 1991) comparing the prophylactic use of LMW-heparin against moderate doses of subcutaneous heparin showed that LMW-heparin was significantly less haemorrhagic for an apparent equivalent anti-thrombotic effect. Whether this reflects an intrinsic property of LMW-heparin or is due to a dose effect is uncertain (Hull and Raskob, 1991). Further comparisons of LMW-heparin with varying dosage regimens will be necessary before firm conclusions can be made (Hull and Raskob, 1991).

Multiple randomised clinical trials (Collaborative European Multicentre Study, 1991; Albada et al, 1989; Bratt, 1985; Bratt 1987; Bratt 1990; Handeland et al, 1990; Harenberg et al, 1990; Holm et al, 1986; Huet et al, 1990; Janvier et al, 1987; Lockner et al, 1986; Prandoni, 1991; Hull 1992) have evaluated LMW-heparin for the initial treatment of patients with venous thrombosis. These data suggest that LMW-heparin administered subcutaneously twice a day is as effective and safe as continuous intravenous heparin. These findings (Collaborative European Multicentre Study, 1991; Albada et al, 1989; Bratt et al, 1985; Bratt et al, 1987; Bratt et al, 1990; Handeland et al, 1990; Harenberg et al, 1990; Holm et al, 1986; Huet et al, 1990; Janvier et al, 1987; Lockner et al, 1986) are largely based on venographic observations rather than clinical outcome.

Two studies (Prandoni, 1991; Prandoni et al, 1992; Hull et al, 1992) evaluating objectively documented clinical outcomes (Rabinov and Paulin, 1972; Dalen et al, 1971; Wheeler et al, 1974; Hull et al, 1977; Hull et al, 1983) provide firm conclusions as to the role of fixed-dose subcutaneous LMW-heparin therapy in patients with venous thrombosis.

An open label randomised trial was recently reported in consecutive symptomatic patients with proximal vein thrombosis comparing the relative effectiveness and risk of bleeding of fixed-dose LMW-heparin (Fraxiparine) with adjusted-dose intravenous unfractionated heparin for 10 days followed by oral warfarin sodium for three months (Prandoni et al, 1992). Patients in the LMW-heparin group received subcutaneous injections every twelve hours according to body weight (12,500 aXa Institute Choay (IC) units for patients under 55 kg; 15,000 aXa IC U for patients between 55 and 80 kg; and 17,500 aXa IC U for patients over 80 kg). Patients in the adjusted-dose intravenous heparin group received a continuous infusion to maintain the APTT within 1.5-2.0 times the mean normal control value, (Hull et al, 1992). All patients had baseline perfusion lung scans and chest X-rays. In these studies also contrast venography was repeated on day 10 or earlier if new symptoms developed. The principal end-point for the assessment of efficacy was symptomatic recurrent venous thrombosis or symptomatic pulmonary embolism. Secondary end points for efficacy assessment were changes between day 0 and 10 in the venograms and perfusion lung scans. The frequency of objectively diagnosed recurrent venous thromboembolism was comparable between the unfractionated heparin and the LMW-heparin groups 12(14%) versus 6(7%), difference 7%; 95% confidence interval -3% to 15%; p = 0.13. Clinically evident bleeding occurred in 3.5% of patients receiving unfractionated heparin versus 1.1% of those receiving LMW-heparin; p>0.2. In the six-month follow-up period there were 12 deaths in the unfractionated heparin group versus six in the CY 216 group and this difference was largely due to cancer deaths (8 of 18 in the unfractionated heparin group versus 1 of 15 in the LMW-heparin group).

In a multi-centre double-blind clinical trial, fixed-dose subcutaneous LMW-heparin (Logiparin) (175 factor Xa IU/kg) was compared with intravenous heparin by continued infusion adjusted to maintain an APTT of 1.5-2.5 times the mean normal control value (Hull et al, 1992). All patients had venographically proven proximal venous thrombosis and at the time of entry had ventilation perfusion lung scans, chest radiographs and impedance plethysmography. Outcome events included objectively documented venous thromboembolism (recurrence or extension of deep-vein thrombosis or pulmonary embolism), major or minor bleeding, thrombocytopenia and death. New episodes of venous thromboembolism were seen in six of 213 patients receiving LMW-heparin (2.8%) and 15 of 219 patients receiving intravenous unfractionated heparin (6.9%) (p = 0.07; 95% confidence interval for the difference 0.02% to 8.1%). Major bleeding associated with initial therapy occurred in one patient receiving LMW-heparin (0.5%) and in all patients receiving intravenous unfractionated heparin (5.0%), a reduction in risk of 95% (p = 0.008). During long-term warfarin therapy major haemorrhage was seen in five patients who had received LMW-heparin (2.3%) and in none of those receiving intravenous heparin (p = 0.028). Ten patients who received LMW-heparin (4.7%) died, as compared to 21 patients who received intravenous unfractionated heparin (9.6%), a risk reduction of 51%, p = 0.049. The most striking difference was in abrupt deaths in patients with metastatic carcinoma and the majority of these deaths occurred within the first three weeks. It is possible that the long-term use of LMW-heparin in place of warfarin sodium may have a greater impact on recurrent thromboembolic events, bleeding and death, particularly in patients with metastatic carcinoma.

Taken together, the results of these studies provide strong evidence that LMW-heparin given subcutaneously is as effective and as safe as unfractionated heparin in the treatment of proximal venous thrombosis. The decreased mortality rate, particularly in patients with metastatic carcinoma was unexpected and requires confirmation in further prospective randomised trials (Green et al, 1992).

In conclusion, the accumulating evidence indicates that certain LMW-heparins administered subcutaneously may replace classic intravenous heparin therapy. Certain of these subcutaneously administered LMW-heparins do not require monitoring. The simplified care offered by LMW-heparin therapy offers the possibility of transferring care from in-hospital to out of hospital in uncomplicated patients with deep vein thrombosis. The advantages to the patient of avoiding in-hospital care and its associated hazards are obvious. Outpatient LMW-heparin therapy will likely prove to be highly cost-effective. It is uncertain at present whether the findings associated with an individual LMW-heparin preparation can be extrapolated to a different LMW-heparin. For this reason the findings of clinical trials apply only to the particular LMW-heparin evaluated and cannot be generalised to the LMW-heparins at large.

# References

Aiach M, Michaud A, Balian JL et al. A new molecular weight heparin derivative, in vitro and in vivo studies. Thromb Res. 31:611, 1983

Albada J, Nieuwenhuis HK, Sixma JJ. Treatment of acute venous thromboembolism with low molecular weight heparin (Fragmin). Results of a double-blind randomised study. Circulation 80:935, 1989

Andersson G, Fagrell B, Holmgren K et al. Subcutaneous administration of heparin: a randomized comparison with intravenous administration of heparin to patients with deep vein thrombosis. Thromb Res 27:631, 1982

Arneson KE, Handeland GF, Abildgaard U et al. What is the optimal dosage of LMW heparin in the subcutaneous treatment of deep vein thrombosis? Thromb Haemost. 58:214 (abstract 794), 1987.

Babcock RB, Dumper CW, Scharfman WB. Heparin-induced immune thrombocytopenia. N Engl J Med. 295:237, 1976.

Bara L, Billand E, Gramond G et al. Comparative pharmacokinetics of a low molecular weight heparin and unfractionated heparin after intravenous and subcutaneous administration. Thromb Res 39:631, 1985

Basu D, Gallus A, Hirsh J, Cade J. A prospective study of the value of monitoring heparin treatment with the activated partial thromboplastin time. N Engl J Med 287:324, 1972

Bell RG. Metabolism of vitamin K and prothrombin synthesis: Anticoagulants and the vitamin K-epoxide cycle. Fed Proc. 37:2599, 1978

Bell WR, Royall RM. Heparin-associated thrombocytopenia: a comparison of three heparin preparations. N Engl J Med. 303:902, 1980.

Bergqvist D, Hedner U, Sjorin E et al. Anticoagulant effects of two types of low molecular weight heparin administered subcutaneously. Thromb Res 32:381, 1983

Boston Area Anticoagulation Trial for Atrial Fibrillation Investigators: The effect of low-dose warfarin on the risk of stroke in patients with nonrheumatic atrial fibrillation. N Engl J Med 323:1505, 1990

Bratt G, Aberg W, Johansson M et al. Two daily subcutaneous injections of Fragmin as compared with intravenous standard heparin in the treatment of deep venous thrombosis (DVT). Thromb Haemost 64:506, 1990

Bratt G, Aberg W, Tornebohm E et al. Subcutaneous KABI 2165 in the treatment of deep venous thrombosis of the leg. Thromb Res Suppl VII 24 (Abstract 20) 1987.

Bratt G, Tornebohm E, Granqvist S et al. A comparison between low molecular weight heparin [KABI 2165] and standard heparin in the intravenous treatment of deep venous thrombosis. Thromb Haemost 54:813, 1985

Bratt G, Tornebohm E, Widlund L et al. Low molecular weight heparin (Kabi 2165; Fragmin): pharmacokinetics after intravenous and subcutaneous administration in human volunteers. Thromb Res 42:613, 1986

Cade JF, Buchanon MR, Boneau B et al. A comparison of the antithrombotic and haemorrhagic effects of low molecular weight heparin fractions: The influence of the method of preparation. Thromb Res. 35:613, 1984

Carter CJ, Kelton JG, Hirsh J et al. Relationship between the antithrombotic and anticoagulant effects of low molecular weight heparin. Thromb Res. 21:169, 1981

Carter CJ, Kelton JG, Hirsh J et al. The relationship between the hemorrhagic and antithrombotic properties of low molecular weight heparin in rabbits. Blood 59:1239, 1982

Cimo PL, Moake JL, Weinger RS et al. Heparin-induced thrombocytopenia: association with a platelet aggregating factor and arterial thromboses. Am J Hematol. 6:125, 1979

Cines DB, Kaywin P, Bina M et al. Heparin-associated thrombocytopenia. N Engl J Med 303:788, 1980

Clouse LH, Comp PC. The regulation of hemostasis: The protein C system. N Engl J Med 314:1298, 1986

A Collaborative European Multicentre Study. A randomised trial of subcutaneous low molecular weight heparin (CY 216) compared with intravenous unfractionated heparin in the treatment of deep vein thrombosis. Thromb Haemost 65:251, 1991

Coon WW, Willis PW III, Symons MJ. Assessment of anticoagulant treatment of venous thromboembolism. Ann Surg 170:559, 1969

Dalen JE, Brooks HL, Johnson LW et al. Pulmonary angiography in acute pulmonary embolism: indications, techniques, and results in 367 patients. Am Heart J 81:175, 1971

Doyle DJ, Turpie AGG, Hirsh J et al. Adjusted subcutaneous heparin or continuous intravenous heparin in patients with acute deep-vein thrombosis: a randomized trial. Ann Intern Med 107:441, 1987

Frydman AM, Bara L, LeRoux Y et al. The antithrombotic activity and pharmacokinetics of enoxaparine, a low molecular weight heparin, in humans given single subcutaneous doses of 20 to 80 mg. J Clin Pharmacol 28:609, 1988

Gallus AS, Jackaman J, Tillett J, Mills W, Wycherley A. Safety and efficacy of warfarin started early after submassive venous thrombosis or pulmonary embolism. Lancet 2:1293, 1986

Glazier RL, Crowell EB. Randomized prospective trial of continuous vs intermittent heparin therapy. JAMA 236:1365, 1976

Green D, Hull RD, Brant R, Pineo GF. Lower mortality in cancer patients treated with low-molecular-weight versus standard heparin. Lancet 339:1476, 1992.

Green D, Lee MY, Lim AC et al. Prevention of thromboembolism after spinal cord injury using low-molecular-weight heparin. Ann Intern Med 113:571, 1990

Green D, Martin GJ, Shoichet SH, de Backer N, Boalski JS, Lind RN. Thrombocytopenia in a prospective randomized double-blind trial of bovine and porcine heparin. Am J Med Sci 288:60, 1984

Handeland GF, Abildgaard U, Holm HA et al. Dose adjusted heparin treatment of deep venous thrombosis: a comparison of unfractionated and low molecular weight heparin. Eur J Clin Pharmacol 39:107, 1990

Harenberg J, Huck K, Bratsch H et al. Therapeutic application of subcutaneous low-molecular-weight heparin in acute venous thrombosis. Haemostasis 20 Suppl 1:205, 1990

Harenberg J, Wurzner B, Zimmermann R et al. Bioavailability and antagonization of the low molecular weight heparin CY216 in man. Thromb Res 44:549, 1986

Hirsh J. From unfractionated heparins to low molecular weight heparins. Acta Chir Scand Suppl. 556:42, 1990

Hirsh J, Poller L, Deykin D et al. Optimal therapeutic range for oral anticoagulants. Chest, 95:5S, 1986

Holm HA, Ly B, Handeland GF et al. Subcutaneous heparin treatment of deep venous thrombosis: a comparison of unfractionated and low molecular weight heparin. Haemostasis 16:30, 1986

Holmer E, Mattsson C, Nilsson S. Anticoagulant and antithrombotic effects of heparin and low molecular weight heparin fragments in rabbits. Thromb Res 25:475, 1982

Hommes DW, Bura A, Mazzolat L, Buller HR, Cate JW. Subcutaneous heparin compared to continuous intravenous heparin administration in the initial treatment of deep vein thrombosis: A systemic overview and meta-analysis. Thromb Haemost 65:753 (abstract 305), 1991.

Huet Y, Janvier G, Bendriss PH et al. Treatment of established venous thromboembolism with enoxaparin: preliminary report. Acta Chir Scand Suppl 556:116, 1990

Huisman MV, Buller HR, ten Cate JW, Vreeken J. Serial impedance plethysmography for suspected deep venous thrombosis in outpatients: the Amsterdam General Practitioner Study. N Eng J Med 314:823, 1986

Hull RD, Carter CJ, Jay RM et al. The diagnosis of acute, recurrent, deep-vein thrombosis: a diagnostic challenge. Circulation 67:901, 1983.

Hull R, Delmore T. Carter C et al. Adjusted subcutaneous heparin versus warfarin sodium in the long-term treatment of venous thrombosis. N Engl J Med. 306:189, 1982.

Hull R, Delmore T, Genton E et al. Warfarin sodium versus low dose heparin in the long-tem treatment of venous thrombosis. N Engl J Med 301:855, 1979

Hull RD, Hirsh J, Carter C et al. Diagnostic efficacy of impedance plethysmography for clinically suspected deep-vein thrombosis. Ann Intern Med 102:21, 1985

Hull RD, Hirsh J, Jay R et al. Different intensities of oral anticoagulant therapy in the treatment of proximal-vein thrombosis. N Engl J Med 307:1676, 1982a

Hull R, Hirsh J, Sackett DL et al. Combined use of leg scanning and impedance plethysmography in suspected venous thrombosis: an alternative to venography. N Engl J Med 296:1497, 1 296:1497, 1977

Hull RD, Raskob GE. Low molecular weight heparin for deep vein thrombosis [letter] Ann Intern Med 115:231, 1991

Hull RD, Raskob GE, Hirsh J et al. Continuous intravenous heparin compared with intermittent subcutaneous heparin in the initial treatment of proximal vein thrombosis. N Engl J Med 315:1109, 1988

Hull RD, Raskob GE, Pineo GF et al. Subcutaneous low-molecular weight heparin compared with continuous intravenous heparin in the treatment of proximal vein thrombosis. N Engl J Med 326:975, 1992

Hull RD, Raskob GE, Rosenbloom D et al. Heparin for 5 days as compared with 10 days in the initial treatment of proximal venous thrombosis. N Engl J Med 322:1260, 1990

Hull RD, Raskob GE, Rosenbloom D et al. Optimal therapeutic level of heparin therapy in patients with venous thrombosis. Arch Intern Med. 152:1589, 1992.

Hyers TM, Hull RD, Weg JG. Antithrombotic therapy for venous thromboembolic disease. Chest 102 October Suppl:408S, 1992

Janvier G, Winnock S, Dugrais G et al. Treatment of deep venous thrombosis with a very low molecular weight heparin fragment (CY 222). Haemostasis 7:49, 1987

Kakkar VV, Flanc C, Howe CT et al. Natural history of postoperative deep-vein thrombosis. Lancet ii:230, 1969

Kakkar VV, Murray WJG. Efficacy and safety of low molecular weight heparin (CY216) in preventing postoperative venous thromboembolism: a co-operative study. Br J Surg 72:786, 1985

Kernohan RJ, Todd C. Heparin therapy in thromboembolic disease. Lancet i:621, 1966

Lagerstedt CI, Fagher BO, Olsson CG, Oquist BW, Albrechtsson U. Need for long-term anticoagulant treatment in symptomatic calf- vein thrombosis. Lancet ii:515, 1985

Levine MN, Hirsh J, Gent M et al. Prevention of deep-vein thrombosis after elective hip surgery. A randomized trial comparing low molecular weight heparin with standard unfractionated heparin. Ann Intern Med 114:545, 1991

Lockner D, Bratt G, Tornebohm E et al. Intravenous and subcutaneous administration of Fragmin in deep venous thrombosis. Haemostasis 16:25, 1986

Mant MJ, O'Brien BD, Thong KL et al. Haemorrhagic complications of heparin therapy. Lancet 1:1133, 1977

Mätzch T, Bergqvist D, Hedner U et al. Effects of an enzymatically depolymerized heparin as compared with conventional heparin in healthy volunteers. Thromb Haemost 57:97, 1987

Moser KM, LeMoine JR. Is embolic risk conditioned by location of deep venous thrombosis? Ann Intern Med 94:439, 1981

O'Reilly RA, Aggeler PM. Studies on coumarin anticoagulant drugs: Initiation of warfarin therapy without a loading dose. Circulation 38:169, 1968

Prandoni P. Fixed dose LMW heparin (CY 216) as compared with adjusted dose intravenous heparin in the initial treatment of symptomatic proximal venous thrombosis. Thromb Haemost 65:872 (abstract 61B) 1991

Prandoni P, Lensing AW, Buller HR et al. Comparison of subcutaneous low molecular weight heparin with intravenous standard heparin in proximal deep-vein thrombosis. Lancet 339:441, 1992.

Rabinov K, Paulin S, Roentgen diagnosis of venous thrombosis in the leg. Arch Surg 104:134, 1972

Rooke TW, Osmundson PJ. Heparin and the in-hospital management of deep-venous thrombosis: cost considerations. Mayo Clin Proc 61:198, 1986

Rosendaal FR, Nurmohamed MT, Buller HR et al. Low molecular weight heparin in the prophylaxis of venous thrombosis: a meta-analysis. Thromb Haemost 65:927, 1991

Sackler JP, Liu L. Heparin-induced osteoporosis. Br J Radiol 46:548, 1973

Salzman EW. Low molecular weight heparin. Is small beautiful? N Engl J Med 315:957, 1986

Salzman EW, Deykin D, Shapiro RM, Rosenberg R. Management of heparin therapy: controlled prospective trial. N Engl J Med 292:1046, 1975

Saour JN, Seck JO, Mamo LAR et al. Trial of different intensities of anticoagulation in patients with prosthetic heart valves. N Engl J Med 322:428, 1990

Squires JW, Pinch LW. Heparin-induced spinal fractures. JAMA 241:2417. 1979.

Turpie AGG, Gunstensen J, Hirsh J et al. Randomized comparison of two intensities of oral anticoagulant therapy after tissue heart valve replacement. Lancet 1:1242, 1988

Turpie AGG, Levine MN, Hirsh J et al. A randomised controlled trial of a low molecular-weight heparin (enoxaparin) to prevent deep-vein thrombosis in patients undergoing elective hip surgery. N. Engl J Med 315:925, 1986

Verstraete M. Pharmacotherapeutic aspects of unfractionated and low molecular weight heparin. Drugs 40:498, 1990

Walker AM, Jick H. Predictors of bleeding during heparin therapy. JAMA 244:1209, 1980

Wheeler HB, O'Donnell JA, Anderson FA Jr et al. Occlusive impedance phlebography: a diagnostic procedure for venous thrombosis and pulmonary embolism. Prog Cardiovasc Dis 17:199, 1974

White RH, McGahan P, Daschback MM, Harting RP. Diagnosis of deep-vein thrombosis using duplex ultrasound. Ann Intern Med 111:297, 1989

Wilson JR, Lampman J. Heparin therapy: a randomized prospective study. Am Heart J 97:155, 1979

Wise PH, Hall AJ. Heparin-induced osteopenia in pregnancy. BMJ 281:110. 1980

PART V

# European Consensus Statement

CHAPTER 41

# Prevention of thromboembolism: European Consensus Statement

CHAIRMAN: AN Nicolaides* (UK)
FACULTY: G Belcaro (Italy)   D Bergqvist (Sweden)**
LC Borris (Denmark)   HR Buller (The Netherlands)
JA Caprini (USA)   D Christopoulos (Greece)
D Clarke-Pearson (USA)**   D Clement (Belgium)
GA Colditz (USA)   P Coleridge-Smith (UK)
AJ Comerota (USA)**   ED Cooke (UK)   B Eklof (Sweden)**
C Fisher (Australia)   LJ Greenfield (USA)   S Haas (Germany)
R Hull (Canada)**   VV Kakkar (UK)***   E Kalodiki (Cyprus)
MR Lassen (Denmark)   J Leclerc (Canada)   A Planes (France)
M Samama (France)**   A Sasahara (USA)   JH Scurr (UK)**
GW ten Cate (The Netherlands)**   AG Turpie (Canada)**
L Widmer (Switzerland)

## The problem and need for prevention

Deep vein thrombosis (DVT) and pulmonary embolism (PE) are major health problems with two serious outcomes. In the immediate course, PE may be fatal. In the long term perspective there is the risk of the development of pulmonary hypertension from recurrent embolism and post-thrombotic venous insufficiency. Both have a great impact on health care costs. Epidemiological data indicate the rate of DVT each year to be around 160 per 100,000 in the general population with the rate of fatal PE 60 per 100,000. Although the

---

The European Consensus Statement was developed at Oakley Court Hotel, Windsor, UK, 1-5 November 1991, under the patronage of the European Commissioner, Mrs Vasso Papandreou, and the auspices of the Cardiovascular Disease Educational and Research Trust and St Mary's Hospital Medical School.
*Editorial committe   **Chairmen of consensus statement groups   ***Chief executive — CDER trust

**Table 1**
Risk groups in trauma and surgery in approximate order of decreasing frequency of DVT*

| | |
|---|---|
| Spinal cord injury | 75-80% |
| Knee arthroplasty | |
| Leg amputation | |
| Hip fracture surgery | |
| Hip arthroplasty | |
| Lower limb fracture | |
| Open prostatectomy | |
| General abdominal surgery | |
| Gynaecological surgery | |
| Kidney transplantation | |
| Non-cardiac thoracic surgery | |
| Neurosurgery | |
| Open meniscectomy | 20-25% |

*The order is true for the total groups of patients. The presence of additional risk factors indicated in the text may change the risk of thromboembolism for individual patients

number of venous ulcers is 200 per 100,000 population, the proportion due to DVT is unknown. Thus, a most important task for the medical profession is to prevent DVT and its complications. In this task, knowledge in epidemiology and diagnostic methodology is important so as to be able to define the risk groups where intervention must be considered.

The attitudes and beliefs towards prophylaxis show great regional variations. This is true for the definition of high risk groups, the proportion of patients receiving prophylaxis and the prophylactic methodology chosen.

### Surgical patients
Patients who sustain major trauma or undergo prolonged operative procedures are at risk of developing venous thromboembolic disease (Table 1).

The degree of risk is increased by age, obesity, malignancy, prior history of venous thrombosis, varicose veins, recent operative procedures and thrombophilic states. These factors are further modified by general care including operative duration, type of anaesthesia, pre- and post-operative immobility, level of hydration and the presence of sepsis.

The risk of venous thromboembolism may continue beyond the period of hospitalisation. This risk needs to be assessed in appropriate prospective studies.

### Medical patients
There are less data available in medical than in surgical patients. However, an increased risk of venous thromboembolism has been shown by prospective studies in patients with acute myocardial infarction, cerebrovascular accidents and immobilised general medical patients.

### Gynaecology and obstetrics
The reported overall incidence of thromboembolic complications in gynaecologic surgery is of the same order of magnitude as in general surgery. Pulmonary embolism is a leading cause of death following gynaecological cancer surgery.

In pregnancy, DVT occurs in 0.13-0.5/1000 in the ante-partum period and 0.61-1.5/1000 in postpartum patients. PE is a leading cause of maternal mortality.

Risk factors associated with DVT are similar to those included in the surgical section. Case control studies show that there is an increased risk of venous thrombosis in women taking oral contraceptives containing 50 micrograms or more of oestrogen. However, there are no data regarding current low dose oral contraceptives.

Other risk factors associated with DVT/PE in pregnancy include Caesarean section, advanced maternal age and thrombophilic states.

# Predisposing haematological changes and indications for screening

Congenital predisposition to thrombosis (thrombophilia) is a rare condition but should be seriously considered in patients defined as having had a documented unexplained thrombotic episode below the age of 40, recurrent DVT and a positive family history. The frequency of congenital thrombophilia in consecutive patients with confirmed venous thrombosis is approximately 8%. In addition, a number of acquired haematological abnormalities such as lupus anticoagulant, anticardiolipin antibodies and myeloproliferative disease are associated with a predisposition to venous thromboembolism.

The recommended screening tests are:
*General:* Complete blood count including platelets.
*For congenital conditions:* Antithrombin III, Protein C, Protein S and fibrinogen/thrombin clotting time for dysfibrinogenaemia.
*For acquired conditions:* Activated partial thromboplastin time (APTT), anticardiolipin antibody.

Plasminogen, plasminogen activator inhibitor activity, tissue plasminogen activator activity, pre- and post-stress lysis may be considered to rule out an abnormality in the fibrinolytic system if the above tests are normal, but the clinical relevance of abnormalities in the fibrinolytic system are uncertain.

Patients with congenital thrombophilia should be considered at high risk of thromboembolism and should receive appropriate prophylaxis according to the clinical setting.

In symptomatic patients the optimal duration of the treatment is unknown and should be considered case by case taking into account the benefit/risk ratio for each individual.

In asymptomatic patients with congenital thrombophilia the value of primary prophylaxis is not yet known, but patients should be protected during surgery or during any medical condition associated with an increased risk of thrombosis.

Pregnant women with thrombophilia belong to a special group and are at risk throughout pregnancy. They should be considered for thrombo-prophylaxis. The period of risk may begin early in the first trimester, particularly in those with anti-thrombin III deficiency.

In patients with acquired haematological abnormalities, the decision regarding primary prophylaxis should be made on an individual basis.

The oestrogen-containing oral contraceptive pills are contraindicated in patients with thrombophilia since there is epidemiological evidence, as stated above, to suggest a relationship between oestrogen containing oral contraceptives and venous thromboembolism.

## Routine screening for thromboembolism

Routine screening for asymptomatic pulmonary emboli is neither necessary nor cost-effective.

It is well documented that the majority of pulmonary emboli and the majority of fatal pulmonary emboli occur following asymptomatic DVT. Therefore, it is important to diagnose asymptomatic calf and proximal DVT. However, in low- and medium-risk patients who are protected by an established prophylactic method, there is insufficient evidence that routine screening for DVT is needed. Furthermore, screening is not cost-effective in these categories. In high-risk patients, even with established prophylaxis, the incidence of asymptomatic DVT is significant, and therefore screening for DVT may be beneficial.

At present there does not appear to be a better alternative to contrast venography which can be recommended for documenting asymptomatic venous thrombi, although it is recognised that venography, too, has limitations. Therefore, it would be desirable to have a reliable, simple and practical method for the screening of high-risk patients. Thus, there is an urgent need to define better practices for the assessment of new non-invasive diagnostic tests. The protocol should include the following:–
a) A priori diagnostic criteria defining positive and negative tests.
b) Studies should be prospective, and include consecutive patients.
c) Results of the new methods should be compared to the reference test in an independent and blinded fashion.

There is also an urgent need to document the possible improved accuracy of B-mode, duplex or colour Doppler ultrasonography above existing noninvasive tests for the diagnosis of asymptomatic venous thrombosis.

## Risk categories

Known clinical risk factors allow the classification of patients into low, medium and high risk of developing thromboembolism (Tables 2-4).

## Prophylaxis in general surgery, urology

There is compelling evidence that low dose heparin is effective in reducing both DVT and fatal PE.

Low molecular weight heparins have been shown to be effective in general surgical patients in reducing the incidence of DVT. There are no data regarding the effect on fatal PE.

Dextran has been shown to be effective in reducing fatal pulmonary embolism. There is only weak evidence to suggest it reduces DVT. It has inherent risks of fluid overload and anaphylactoid reactions. Preinfusion hapten injection reduces this risk.

Intermittent pneumatic compression has been shown to be effective in reducing the incidence of DVT. There are insufficient data covering other methods of mechanical prophylaxis to assess their efficacy.

There is some evidence that graduated compression stockings are effective in reducing the incidence of DVT.

There is no evidence that antiplatelet agents are effective in reducing the incidence of venous thromboembolism.

**Table 2**
Risk categories in surgical patients

| Risk category | Risk of venous thromboembolism (Assessed by objective tests) | | |
|---|---|---|---|
| | Calf-vein thrombosis | Proximal-vein thrombosis | Fatal pulmonary embolism |
| *HIGH RISK* | | | |
| General and urological surgery in patients over 40 yrs with recent history of DVT or PE | 40-80% | 10-30% | 1-5% |
| Extensive pelvic or abdominal surgery for malignant disease | | | |
| Major orthopaedic surgery of lower limbs | | | |
| *MODERATE RISK*[*] | | | |
| General surgery in patients over 40 years lasting 30 minutes or more and in patients below 40 years on oral contraceptives | 10-40% | 2-10% | 0.1-0.7% |
| *LOW RISK* | | | |
| Uncomplicated surgery in patients under 40 years without additional risk factors | <10% | <1% | <0.01% |
| Minor surgery (i.e. less than 30 minutes) in patients over 40 years without additional risk factors | | | |

[*]The risk is increased by additional factors (see page 446)


**Table 3**
Risk categories in gynaecology and obstetrics

| | Gynaecology | Obstetrics[*] |
|---|---|---|
| High risk | History of previous DVT/PE | History of previous DVT/PE |
| | Age >60 | |
| | Cancer | |
| | Thrombophilic condition | Thrombophilic condition |
| Moderate risk | Patients over 40 years with major surgery | Patients over 40 years |
| | Patients below 40 years on oral contraceptives with major surgery | |
| Low risk | Uncomplicated surgery <40 years without additional risk factors | |
| | Minor surgery (<30 min) in patients over 40 years without additional risk factors | |

[*]The risk of DVT in obstetric patients with pre-eclampsia and other risk factors is unknown but prophylaxis should be considered (see page 447)

**Table 4**
Risk categories in medical patients

| | |
|---|---|
| High risk | Stroke |
| | Congestive heart failure |
| | Thrombophilia with additional disease |
| Moderate/low risk | All immobilised patients with active disease |

The risk is increased by infectious diseases, malignancy, and other risk factors: see page 446)

There are insufficient data to support the use of oral anticoagulants for thromboembolism prophylaxis.

There are insufficient data on the use of heparinoids in general surgery.

Combinations of mechanical and pharmacological methods may be more effective.

**Low risk** patients may receive prophylaxis. On the basis of risk/benefit ratio it is local routine practice in some countries to use graduated compression stockings. The data are insufficient to make this a mandatory requirement.

In all **moderate risk** patients the use of low dose heparin/low molecular weight heparin is recommended. An alternative recommendation may be intermittent pneumatic compression used continuously until the patient is ambulant. There is insufficient evidence that the addition of graduated compression stockings further reduces the frequency of venous thrombosis in patients in this risk group. However, it is routine clinical practice in some countries, to combine pharmacological methods with graded compression stockings in selected patients.

The most urgently needed direct comparison in moderate risk patients is fixed low dose heparin with low molecular weight heparin with respect to total mortality and confirmed fatal pulmonary embolism.

Further studies are needed to see if graduated compression stockings/intermittent pneumatic compression enhance the efficacy of pharmacological methods.

All **high risk** patients should receive prophylaxis. Apart from single modalities that have been demonstrated to be effective and safe such as low dose heparin, and low molecular weight heparin, combined modalities of pharmacological and mechanical methods may be considered.

Prophylaxis should be initiated before operation in all groups. The current recommendation is to continue prophylaxis for 7 to 10 days after operation. Although the evidence is weak, consideration should be given to extending prophylaxis when the hospital stay is prolonged or the risk continues.

There is an urgent need for a proper randomised comparison of the pre- and post-operative commencement of pharmacological prophylactic modalities.

The efficacy of continued prophylaxis beyond the period of hospitalisation deserves investigation.

For women taking the oestrogen-containing contraceptive pills, if the latter are not stopped 4-6 weeks before surgery then consideration should be given to prophylaxis.

Patients with a high risk of bleeding either from known systemic bleeding disease or from specific surgical procedures should receive mechanical methods of prophylaxis.

## Neurosurgery

Neurosurgical patients should be considered for receiving mechanical methods of prophylaxis.

## Orthopaedic surgery and trauma

Patients undergoing elective or emergency operations are at a "high risk" of developing postoperative venous thromboembolism. Total hip replacement without prophylaxis is associated with a high incidence of deep vein thrombosis (DVT) of about 50% and pulmonary embolism which in 1 to 3% is fatal. In addition, they are also at risk of developing late sequelae of DVT — "the post-phlebitic syndrome" the incidence of which has been estimated to be approximately 50% five years after an episode of thrombosis. These observations emphasise the need for a routine effective prophylactic method.

Methods of prophylaxis which have been investigated in this particular high risk group include aspirin, dextran, fixed low dose unfractionated heparin (FLDUH), adjusted dose heparin, addition of dihydroergotamine to fixed low dose unfractionated heparin, fixed mini-dose and adjusted dose of oral anticoagulant therapy, external pneumatic compression, low molecular weight heparin and heparinoid.

The following recommendations are made:

**Elective surgery**

There is insufficient evidence to recommend the use of antiplatelet drugs for prophylaxis.

Dextran is only moderately effective and has inherent risks such as fluid overload and anaphylactoid reactions, the latter being minimised by hapten inhibition.

Fixed low dose unfractionated heparin prophylaxis (5000 bid/tid) is moderately effective.

Increasing the fixed heparin dosage enhances the bleeding risk.

Adjusting the heparin dosage to the results of a coagulation assay, is more effective, but difficult to manage.

The addition of dihydroergotamine to fixed low dose unfractionated heparin enhances efficacy, but has the inherent risk of vasospasm.

Fixed mini dose of oral anticoagulant therapy is ineffective and is not recommended.

Adjusting the dose of oral anticoagulants to a desired international normalised ratio (INR) improves efficacy, but adds to management procedures.

External pneumatic compression with and without graduated elastic stockings is effective, but has practical limitations.

Fixed dose low molecular weight heparins and one heparinoid are currently the most effective. However, the efficacy and safety of each product need to be documented separately.

Prophylaxis should preferably be started before operation and continued for 7-10 days after operation or until fully ambulant. No data are available to make recommendations for patients discharged from hospital.

The extensive experience with fixed low dose heparin indicates that there is no evidence that the pre-operative start of prophylaxis does not enhance the risk of haemorrhage associated with spinal or epidural anaesthesia.

A prospective registration (post-marketing surveillance) on the prevalence of spinal/epidural anaesthesia induced haemorrhage in patients pretreated with thrombosis prophylactic anticoagulant agents is needed.

The limited number of studies in patients undergoing knee replacement does not permit a firm recommendation about the preferred methods of prophylaxis. However, the modalities effective in patients undergoing elective hip replacement can be applied in this category until more information becomes available.

**Emergency surgery**
The prophylactic modalities for hip fracture should be started as soon as possible and are comparable to those for elective hip surgery, with the exception of DHE/heparin which is contra-indicated and adjusted dose heparin for which no studies exist. The comparison of efficacy and safety between fixed low dose unfractionated heparin, low molecular weight heparins and low molecular weight heparinoid needs to be investigated.

# Obstetrics and gynaecology

**Gynaecological surgery**
*Low risk patients*
Low risk patients may receive prophylaxis. On the basis of risk-benefit ratio, it is routine local practice in some countries to use graduated compression stockings. The data are insufficient to make this a mandatory requirement.

*Moderate risk patients*
Low dose heparin (5000 units 12 hourly) has been demonstrated to be an effective prophylaxis in medium risk gynaecologic surgery patients. Intermittent pneumatic compression might also be considered since it has been shown to be effective in higher risk patients.

Dextran and adjusted dose warfarin are not recommended on the basis of cost-benefit for routine prophylaxis but may have a role when low dose heparin is contraindicated.

Data evaluating low molecular weight heparin, and/or graduated compression stockings in moderate risk gynaecological surgery are insufficient to make a recommendation at present.

The use of combination oestrogen containing oral contraceptives may be associated with increased risk of DVT in patients undergoing gynaecological surgery. Discontinuation of oral contraceptives 4-6 weeks before surgery should be considered. If oral contraceptives have not been discontinued, prophylaxis should be provided.

*High risk patients*
In high risk patients undergoing gynaecological surgery, low dose heparin (5,000 units 8 hourly) or intermittent pneumatic compression used continuously for at least 5 days provide effective prophylaxis.

Prophylaxis with combined methods and for extended periods need to be studied further. Data evaluating low molecular weight heparin and graduated compression stockings in high risk gynaecological surgery patients are insufficient.

## Pregnancy

Low dose heparin prophylaxis is commonly used in pregnant patients at high risk of DVT and pulmonary embolism, although data of efficacy from controlled trials are lacking. There are insufficient data on both the optimum timing and dosing schedule of low dose heparin prophylaxis.

Oral anticoagulants are contraindicated in the first trimester (due to the risk of embryopathies) and available data indicate that they are associated with fetopathy in the second trimester and increased maternal-fetal bleeding in the second and third trimester.

The benefits of prophylaxis have not been demonstrated in patients undergoing Caesarean Section who have no additional risk factors. Perioperative and postpartum prophylaxis may be seriously considered in the presence of additional risk factors.

There are insufficient data on the use of low molecular weight heparins or mechanical methods in pregnancy. There is an urgent need for a multicentre trial comparing standard heparin with low molecular weight heparin in high risk pregnant patients assessing efficacy, safety and side effects such as osteoporosis.

Women who develop thromboembolism during pregnancy should be treated with therapeutic levels of heparin. Heparin should be continued throughout the duration of pregnancy, labour and delivery. Anticoagulation is usually continued for at least 4 to 6 weeks postpartum, although the optimal duration of this therapy has not been established.

Patients who develop thromboembolism during pregnancy or the puerperium should be referred for haematological screening.

The management of thrombophilic conditions throughout pregnancy is under investigation.

# Prophylaxis in medical patients

There are less data available in medical than in surgical patients. However, an increased risk of venous thromboembolism has been shown by prospective studies in patients with acute myocardial infarction, cerebrovascular accident and in immobilised general medical patients.

The following recommendations are based on experience from level one clinical trials.

### Acute myocardial infarction

Patients not receiving anticoagulant therapy as primary treatment of acute myocardial infarction are at risk for venous thromboembolism. They should receive low-dose heparin.

### Stroke

Patients with ischaemic stroke are at high risk for venous thromboembolism. They should receive low dose heparin or low molecular weight heparinoid.

### Immobilised general medical patients

The following recommendations are based on extrapolation of data from trials in other high-risk patient groups. Patients at risk should receive prophylaxis.

The following modalities could be considered:
- Graduated compression stockings
- Intermittent pneumatic compression
- Low-dose heparin

- Low molecular weight heparin
- Low molecular weight heparinoid
- Oral anticoagulants

## Cost-effectiveness for all groups

In discussing prophylactic methods used in prevention of thromboembolism it is important to consider health economics. Primary prevention is more cost effective than secondary prevention through routine screening of postoperative patients.

In medium and high risk patients, the costs of screening, diagnosis and treatment of thromboembolism are so high that the currently recommended methods of primary prophylaxis are cost effective (i.e. optimise the use of available resources).

In low risk patients no data are available at present concerning the cost effectiveness of the current recommended prophylactic methods.

International variations in the structure of health services preclude a ranking of relative cost effectiveness. However, relative cost effectiveness should be considered when choosing between different forms of prophylaxis.

## Combined methods of prevention

**Surgery**
*High risk patients*
All high risk patients should receive prophylaxis. Apart from single modalities that have been demonstrated to be effective and safe, such as low dose heparin and low molecular weight heparin, combined modalities may be considered for local practice, i.e. combinations of pharmacological and mechanical methods such as low dose heparin/low molecular weight heparin combined with mechanical methods.
*Moderate risk patients*
Combined mechanical methods may be applied as an alternative to low dose heparin/low molecular weight heparin.
*Gynaecology patients*
Combinations of prophylaxis have not been evaluated properly in these patients. Based on results of other surgical trials, combined prophylaxis may be considered.
*Medical patients*
In each of these risk categories, and particularly in high risk patients, there is a lack of studies employing combined methods in the prevention of deep vein thrombosis. Hence, no specific recommendations regarding the application of combined prevention modalities can be offered.

## Secondary prevention

The objectives of the treatment of thromboembolism are to prevent extension of thrombus, progressive swelling of the leg resulting in increased compartmental pressure which can lead to phlegmasia cerulea dolens, venous gangrene and limb loss, symptomatic recurrence of thrombosis, pulmonary embolism, which can be fatal or later lead to chronic pulmonary hypertension, and severe post-thrombotic syndrome by preservation of the venous outflow and functional valves.

**Anticoagulants**
There is strong evidence to support the statement that *anticoagulation* is necessary for the prevention of morbidity and mortality if deep vein thrombosis. Anticoagulation should be started either with an initial course of intravenous adjusted-dose standard (unfractionated) heparin given by continuous infusion (preceded by an i.v. bolus injection) or with subcutaneous adjusted-dose standard heparin. It is important that a therapeutic level is reached within the first 24 hours. APTT should be at least 1.5 times the patient's control value. APTT measurements in patients treated with subcutaneous heparin should be done in the mid-interval of two injections. The upper limit for APTT varies according to local practice and is not well defined. The heparin regimen should be continued for a minimum period of 5-7 days.

It is acceptable to start oral anticoagulant therapy on the first day of heparin therapy or on subsequent days. Under normal circumstances, heparin treatment should be discontinued when the patient's INR is within the therapeutic range (i.e., 2-3) for at least two days. Oral anticoagulant therapy should be continued for a period of at least three months in patients with a first episode of venous thrombosis and no continuing risk factors. However, the optimal duration of therapy is not known.

Patients presenting with a recurrent episode of venous thrombosis should be treated with heparin with a similar therapeutic regimen as for patients with a first episode of DVT. However, the optimal duration of oral anticoagulant therapy is not known.

Adjusted doses of subcutaneous heparin may be used as secondary prophylaxis in special clinical conditions such as pregnancy where oral anticoagulant therapy is contraindicated.

Low molecular weight heparins given subcutaneously have been shown to be as safe and effective as standard heparin therapy for the initial treatment of DVT in terms of reduction of the thrombus size as assessed by repeat venography. Preliminary results demonstrate that fixed dose body weight adjusted unmonitored low molecular weight heparins are as effective as adjusted dose intravenous standard heparin in the prevention of symptomatic recurrent venous thromboembolism during long-term follow-up.

**Thrombolytic therapy**
There is good evidence that thrombolytic therapy produces a more effective lysis in proximal DVT than unfractionated heparin. However, its use is limited because the benefit/risk ratio of this treatment as compared with unfractionated heparin has not yet been established. Therefore, at present it cannot be recommended that all patients with DVT receive thrombolytic therapy. Anecdotal evidence suggests that thrombolytic treatment may be considered in selected patients who sustain acute recent massive vein thrombosis, in the absence of contraindications to thrombolytic therapy.

**Thrombectomy**
Thrombectomy is indicated for limb salvage, (e.g., in impending venous gangrene in patients with iliofemoral DVT) but its use under other circumstances is still limited. Long term follow-up information is required.

**Inferior vena cava filters**
A filter device should be inserted in the inferior vena cava when anticoagulation is contraindicated in the management of pulmonary embolism or venous thrombosis above the knee, or when adequate anticoagulation fails to prevent recurrent embolism. For thrombosis extending to, or involving the renal veins and in pregnant patients, only a proven device (Greenfield filter) should be placed above the level of the renal veins. Expanded indications for filter insertion are under clinical investigation.

# Key questions to be answered

The statements and recommendations made in this consensus have been based on different levels of evidence. When the evidence for a particular recommendation was compelling, such as that provided by level one studies, the term "mandatory" was used. Where the evidence was weak, insufficient or lacking, this was also stated. During this process, a number of key questions that need to be urgently addressed by future research have been identified. They are repeated in this final section.

The risk for venous thromboembolism may continue beyond the period of hospitalisation. This risk needs to be assessed in prospective trials.

The efficacy of continued prophylaxis beyond the period of hospitalisation deserves investigation.

A proper randomised comparison of pre- and post-operative commencement of pharmacological prophylactic modalities is necessary.

An urgently needed study in moderate risk patients is a direct comparison of fixed low dose heparin with low molecular weight heparin with respect to total mortality and confirmed fatal pulmonary embolism.

Further studies are needed to determine if graduated compression stockings and/or intermittent pneumatic compression enhance the efficacy of pharmacological methods.

A prospective registration (post-marketing surveillance) on the prevalence of spinal/epidural anaesthesia induced haemorrhage in patients pretreated with prophylactic anticoagulant agents is needed.

The risk of DVT in the new minimally invasive abdominal surgical procedures needs to be established.

A multicentre trial comparing standard heparin with low molecular weight heparin in high risk pregnant patients assessing efficacy, safety and the incidence of side effects such as osteoporosis is also needed.

The possible improved accuracy of B-mode, duplex or colour Doppler ultrasonography above existing noninvasive tests for the diagnosis of asymptomatic venous thrombosis needs to be documented.

# Index

Air plethysmography, 381-389
Anaesthesia, 57
   general and venous flow, 57
   spinal and venous flow, 57
Anticoagulant therapy,
   continuous iv heparin, and, 429
   oral, 42, 433, 434
      INR, 434
      laboratory monitoring, 43
      WHO reference thromboplastin, 434
   recurrent DVT, in, 429
Anticoagulants
   contraindications to, 435
   postthrombotic syndrome
      incidence of, 17
Antiplatelet agents, 201
   general surgery, in, 201
   orthopaedics, in, 201
   trauma, in, 201
AV fistula, thrombectomy in, 359

Birds nest filter, 397

Calf DVT, untreated, 430
Coagulation abnormalities
   DVT, and, 43
   thrombosis, and, 47
Coagulation
   new markers of activation, 49
Colour coded Doppler
   predictive value of, 84
   sensitivity, 84
   specificity, 84
Colour flow imaging
   asymptomatic vs symptomatic patients, 99
   comparison with B-mode, 95
   comparative studies in symptomatic calf DVT, 97
   methodology, 94
   postoperative surveillance, 98
      calf veins, 98
      femoropopliteal segment, 98
      hip arthroplasty
         calf veins, 99
         femoral veins, 98
         popliteal veins, 98
Combined methods of prevention
   DHE and LDH, 228
   GEC and LDH, 229
   in hip surgery, 228
   studies in, 228
Contact factors and DVT, 47

D-dimer assays, 51
Deficiency in, 48
   At-III, 48
   HC II, 48
   Protein C, 48
   Protein S, 48
Dextran
   clinical indications for, 182
   combined with anticoagulants, 187
   combined with other methods, 185
   dosage and timing, 190
   DVT prevention, and, 184
   historical background, 181
   mechanism of action, 182, 183
      and Factor VIII, 183
      and haemostatic system, 183
      and haemodynamics, 182
      and platelet adhesiveness, 183
   metabolism, 182
      PE, prevention of, 186
   side effects, 191, 192
      anaphylactoid reactions, 191
      cardiac overload, 191
      haemorrhagic complications, 191
      metabolic acidosis, 191
      renal dysfunction, 192
      vs anticoagulants, 189
      vs controls, 186
Diagnostic efficacy indices, 75
Duplex scanning
   compared with venography, 353
   compared with LCT, 364
   sensitivity, 67, 353
   specificity, 353

DVT
- amputation, frequency after, 8
- and post-thrombotic syndrome, 21
- and thrombolysis, 18
- and venous dilatation, 34
- oaortoiliac reconstruction, frequency after, 8
- coagulation abnormalities, and, 43
- colour flow imaging and, 93
- diagnostic tests in, 63-65, 73
- early studies, 8
- endothelial damage, and, 32
- extent of leg ulcers, and, 23
- extent of, and mortality, 22
- femoropopliteal reconstruction, and, 8
- five-year follow-up, 20
- frequency after hip fracture, 10
- incidence of
  - and contraceptive medication, 6
  - in general surgery, 111
  - in gynaecological surgery, 111
  - in myocardial infarction, 6
  - in non-surgical patients, 6
  - in oestrogen therapy, 6
  - in orthopaedic surgery, 112
  - in pregnancy, 6
  - in thoracic surgery, 111
  - in urological surgery, 111
  - in vascular surgery, 112
- late sequelae
  - incidence of, 12
  - incidence of after thrombolysis, 17
  - incidence of after anticoagulation, 17
  - interval treatment, and, 26
  - risk factors for, 27
  - socio-economic consequences of, 27
- leg fracture and frequency of, 8
- leg ulcer, and, 20
- meniscectomy after, 8
- natural history of
  - asymptomatic, 109
  - collateral blood supply, and, 110
  - fatal, 109
  - liposclerotic eczema, and, 109
  - meta-analyses, and, 111
  - non-fatal, 109
  - pathology and symptoms, 109
  - post-thrombotic syndrome, and, 109
  - pulmonary embolism, and, 109
  - sequelae, and
    - alveolar hyperventilation, 111
    - hypoxaemia, 111
    - pulmonary oedema, 111
    - V/Q abnormalities, 111
  - spontaneous thrombolysis, 110
  - symptomatic, 109
  - valve cusp impairment, 110
  - venous valve, destruction of, 109
- non-operated groups, in, 6
- operative venodilatation, and, 35
- oral contraceptives, and, 7
- postoperative
  - after cardiothoracic surgery, 7
  - after general surgery, 7
  - after gynaecological surgery, 7
  - after herniorrhaphy, 7
  - after hip surgery, 7
  - after knee surgery, 7
  - after neurologic surgery, 7
  - after prostatectomy, 7
  - detection of
    - by AT-III, 237
    - by D-Dimer, 237
  - frequency of, 7, 235
  - PAI-levels, 237
  - and risk-factors
    - age, 235
    - malignancy, 235
    - obesity, 235
- prophylaxis, costeffectiveness of, 236
- risk categories, and, 146
- risk factor indices, and, 236
  - age, 236
  - malignancy, 236
  - obesity, 236
  - operation type, 236
  - platelet adhesiveness, 236
  - previous history of DVT, 236
  - varicose veins, 236
- venous dilatation, and, 31
- prevention, costeffectiveness of, 405
- primary prevention, 406
  - combined methods, 225
  - graduated compression, 203, 204
    - efficacy of, 205, 206
    - mode of action, 203

studies in, 204
hip surgery, in, 271
intermittent pneumatic compression
LDH
  and DHE, 131, 132, 137, 138
  complications of, 136
  in malignancy, 134
  in neurosurgery, 135
  in spinal cord injury, 135
  in total hip replacement, 134
  pulmonary embolism, fatal, 135
  pulmonary embolism, non-fatal, 135
LMWH
  and DHE, 139
  anti-IIa activity, and, 150
  anti-Xa activity, and, 150
  comparative studies, 150-156
  complications of, 158
  dosage, 144-157
  efficacy of, 149
  mode of action, 143, 144
prophylaxis
  approaches to, 423
  compliance, 426
  cost effectiveness, 415-418
  cost of, 413, 414
  cost of diagnosis, 414
  cost of treatment, 414
  cost per patient, 414
  cost and estimated savings, 418
  DHE, use of, 35
  ease of administration, 426
  elastic stockings, 35, 203, 204
  general model, 413
  ideal method, 427
  intermittent pneumatic compression, 35, 209
  laboratory monitoring, 426
  relative effectiveness, 425
  relative safety, 425
recurrence of, 116
renal transplantation, after, 8
risk factors, and, 10
  anaesthesia, type of, 10
  geographic differences, 10
role of previous DVT, and, 47
secondary prevention, 406
  duplex scanning, 350

LCT, 349
  thrombectomy, 357
sequelae
  acute phase treatment, and, 25
  late
    heparin, and, 25
    randomised studies, and, 26
    streptokinase, and, 26
  methodological difficulties, 24
  spinal cord injury, after

Endothelial damage and DVT, 32, 33
European Consensus Statement, 444

FDP assays, 51
Fibrinogen alterations and DVT, 46
Fibrinolysis
  activation of, 50
  alterations and DVT, 46
  in secondary prevention, 373, 374
  treatment objectives, 374
Fibrinolytic system and DVT, 43
FUT
  accuracy, 77
  and IPG 68, 80, 81
  calf vein DVT, and, 85
  in orthopaedic surgery, 76
  proximal DVT, and, 85
  positive predictive value, 79
  sensitivity, 79
  specificity, 86

Graduated compression, 225, 226
  in primary DVT prevention, 203
Greenfield filter, 396
Gynaecologic surgery
  Dextran, use of, 257, 258
  mechanical methods of prophylaxis, 260-263
    compression, 261
    IPC, 262, 263
    summary of studies, 261
    vena cava interruption, and, 263
  pelvic vein thrombosis, 263
  pharmacological methods of prophylaxis, 258-260

Heparin
  adjusted subcutaneous, 435

adverse effects of, 432
initial i.v. therapy, 430
risks of use, 255
use in pregnancy, 256, 257
Hip fracture
anaesthesia and, 289
postoperative venography, and, 11
prophylaxis of DVT, and, 281-287
Hip surgery
combined modalities in prevention, 297-303
DVT, natural history of, 271
elective, prophylaxis in, 271-276
recent studies, 58,59
venous stasis, and, 57
Hormonal treatment and DVT, 49
Hypercoagulable state
acquired risk factors, 44
inherited risk factors, 44
stasis, and, 44

Iliofemoral thrombosis
surgical management, 359-361
thrombectomy, and, 359
Impedance plethysmography, 67
IVC filters, 393-395
Inherited risk factors and DVT, 43
Antithrombin III, 43
Protein C, 43
Protein S, 43
Heparin Cofactor II, 43
Intermittent pneumatic compression (IPC)
IPC
advantages of, 209, 214
contraindications, 218
cost-effectiveness, 219
DVT, incidence of, and, 213, 215, 227
effectiveness, 211, 212
GEC, comparison with, 214
indications for, 218
optimal period of application, 214
pharmacological modalities, combined with, 214, 216, 217
rationale, 211
safety, 211
sensitivity, 85
specificity, 82

thrombogenic factors, improvement in, 210
Knee surgery
primary prophylaxis
anaesthesia and, 315
dosage regimens, 315
incidence of DVT, 309, 310
modalities, 311-314
prospective studies of, 312, 313
risk factors, and, 311
side effects, and, 311
use of tourniquet, and, 315, 316

Liquid crystal thermography (LCT)
LCT
compared with venography, 352
cost-effectiveness, 352
duplex scanning, comparison with, 354, 355
sensitivity, 353
specificity, 353
Lupus anticoagulant, 48
LMWH
Orgaran, and, 175-179
standard heparin, and, 163-165
unfractionated heparins, and, 166-170

Maternal mortality and PE, 254
Medical patients and primary prophylaxis, 319-327

Neurosurgical patients and primary prophylaxis, 327
Noninvasive tests in asymptomatic patients, 69

Obstetrics and DVT prophylaxis, 256
Obstetrics and low dose heparin, 257
Operative venodilatation, 35
and DVT, 37-40
Oral contraceptives and operation, 49
Oral anticoagulants, 199, 200

PAI and DVT, 238
Pelvic vein thrombosis, 263
Phleborheography, 67, 68
Platelet abnormalities and DVT, 45
Post-thrombotic syndrome
and leg ulcers, 23

# INDEX

natural history of, 115
Pregnant patients and DVT, 256
Prevention of postoperative DVT
    general surgery, in, 244-246
    obstetrics and gynaecology, in, 249-251
    PE, and incidence of, 246
Primary prevention of DVT, 123-129
Prognostic indices for DVT, 239
Prophylaxis, selective, 239
Protocol plan for DVT prevention, 339-344
Pulmonary embolism
    angiography, and, 4
    antepartum patients, in, 249
    fatal, frequency of, 8,9
    maternal mortality, and, 254
    natural history of, 113
    non-fatal, frequency of, 8,9
    PIOPED Study, 4
    post-partum patients, in, 249
    prevention, cost effectiveness of, 407
    scintigraphy, and, 4

Reflux, incidence of, 116
Risk factor indices, 240

Streptokinase therapy, 18
Stroke patients, primary prophylaxis in, 327-329
Surgical patients, risk categories, 422

T-AT assays, 51
T-AT complexes, 51
Thrombectomy
    AV-fistula, 359
        closure of, 362
        role of, 362
    clinical success of, 363-365
    indications for, 367
    post-thrombotic syndrome, and, 366
    results
        early, 362
        late, 364
        value of, 357
        with AV-fistula, 362
        without AV-fistula, 364
Thrombin interaction with fibrinogen, 50
Thromboembolism
    economic outcomes, 408
    Key questions, 421

LMWH, and, 435
    risk classification, and, 421
    risk factors, and, 421
Thrombolysis
    cause of death in, 20
    complete and post-thrombotic syndrome, 23
    drug administration, 379
        new treatment strategies, 379
        r-TPA, 379
        streptokinase, 379
        urokinase, 379
    DVT recurrence, in, 20
    factors influencing efficacy, 374, 375
    five-year follow up, after, 20
    haemorrhagic events, and, 18
    intracranial haemorrhage, and, 19
    mortality, and, 20
    post-thrombotic syndrome, 20, 21
    pulmonary emoblism, for, 376, 378
    pulmonary vasculature, restoration of, 376
    severe complications of, 19
    success, 19
    venous insufficiency, and, 375
Thrombosis, idiopathic, 44

Ultrasonography and DVT
    predictive value, 843
    sensitivity, 83
    specificity, 83
Urokinase therapy, 18
Urologic surgery, prophylaxis, 333-335

Vena cava filters, 394-400
    Birds nest filter, 399
    complications of, 394
    efficacy of, 396
    following PE, 395
    in special circumstances, 395
    Nitinol filter, 399
    prophylactic, 394
    results reported, 398
    Titanium Greenfield, 401
    Venatech filter, 400
Venography
    interobserver variation, 84
    positive predictive value, 80
Venous stasis and anaesthesia, 57

Venous thromboembolism
   diagnosis of, 5
   medical patients, in, 3
   problem, the, 5
   surgical patients, in, 3
Virchow's triad, 31